Articulation
and
Phonological Disorders

third edition

ARTICULATION
AND
PHONOLOGICAL DISORDERS

John E. Bernthal
University of Nebraska–Lincoln

Nicholas W. Bankson
Boston University

Prentice Hall, Englewood Cliffs, New Jersey 07632

Library of Congress Cataloging-in-Publication Data

Bernthal, John E.
    Articulation and phonological disorders / John E. Bernthal,
  Nicholas W. Bankson. -- 3rd ed.
        p.   cm.
    Includes bibliographical references and indexes.
    ISBN 0-13-052408-5
    1. Articulation disorders.   I. Bankson, Nicholas W.   II. Title.
  RC424.7.B47   1993
  618.92'855--dc20   92-22821
                                                           CIP

Editorial/production supervision
  and interior design: Joan E. Foley
Acquisitions editor: Julie Berrisford
Editorial assistant: Nicole Signoretti
Copy editor: Nancy Savio-Marcello
Cover designer: Joe DiDomenico
Prepress buyer: Kelly Behr
Manufacturing buyer: Mary Ann Gloriande

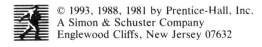 © 1993, 1988, 1981 by Prentice-Hall, Inc.
A Simon & Schuster Company
Englewood Cliffs, New Jersey 07632

Previously published under the title of *Articulation Disorders*

Printed in the United States of America

10 9 8 7 6

ISBN 0-13-052408-5

Prentice-Hall International (UK) Limited, *London*
Prentice-Hall of Australia Pty. Limited, *Sydney*
Prentice-Hall Canada Inc., *Toronto*
Prentice-Hall Hispanoamericana, S.A., *Mexico*
Prentice-Hall of India Private Limited, *New Delhi*
Prentice-Hall of Japan, Inc., *Tokyo*
Simon & Schuster Asia Pte. Ltd., *Singapore*
Editora Prentice-Hall do Brasil, Ltda., *Rio de Janeiro*

Contents

Preface

This edition reflects our ongoing efforts to teach students about the nature and treatment of disorders of the speech sound system. Since submission of our second edition for publication, new ideas, concepts, and issues have been advanced in the area of clinical phonology and we have tried to reflect them.

This book presents both theoretical and practical information, recognizing that elements of both are essential to the understanding of the literature and to clinical practice. We have attempted to organize and synthesize the literature so that the student may view clinical phonology from a broad perspective. We have again adopted an "eclectic" perspective relative to the natures and treatment of phonological disorders, since our readers have indicated that this is of value when acquiring the foundation of knowledge that is necessary for more advanced study in the area. In the assessment and intervention chapters, you will again see some of our own biases regarding clinical management; however, in general we have deferred to clinician judgment in deciding which assessment and management tools may be most useful. Throughout the text we have attempted to identify unresolved issues regarding the topics that are discussed.

While it would be impossible to acknowledge everyone who has contributed either directly or indirectly to the writing of this book, there are several people who have contributed immeasurably to this effort. Of special assistance has been the revision by Ray Kent of Chapter 1, and Chapters 2 and 3 by Marilyn Vihman. There are two new chapters that were added to this edition. Chapter 4, co-authored by Aquiles Iglesias and Noma Anderson, deals with phonological characteristics associated with Black English Vernacular and Spanish/Spanish-influenced English. While multicultural aspects of communication are typically included in the master's degree curriculum in speech-language pathology, we thought that it was more than timely that specific information concerning phonological characteristics of two frequently encountered linguistic populations be integrated into this text. The information presented herein is, however, only an introduction to this area. The second addition to this edition is Chapter 8, dealing with computerized phonological analysis, co-authored by Julie Masterson and Steven Long. They present several computerized phonological analysis systems through their identification of a framework through which clinicians can determine whether particular computer software will meet their needs. In the process, they also present a detailed review of several of the major process analysis systems.

The advice and suggestions we have received from the users of our previous work have been invaluable and we hope that this effort reflects a step forward in the presentation of this information. We encourage the users of this text to communicate directly with us concerning their suggestions for changes. This manuscript has again been enhanced by comments and discussions with many individuals, especially the individuals who frequent the Midwest Phonology Conference. We also gratefully acknowledge the following reviewers: Richard A. Forcucci, Edinboro University of Pennsylvania; Julie Masterson, Arizona State University; Karen E. Pollock, Memphis State University; and Virginia G. Walker, Florida State University. However, we alone assume responsibility for errors, oversights, and misperceptions that may appear in this book. We also wish to express our gratitude for the efforts of Evie Reiners, our primary typist. Her diligence, patience, proofreading, and assistance very much contributed to the completion of this work in a timely manner.

We dedicate this edition to our past and current students, some of whom convinced us that a book of this nature was needed. Not in our wildest dreams, however, did we think we would still be collaborating on revisions for more than a decade!

J.E.B. and N.W.B.

Introduction

At one time or another, you have likely encountered a person who seemed to have difficulty saying one or more of the sounds of American English. It may have been a child who was unintelligible, a teenager with a lisp, or someone who somehow "didn't say his sounds right." Producing and using the speech sounds of one's linguistic community is a critical communication skill. When a speaker has difficulty being understood, or when sounds are consistently produced at variance with cultural or age expectations and norms, an individual may be said to evidence a phonological disorder or delay. This book presents an overview of clinical phonology. It includes an introduction to the normal aspects of speech sound articulation and the sound system, phonological development, possible factors related to the presence of phonological disorders, and the assessment and remediation of phonological disorders.

In their study of the prevalence of communication disorders, Hull, Mielke, Timmons, and Willeford (1971) reported that 2 percent of the school-age population evidenced "extreme deviation" in the production of English speech sounds. They also found that speech sound deviations constituted the most prevalent type of communication disorder in school-age children. The caseloads of speech-language pathologists typically include many individuals with phonological disorders.

This text is primarily concerned with those phonological disorders not etiologically associated with known or obvious sensory, structural, or neuromotor deficits. Such disorders traditionally have been labeled *functional* articulation disorders, a category that has come to be viewed clinically as a catch-all, frequently including all individuals with phonological errors of unknown causes. A phonological disorder of unknown etiology may be caused by one or more subtle organic, learning, or environmental factors.

Those individuals acquainted with the last edition of this text will notice several changes and additions in this version. Most obvious are the new chapters on "Dialectal Variations" and "Computerized Phonological Analysis." These topics represent two areas in which interest and knowledge in the area of phonology is advancing. Our increasingly multicultural society reflects phonological variety about which clinicians are called upon to be knowledgeable. Additionally, modern technology affords the tools to analyze phonological samples more efficiently and more thoroughly than we have in the past. It was our perception that students would be well served by more in-depth discussions of these topic areas than were included in previous editions—thus the new chapters.

Other chapters of the text reflect updating and reorganization. Our knowledge is expanding in areas such as details of the normal phonological acquisition process, descriptions of disorders and etiological subgroups, effectiveness of clinical management procedures, and the implications of management outcomes to our understanding of the nature of phonological behavior. In this book we have attempted once again to synthesize the literature and present it in a manner meaningful to a student studying clinical phonology.

The book has been divided into ten chapters. Chapter 1 reviews normal aspects of articulation and provides an introduction to the phonological system of American English. This information is sometimes covered in courses other than clinical phonology; however, for those lacking such coursework or in need of review, this content is presented.

Chapters 2 and 3 focus on normal phonological acquisition in children and review the process through which children develop production and perceptual skills at both the prelinguistic and linguistic levels. Since speech-language pathologists must distinguish delayed or deviant phonological development from normal development, they must recognize and understand normal phonological development.

Chapter 4 is a new addition to this text, and as stated above, reflects our growing awareness of the multicultural nature of our society and the fact that the linguistic systems of our clients are often reflective of other than "Standard American English." Two major dialectal variations found in our society are reviewed in this chapter: Black English Vernacular and Spanish-influenced English.

Chapter 5 reviews factors related to the development of normal and disordered phonology. Since this text is primarily focused on disorders of unknown or functional etiology, review of cognitive-linguistic as well as psychosocial factors as they relate to phonological disorders is presented. In addition, potential etiological variables, both major and minor, arising from impairments of the speech and hearing mechanism are reviewed.

Chapter 6 is concerned with procedures for obtaining samples of phonological behavior. Both theoretical and practical aspects related to various types of testing procedures are presented.

Chapter 7 continues the assessment presentation begun in Chapter 6 by focusing on the analysis and interpretation of data obtained during phonological assessment. Included in this discussion are rationale and procedures related to case selection, identification of treatment targets, and determination of appropriate treatment approaches.

Chapter 8 is another new addition to the text and reflects the growing use of computer instrumentation to analyze phonological samples. Computer programs can enhance the breadth and depth of phonological analyses. Hopefully this chapter will provide a better understanding of just what programs may or may not do, and thereby increase the clinician's "comfort level" with this form of technical assistance.

Chapter 9 looks at the remediation of phonological disorders. The treatment process is presented as a treatment continuum consisting of three phases—establishment, generalization, and maintenance. This continuum constitutes a framework for a variety of treatment techniques and procedures. Included in this chapter is a review of pertinent literature and a discussion of remediation issues.

Chapter 10 describes selected treatment programs and approaches that represent a number of different clinical and theoretical points of view. These approaches are organized under two broad categories of remediation—motor approaches and cognitive-linguistic approaches.

This text is designed to introduce the student to the clinical management of individuals with phonological disorders. Although the reader does not need an extensive background in speech-language pathology to understand this presentation, knowledge of phonetic transcription, basic anatomy and physiology of the speech mechanism, and language acquisition is useful.

REFERENCE

Hull, F., P. Mielke, R. Timmons, and J. Willeford, "The national speech and hearing survey: preliminary results." *ASHA, 13* (1971): 501–509.

chapter

1

Normal Aspects of Articulation

Ray Kent, University of Wisconsin–Madison

INTRODUCTION

Speech has been defined as *a system that relates meaning with sound*. Meaning itself arises in **language**. A *language* is *an arbitrary system of signs or symbols used according to prescribed rules to convey meaning within a linguistic community*. Of course, once an arbitrary association of symbol with meaning has been made, the users of that language must be consistent in this association if they want to communicate with one another. The word *dog* has a meaning in the English language, but this word can be communicated to other users of English by speaking, by writing, or by signing it with the manual symbols used by the deaf. Speech is but one modality for the expression of language; however, speech has special importance because it is the primary, first-learned modality for normal language users. Speech is a system in the sense that it consistently and usefully relates the meanings of a language with the sounds by which the language is communicated.

Not all sound variations in speech are related to meaning. When a person suffers from a cold, he or she has a different way of talking, but so long as the cold is not so severe as to make speech unintelligible, the relation of sound to meaning is basically the same as when the person is healthy. The acoustic signal of speech—that is, the vibrations of air molecules in response to the energy source of human speech—carries more information than just the expression of meaning. As we listen to a speaker, we often make judgments not only about the intended meaning but also about the speaker's age and sex (if the speaker isn't visible), the speaker's mood, the speaker's state of health, and perhaps even the speaker's dialectal background. Thus, on hearing a simple question—"Could you tell me the time, please?''—we might deduce that the speaker is a young southern woman in a hurry, an elderly British gentleman in a cheerful mood, or a young boy quite out of breath.

STRUCTURE OF LANGUAGE

To derive a speaker's meaning, the listener is basically concerned with the **phonemes** in the speech message. From a linguistic perspective, phonemes are sound units related to decisions about meaning. In the list, *cat hat mat bat sat fat that chat*, each word rhymes with every other word because all end with the same sound. However, the words differ in their initial sounds, and these differences can change the meaning of the syllables. In fact, the linguist identifies the phonemes in a given language by assembling lists of words and then determining the sound differences that form units of meaning. The layman usually thinks of words as the units of meaning, but the linguist recognizes a smaller form called the **morpheme**. For example, the linguist describes the words *walked* and *books* as having two morphemes: *walk* + *past tense* for *walked*, and *book* + *plural* for *books*. If two sounds can be interchanged without changing word meaning, or if they never occur in exactly the same combination with other sounds, then they are not different phonemes. Hence, phonemes are the minimal sound elements that represent and distinguish language units (words or morphemes).

A **phonemic transcription** (which is always enclosed in virgules / /) is less detailed than a **phonetic transcription** (which is enclosed in brackets [ ]). A phonetic transcription is sensitive to sound variations within a phoneme class. An individual variant of this kind is called an *allophone*. Thus, a phoneme is a family of allophones. Phonemes are the minimal set of sound classes needed to specify the meaningful units (words or morphemes) of the language. Allophones are a more numerous set of distinct sounds, some of which may belong to the same phoneme family. As a very simple example, the word *pop* begins and ends with the same phoneme but often begins and ends with a different allophone. If the final /p/ is produced by holding the lips together after they close, then this sound is the unreleased allophone of the /p/ phoneme. However, the initial /p/ must be released before the vowel is formed, so this sound is the released allophone of the /p/ phoneme. The /p/ phoneme also includes a number of other allophones, though perhaps not as obvious as these two.

To understand more clearly the difference between phonemes and allophones, say the following word-pairs to yourself as you try to detect a difference in the production of the italicized sounds.

*k*eep – *c*oop	(phoneme /k/)
m*a*n – b*a*t	(phoneme /æ/)
te*n* – te*n*th	(phoneme /n/)

In the first pair of words, the phoneme /k/ is articulated toward the front of the mouth in the first word and toward the back of the mouth in the second. Despite the differences in the place of tongue contact, the two sounds are heard by speakers of English to be the same phoneme. Speakers of other languages, such as Arabic, may hear the two sounds as different phonemes. The tongue-front and tongue-back versions are allophones of the /k/ phoneme.

In the next pair of words, *man* and *bat*, the pertinent difference might be

Normal Aspects of Articulation

more easily heard than felt through articulation. In the word *man*, the vowel is nasalized (produced with sound transmission through the nose) owing to the influence of the surrounding nasal consonants. But in the word *bat*, the vowel /æ/ is not normally nasalized. The phonetic environment of the vowel—that is, its surrounding sounds—determines whether or not the vowel is nasalized. The nasal and nonnasal versions of the vowel are allophones of the /æ/ phoneme.

Finally, in comparing /n/ in the words *ten* and *tenth*, you might notice that your tongue is more toward the front (just behind the upper front teeth) in the word *tenth*. The final *th* sound exerts an articulatory influence on the preceding /n/, causing it to be dentalized or produced at the teeth. Again, the two types of /n/ are simply allophones of the /n/ phoneme.

Allophonic variation is of two types: *complementary distribution* and *free variation*. In complementary distribution, two (or more) allophones never occur in exactly the same phonetic environment, so that the occurrence of one is complementary (non-overlapping) to the occurrence of the other. For example, the front and back /k/ discussed above are in complementary distribution. The front /k/ occurs in the environment of vowels made in the front of the mouth and the back /k/ occurs in the environment of vowels made in the back of the mouth. Similarly, the nasal and nonnasal allophones of /æ/ are in complementary distribution, determined by the presence or absence of nasals in the phonetic environment. The nasalized /æ/ occurs only when this vowel is preceded or followed by nasal sounds. Allophones are said to be in free variation when they can occur in the same phonetic context. For example, the released /p/ and the unreleased /p/ are in free variation in word-final position in words like *pop* or *map*. As indicated above, the final /p/ can be released audibly with a small burst as the lips open or it can be unreleased if the lip closure is maintained.

The discipline of linguistics is concerned primarily with the structure of language. The disciplines of psychology and speech pathology are concerned primarily with the processing of language—with its formulation and its reception. The linguistic study of language structure has influenced the study of language processing, and, to some degree, the reverse is true as well. Descriptions of language processing often use terms, such as syntax, semantics, phonology, and phonetics, that denote traditional areas of linguistic study. These terms have come to have a dual usage, one referring to structure and another to processing.

Figure 1–1 is a diagram of an information processing model of verbal formulation and utterance production. The diagram attempts to show how different types of information are processed in the act of speaking. The cognitive level is where a thought is initiated. This is a prelinguistic, propositional level that involves decisions such as the identification of participants and actions. For example, the cognitive processing that preceded formulation of the sentence, *the dog chased the cat*, involved the identification of a dog and a cat as participants and chasing or pursuit as an action. However, the words *dog, cat,* and *chased* were not actually selected. Rather, propositions or relations associated with these words were established.

Information from the cognitive level is used to make decisions at the syntactic and semantic levels. Syntax involves the ordering of words in a sentence and semantics involves the selection of words. Research on verbal formulation indicates that syntactic and semantic processing are interactive (hence, the arrows

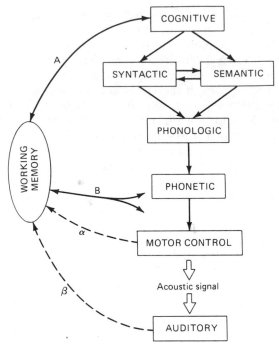

FIGURE 1–1. **Information processing model of verbal formulation and utterance production.** Adapted from J.K. Bock, "Toward a cognitive psychology of syntax: Information processing contributions to sentence formulation." *Psychological Review,* 89 (1982): 1–47.

between them in the diagram). Deciding upon a particular syntactic structure for a sentence can influence word selection, and selection of particular words can limit or direct syntactic decisions. The semantic level is sometimes called lexicalization, or the choice of lexical units. Lexicalization appears to be a two-stage process. The first stage is selection of a lexical concept, not a phonologically complete word. Phonologic specification, that is, specification of the word's sound pattern, is accomplished in the second stage of the process. The phonologic level in Figure 1–1 is the level at which the evolving sentence comes to have phonologic structure. Various decisions are made at this level to insure that a sound pattern accurately represents the syntactic and semantic decisions made earlier. The phonologic information then directs decisions at the phonetic level, where the details of the sound pattern are worked out. We might think of the phonetic level as producing a detailed phonetic representation of the utterance.

The output of the phonetic level is sufficient to specify the phonetic goals to be satisfied in speech production. Actual motor instructions are determined by a motor control level. This level selects the muscles to be activated and controls the timing and strength of the muscle contractions. This is no small task. Speech requires rapid changes in the activation of about 100 muscles. Once the muscles have done their work, the acoustic speech signal is produced. This signal is then processed by the speaker and the listener(s) as auditory information. For the speaker, the auditory processing completes a feedback loop.

One component that remains to be explained in Figure 1–1 is working mem-

Normal Aspects of Articulation

ory and its connections to other parts of the diagram. Working memory is a speaker's operational memory, the memory that is used to keep track of the information involved in sentence production. But this memory is limited, so it is in the interest of efficient processing to minimize demands on it. Therefore, the theory goes, two kinds of processing are involved in utterance production. One is **controlled processing**; this kind makes demands on working memory. The other is **automatic processing**, which does not require allocation of working memory. Verbal formulation is performed with both controlled processing and automatic processing. Controlled processing can be identified in Figure 1–1 by the arrows labeled A and B. Note that syntactic, semantic, and phonologic processing are automatic; that is, the speaker does not have direct access to these operations. It is for this reason that slips of the tongue are not detected until they are actually spoken.

Feedback is provided by two channels, labeled α and β in Figure 1–1. Channel α represents information from touch and movement. Channel β represents auditory feedback.

Researchers have concluded that when we ordinarily produce a sentence, we don't make all of the syntactic, semantic, and phonologic decisions before beginning to speak. Rather, it is likely that we will utter a few words and then formulate the remainder of the utterance.

According to this view of verbal formulation, producing a sentence involves highly interactive levels of processing and a complex time pattern for this processing. It would not be surprising, then, to discover that articulation is affected by syntactic, semantic and phonologic variables.

The following discussion of articulatory phonetics presents basic information on speech sound production. For the student who has had a course in phonetics, this chapter should be a summary review. The student without such background should be able to acquire at least the basics of articulatory phonetics. The topics to be discussed are these:

The Speech Mechanism
Vowels
   Monophthongs (single vowels)
   Diphthongs
Consonants
   Stops
   Nasals
   Fricatives
   Affricates
   Liquids
   Glides
Suprasegmentals
Coarticulation
Aerodynamics
Acoustics
Afference
Sensory Information
Phonology

FUNDAMENTALS OF ARTICULATORY PHONETICS

THE SPEECH MECHANISM

The anatomy of the speech production system is not within the scope of this chapter, but some general anatomical descriptions are needed to discuss the fundamentals of articulatory phonetics. The basic aspects of speech production can be understood by an examination of six principal organs or subsystems, illustrated in Figure 1–2. The *respiratory system*, consisting of the lungs, airway, rib cage, diaphragm, and associated structures, provides the basic air supply for generating sound. The *larynx*, composed of various cartilages and muscles, generates the voiced sounds of speech by vibration of the vocal folds, or it allows air to pass from lungs to the vocal tract (the oral and nasal cavities) for voiceless sounds. The *velopharynx*—the soft palate (or velum) and associated structures of the velopharyngeal port—joins or separates the oral and nasal cavities so that air passes through the oral cavity, the nasal cavity, or both. The *tongue*, primarily a complex of muscles, is the principal articulator of the oral cavity; it is capable of assuming a variety of shapes and positions in vowel and consonant articulation. For articulatory purposes, the tongue is divided into five major parts: the tip or apex, the blade, the back or dorsum, the root, and the body. These divisions are illustrated in Figure 1–3. The *lips*, along with the jaw, are the most visible of the articulators; they are involved in the production of vowels and consonants. The *jaw*, the massive bony structure and its associated muscles, supports the soft

FIGURE 1–2. **Organs of speech production.**

FIGURE 1-3. Divisions of tongue into five functional parts for speech articulation.

tissues of both tongue and lower lip. It participates in speech production by aiding tongue and lip movements and by providing skeletal support for these organs.

Other anatomical features shown in Figure 1–2 provide general orientation or are relevant in a significant way to the processes of speech and hearing.

The respiratory system and larynx work together to provide the upper airway with two major types of air flow: a series of pulses of air created by the action of the vibrating vocal folds (for voiced sounds like the sounds in the word *buzz*), and a continuous flow of air that can be used to generate noise energy in the vocal tract (for voiceless sounds like the *s* in *see*). The basic function of the respiratory system in speech is to push air into the airway composed of the larynx and the oral and nasal cavities. The basic function of the larynx is to regulate the air flow from the lungs to create both voiced and voiceless segments. The upper airway, often called the vocal tract, runs from the larynx to the mouth or nose and is the site of what is commonly called speech articulation. For the most part, this process is accomplished by movements of the *articulators:* tongue, lips, jaw, and velopharynx. The vocal tract may be viewed as a flexible tube that can be lengthened or shortened (by moving the larynx up and down in the neck or by protruding and retracting the lips) and constricted at many points along its length by actions of tongue, velopharynx, and lips. Speech articulation is thus a matter of lengthening, shortening, and constricting the tube known as the vocal tract.

This entire process is controlled by the nervous system, which must translate the message to be communicated into a pattern of signals that run to the various muscles of the speech mechanism. As these muscles contract, a variety of things can happen: Air may be pushed out of the lungs, the vocal folds may start to vibrate, the velopharynx may close, the jaw may lower, or the lips may protrude. The brain has the task of coordinating all the different muscles so that they contract in the proper sequence to produce the required phonetic result. The margin for error is small; sometimes an error of just a few milliseconds in the timing of a muscle contraction can result in a misarticulation.

It is appealing to suppose that speech production is controlled at some relatively high level of the brain by discrete units, such as phonemes. However, a major problem in the description of speech articulation is to relate the discrete linguistic units that operate at a high level of the brain to the muscle contractions that result in articulatory movements. For example, to say the word *stop*, a speaker's brain must send nervous instructions, in the proper sequence, to the muscles of the respiratory system, larynx, tongue, lips, and velopharynx. The full understanding of speech production therefore involves a knowledge of **phonology** (the study of how sounds are put together to form words and other linguistic units), **articulatory phonetics** (the study of how the articulators make individual sounds), **acoustic phonetics** (the study of the relationship between articulation and the acoustic signal of speech), and **speech perception** (the study of how phonetic decisions are made from the acoustic signal).

Vowel Articulation: Traditional Phonetic Description

A vowel sound is usually formed as sound energy from the vibrating vocal folds escapes through a relatively open vocal tract of a particular shape. Because a syllable must contain a vowel or vowel-like sound, vowels sometimes are called *syllable nuclei*. Each vowel has a characteristic vocal tract shape that is determined by the position of the tongue, jaw, and lips. Although other parts of the vocal tract, like the velum, pharyngeal walls, and cheeks, may vary somewhat with different vowels, the positions of the tongue, jaw, and lips are of primary consequence. Therefore, individual vowels can be described by specifying the articulatory positions of tongue, jaw, and lips. Furthermore, because the jaw and tongue usually work together to increase or reduce the mouth opening (Figure 1–4), for general phonetic purposes vowel production can be described by specifying the positions of just two articulators, tongue and lips. Usually, the vocal folds vibrate to produce voicing for vowels, but exceptions, such as whispered speech, do occur.

    The two basic lip articulations can be demonstrated with the vowels in the words *he* and *who*. Press your finger against your lips as you say first *he* and then

FIGURE 1–4. **Variations in mouth opening (darkened area) related to lowering of jaw and tongue.**

Normal Aspects of Articulation

FIGURE 1–5. Vocal tract configurations for /i/ and /u/. Note lip rounding for /u/.

FIGURE 1–6. The two major dimensions of tongue position, front-back and high-low.

who. You should feel the lips push against your finger as you say *who*. The vowel in this word is a rounded vowel, meaning that the lips assume a rounded, protruded posture. Vowels in English are described as being either rounded, like the vowel in *who*, or unrounded, like the vowel in *he*. Figure 1–5 illustrates the lip configuration for these two vowels.

The tongue moves in essentially two dimensions within the oral cavity, as shown in Figure 1–6. One dimension, front-back, is represented by the motion the tongue makes as you alternately say *he, who* or *map, mop*. The other dimension, high-low, is represented by the motion the tongue makes as you say *heave-have* or *who-ha*. With these two dimensions of tongue movement, we can define four extreme positions of the tongue within the oral cavity, as shown in Figure 1–7. The phonetic symbols for these four vowels also are shown in the illustration. With the tongue high and forward in the mouth, the high-front vowel /i/ as in *he* is produced. When the tongue is low and forward in the mouth, the low-front vowel /æ/ as in *have* is produced. A tongue position that is high and back in the mouth yields the high-back vowel /u/. Finally, when the tongue is low and back in the mouth, the vowel is the low-back /ɑ/. The four vowels, /i/, /æ/, /u/, and /ɑ/, define four points which establish the *vowel quadrilateral*, a four-sided figure against which tongue position for vowels can be described. In Figure 1–8, the vowels of English have been plotted by phonetic symbol and key word

FIGURE 1–7. **The four corner vowels /i/, /u/, /ɑ/, and /æ/ are shown at the top as tongue positions in the oral cavity and at the bottom as points of a quadrilateral.**

Normal Aspects of Articulation

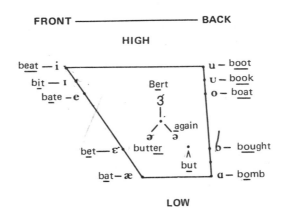

FIGURE 1–8. **English vowels, identified by phonetic symbol and key word and plotted within vowel quadrilateral.**

within the quadrilateral. As an example, notice the vowel /ɪ/ as in *bit* has a tongue position that is forward in the mouth and not quite as high as that for /i/. The tongue position for any one vowel can be specified with terms such as low-high, front for /ɪ/ as in *bit*, low-mid, front for /ɛ/ as in *bet*, mid-central for /ɜ/ as in *Bert*, and low-mid, back for /ɔ/ as in *bought*.

The vowels of English can be categorized as follows with respect to tongue position:

Front vowels: /i/ /ɪ/ /e/ /ɛ/ /æ/
Central vowels: /ɜ/ /ʌ/ /ɚ/ /ə/
Back vowels: /u/ /ʊ/ /o/ /ɔ/ /ɑ/
High vowels: /i/ /ɪ/ /u/ /ʊ/
Mid vowels: /e/ /ɛ/ /ɜ/ /ʌ/ /ɚ/ /ə/ /o/ /ɔ/
Low vowels: /æ/ /ɑ/

The vowels can also be categorized with respect to lip rounding, with the following being rounded: /u/, /ʊ/, /o/, /ɔ/, and /ɜ/. All other vowels are unrounded. Notice that, in English, the rounded vowels are either back or central vowels; front rounded vowels do not occur.

Vowel production is also commonly described as *tense (long)* or *lax (short)*. Tense vowels are longer in duration and supposedly involve a greater degree of muscular tension. Lax vowels are relatively short and involve less muscular effort. One way of demonstrating the distinction between tense and lax is to feel the fleshy undersurface of your jaw as you say /i/ as in *he* and /ɪ/ as in *him*. Most people can feel a greater tension for /i/ (a tense vowel) than for /ɪ/ (a lax vowel). The tense vowels are /i/, /e/, /ɜ/, /u/, /o/, /ɔ/ and /ɑ/. The remaining vowels are considered lax, but opinion is divided for the vowel /æ/ as in *bat*.

In standard production, all English vowels are voiced (associated with vibrating vocal folds) and nonnasal (having no escape of sound energy through the nose). Therefore, the descriptors *voiced* and *nonnasal* usually are omitted. However, it should be remembered that vowels are sometimes devoiced, as in whispering, and nasalized, as when they precede or follow nasal consonants. For phonetic purposes it is usually sufficient to describe a vowel in terms of the three major characteristics of tenseness–laxness, lip configuration, and tongue position. Examples of vowel description are given as follows.

/i/   tense, unrounded, high-front
/o/   tense, rounded, high-mid, back
/ɝ/   tense, rounded, mid-central
/ʊ/   lax, rounded, low-high, back

Closely related to the vowels are the *diphthongs*, which, like vowels, are produced with an open vocal tract and serve as the nuclei for syllables. But unlike vowels, diphthongs are formed with an articulation that gradually changes during production of the sound. Diphthongs are dynamic sounds, because they involve a progressive change in vocal tract shape. An example of the articulation of /aɪ/ is shown in Figure 1–9. Many phoneticians regard diphthongs as combinations of two vowels, one called the *onglide* portion and the other called the *offglide* portion. This vowel + vowel description underlies the phonetic symbols for the diphthongs, which have the *digraph* (two-element) symbols /aɪ/, /aʊ/, /ɔɪ/, /eɪ/, and /oʊ/. Key words for these sounds are as follows:

/aɪ/   *I, buy, why, ice, night*
/aʊ/   *ow, bough, trout, down, owl*
/ɔɪ/   *boy, oil, loin, hoist*
/eɪ/   *bay, daze, rain, stay*
/oʊ/   *bow, no, load, bone*

Whereas the diphthongs /aɪ/, /aʊ/, and /ɔɪ/ are truly phonemic diphthongs, /eɪ/ and /oʊ/ are not; they are variants of the vowels /e/ and /o/, respectively. The diphthongal forms /eɪ/ and /oʊ/ occur in strongly stressed syllables, whereas the monophthongal (single-vowel) forms /e/ and /o/ tend to occur in weakly stressed syllables. For example, in the word *vacation*, the first syllable (weakly stressed) is produced with /e/ and the second syllable (strongly stressed) is produced with

FIGURE 1–9. **Articulation of diphthong /aɪ/ (as in *eye*), represented as onglide (/a/) and offglide (/ɪ/) configurations.**

Normal Aspects of Articulation

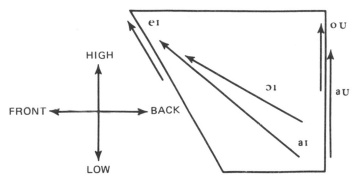

FIGURE 1–10. Diphthong articulation shown as onglide to offglide arrows in the vowel quadrilateral.

/eɪ/. Stressed syllables tend to be long in duration and therefore allow time for the articulatory movement of the diphthong. The diphthongs /aɪ/, /aʊ/, and /ɔɪ/ do not alternate with monophthongal forms. To produce a recognizable /aɪ/, /aʊ/, or /ɔɪ/, a speaker must use a diphthongal movement.

As shown in Figure 1–10, the onglide and offglide segments of the diphthongs are roughly located by the positions of the digraph symbols on the vowel quadrilateral. For example, in diphthong /aɪ/, the tongue moves from a low-back to nearly a high-front position. However, it should be noted that these onglide and offglide positions are only approximate and that substantial variation occurs across speakers and speaking conditions.

VOWEL ARTICULATION: DESCRIPTION BY DISTINCTIVE FEATURES

The phonetic descriptions considered to this point are one method of classifying vowel sounds. An alternative is a method relying on *distinctive features*, as defined by the linguists Noam Chomsky and Morris Halle (1968). The distinctive features are a set of binary (two-valued) features designed to describe the phonemes in all languages of the world. A convenient example of a binary feature is nasality. In general terms, a given speech sound is either nasal or nonnasal, meaning that sound energy is transmitted through the nose (nasal) or is not (nonnasal). If nasality is described as a binary feature, then sounds can be classified as + nasal (indicating the nasal transmission of sound) or − nasal (indicating the absence of nasal transmission). Hence, a positive value (+ nasal) means that the property is not present or is not relevant to description of the sound. In some ways, distinctive feature analysis is similar to the guessing game of Twenty Questions in which the participants have to identify an object by asking questions that can be answered with only yes or no. Chomsky and Halle proposed a set of 13 binary features, which, given the appropriate yes (+) or no (−) answers, can describe all phonemes used in the languages of the world.

In the Chomsky-Halle system, the voiced vowels are specified primarily with the features shown in Table 1–1. First, notice the three major class features of *sonorant*, *vocalic*, and *consonantal*. A sonorant sound is produced with a vocal cavity configuration in which spontaneous voicing is possible. Essentially, the vocal tract above the larynx is sufficiently open so that no special laryngeal adjustments are needed to initiate voicing. For nonsonorants, or *obstruents*, the

TABLE 1–1. **Distinctive Features for Selected Vowel Sounds. The Class Features Distinguish Vowels from Various Consonants; Therefore, All Vowels Have the Same Values for These Features.**

CLASS FEATURES	i	ɪ	ɛ	æ	ʌ	ɝ	u	ʊ	ɔ	ɑ
Sonorant	+	+	+	+	+	+	+	+	+	+
Vocalic	+	+	+	+	+	+	+	+	+	+
Consonantal	–	–	–	–	–	–	–	–	–	–
CAVITY FEATURES										
High	+	+	–	–	–	–	+	+	–	–
Low	–	–	–	+	–	–	–	–	+	+
Back	–	–	–	–	–	–	+	+	+	+
Rounded	–	–	–	–	–	+	+	+	+	–
Nasal	–	–	–	–	–	–	–	–	–	–
MANNER OF ARTICULATION FEATURE										
Tense	+	–	–	+	–	+	+	–	+	+

cavity configuration does not allow spontaneous voicing. Special mechanisms must be used to produce voicing during the nonsonorant sounds. Vocalic sounds are produced with an oral cavity shape in which the greatest constriction does not exceed that associated with the high vowels /i/ and /u/ and with vocal folds that are adjusted so as to allow spontaneous voicing. This feature, then, describes the degree of opening of the oral cavity together with the vocal fold adjustment. Finally, consonantal sounds have a definite constriction in the *midsagittal*, or midline, region of the vocal tract; nonconsonantal sounds do not. Vowels are described as +sonorant, +vocalic, and –consonantal. Taken together, these three features indicate that vowels are produced with a relatively open oral cavity, with no severe constriction in the midsagittal plane, and with a vocal fold adjustment that allows for spontaneous vocal fold vibration.

Vowels are also described with respect to cavity features and manner of articulation features, some of which are shown in Table 1–1 (the others will be discussed with respect to consonants later in this chapter). The cavity features of primary concern in vowel description are:

> Tongue Body Features: High–Nonhigh; Low–Nonlow; Back–Nonback (see Figure 1–11a, b, c)
> High sounds are produced by raising the body of the tongue above the level that it occupies in the neutral (or resting) position, as shown in Figure 1–11(a).
> Low sounds are produced by lowering the body of the tongue below the level that it occupies in the neutral position; see Figure 1–11(b).
> Back sounds are produced by retracting the body of the tongue from the neutral position, as shown in Figure 1–11(c).
>
> Rounded–Nonrounded
> Rounded sounds have a narrowing or protrusion of the lips.
>
> Nasal–Nonnasal
> Nasal sounds are produced with a lowered *velum*, so that sound energy escapes through the nose.

Table 1–1 shows that most vowels can be distinguished using the cavity features. For example, /i/ and /u/ differ in the back and rounded features, and /æ/ and /i/ differ in the high and low features. Most other distinctions can be made by referring

Normal Aspects of Articulation

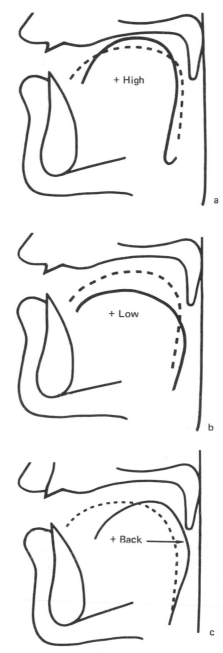

FIGURE 1–11 (a, b, and c). **Vocal tract drawings illustrating the tongue body features high, low, and back relative to the neutral tongue position (broken line).**

to a manner of articulation called tense–nontense. Tense sounds are produced with a deliberate, accurate, maximally distinct gesture that involves considerable muscular effort. The tense-nontense distinction is best illustrated with the vowel pairs /i/–/ɪ/ and /u/–/ʊ/. Vowels /i/ and /u/ are tense vowels because they are lengthened and are produced with marked muscular effort. As mentioned earlier, the difference in muscular effort can be felt by placing your fingers in the fleshy area just under the chin, saying alternately /i/–/ɪ/. A greater tension occurs during production of the tense vowel /i/ than during the nontense vowel /ɪ/.

CONSONANT ARTICULATION: TRADITIONAL PHONETIC DESCRIPTION

The consonants generally differ from the vowels in terms of the relative openness of the vocal tract and the function within the syllable. Vowels are produced with an open vocal tract; most consonants are made with a complete or partially constricted vocal tract. Within a syllable, vowels serve as a nucleus, meaning that a syllable must contain one and only one vowel (the only exceptions to this rule are the diphthongs, which are like vowels plus vowel glides, and certain syllabic consonants to be discussed later). Consonants are added to the vowel nucleus to form different syllable shapes, such as the following, where V represents a vowel and C represents a consonant.

VC shape:	*on, add, in*
CV shape:	*do, be, too*
CVC shape:	*dog, cat, man*
CCVC shape:	*truck, skin, clap*
CCVCC shape:	*screams, squint, scratched*

Consonants are described by degree or type of closure and by the location at which the complete or partial closure occurs. The *manner* of consonant articulation refers to the degree or type of closure, and the *place* of consonant articulation refers to the location of the constriction. In addition, consonants are described as *voiced* when the vocal folds are vibrating and *voiceless* when the vocal folds are not vibrating. Thus, an individual consonant can be specified by using three terms: one to describe *voicing*, one to describe *place*, and one to describe *manner*. Tables 1–2 and 1–3 show combinations of these terms used to specify the consonants of English.

Table 1–2 contains four columns, showing place of articulation, phonetic symbol and key word, manner of articulation, and voicing. The terms for place of articulation usually signify two opposing structures that accomplish a localized constriction of the vocal tract. Notice in the following definitions the two structures involved for the place terms.

Bilabial: two lips (*bi = two* and *labia = lip*)

Labial/velar: lips, and also a constriction between the *dorsum* or back of the tongue and the velum

Labiodental: lower lip and upper teeth

Linguadental or interdental: tip of tongue and upper teeth (*lingua = tongue*)

Lingua-alveolar: tip of tongue and the *alveolar ridge*

Linguapalatal: blade of tongue and palatal area behind the alveolar ridge

TABLE 1-2. **Classification of Consonants by Manner and Voicing within Place.**

PLACE OF ARTICULATION	PHONETIC SYMBOL AND KEY WORD	MANNER OF ARTICULATION	VOICING
Bilabial	/p/ (pay)	Stop	−
	/b/ (bay)	Stop	+
	/m/ (may)	Nasal	+
Labial/velar	/ʍ/ (which)	Glide (semivowel)	−
	/w/ (witch)	Glide (semivowel)	+
Labiodental	/f/ (fan)	Fricative	−
	/v/ (van)	Fricative	+
Linguadental	/θ/ (thin)	Fricative	−
(interdental)	/ð/ (this)	Fricative	+
	/t/ (two)	Stop	−
	/d/ (do)	Stop	+
	/s/ (sue)	Fricative	−
Lingua-alveolar	/z/ (zoo)	Fricative	+
	/n/ (new)	Nasal	+
	/l/ (Lou)	Lateral	+
	/ɾ/ (butter)	Flap	+
Linguapalatal	/ʃ/ (shoe)	Fricative	−
	/ʒ/ (rouge)	Fricative	+
	/tʃ/ (chin)	Affricate	−
	/dʒ/ (gin)	Affricate	+
	/j/ (you)	Glide (semivowel)	+
	/r/ (rue)	Rhotic	+
Linguavelar	/k/ (back)	Stop	−
	/g/ (bag)	Stop	+
	/ŋ/ (bang)	Nasal	+
Glottal (laryngeal)	/h/ (who)	Fricative	−
	/ʔ/ —	Stop	+(−)

    Linguavelar: dorsum or back of tongue and roof of mouth in the velar area
    Glottal: the two vocal folds

Each of these places of articulation is discussed more fully below. To get a feeling for these different places of consonant articulation, concentrate on the first sounds in each word as you say the sequence: *pie, why, vie, thigh, tie, shy, guy, hi.* Notice from Figure 1-12 that the initial sounds constitute a progression from front to back in place of articulation.

Table 1-3 provides a breakdown of English consonants by place and voicing within manner classes. The manner of production associated with complete closure is the *stop*, which is formed when two structures completely block the passage of air from the vocal tract, building up air pressure behind the closure. Usually, when the closure is released, the air pressure built up behind the constriction causes a burst of escaping air. The burst is audible in words like *pie* and *two.*

Fricatives, like the initial sounds in *sue* and *zoo*, are made with a narrow constriction so that the air creates a noisy sound as it rushes through the narrowed passage.

Affricates, as in *church* and *judge*, are combinations of stop and fricative segments; that is, a period of complete closure is followed by a brief fricative segment. The stop + fricative nature of the affricates explain why these sounds are represented by the digraph symbols /tʃ/ and /dʒ/.

Nasals, as in the word *meaning* /miniŋ/, are like stops in having a complete

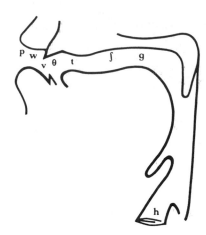

FIGURE 1–12. **Places of articulation are marked by location of the phonetic symbols for the initial sounds in** *pie, why, vie, thigh, tie, shy, guy, hi.*

oral closure (bilabial, lingua-alevolar, or linguavelar) but are unlike stops in having an open velopharyngeal port so that sound energy passes through the nose rather than the mouth.

The *lateral* /l/ as in *lay* is formed by making a lingua-alveolar closure in the midline but with no closure at the sides of the tongue. Therefore, the sound energy from the vibrating folds escapes laterally, or through the sides of the mouth cavity.

The *rhotic* (or *rhotacized*) /r/ as in *ray* is a complex phoneme sometimes called *retroflex* in the phonetic literature. Retroflex literally means *turning* or *turned back* and refers to the appearance of the tongue tip, as viewed in X-ray films, for some /r/ productions. But in other productions of /r/, the tongue has a bunched appearance in the center or near the front of the mouth cavity. Because

TABLE 1–3. **Classification of Consonants by Place and Voicing within Manner.**

MANNER	PLACE	VOICED	VOICELESS
Stop	Bilabial	b	p
	Alveolar	d	t
	Velar	g	k
	Glottal	-----ʔ-----------------	
Fricative	Labiodental	v	f
	Linguadental	ð	θ
	Alveolar	z	s
	Palatal	ʒ	ʃ
	Glottal		h
Affricate	Palatal	dʒ	tʃ
Nasal	Bilabial	m	
	Alveolar	n	
	Velar	ŋ	
Lateral	Alveolar	l	
Rhotic	Palatal	r	
Glide	Palatal	j	
	Labial/Velar	w	ʍ

/r/ is produced in at least these two basic ways, the general term *rhotic* (Ladefoged, 1975) is preferable to the narrower term *retroflex*. This issue is discussed in more detail below.

The /ʍ/, /w/, and /j/ sounds are said to have a *glide* (semivowel) manner of production. These sounds are characterized by a gliding, or gradually changing, articulatory shape. For example, in /ʍ/ and its voiced counterpart /w/, the lips gradually move from a rounded and narrowed configuration to the lip shape required by the following vowel simultaneously with a change in tongue position from high-back (like that for /u/) to the position for the following vowel. The glides always are followed by vowels.

In the following summary, manner of articulation is discussed for different places of articulation, proceeding from front to back.

Bilabial Sounds. In American English, the only consonant phonemes produced with a complete or partial labial closure (bilabial production) are the voiceless and voiced stops /p/ as in *pay* and /b/ as in *bay*, the nasal /m/ as in *may*, and the voiced and voiceless glides /w/ as in *witch* and /ʍ/ as in *which*. The vocal tract configurations for /p/, /b/, and /m/ are shown in Figure 1–13. These three sounds share a bilabial closure but differ in voicing and nasality. The stops /p/ and /b/ are called voiced and voiceless *cognates*, which means that they differ only in voicing. The production of these bilabial sounds is usually marked by a closed jaw position because the jaw closes somewhat to assist the constriction at the lips. The tongue is virtually unconstrained for /p/, /b/, and /m/, so that these bilabial sounds often are made simultaneously with the tongue position for preceding or following vowels. In other words, when we say words like *bee*, *pa*, and

FIGURE 1–13. Vocal tract configurations for /p/, /b/, and /m/. Note labial closure for all three sounds and the open velopharynx for /m/.

FIGURE 1–14. Variation in tongue position during a bilabial closure. Top: tongue position during *pea;* bottom: tongue position for *pa.*

moo, the tongue is free to assume the required shape for the vowel during the closure for the bilabial, as illustrated in Figure 1–14.

The glides /w/ and /ʍ/ have a specified tongue position, roughly like that for the high-back vowel /u/, so these sounds cannot interact as freely with preceding or following sounds. Students (and even some practicing clinicians) sometimes fail to appreciate the importance of tongue articulation for /w/ and /ʍ/; for these sounds, both the tongue and lips execute gliding movements, as shown for the word *we* in Figure 1–15.

Labiodental Sounds. The voiceless and voiced *fricatives* /f/ as in *fan* and /v/ as in *van* are the only labiodental sounds in American English. The articulation is illustrated in Figure 1–16. Frication noise is generated by forcing air through the constriction formed by the lower lip and the upper teeth, principally the incisors. The noise is quite weak, very nearly the weakest of the fricatives. Like the labial sounds /p/, /b/, and /m/, the labiodentals allow the tongue to assume its position for preceding or following sounds. The jaw tends to close to aid the lower lip in its constricting gesture.

Interdental Sounds. There are only two interdentals, both fricatives: the voiceless /θ/ (e.g., *thaw*) and voiced /ð/ (e.g., *the*). They are illustrated in Figure 1–17. The frication noise is generated as air flows through the narrow constriction created by the tongue tip and the edge of the incisors. The weak frication noise

Normal Aspects of Articulation

FIGURE 1–15. **Illustration of gliding motion of tongue and lips for the word** *we* **(/wi/).**

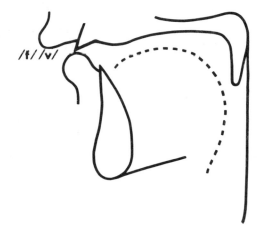

FIGURE 1–16. **Vocal tract configuration for /f/ and /v/. Note labiodental constriction.**

FIGURE 1–17. **Vocal tract configuration for /θ/ and /ð/. Note linguadental constriction.**

is not much different from that for /f/ or /v/. The weak intensity of these sounds should be remembered in articulation testing, and the clinician should include both visual and auditory information in evaluating this pair of sounds. Jaw position for /θ/ and /ð/ usually is closed to aid the tongue in making its constriction. These sounds may be produced with either an interdental projection of the tongue or tongue contact behind the teeth.

Alveolar Sounds. The alveolar place of production is used for two stops: the voiceless /t/ (e.g., *too*) and the voiced /d/ (e.g., *do*); a nasal: /n/ (e.g., *new*); a lateral: /l/ (e.g., *Lou*); and two fricatives: the voiceless /s/ (e.g., *sue*) and the voiced /z/ (e.g., *zoo*). Not surprisingly, given the frequent and diverse movements of the tongue tip in the alveolar region, motions of the tongue tip are among the fastest articulatory movements. For example, the major closing and release movement for the stops /t/ and /d/ is made within about 50 milliseconds, or a twentieth of a second. For /t/ and /d/, an airtight chamber is created as the tongue tip closes firmly against the alveolar ridge and the sides of the tongue seal against the lateral oral regions. The site of tongue tip closure actually varies to a limited degree with phonetic context. When /t/ or /d/ are produced before the dental fricatives /θ/ and /ð/, the stop closure is made in the dental region. This context-dependent modification of alveolar consonant production is termed *dentalization* and is illustrated for /t/ in Figure 1–18.

The nasal /n/ is similar in basic tongue shape and movement to the stops /t/ and /d/. But /n/ differs from both /t/ and /d/ in having an open velopharyngeal port, making /n/ nasalized. /n/ further differs from /t/ in that /n/ is voiced; /t/ is not. Because /n/ and /d/ are very similar in lingual articulation and voicing, failure to close the velopharyngeal port for /d/, as might happen with some speech disorders, results in /n/. Like /t/ and /d/, /n/ is dentalized when produced in the same syllable and adjacent to a dental sound like /θ/; compare, for example, the /n/ in *nine* /naɪn/ with the /n/ in *ninth* /naɪnθ/.

The lateral /l/ is a *liquid* formed with midline closure and a lateral opening, usually at both sides of the mouth (see Figure 1–19). Because of the midline closure made by the tongue tip against the alveolar ridge, sound energy escapes through

FIGURE 1–18. Dentalization of /t/. The normal alveolar closure is shown by the solid line and the dental closure is shown by the broken line.

Normal Aspects of Articulation

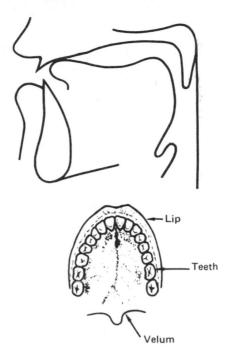

FIGURE 1–19. Articulation of /l/, shown in side view of a midline section (top) and as regions of tongue closure (shaded areas) against roof of mouth.

the sides of the oral cavity. Although /l/ is the only lateral sound in English, there are at least two major allophones. Historically, these allophones are termed *light* and *dark*, but phoneticians disagree as to exactly how these allophones are formed. Wise (1957a, 1957b) explained that the light /l/ is made with linguadental contact whereas the dark /l/ is made with a lingua-alveolar contact. However, Kantner and West (1960) contend that the light /l/ has a greater lip spread and a lower and flatter tongue position than the dark /l/. An important feature of /l/, presumably, is a raising of the tongue toward the velum or palate. Giles (1971) concluded from X-ray pictures of speech that for allophonic variations of /l/, the position of the tongue dorsum falls into three general groups regardless of phonetic context: prevocalic, postvocalic, and syllabic (with syllabic being similar to postvocalic /l/). The postvocalic allophones had a more posterior dorsal position than the prevocalic allophones. Tongue tip contact occasionally was not achieved for the postvocalic allophones in words like *Paul*. Otherwise, the only variation in tongue tip articulation was dentalization influenced by a following dental sound. Apparently, then, /l/ can be produced with either a relatively front (light /l/) or back (dark /l/) dorsal position, but the light and dark variants are perhaps just as well termed prevocalic and postvocalic. Lingua-alveolar contact is not essential at least for /l/ in postvocalic position, which explains why postvocalic /l/ in words like *seal* may sound like /o/ or /ʊ/. The fricatives /s/ and /z/ are made with a narrow constriction between the tongue tip and the alveolar ridge (Figure 1–20).

Palatal Sounds. The palatal sounds include the voiceless and voiced fricatives /ʃ/ (e.g., *shoe*) and /ʒ/ (e.g., *rouge*), the voiceless and voiced affricates /tʃ/ (e.g., *chin*) and /dʒ/ (e.g., *gin*), the glide /j/ (e.g., *you*), and the rhotic or retroflex

FIGURE 1–20. Vocal tract configuration for /s/ and /z/. Note lingua-alveolar constriction.

/r/ (e.g., *rue*). For these sounds, the blade or tip of the tongue makes a constriction in the palatal region, the area just behind the alveolar ridge (see Figure 1–21).

   The fricatives /ʃ/ and /ʒ/, like /s/ and /z/, are sibilants associated with intense noisy energy. For /ʃ/ and /ʒ/, this noise is generated as air moves rapidly through a constriction formed between the blade of the tongue and the front palate. Similarly, the affricates /tʃ/ and /dʒ/ are made in the palatal area as stop + fricative combinations. The air stream is first interrupted during the stop phase and then released during the fricative phase that immediately follows. In English, the only affricates are the palatal /tʃ/ and /dʒ/.

   The glide /j/ is similar to the high-front vowel /i/ (as in *he*). The tongue is initially far forward and high in the mouth and subsequently moves toward the position for the following vowel. The similarity between /j/ and /i/ can be demonstrated by saying the biblical pronoun *ye* while noting the tongue position. Because the glide /j/ must be followed by a vowel, its articulation involves a gliding motion from the high-front position to some other vowel shape. The gliding motion can be felt during articulation of the words *you, yea, ya.*

   As mentioned briefly above, the articulation of /r/ is highly variable. It some-

FIGURE 1–21. Vocal tract configuration for /ʃ/ and /ʒ/. Note linguapalatal constriction.

Normal Aspects of Articulation

FIGURE 1–22. The two major articulations of /r/: *left,* the retroflexed articulation; *right,* the bunched articulation.

times is produced as a retroflexed consonant, in which case the tongue tip points upward and slightly backward in the oral cavity. But /r/ also can be produced with a bunching of the tongue, either in the middle of the mouth or near the front of the mouth. These basic articulations are illustrated in Figure 1–22. Some speakers also round their lips for /r/, and some constrict the lower pharynx by pulling the root of the tongue backward. Because /r/ is variably produced, it seems advisable to use *rhotic* or *rhotacized* (Ladefoged, 1975) rather than *retroflex* as a general articulatory descriptor. Given the complicated articulation of /r/, it is not surprising that it should present a major problem to children learning to talk. The variation in tongue shape and position also complicates a speech clinician's attempts to teach /r/ articulations to a child who misarticulates the sound.

Velar Sounds. A velar constriction, formed by elevation of the tongue dorsum toward the roof of the mouth, occurs for the voiceless and voiced stops /k/ and /g/ and for the nasal /ŋ/. This articulation is illustrated in Figure 1–23, which

FIGURE 1–23. Vocal tract configurations for velar consonants. Note variation in site of closure.

shows that the constriction can be made with the tongue relatively toward the front or relatively toward the back. The tongue placement is generally determined by the vowel context, with a front placement for velars adjacent to front vowels (e.g., /g/ in *geese*) and a back placement for velars adjacent to back vowels (e.g., /g/ in *goose*). The nasal /ŋ/ has a tongue constriction similar to that for /k/ and /g/ but has an open velopharyngeal port for nasalization. The velar and bilabial places of articulation are similar in that both are used in English only for stops and nasals.

Glottal Sounds. The glottis, or chink between the vocal folds, is primarily involved only with two sounds, the voiceless fricative /h/ and the stop /ʔ/ (a stoppage of air at the vocal folds). The fricative is produced with an opening of the vocal folds so that a fricative noise is generated as air moves at high speed through the glottis. A similar vocal fold adjustment is used in whisper.

It can be seen from Tables 1–2 and 1–3 that more types of sounds are made at some places of articulation than at others. Moreover, some sounds occur more frequently in the English language than others, contributing to a further imbalance in the use of places of articulation. Actual data on the frequency of occurrence of English consonants, grouped by place of articulation, are shown in Figure 1–24. In this circle graph, based on data from Dewey (1923), the relative frequencies of occurrence of different places of articulation are shown by the relative sizes of the pieces of the graph. Notice that alveolar sounds account for almost 50 percent of the sounds in English. The rank order of frequency of occurrence for place of articulation, from most to least frequent, is: alveolar, palatal, bilabial, velar, labiodental, interdental, and glottal. Within each place-of-articulation seg-

FIGURE 1–24. Circle graph showing relative frequency of occurrence of consonants made at different places of articulation Based on data from Dewey (1923).

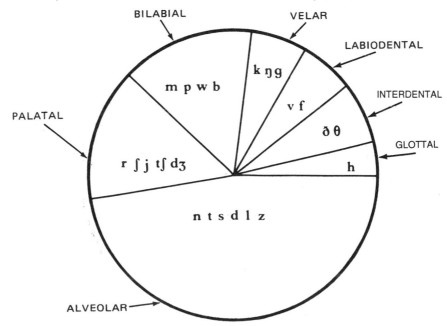

Normal Aspects of Articulation

ment in Figure 1–24, the individual consonants are listed in rank order of frequency of occurrence. For example, /n/ is the most frequently occurring alveolar consonant (in fact, it is the most frequently occurring of all consonants). Because of the differences in frequency of occurrence of consonants, a misarticulation affecting one place of articulation can be far more conspicuous than a misarticulation affecting another place. Therefore, statistical properties of the language are one consideration in the assessment and management of articulation disorders.

CONSONANT ARTICULATION: DESCRIPTION BY DISTINCTIVE FEATURES

Distinctive features, discussed earlier with respect to vowels, can be used as an alternative to the place-manner chart to describe consonants. One simple example is the feature of voiced: All voiced consonants can be assigned the feature value of + voiced, and all voiceless consonants can be assigned the value of − voiced. Some important features for consonants are defined briefly below and are used for consonant classification in Table 1–4. These definitions are based on Chomsky and Halle (1968).

> *Consonantal* sounds have a radical or marked constriction in the midsagittal region of the vocal tract. This feature distinguishes the "true" consonants from vowels and glides.
>
> *Vocalic* sounds do not have a radical or marked constriction of the vocal tract and are associated with spontaneous voicing. The voiced vowels and liquids are vocalic; the voiceless vowels and liquids, glides, nasal consonants, and obstruents (stops, fricatives, and affricates) are *nonvocalic* (that is, − vocalic).
>
> *Sonorant* sounds have a vocal configuration that permits spontaneous voicing, which means that the airstream can pass virtually unimpeded through the oral or nasal cavity. This feature distinguishes the vowels, glides, nasal consonants, and lateral and rhotacized consonants from the stops, fricatives and affricates (the class of obstruents).

TABLE 1–4. **Distinctive Feature Classifications for Selected Consonants.**

CONSONANTS										
Feature	p	b	m	t	d	n	s	l	θ	k
Consonantal	+	+	+	+	+	+	+	+	+	+
Vocalic	−	−	−	−	−	−	−	−	−	−
Sonorant	−	−	+	−	−	+	−	+	−	−
Interrupted	+	+	−	+	+	−	−	−	−	+
Strident	−	−	−	−	−	−	+	−	−	−
High	(−)	(−)	(−)*	−	−	−	−	−	−	+
Low	(−)	(−)	(−)	−	−	−	−	−	−	−
Back	(−)	(−)	(−)	−	−	−	−	−	−	+
Anterior	+	+	+	+	+	+	+	+	+	−
Coronal	−	−	−	+	+	+	+	+	+	−
Rounded	−	−	−	−	−	−	−	−	−	−
Distributed	+	+	+	−	−	−	−	−	+	−
Lateral	−	−	−	−	−	−	−	+	−	−
Nasal	−	−	+	−	−	+	−	−	−	−
Voiced	−	+	+	−	+	+	−	+	−	−

* Feature values enclosed in parentheses indicate that the feature in question may not be specified for this sound. For example, tongue position for /p/, /b/, and /m/ is not really specified, as it is free to assume the position required for the following vowel.

Interrupted sounds have a complete blockage of the airstream during a part of their articulation. Stops and affricates are + interrupted, which distinguishes them from fricatives, nasals, liquids, and glides. Sometimes the feature *continuant* is used rather than interrupted, with opposite values assigned, that is, + continuant sounds are − interrupted and vice versa.

Strident sounds are those fricatives and affricates produced with intense noise: /s/, /z/, /ʃ/, /ʒ/, /tʃ/, /dʒ/. The amount of noise produced depends on characteristics of the constriction, including roughness of the articulatory surface, rate of air flow over it, and angle of incidence between the articulatory surfaces.

High sounds are made with the tongue elevated above its neutral (resting) position (see Figure 1–11a).

Low sounds are made with the tongue lowered below its neutral position (see Figure 1–11b).

Back sounds are made with the tongue retracted from its neutral position (see Figure 1–11c).

Anterior sounds have an obstruction that is farther forward than that for the palatal /ʃ/. Anterior sounds include the bilabials, labiodentals, linguadentals, and lingua-alveolars.

Coronal sounds have a tongue blade position above the neutral state. In general, consonants made with an elevated tongue tip or blade are + coronal.

Rounded sounds have narrowed or protruded lip configuration.

Distributed sounds have a constriction extending over a relatively long portion of the vocal tract (from back to front). For English, this feature is particularly important to distinguish the dental fricatives /θ/ and /ð/ from the alveolars /s/ and /z/.

Lateral sounds are coronal consonants made with midline closure and lateral opening.

Nasal sounds have an open velopharynx allowing air to pass through the nose.

Voiced sounds are produced with vibrating vocal folds.

The feature assignments in Table 1–4 are for general illustration of the use of features. The features should be viewed with some skepticism, as several different feature systems have been proposed, and any one system is subject to modification. It should be understood that distinctive features are one type of classification system. It should also be realized that distinctive features have an intended linguistic function that may not always be compatible with their application to the study of articulation disorders. The issue is beyond the scope of this chapter, but the interested reader is referred to Walsh (1974) and Parker (1976).

The relationship between the traditional place terms of phonetic description and the distinctive features is summarized below. For each traditional place term, the associated features are listed. As an example, a bilabial stop is + anterior, − coronal, and + distributed. (The placement of both features within brackets indicates that they are considered together in sound description.)

$$
\text{Bilabial} \quad \begin{bmatrix} +\text{anterior} \\ -\text{coronal} \\ +\text{distributed} \end{bmatrix}
$$

$$
\text{Labiodental} \quad \begin{bmatrix} +\text{anterior} \\ -\text{coronal} \\ -\text{distributed} \end{bmatrix}
$$

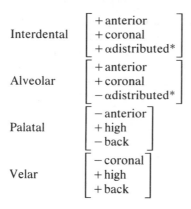

Interdental	$\begin{bmatrix} + \text{anterior} \\ + \text{coronal} \\ + \alpha\text{distributed*} \end{bmatrix}$
Alveolar	$\begin{bmatrix} + \text{anterior} \\ + \text{coronal} \\ - \alpha\text{distributed*} \end{bmatrix}$
Palatal	$\begin{bmatrix} - \text{anterior} \\ + \text{high} \\ - \text{back} \end{bmatrix}$
Velar	$\begin{bmatrix} - \text{coronal} \\ + \text{high} \\ + \text{back} \end{bmatrix}$

SUPRASEGMENTALS

The phonetic characteristics discussed to this point are *segmental*, which means that the units involved in the description are the size of phonemes or phonetic segments. *Suprasegmentals* are characteristics of speech that involve larger units, such as syllables, words, phrases, or sentences. Among the suprasegmentals are stress, intonation, loudness, pitch level, juncture, and speaking rate. Briefly defined, the suprasegmentals, also called *prosodies*, or *prosodic features*, are properties of speech that have a domain larger than a single segment. This definition does not mean that a single segment cannot, at times, carry the bulk of information for a given suprasegmental; on occasion, a segment, like a vowel, can convey most of the relevant information. Most suprasegmental information in speech can be described by the basic physical quantities of amplitude (or intensity), duration, and fundamental frequency (f_0) of the voice. Stated briefly, amplitude refers to the perceptual attribute of loudness; duration, to the perceptual attribute of length; and fundamental frequency, to the perceptual attribute of vocal pitch.

Stress. *Stress* refers to the degree of effort, prominence, or importance given to some part of an utterance. For example, if a speaker wishes to emphasize that someone should take the red car (as opposed to a blue or green one), the speaker might say "Be sure to take the *red* car," stressing *red* to signify the emphasis. There are several varieties of stress, but all generally involve something akin to the graphic underline used to denote emphasis in writing. Although underlining is seldom used in writing, stress is almost continually used in speech. In fact, any utterance of two or more syllables may be described in terms of its stress pattern. Because stress has influences that extend beyond the segment, stress usually is discussed with respect to syllables. The pronouncing guide of a dictionary places special marks after individual syllables to indicate stress. For example, the word *ionosphere* is rendered as (ı-*an'ə-sfer'*), with the marks ' and ' signifying the primary and secondary stress for the syllables.

The International Phonetic Alphabet (IPA) uses a different stress notation from that commonly found in dictionaries. In IPA the stress mark precedes the

---

*The symbol α is a "dummy variable" and is used here to indicate that the Chomsky-Halle features can distinguish the interdental and alveolar consonants only if they differ with respect to the feature *distributed*. Thus, if interdentals are regarded as − distributed, then alveolars must be + distributed. (See Ladefoged, 1971 for development of this issue.)

syllable to which it refers, and the degree of stress is indicated by whether *any* stress mark is used and by the *location* of the stress mark in the *vertical* dimension. The strongest degree of stress is indicated by a mark above the symbol line: ′ɑn (rather like a superscript); the second degree of stress is indicated by a mark below the symbol line: ‚aɪ (like a subscript); and the third degree of stress is simply unmarked: ə. The word *ionosphere* is rendered as /‚aɪ′ɑn ə ‚sfir/, with three degrees of stress marked.

Acoustically, stress is carried primarily by the vowel segment within a syllable. The acoustic correlates, roughly in order of importance, are fundamental frequency (especially with a rise in fundamental frequency on or near the stressed syllable), vowel duration (greater duration with increased stress), relative intensity (greater intensity with increased stress), sound quality (reduction of a vowel to a weaker, unstressed form, like /ɑ/ to /ə/, vowel substitution, and consonant changes), and disjuncture (pauses or intervals of silence) (Rabiner, Levitt, and Rosenberg, 1969).

Another form of unstressed (or weakly stressed) syllable is the syllabic consonant. This type of consonant, usually an /l/, /m/, or /n/ (but infrequently /r/), acts like a vowel in forming a syllable nucleus. Examples of syllabic consonants are the final sounds in the words *battle* /bætl̩/, *something* /sʌmʔm̩/, and *button* /bʌtn̩/. The syllabic function of a consonant is designated by a small vertical mark placed under the phonetic symbol. Syllabic consonants are most likely to occur when the consonant is *homorganic* (shares place of articulation) with a preceding consonant because it is economical or efficient simply to maintain the articulatory contact for both sounds. Additional information on stress will be provided following some basic definitions of related terms.

Intonation. Intonation is the vocal pitch contour of an utterance, that is, the way in which the fundamental frequency changes from syllable to syllable and even from segment to segment. Fundamental frequency can be affected by several factors, including the stress pattern of an utterance, tongue position of a vowel (high vowels have a higher f_0), and the speaker's emotional state.

Loudness. Loudness is related to sound intensity or to the amount of vocal effort that a speaker uses. Although loudness is ordinarily thought to be related to the amplitude or intensity of a sound, some evidence suggests that a listener's judgments of loudness of speech are related more directly to the perceived vocal effort, essentially the amount of work that a speaker does (Cavagna and Margaria, 1968). There is some evidence (Hixon, 1971; MacNeilage, 1972) that intensity variations in speech result mostly from respiratory activity, but variations of f_0 are easily accomplished at the level of the vocal folds.

Pitch Level. Pitch level is the average pitch of a speaker's voice and relates to the mean f_0 of an utterance. A speaker may be described as having a high, low, or medium pitch.

Juncture. Juncture, sometimes called "vocal punctuation," is a combination of intonation, pausing, and other suprasegmentals to mark special distinctions in speech or to express certain grammatical divisions. For example, the written sentence "Let's eat, Grandma," has a much different meaning than the same sentence without the comma, "Let's eat Grandma!" A speaker can mark a comma vocally with a short pause and an adjustment in intonation. Juncture is also used to make distinctions between similar articulations, such as between the word *nitrate* and the phrase *night rate.* Intonation and pausing enable a speaker to indicate which alternative he or she wants to express.

Speaking Rate. The rate of speaking is usually measured in words per second, syllables per second, or phonemes per second. As speaking rate increases, segment durations generally become shorter, with some segments affected more than others. The segments most vulnerable to contraction as a speaker talks more rapidly are pauses, vowels, and consonant segments involving a sustained articulation (like fricatives). Apparently, most speakers do not really increase the rate of individual articulatory movement as they increase their rate of speaking. Rather, they reduce the duration of some segments and reduce the overall range of articulatory movement (Lindblom, 1963). As a result, the articulatory positions normally assumed during a slow rate of speaking may be missed at a faster rate. The ''missing'' of articulatory positions as speaking rate increases is called *undershoot.* This is why a speaker's words are apt to sound less distinct to you as the rate of speaking increases.

Vowel Reduction. Vowels are particularly susceptible to articulatory change as speaking rate is increased or stress is decreased. Such articulatory alterations are termed *reduction* and are schematized in Figure 1–25. The arrows between pairs of vowels show directions of reduction; for example, /i/ reduces first to /ɪ/ and then to /ə/, the ultimate reduced vowel. The schema shows that, with reduction, all vowels tend toward /ə/ or /ʌ/.

Clear versus Conversational Speech. There is considerable evidence to show that speakers alter their patterns of speech production depending on situation and listener. One variation is clear versus conversational speech. Clear speech is what speakers use when they are trying to be as intelligible as possible. Compared to more casual conversational speech, clear speech is (1) slower (with longer pauses between words and a lengthening of some speech sounds), (2) more likely to avoid modified or reduced forms of consonant and vowel segments (such as the vowel reduction described earlier), and (3) characterized by a greater intensity of obstruent sounds, particularly stop consonants (Picheny, Durlach, and Braida, 1986). When talkers want to be easily understood, they modify their speech to make it slower and more acoustically distinctive. Whereas vowels in conversational speech often are modified or reduced, therefore losing some of their acoustic

FIGURE 1–25. A scheme of vowel reduction. The arrows between vowel symbols show vowel changes resulting from reduction. For example, /i/ and /e/ reduce to /ɪ/, and /ɪ/ reduces to /ə/, which is the ultimate reduced vowel. Note that these changes occur within the quadrilateral defined by the corner vowels /i/, /æ/, /ɑ/, and /u/.

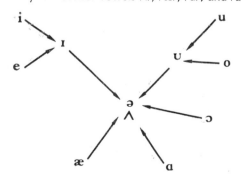

distinctiveness, these sounds in clear speech are produced in distinctive forms. Similarly, word-final stops in conversational speech frequently are not released, so that the burst cue for their perception is eliminated. But in clear speech, stop consonants (and consonants in general) tend to be released and this feature enhances their perception.

These differences are central to a recent hypothesis proposed by Lindblom (1990) that speakers vary their speech output along a continuum from *hypospeech* to *hyperspeech* (the H&H hypothesis). The basic idea is that speakers adapt to the various circumstances of communication, to match their production patterns to communicative and situational factors. When a speaker believes that special care is required to be understood, he or she alters articulation accordingly. In Lindblom's view, clear speech (hyperspeech in his H&H hypothesis) is not simply loud speech but reflects an articulatory reorganization (Moon and Lindblom, 1989). Adams (1990), however, reported contrary evidence. He concluded from an X-ray microbeam study of speech movements that changes in speech clarity did not seem to reflect a reorganization of speech motor control. Adams observed that in clear speech, articulatory movements tended to be both larger and faster but there was no general indication that the speech patterns were organized differently than in conversational speech. The important point for clinical purposes is that speech articulation can be controlled by a speaker to enhance intelligibility when conditions warrant such deliberate effort. The primary articulatory change appears to be in the magnitude and speed of movement.

New versus Given Information. New information in a discourse is information that the listener would not be expected to know from the previous conversation or from the situation. Given information is predictable, either from the previous discourse or from the general situation. New information often is highlighted prosodically. For example, Behne (1989) studied prosody in a mini-discourse such as the following:

"Someone painted the fence."
"Who painted the fence?"
"Pete painted the fence."

In this exchange, the new information ("Pete") is lengthened and produced with a higher fundamental frequency. In effect, the speaker uses prosody to highlight the new information.

Contrastive Stress in Discourse. Another discourse-related prosodic effect is *contrastive stress*. Such stress can be given to almost any word, phrase, or clause which the speaker considers to contradict or contrast with one that was previously expressed or implied. For instance, a speaker who wants to emphasize that she took the red ball rather than the green or blue one, might say, "I took the *red* ball" (where the italicized word receives contrastive stress). Contrastive stress is sometimes used clinically to give prosodic variation to an utterance or to elicit a stressed form of a target element.

Phrase-Final Lengthening. At the syntactic level, juncture and pause phenomena are used to mark multiword units. For example, in English, *phrase-final lengthening* operates to lengthen the last stressable syllable in a major syntactic phrase or clause. For example, if we contrast the following two sentences:

Normal Aspects of Articulation

1. Red, green, and blue are my favorite colors.
2. Green, blue, and red are my favorite colors.

the word *blue* will be longer in (1) than in (2) because in the former this word is at the end of the subject noun phrase and is therefore subject to phrase-final lengthening. This regularity can be exploited clinically to obtain durational adjustments for a target word. In addition, Read and Schreiber (1982) showed that phrase-final lengthening is helpful to listeners in parsing (that is, to recognize the structure of) spoken sentences. They also suggested that children rely more on this cue than adults do, and, moreover, that prosody assists the language-learner by providing structural guides to the complex syntactic structures of language.

Declination. Another effect at the syntactic level is *declination*, or the effect in which the vocal fundamental frequency contour typically declines across clauses or comparable units. Why this tilt in the overall fundamental frequency pattern occurs is a matter of debate (Cohen, Collier, and t'Hart, 1982), but it is a robust feature of prosody at the sentence or clause level. This pattern is helpful to listeners in recognizing the structure of discourse, such as in identifying sentence units.

Lexical Stress Effects. These effects operate at the level of the word. For example, English has many noun–verb pairs like *'import* versus *im'port*, or *'contrast* versus *con'trast*, in which the difference between the members of a pair is signaled primarily by stress pattern. Another common effect at the word level occurs with a distinction between compounds and phrases. For example, the compound noun *'blackbird* contrasts with the noun phrase *black 'bird* (a bird that is black).

Although the lay listener often thinks stress in English is just a matter of giving greater intensity to part of an utterance, laboratory studies have shown that stress is signaled by duration, intensity, fundamental frequency, and various phonetic effects (Fry, 1955). It is important to remember that stress affects segmental properties such as the articulation of vowels and consonants (Kent and Netsell, 1972; de Jong, 1991). Segments in stressed syllables tend to have larger and faster articulatory movements than similar segments in unstressed syllables. For this reason, stressed syllables often are favored in some phases of articulation therapy.

TOWARD A UNIFIED THEORY OF STRESS

The various stress effects summarized in the foregoing may appear to be a formidable collection of phenomena that the speaker somehow has to manage during the production of an utterance. Indeed, the list is imposing and belies the apparent ease with which most people can say something like, "But I didn't say *alveolar*, I said *velar* stop," which is produced with an overall pattern of declining fundamental frequency but with prosodic adjustments to place contrastive stress on the words *alveolar* and *velar*. The stressed words must be produced in accord with the lexical stress patterns, so that, for example, *velar* is spoken as *'velar* and not *ve'lar* or *'ve'lar*.

Some of the stress effects outlined in the previous section may be unified in a recent theory described by Beckman (1986) and Beckman and Edwards (1991). They propose a unified representation with four levels:

Level 1. Syllables with reduced nuclei, such as the second syllable in *vita*.

Level 2. Syllables similar to those above except that they have full vowels, e.g., *veto*.

Level 3. Syllables may be selectively given more stress by assigning to them a pitch accent.

Level 4. Syllables can receive a marking called *nuclear accent* (or *phrase accent*) in which the last accented item in a phonological grouping assumes the most prominent accent.

This proposal illustrates both the complexity of stress and a solution for its representation. Consider a speaker who wants to place pitch accent on the word *tuba*. The accent cannot be placed on the second syllable, which is a reduced nucleus. Rather, the accent must be placed on the stressed syllable. The levels discussed above help to show how various levels of the stress representation interact without destroying essential phonological patterns.

Because suprasegmentals like stress and speaking rate influence the nature of segmental articulation, some care should be taken to control suprasegmental variables in articulation tests and speech materials used in treatment. Vowels carry much of the suprasegmental information in speech, but stress, speaking rate, and other suprasegmentals can influence consonant articulation as well. The suprasegmental features of speech have been discussed by Crystal (1973), Lehiste (1970), and Lieberman (1967), and the reader is referred to these accounts for a more detailed consideration of this complex area.

COARTICULATION: INTERACTIONS AMONG SOUNDS IN CONTEXT

Convenient though it might be to consider phonemes as independent, invariant units that are simply linked together to produce speech, this simplistic approach does not really fit the facts. When sounds are put together to form syllables, words, phrases, and sentences, they interact in complex ways and sometimes appear to lose their separate identity. The influence that sounds exert on one another is called *coarticulation*, which means that the articulation of any one sound is influenced by a preceding or following sound. Coarticulation makes it impossible to divide the speech stream into neat segments that correspond to phonemes. Coarticulation implies nonsegmentation, or, at least, interaction of the presumed linguistic segments. Hockett provided a colorful illustration of the transformation from phoneme to articulation:

> Imagine a row of Easter eggs carried along a moving belt; the eggs are of various sizes, and variously colored, but not boiled. At a certain point, the belt carries the row of eggs between the two rollers of a wringer, which quite effectively smash them and rub them more or less into each other. The flow of eggs before the wringer represents the series of impulses from the phoneme source. The mess that emerges from the wringer represents the output of the speech transmitter (1955; 210).

Although this analogy makes the process of articulation sound completely disorganized, in fact the process must be quite well organized if it is to be used for communication. Phoneme-sized segments may not be carried intact into the various contractions of the speech muscles, but some highly systematic links between articulation and phonemes are maintained. Research on speech articulation has

Normal Aspects of Articulation

provided a clearer understanding of what the links are although the total process is far from being completely understood.

It often is possible to describe coarticulation in terms of articulatory characteristics that spread from one segment to another. Examine the following examples of coarticulation:

1a. He sneezed   /h i s n i z d/ (unrounded /s/ and /n/)
1b. He snoozed   /h i s n u z d/ (rounded /s/ and /n/)
2a. He asked   /h i æ s k t/ (nonnasal /æ/)
2b. He answered   /h i æ n s ɝ d/ (nasal /æ/)

The only phonemic difference between the first two items is the appearance of the unrounded vowel /i/ in 1a and the appearance of the rounded vowel /u/ in 1b. The lip rounding for /u/ in *He snoozed* usually begins to form during the articulation of the /s/. You might be able to feel this anticipatory lip rounding as you alternately say *sneeze* and *snooze* with your finger lightly touching your lips. In articulatory terms, the feature of lip rounding for the vowel is assumed during the /sn/ consonant cluster as the consequence of anticipating the rounding. The contrast between *sneeze* and *snooze* shows that the /sn/ cluster acquires lip rounding only if it is followed by a rounded vowel. This example of sound interaction is termed *anticipatory lip rounding* because the articulatory feature of rounding is evident before the rounded vowel /u/ is fully articulated as a segment.

Another form of anticipatory coarticulation occurs in 2b. Perhaps you can detect a difference in the quality of the /æ/ vowel in the phrases *He asked* and *He answered.* You should be able to detect a nasal quality in the latter because the vowel tends to assume the nasal resonance required for the following nasal consonant /n/. In this case, we can say that the articulatory feature of velopharyngeal opening (required for nasal resonance) is anticipated during the vowel /æ/. Normally, of course, this vowel is not nasalized. The contrasts between 1a and 1b and between 2a and 2b illustrate a type of coarticulation called *anticipatory.* Another type, *retentive*, applies to situations in which an articulatory feature is retained after its required appearance. For example, in the word *me* the vowel /i/ tends to be nasalized because of a carry-over velopharyngeal opening from the nasal consonant /m/. The essential lesson to be learned is that coarticulation occurs frequently in speech, so frequently in fact that the study of articulation is largely a study of coarticulation.

Phonetic context is highly important in understanding allophonic variation. For example, you should be able to detect a difference in the location of linguavelar closure for the /k/ sounds in the two columns of words below.

keen   *coon*
kin   *cone*
can   *con*

The point of closure tends to be more to the front of the oral cavity for the words in the first column than it is for the words in the second column. This variation occurs because, in English, the velar stops /k/ and /g/ do not have a narrowly defined place of articulation; all that is required is that the dorsum, or back, of the tongue touch the ceiling of the mouth. Therefore, the tongue is simply elevated at the position needed for the following vowel. When the tongue is in the front of the mouth (note that the vowels in the left column are front vowels), the dorsal closure is made in the front of the mouth, and when the tongue is in the back of the mouth (as it would be for the vowels in the right column), the point of closure is to the back of the velar surface.

Coarticulation arises for different reasons, some having to do with the phonology of a particular language, some with the basic mechanical or physiological constraints of the speech apparatus. Hence, some coarticulations are learned and others are the inevitable consequences of muscles, ligaments, and bones of the speech apparatus that are linked together and unable to move with infinite speed. Consider, for example, the closing and opening of the velopharyngeal port. This articulatory gesture is rather sluggish (compared to movements of the tongue tip), so it is not surprising that the velopharyngeal opening for a nasal consonant carries over to a following vowel, as in the word *no*. The extent of this carry-over nasalization, however, varies with the phonologic characteristics of a particular language. In French, vowel nasalization is phonemic (that is, it can make a difference in meaning), but in English, vowel nasalization is only allophonic. Some aspects of coarticulation reflect universal properties of the human speech mechanism and hence affect all languages. Other coarticulations are governed by the phonemic structure of a particular language and are therefore learned with that language. Many coarticulatory effects are assimilatory in that a feature from one segment is adopted by an adjacent segment. For example, the nasalization of vowels by neighboring nasal consonants is nasal assimilation. Such effects may make speech production easier and faster because articulatory movements can be adapted to a particular phonetic and motor sequence. Assimilation is a general process in spoken language and will be taken up later in discussions of phonology.

Another aspect of coarticulation is the overlapping of articulations for consonants in clusters. Quite often, the articulation for one consonant is made *before* the release of a preceding consonant in any two-consonant cluster. For example, in the word *spy* /spaɪ/, the bilabial closure for /p/ is accomplished shortly (about 10 to 20 msec) before the release of the constriction for /s/. This overlapping of consonant articulations makes the overall duration of the cluster shorter than the sum of the consonant durations as they occur singly; that is, the duration of /sp/ in *spy* is shorter than the sum of the durations of /s/ in *sigh* /s aɪ/ and /p/ in *pie* /p aɪ/. The overlapping of articulation contributes to the articulatory flow of speech by eliminating interruptions. The temporal structure of an /spr/ cluster, as in the word *spray*, is pictured schematically in Figure 1–26. Notice that the constrictions for /s/ and /p/ overlap by 10 to 20 milliseconds and that the closure for /p/ overlaps

FIGURE 1–26. **Schematic drawing of the articulatory organization of a /spr/ consonant cluster (as in the word *spray*), showing overlapping of consonantal articulations. Based on data from Kent and Moll (1975).**

Normal Aspects of Articulation

with the tongue position for /r/ by a similar amount. Because consonants in clusters frequently present special difficulties to children (and adults) with articulation disorders, clinicians must know how such clusters are formed. Because clusters have overlapping articulations of the constituent consonants, in general, the cluster is a tightly organized sequence of articulatory gestures. The articulation of clusters is further complicated by allophonic variations, such as those listed in Table 1–5. In English, unaspirated released stops occur only when stops follow /s/, as in the words *spy*, *stay*, and *ski*. Otherwise, released stops are aspirated, meaning that the release is followed by a brief interval of glottal frication (an /h/-like noise). Similarly, the devoiced /l/ and /r/ normally occur only after voiceless consonants, as in the words *play* and *try*.

The examples of context-dependent articulatory modifications in Table 1–5 show the variety of influences that sounds exert on adjacent sounds. For a given sound, place of articulation, duration, voicing, nasalization, and rounding may vary with phonetic context, and these variations are noted with the special marks shown in Table 1–5.

Some aspects of coarticulation can be understood by knowing the extent to which individual sounds restrict the positions of the various articulators. Table 1–6 summarizes degrees of restriction on lips, jaw, and parts of the tongue for the different places of consonant articulation. A strong restriction is indicated by an X, a slight to moderate restriction by a —, and a minimal restriction by an O. Because this table shows which parts of the vocal tract are free to vary during articulation of a given consonant, it can be used to predict certain aspects of coarticulation. For example, because bilabial sounds do not restrict the tongue as long as it does not close off the tract, Os are indicated for all parts of the tongue.

TABLE 1–5. **Examples of Context-Dependent Modifications of Phonetic Segments.**

MODIFICATION	CONTEXT DESCRIPTION
Nasalization of vowel	Vowel is preceded or followed by a nasal, e.g., [ɜ̃n]—*on* and [mæ̃n]—*man*
Rounding of consonant	Consonant precedes a rounded sound, e.g., [kʷwin]—*queen* and [tʷru]—*true*
Palatalization of consonant	Consonant precedes a palatal sound, e.g., [kɪʃ ju]—*kiss you*
Devoicing of obstruent	Word-final position of voiced consonant, e.g., [dɔg̊]—*dog* and [liɣ̊]—*leave*
Devoicing of liquid	Liquid follows word-initial voiceless sound, e.g., [pl̥eɪ]—*play* and [tr̥i]—*tree*
Dentalization of coronal	Normally alveolar sound precedes a dental sound, e.g., [wɪd̪θ]—*width* and [naɪn̪θ]—*ninth*
Retroflexion of fricative	Fricative occurs in context of retroflex sounds, e.g., [har ʂ ɚ]—*harsher* and [pɝʂɚ]—*purser*
Devoicing of sound	Consonant or vowel in voiceless context, e.g., [sl̥stɚ]—*sister*
Lengthening of vowel	Vowel preceding voiced sound, especially in stressed syllable, e.g., [ni : d]—*need*
Reduction of vowel	Vowel in unstressed (weak) syllable, e.g., [t æ bjuleɪt] [t æ bjəleɪt]—*tabulate*
Voicing of sound	Voiceless in voiced context, e.g., [æbʐ̬ɝd]—*absurd*
Deaspiration of stop	Stop follows /s/, e.g., [sp=aɪ]—*spy* vs. [pʰaɪ]—*pie*

TABLE 1–6. Coarticulation Matrix, Showing for Each Place of Consonant Articulation Those Articulators That Have Strong Restrictions on Position (Marked with X), Those That Have Some Restriction on Position (Marked with —), and Those That Are Minimally Restricted (Marked with O). For Example, the Bilabials /b/, /p/, and /m/ Strongly Restrict the Lips, Moderately Restrict the Jaw, and Leave the Tongue Essentially Free to Vary. The Glides /w/ and /ʍ/ Are Not Included because They Involve Secondary Articulations. Lip Rounding, as Often Occurs for /r/, Has Been Neglected.

Place	Lip	Jaw	TONGUE Tip	Blade	Dorsum	Body
Bilabial /bpm/	X	—	O	O	O	O
Labiodental /vf/	X	—	O	O	O	O
Interdental /ðθ/	O	—	X	X	—	—
Alveolar /dtzsln/	O	—	X	X	—	—
Palatal /ʃ ʒ dʒ tʃ j r/	O	—	—	X	X	X
Velar /gkŋ/	O	O	O	—	X	X
Glottal /h/	O	O	O	O	O	O

Jaw position is shown as moderately restricted for most places of articulation because some degree of jaw closing usually aids consonant formation. The ability of jaw movement to aid tongue movement declines as place of articulation moves back in the mouth, so a velar consonant may not restrict jaw position as much as more frontal articulation (Kent and Moll, 1972). The only sound that allows essentially unrestricted coarticulation is the glottal /h/. Thus, /h/ usually is made with a vocal-tract configuration adjusted to an adjacent sound, such as the following vowel in the words *he* /hi/, *who* /hu/, *ham* /hæm/, and *hop* /hɑp/.

Investigators of speech articulation (Daniloff and Moll, 1968; Moll and Daniloff, 1971; Kent and Minifie, 1977) have shown extensive overlapping of articulatory gestures across phoneme-sized segments, causing debate about the size of unit that governs behavior. Some investigators propose that the decision unit is an allophone, others argue for the phoneme, and still others for the syllable. A popular syllable-unit hypothesis is one based on CV (consonant-vowel) syllables, with allowance for consonant clustering (CCV, CCCV, and so on). This hypothesis states that articulatory movements are organized in sequences of the form CV, CCV, CCCV, and the like, so that a word like *construct* would be organized as the articulatory syllables /kɑ/ + /nstrʌkt/. Notice the odd assembly of the second syllable. This issue is of more than academic importance. Discovery of the basic decision unit would have implications for speech remediation; for example, enabling a speech clinician to choose the most efficient training and practice items for correcting an error sound. In addition, syllabic structures may explain certain features of speech and language development as discussed by Branigan (1976).

Normal Aspects of Articulation

Coarticulation also has clinical relevance, in that a sound might be more easily learned or more easily produced correctly in one context than in others. In other words, the phonetic context of a sound can facilitate or even interfere with correct production of the sound. The effect of phonetic context could explain why misarticulations are often inconsistent, with correct production on certain occasions and incorrect productions on others. By judiciously selecting the phonetic context where an error sound is initially corrected, the clinician can sometimes enhance the efficiency of speech remediation. Such examples show why a thorough knowledge of articulatory phonetics is important to decisions in the management of articulation disorders.

There is considerable theoretical controversy about how speech is organized as a motor behavior. Figure 1–27, which illustrates the controversy, depicts three levels of speech organization. (Actually, some contributors to the debate do not agree that these three levels are required; however, since most writers recognize them, they are used here.) The highest level is a sequence of units. This sequence may take the form of a psychological network of conceptual dependencies, a surface-structure representation of words (as suggested by Chomsky), or a syntagma (a rhythmic organization of syllables).

Most experts (it is hard to think of an exception) recognize the existence of some basic speech unit, the second level of Figure 1–27, but they disagree about the nature of this unit. Some prefer the syllable, others the phoneme, others the allophone, and still others the phonetic feature. Moreover, some think all of these

FIGURE 1–27. **Some alternative representations at three levels of organization of speech production. The top level is one of networks or strings, the middle level refers to a basic unit of speech production, and the third level pertains to the direct motor control of speech.**

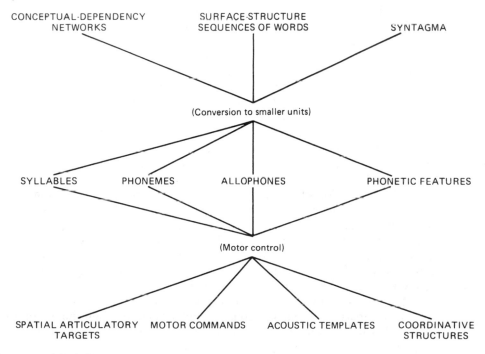

units are involved in a hierarchical organization, with syllables branching into phonemes, phonemes into allophones, and allophones into features.

The third level is motor control—the level at which the basic unit described above is converted into instructions that tell the muscles of speech what to do. One candidate for this level is a spatial articulatory target, a kind of snapshot of what the total vocal tract configuration should be. A second candidate is the motor command, presumed to be identical for each occurrence of the basic control unit (whatever that may be!). For those experts who believe the speech system tries to produce patterns that fit the acoustic goals of speech, the third candidate is an acoustic template. And finally, a relatively recent view identifies this level as a coordinative structure, an assembly of elementary movements that defines a basic unit of action. Obviously, there is no lack of theory!

AERODYNAMIC CONSIDERATIONS IN SPEECH PRODUCTION

Because the production of speech depends on the supply and valving of air, a knowledge of air pressure, flow, and volume is essential to an understanding of both normal and disordered speech. Many abnormalities of speech production are caused by irregularities or deficiencies in the supply and valving of air, and a number of clinical assessment techniques rely on measures of air pressure, flow, or volume. To understand the regulation of air pressures and flows in speech, it is important to recognize that (1) air flows only in one direction—from a region of greater pressure to one of lesser pressure; and (2) whenever the vocal tract is closed at some point, the potential exists for the buildup of air pressure behind the closure.

English speech sounds are normally *regressive*, meaning that, in sound production, air flows from the inside (usually the lungs) to the outside (the air around us). The basic energy needed to produce sound is developed in the lungs. After air is inspired by enlargement of the lung cavity, the muscle activation changes so that the lung cavity returns to a smaller size. If the airway above is closed, the same volume of air is enclosed in a smaller space. Because the same amount of air is contained in a smaller cavity, the air pressure within the lungs increases. This overpressure (relative to atmosphere) in the lungs is the source of the regressive air flow for all speech sounds. It is a fact of clinical importance that the air flow requirements for speech are not much greater than the requirements for ordinary breathing; that is, the volume of air inspired and expired in speaking is not much different from that in quiet respiration.

The regulation of air pressure and flow for speech is diagrammed in Figure 1–28, a simple model of the vocal tract. This model, in the form of the letter F, shows the three general areas where constriction (narrowing or closure) can occur: the laryngeal, oral, and nasal sections. The first site of constriction for egressive air is in the larynx. If the vocal folds close tightly, no air can escape from the lungs. If the folds are maximally open, then air passes through the larynx readily. If the folds are closed with a moderate tension, then the buildup of air pressure beneath them eventually blows them apart, releasing a pulse of air. After the folds are blown apart, they quickly come together again through the action of various physical restoring forces. This alternation of closed and open states, occurring

Normal Aspects of Articulation

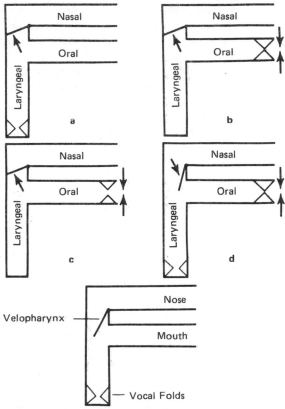

FIGURE 1–28. Simple models of vocal tract for major sound classes: a — vowels, liquids, and glides; b — voiceless stops; c — voiceless fricatives; d — nasals. The major parts of the model are shown at the bottom of the figure.

many times per second, is called voicing. Successive pulses of air from the vocal folds are a source of acoustic energy for all voiced sounds, such as vowels.

The F-shaped vocal tract model shown in Figure 1–28a illustrates the air flow for vowel sounds. The vocal folds are shown as being partly closed to represent the vibratory pattern of opening and closing. The nasal tube is tightly closed because vowels in English are nonnasal unless they precede or follow nasal consonants. The oral tube is widely open to represent the open oral cavity in vowel articulation. Because the nasal tube is closed, the acoustic energy from the vibrating vocal folds passes through the oral tube.

The configuration of the vocal tract for a voiceless stop like /p/, /t/, or /k/ is diagrammed in Figure 1–28b. The constriction at the larynx is shown as completely open because air from the lungs passes readily through the larynx and into the oral cavity. The constriction at the velopharynx is shown as closed to indicate that no air flows through the nasal tube. The oral constriction is closed to represent the period of stop closure. After this period, the oral constriction opens rapidly to allow a burst of air to escape from the oral pressure chamber. Assuming a stop closure of suitable duration, the air pressure developed within the oral cavity can be nearly equal to that in the lungs because the open vocal folds permit an equalization of air pressure in the airway reaching from the lungs up to the oral cavity. Therefore, voiceless stops have high intraoral air pressures. Also, it should be noted that children may use *greater* intraoral air pressures than adults (Subtelny, Worth, and Sakuda, 1966; Bernthal and Beukelman, 1978).

The model for voiceless fricatives in Figure 1–28c is like that for voiceless stops, but instead of a complete oral constriction, the model has a very narrow constriction, required for fricative noise. Because the velopharyngeal constriction is tightly closed and the laryngeal constriction is open, voiceless fricatives like /s/ and /ʃ/ have high intraoral air pressures. The voiceless stops and fricatives are sometimes called *pressure consonants*.

Voiced stops and fricatives differ from voiceless stops and fricatives in having vibrating vocal folds. Therefore, the models in Figure 1–28b and 1–28c would have a partial laryngeal constriction to represent voicing of these sounds. Because a certain amount of air pressure is lost in keeping the vocal folds vibrating (that is, pressure across the glottis drops), the voiced stops and fricatives have smaller intraoral air pressures than their voiceless cognates.

Finally, the model for nasal consonants is depicted in Figure 1–28d. A partial constriction at the larynx represents the vibrating vocal folds, and a complete oral constriction represents the stop-like closure in the oral section of the vocal tract. For nasal consonants, the acoustic energy of voicing is directed through the nasal cavity. Very little air pressure builds up within the oral chamber.

Liquids and glides can be modeled in essentially the same way as vowels (Figure 1–28a). Because the oral constriction for these sounds is only slightly greater than that for vowels, there is very little intraoral air pressure buildup.

Pressures and flows can be used to describe the function of many parts of the speech system. For example, a normal efficient operation of the larynx can often be distinguished from inefficient pathological states by the excessive air flow in the latter conditions. This excessive flow, or air wastage, may be heard as breathiness or hoarseness. Velopharyngeal incompetence can be identified by recording air flow from the nose during normally nonnasal segments. Frequently, velopharyngeal incompetence is signaled both by inappropriate nasal air flow (for example, air flow during stops or fricatives) and by reduced levels of intraoral air pressure. Sometimes, more than one pressure or flow must be recorded to identify the problem. For example, reduced levels of intraoral air pressure for consonants can be related to at least three factors: (1) respiratory weakness, resulting in insufficient air pressure; (2) velopharyngeal dysfunction, resulting in a loss of air through the nose; or (3) an inadequacy of the oral constriction, allowing excessive air to escape.

Clinically, aerodynamic assessment is especially important when dealing with a structural defect (such as cleft palate) or a physically based control problem (as in cerebral palsy, vocal fold paralysis, and other neurologic disorders). As noted above, young children may use greater intraoral air pressure than adults for consonant production, so normative pressure data obtained from adults should be used with caution in clinical evaluation of children. Moreover, the higher pressures in children's speech mean that children must close the velopharyngeal port even more tightly than adults to prevent nasal loss of air during stop or fricative consonants. Speech and language clinicians who do not possess equipment for aerodynamic recordings of speech should nonetheless be aware of the pressure

Normal Aspects of Articulation

and flow requirements in speech production. These requirements have important implications for the diagnosis and evaluation of communicative problems and for the design of remediation programs.

ACOUSTIC CONSIDERATIONS OF SPEECH

It is far beyond the scope of this chapter to consider in any detail the acoustic structure of speech sounds, but it is possible to draw here a few major conclusions about the acoustic signal of speech. Acoustic signals can be described in terms of three fundamental physical variables—frequency, amplitude, and duration. *Frequency* refers to the rate of vibration of a sound. Generally, the faster the rate of vibration, the higher the pitch heard. In other words, frequency is the most direct physical correlate of pitch. *Amplitude* refers to the strength or magnitude of vibration of a sound. The higher the magnitude of vibration, the louder the sound heard. Amplitude is the most direct physical correlate of loudness. Because the actual amplitude of vibration is minute and, therefore, difficult to measure, sound intensity or sound pressure level is used instead when making actual speech measurements. *Duration* refers to the total time over which a vibration continues. Duration is the most direct physical correlate of perceived length.

Virtually all naturally occurring sounds, speech included, have energy at more than a single frequency. A tuning fork is designed to vibrate at a single frequency and is one of the very few sound sources with this property. The human voice, musical instruments, and animal sounds all have energy at several frequencies. The particular pattern of energy over a frequency range is the *spectrum* of a sound. Speech sounds differ in their *spectra*, and these differences allow us to distinguish sounds perceptually.

Table 1–7 is a summary of the major acoustic properties of several phonetic classes. The table shows the relative sound intensity, the dominant energy region in the spectrum, and the relative sound duration for each class. Vowels are the most intense speech sounds, have most of their energy in the low to mid frequencies, and are longer in duration than other sounds (although the actual duration of vowel sounds may range from about 50 milliseconds to half a second). Because vowels are the most intense sounds, they typically determine the overall loudness of speech. The most intense vowels are the low vowels and the least intense, the high vowels.

The glides and liquids are somewhat less intense than the vowels and have most of their energy in the low to mid frequencies. The duration of the glides /w/ and /j/ tends to be longer than that of the liquids /l/ and /r/.

TABLE 1–7. **Summary of Acoustic Features for Six Phonetic Classes.**

SOUND CLASS	INTENSITY	SPECTRUM	DURATION
Vowels	Very strong	Low frequency dominance	Moderate to long
Glides and liquids	Strong	Low frequency dominance	Short to moderate
Strident fricatives and affricates	Moderate	High frequency dominance	Moderate
Nasals	Moderate	Very low frequency dominance	Short to moderate
Stops	Weak	Varies with place of articulation	Short
Nonstrident fricatives	Weak	Flat	Short to moderate

The strident fricatives and affricates (/s, z, ʃ, ʒ, tʃ, dʒ/) are more intense than other consonants but considerably weaker than vowels. The stridents have energy primarily at the high frequencies and, therefore, are vulnerable to high-frequency hearing loss. A good tape recording of the stridents requires a recorder with a wide frequency response. Stridents tend to be relatively long in duration, especially compared to other consonants, and fricatives typically are longer than affricates.

The nasals are sounds of moderate intensity, low-frequency energy, and brief to moderate duration. The nasals have more energy at very low frequencies than do other sounds.

The stops are relatively weak sounds of brief duration. The burst that results from release of a stop closure can be as short as 10 milliseconds. The primary energy for stops varies over a wide range of frequencies—from low to high; bi-labials have relatively low-frequency energy, while velars and alveolars have most of their energy in, respectively, the mid and mid to high frequencies.

The nonstrident fricatives /f, v, θ, ð/ are weak sounds of typically moderate duration. They tend to have a flat spectrum, meaning that the noise energy is distributed fairly uniformly over the frequency range. Of all sounds, /θ/ usually is the weakest—so weak that it can barely be heard when produced in isolation at any distance from a listener.

Finally, two points should be made concerning acoustic implications for clinical assessment and management. First, the absolute frequency location of energy for speech sounds varies with speaker age and sex. Men have the lowest overall frequencies of sound energy, women somewhat higher frequencies, and young children the highest frequencies. This relationship follows from the acoustic principle that an object's resonance frequency is inversely related to its length. The longest pipe in a pipe organ has a low frequency (or low pitch) and the shortest pipe a high frequency (high pitch); similarly the adult male vocal tract is longer than a woman's or a child's and therefore has resonances of lower frequency. This difference has practical implications. Most acoustic data have been collected for men's speech; much less is known about women's or children's speech, and the data for men may not be directly applicable to either. Moreover, the recording and analysis of women's and children's speech requires a wider frequency range than that suitable for men's speech. This issue can be particularly important for fricatives and affricates.

Second, because speech sounds vary widely in intensity, dominant energy region, and duration, they are not equally discriminable under different listening situations. The acoustic differences summarized in Table 1–7 should be kept in mind when testing articulation or auditory discrimination.

SENSORY INFORMATION IN SPEECH PRODUCTION

As speech is produced, a number of different kinds of sensory information is generated. The types of information include tactile (touch and pressure), pro-prioceptive (position sense), kinesthetic (movement sense), and auditory. The total sensory information is genuinely plurimodal, that is, available in several modalities. Most authorities agree that the rich sensory information associated with speech production is particularly important in speech development and in the management of some speech disorders, as when a child must learn a new articulatory pattern. A clinician therefore should be knowledgeable about the kinds and characteristics of sensory, or afferent, information.

The major characteristics of the sensory systems in speech were reviewed by Hardcastle (1976) and more recently by Kent, Martin, and Sufit (1990). Tactile receptors, which consist of free nerve endings and complex endings (for example, Krause end-bulbs and Meissner corpuscles), supply information to the central nervous system on the nature of contact (including localization, pressure, and onset time) and direction of movement. Remarkably, the oral structures are among the most sensitive regions of the body. The tongue tip is particularly sensitive and can therefore supply detailed sensory information. Tactile receptors belong to a more general class of receptors called mechanoreceptors (which respond to mechanical stimulation). These receptors respond not only to physical contacts of articulatory structures but also to air pressures generated during speech.

The proprioceptive and kinesthetic receptors include the muscle spindles, Golgi tendon organs, and joint receptors. Muscle spindles provide rich information on the length of muscle fibers, degree and velocity of stretch, and the direction of movement of a muscle. Golgi receptors relay information on the change of stretch on a tendon caused by muscular contraction or by other influences, including passive movement. Joint receptors, located in the capsules of joints, inform the central nervous system on the rate, direction, and extent of joint movement. Even a relatively simple movement, such as closing the jaw and raising the tongue, supplies a variety of afference to the central nervous system.

The auditory system supplies information on the acoustic consequences of articulation. Because the purpose of speech is to produce an intelligible acoustic signal, auditory feedback is of particular importance in regulating the processes of articulation. Interestingly, when an adult suffers a sudden and severe loss of hearing, speech articulation usually does not deteriorate immediately, but only gradually. The other types of sensory information are probably sufficient to maintain the accuracy of articulation for some time.

Many tactile receptors are comparatively slow acting because the neural signals travel along relatively small fibers in a multisynaptic pathway (a pathway composed of several neurons). Much of the tactile information is available to the central nervous system after the event to which it pertains. This information is particularly important to articulations that involve contact between articulatory surfaces, such as stops and fricatives. Obviously, prolonging an articulation helps to reinforce its sensory accompaniment. When the mucosal surfaces of the articulators are anesthetized, one of the most disturbed class of sounds is the fricatives.

Proprioceptive and kinesthetic receptors tend to be faster because spindle afferent fibers are large, and neural transmission is monosynaptic (that is, a two-neuron pathway). The relatively short latency of this afference means that some information can reach the central nervous system during the articulatory event.

The auditory system is slower than either the tactile or proprioceptive systems and provides most of its information after the corresponding articulatory event has occurred. Some current theories about sensory information in speech propose that this information is not sampled continuously but rather intermittently. Because speech is a highly rehearsed motor skill, it is not necessary to rely continuously on sensory information for its regulation. Instead, the process only samples the sensory feedback on an occasional basis to insure that the actual sensory information matches the expected sensory information.

GENERATIVE PHONOLOGY

Phonology has been defined as the part of linguistics concerned with "putting sounds together" or "putting sounds into words." Somewhat more precisely, Sloat, Taylor, and Hoard define phonology as "the science of speech sounds and sound patterns" (1978; 1). These authors note that each language has its own sound pattern, which is (1) the set of sounds used by a certain language, (2) the acceptable arrangement of these sounds to form words, and (3) the various processes by which sounds are added, deleted, or changed. Thus, the sound patterns of different languages can differ in the sounds available for use, the permissible ordering of these sounds, and the rules or processes that operate on the sounds. Phonological rules are prescriptions that convert abstract phonological representations into phonetic representations. An example from Hyman (1975) is the pronunciation of the verb *miss*. The word is pronounced /mis/ in the phrase *we miss it* but /mɪʃ/ in the phrase *we miss you*. In English, the /s/ often is palatalized when it is followed by a palatal /j/ (which itself may be deleted). Thus, the morpheme *miss* has these two pronunciations determined by the phonology of English.

Phonological processes are operations that affect sound change, both within individual language users and within the history of a particular language. Some examples of processes are cluster reduction: *snow* /snoʊ/ → /noʊ/; deletion of unstressed syllables: *baloney* /bəloʊnɪ/ → /bloʊnɪ/; and final consonant devoicing: *pig* /pɪg/ → /pɪk/. Other examples will be discussed later in this chapter and in other chapters of this book.

Although this chapter is not directly concerned with linguistics, the student should at least recognize the relevance of some phonological principles to the study of normal and disordered articulation. The study of phonology offers many important insights into the interactions among sound segments and the interactions between speech articulation and higher levels of linguistic organization. In a sense, phonological analysis is a key to the door between articulation and the various levels of language structure. Many aspects of articulation—such as the duration of constriction for an /s/, the duration of a vowel sound, the occurrence of palatalization for consonants, or the devoicing of a normally voiced segment—can be understood through the study of phonology.

Some of the interactions among units in the oral expression of language can be described and perhaps even explained through *phonological rules*. A phonological rule is a formal expression of a regularity that occurs in the phonology of a language or in the phonology of an individual speaker. These rules are either *context-free* or *context-sensitive*. A context-free rule is not dependent on a specific context. For example, if a child always substitutes (replaces) stops for fricatives (e.g., *sees* /siz/ becomes /tid/), we can formulate a rule that states simply that fricatives become stops:

Fricative ⟶ Stop

In this example, the word *fricative* represents the category of fricatives and the word *stop* represents the category of stops and the arrow means "is replaced by." Thus, the rule means that a fricative unit is replaced by a stop unit. Because this change or replacement always occurs, it is not necessary to state any context restriction on its operation.

On the other hand, assume that a child replaces fricatives with stops only in the initial position of a syllable; for example /si/ *(see)* becomes /ti/ and /zu/ *(zoo)* becomes /du/. The restriction to syllable-initial position is a context restriction, or a constraint on the operation of the rule. To formalize this operation, the following rule can be used:

$$\text{Fricative} \longrightarrow \text{Stop} \quad / \quad \# \quad \underline{\quad\quad}$$

This rule states that a fricative unit is replaced by a stop unit if the fricative is in the context such that it initiates a syllable. The slash / means "in the environment such that," the # represents a syllable boundary, and the underline _____ indicates the location of the fricative segment. Hence, the slash-#-underline means that the fricative immediately follows the syllable boundary (that is, begins the syllable).

A general form of a phonological rule is the following:

$$X \longrightarrow Y \quad / \quad a \underline{\quad\quad} b$$

This rule expresses a modification in which X becomes Y whenever X occurs following *a* and preceding *b*. The rule structure is decomposed as follows:

For example, imagine an allophonic modification in which a vowel is nasalized if it occurs between two nasal consonants (as in the word *man*). A rule of the form given above could be used to describe this change as follows:

$$\text{Vowel} \longrightarrow \text{Nasal vowel} \quad / \quad \text{Nasal consonant} \underline{\quad\quad} \text{Nasal consonant}$$

But a nasal consonant can be regarded as a sound having the features +nasal and +consonant. When features such as nasal and consonant apply together, it is convenient to place them in brackets so that the rule above becomes:

$$\text{Vowel} \longrightarrow \begin{bmatrix} +\text{Nasal} \\ +\text{Vowel} \end{bmatrix} \quad / \quad \begin{bmatrix} +\text{Nasal} \\ +\text{Consonant} \end{bmatrix} \underline{\quad\quad} \begin{bmatrix} +\text{Nasal} \\ +\text{Consonant} \end{bmatrix}$$

Some additional examples of rules are given below. By studying these rules, the student should be able at least to interpret phonological rules, if not to devise them. The basic advantage of a phonological rule is that it expresses in a formal or mathematical fashion a regularity of the phonological system and allows for an accurate, compact description of various context dependencies.

Example of deletion rule: Consonants following nasal consonants are deleted.

$$C \longrightarrow \emptyset \quad / \quad \begin{bmatrix} + \text{Nasal} \\ C \end{bmatrix} \underline{\hspace{1cm}} .$$

(Ex.: [ænt] ⟶ [æn])

Explanation: As an abbreviatory convenience, *C* stands for consonant, and a nasal consonant is *C* with the feature + nasal. Deletion is represented by the null element ø so that the rule literally reads "a consonant is replaced by a null element (nothing) when the consonant follows a nasal consonant."

Example of insertion rule: A schwa vowel is inserted following syllable-final voiced stops.

$$\emptyset \longrightarrow /\text{ə}/ \quad / \quad \begin{bmatrix} + \text{Voiced} \\ + \text{Stop} \end{bmatrix} \underline{\hspace{1cm}} \#$$

(Ex.: [dɔg] ⟶ [dɔgə])

Explanation: The rule literally reads "a null element (nothing) is replaced by a schwa vowel when the null element occurs at the end of a syllable following a voiced stop."

Example of feature-changing rule: Syllable-final voiced obstruents are devoiced.

$$\begin{bmatrix} - \text{Sonorant} \\ + \text{Voiced} \end{bmatrix} \longrightarrow [- \text{Voiced}] \quad / \quad \underline{\hspace{1cm}} \#$$

(Ex.: [bɪg] ⟶ [bɪk])

Explanation: Obstruents are stops, fricatives, and affricates, all of which are represented by the feature − sonorant. Thus, the rule states literally that "voiceless nonsonorants (i.e., obstruents) are replaced by their voiceless counterparts at the end of syllables."

Example of feature-assimilation rule: A normally voiceless consonant is voiced when it occurs between two voiced sounds.

$$\begin{bmatrix} C \\ - \text{Voiced} \end{bmatrix} \longrightarrow [+ \text{Voiced}] \quad / \quad [+ \text{Voiced}] \underline{\hspace{1cm}} [+ \text{Voiced}]$$

(Ex.: [æ bsɝd] ⟶ [æ bzɝd])

Explanation: A voiceless consonant becomes voiced if the preceding and following segments are voiced.

NATURAL PHONOLOGY

A topic of considerable interest and importance in phonology is that of *naturalness*. A natural class, property, process, or rule is one that appears to be preferred or is frequently used in phonologic systems (Sloat, Taylor, and Hoard, 1978; Stampe, 1972; Ingram, 1976). Evidence of naturalness is generally taken from

Normal Aspects of Articulation

developmental studies (early appearance or acquisition in a child's language), from cross-linguistic studies (universality across languages), or from studies of sound change in a language. One phonological property is more natural than another if the first appears before the second in language development and if the first is attested to in a greater number of languages. *Markedness* is a term sometimes used in this connection. An *unmarked* sound is one that appears to be natural. Unmarked sounds are acquired earlier than marked sounds in children's language, tend to be established in a language before marked sounds can be added, and tend to occur in different languages more frequently than marked sounds. By these criteria, voiceless stops are an example of unmarked (more natural) sounds, whereas voiced obstruents are marked (less natural).

Studies of natural phonology have shown that certain *assimilatory* and *nonassimilatory* processes occur commonly enough to be regarded as natural (Sloat, Taylor, and Hoard, 1978). An assimilatory process is one in which a sound changes to assimilate (become similar) to another sound. A nonassimilatory process does not appear to be based on similarity between sounds.

Examples of Assimilatory Processes

Voicing changes. These are intervocalic voicing and voicing and devoicing of obstruents. In intervocalic voicing, an obstruent (stop, fricative, or affricate) becomes voiced when it occurs between two vowels (hence, intervocalic). For example, *puppy* /pʌpɪ/ becomes /pʌbɪ/. The voiceless obstruent is assimilated to the voiced elements that surround it. The pattern of obstruent voicing or devoicing varies with languages, but one common process is word-final devoicing, in which an obstruent loses its voicing when it occurs at the end of the word. This change sometimes is considered assimilatory because it is thought that the voiced segment is assimilated to the voiceless pause at the end of the word. For example, *dog* /dɔg/ becomes /dɔk/.

Nasalization. As already discussed in this chapter, vowels and, occasionally, other resonants are assimilated to nasal consonants by becoming nasal themselves. Thus, in the word *lamb* /l æ m/, the vowel often is nasalized.

Nasal assimilation. Nasal consonants tend to assume the place of articulation of a neighboring sound. In English, this process is amply illustrated by the large number of homorganic nasal-stop combinations: *impolite, imbue, improper, indelicate, unturned, endeared, anchor, anger, congress.*

Palatalization. Nonpalatal consonants become palatal when followed by a front vowel or a glide. For example, the /n/ in *news* and the /k/ in *cute* become palatalized when these words are produced with the glide + vowel /ju/ (/njuz/ and /kjut/). As mentioned above, /s/ often is palatalized when it is followed by the glide /j/ in phrases such as *miss you*.

Examples of Nonassimilatory Processes

Deletion or loss of segments. Sometimes a segment or number of segments at the end of a word are dropped in a process known as *apocope*. For example, in the Eastern dialect of English, speakers often drop the /r/ in words such as *car, store,* and *stair*, pronouncing *car* /kar/ as /ka:/. Young children also frequently delete the final consonants of words. Final consonant omission is noted by speech clinicians more often than initial consonant omission. When segments are lost at other than the end of a word, the process is sometimes called *syncope*. Apocope and syncope frequently simplify (or reduce) clusters; *extra*, for example, may become /ɛ ktr ə/ and *asks* may become /æks/.

Insertion of segments. In one type of insertion process, called *prosthesis*, a segment is added in the initial position. In another type, called *epenthesis*, a segment is added elsewhere in the word. Children frequently will break up clusters by inserting vowels (often the schwa /ə/): *blue* becomes /bəlu/ and *clock* becomes /kəlak/.

Metathesis. The order of segments is reversed in this process. For example, a child may say /nets/ for *nest* /nɛst/ and /mjukis/ for *music* /mjusik/ (the second example also involves final-segment devoicing).

Breaking. By this process, long vowels become diphthongs, as in the examples *fast* /fæ ɪ st/, *pass* /pæ ɪ s/, *bag* /bæ ɪ g/, and *cat* /k æ ɪ t/. Breaking often may be heard in the speech of young children.

Natural phonology offers some valuable perspectives on the acquisition of phonology by children. Some authors believe that natural phonological processes are innate or are acquired early and rather easily by children and that whenever a natural process opposes a phonological property of the language the child is learning, some resistance may be expected. Stampe (1969) viewed natural processes as innate processes that simplify the adult target word. One interesting implication of naturalness is that children tend to exhibit strong biases or preferences in their sound formations and sound sequences. It has been proposed that some such preferences are based on phonetic grounds. For example, obstruent devoicing (or the tendency for stops, fricatives, and affricates to be devoiced) may be related to the fact that it is difficult to maintain laryngeal vibrations during a period of vocal tract closure. To maintain voicing during closure of the tract, special measures must be taken to enable air flow to continue through the vocal folds. This can be done through an expansion of the oral air chamber (Perkell, 1969; Kent and Moll, 1969), accomplished by expanding the pharynx or by depressing the larynx. However, not all natural processes have a simple phonetic basis, and, most likely, other factors will have to be considered in reaching a full explanation. Whatever this explanation may be, it behooves the speech clinician to be aware that speech and language learning may be influenced by phonological forces that occur commonly enough to be called natural. Such preferences or predispositions in speech production may be a substrate for the process of acquisition. Furthermore, the maintenance of natural processes beyond their usual survival time in learning a particular phonological system could result in articulation disorders.

NONLINEAR PHONOLOGY

Nonlinear phonology was developed as an alternative to linear generative phonology because the latter was perceived to have certain shortcomings. Some aspects of generative phonology (launched largely through the classic work, *The Sound Pattern of English* by Chomsky and Halle, 1968) were considered earlier. The basic goals of generative phonologies are to (1) describe phonological patterns in natural languages, (2) formulate the rules that account for these systems, and (3) identify universal principles that apply to phonological systems. A particular reason why nonlinear phonologies were introduced was to account for the influence of stress (as in weak and strong clusters in English stress systems) and the description of tone and stress features in levels of representation independent of the segmental representation. Linear generative phonology was regarded by some to be inadequate in dealing with prosodic effects in general. Early generative

Normal Aspects of Articulation

phonologies regarded phonological representation as "linear strings of segments with no hierarchical organization other than that provided by syntactic phrase structure" (Clements and Keyser, 1983; 1). This kind of generative phonology was characterized by rules that operated in a domain of linear strings of segments. But this approach encountered some difficulties in regard to the effects of stress and other prosodic variables. More generally, linear generative phonology failed to account satisfactorily for the relationships among various sizes of units because phonological operations were constrained to act on linear sequences.

There are several different versions of nonlinear phonology, but two particularly influential theories are autosegmental theory (Goldsmith, 1976, 1990; Hayes, 1988) and metrical theory (Goldsmith, 1990; Hayes, 1988). Autosegmental theory divides phonological features into parallel tiers of quasi-independent sequences. The tiers are like interconnected but independent levels. The term *autosegment* refers to a unit in a given tier. An autosegment can be realized in one or more ways; for example, a tonal tier may allow realizations such as high, mid, or low tones. The sequences in each tier are time-aligned with association lines that indicate simultaneity across tiers. In this way, stress and segmental representations are coordinated. A detailed discussion cannot be given here for this complex development in phonological theory, but the central idea is fairly simple: Phonological patterns evolve from connections across different representations, and not, as linear generative phonology maintained, from operations across a single linear sequence of phonological units. Nonlinear phonology is a significant break from an earlier theoretical view. It accommodates interactions across various sizes and types of phonological representation.

Metrical theory organizes phonological units into hierarchies, for example, feet, syllables, and segments. Unlike linear generative phonology, metrical theory gives a special definition to stress. Stress patterns arise from rhythm (an alternating prominence, such as strong–weak) and syllable weight. Stress assignments are made across the various levels of the hierarchy (such as syllables, feet, and words). This treatment of stress is very different from that of linear generative phonology.

Hierarchy also is important to theories of feature geometry, another development in nonlinear phonology. Two influential accounts of feature geometry are McCarthy (1988) and Sagey (1986). In systems such as that shown in Figure 1–29, syllable, consonant, and vowel appear as superordinate nodes that govern other nodes specifying laryngeal and supralaryngeal articulations. That is, the features are arranged hierarchically. Linear phonology, such as that of Chomsky and Halle (1968), typically specified features in a matrix where orthogonality or independence among features was desirable if not always attainable. In contrast, feature geometry exploits nonorthogonality among features. The hierarchical patterns implied by nonorthogonality become organizing principles in feature geometry.

The three phonological theories reviewed here—autosegmental theory, metrical theory and feature geometry—all represent major departures from what had been the standard phonological theory. Not surprisingly, these new theories are now being considered with respect to phonological development (Schwartz, in press; Spencer, 1988) and phonological disorders in children (Bernhardt, 1990; Chiat, 1989; Chin and Dinnsen, in press; Gandour, 1981; Spencer, 1984).

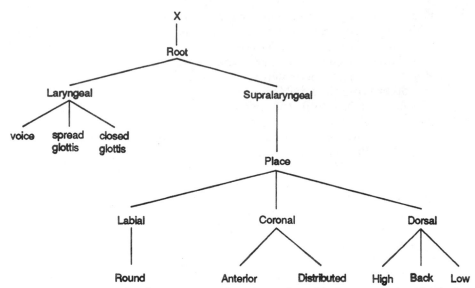

FIGURE 1–29. Hierarchical tree structure for one version of feature geometry. The features under the supralaryngeal node have been defined previously. The features under the laryngeal node refer to vocal fold configurations.

SUMMARY OF LEVELS OF ORGANIZATION OF SPEECH

Various levels of organization of speech are shown in Table 1–8, beginning with the syllable and working down to the acoustic sequence that might be seen on a spectrogram or visual representation of sounds. Although *syllable integrity* is the highest level shown, the table could have begun with an even higher level, such as a phrase or a sentence. However, for our purposes here, it is sufficient to consider only the levels presented in the table. The syllable is an organizational unit that consists of one or more phonemes; in this case, the syllable /p a/ includes the phonemes /p/ and /a/. Because phonemes are abstract, a phonemic description does not touch on a number of details of phonetic organization and speech behavior. Some of these details are shown in the level of *phonetic properties*. The phoneme /p/ has as its phonetic representation the aspirated [pʰ], and the phoneme /a/ has as its phonetic representation the lengthened [a:]. These phonetic representations are, of course, allophones of the /p/ and /a/ phonemes. The English phoneme /p/ is always aspirated in syllable-initial position, and the phoneme /a/ frequently is lengthened when uttered in an open monosyllable (that is, a CV syllable).

Segmental features comprise the next level of the table. These features are phonetic dimensions or attributes by which sounds may be described. For example, the consonant [p] is defined by its inclusion in the classes of *stops*, *labials*, and *consonantals* and by its exclusion from the classes of *nasals* and *voiced sounds*. These features are similar to the distinctive features discussed earlier in this chapter, but they are intended to be more phonetic in character. Even without rigorous definitions of the features suggested, it should be clear that each feature defines an articulatory property of the sound in question; for example, vowel [a]

Normal Aspects of Articulation

TABLE 1–8. **Levels of Organization of Speech.**

SYLLABIC INTEGRITY:	/p a/
	SYL
PHONEMIC COMPOSITON:	/p/ + /a/
PHONETIC PROPERTIES:	[pʰa:]
Note: stop /p/ is aspirated and vowel /a/ is lengthened	
SEGMENTAL FEATURES:	[p] — + Stop
	+ Labial
	+ Consonantal
	− Nasal
	− Voice
	[a] — + Syllabic
	− Consonantal
	− Front
	+ Low
	− Round
	− Nasal
	+ Voice
ARTICULATORY SEQUENCE:	Closure of velopharynx
	Abduction of vocal folds
	Adjustment of tongue for /a/
	Closure of lips
	Opening of lips and jaw
	Adduction of vocal folds
	Final abduction of vocal folds
ACOUSTIC SEQUENCE:	Silent period during /p/ closure
	Noise burst for /p/ release
	Aspiration period as folds close
	Voiced period after folds close, with distinct resonant shaping

is a syllable nucleus, is not a consonant, is low-back and unrounded, and is a voiced nonnasal sound.

The features are less abstract than phonemes but still must be interpreted by the motor control system of the brain to provide proper neural instructions to the speech muscles; that is, the features listed for [p] and [a] must be translated into a pattern of muscle contractions that yields the *articulatory sequence* shown in the next to last level of the table. The −*nasal* feature of [p] requires that the velopharynx be closed, and the −*voice* feature of the same segment requires that the vocal folds be abducted (open). In this way, each feature requirement is given an articulatory interpretation, accomplished by the contraction of muscles.

Finally, as the consequence of muscle contractions, a series of speech sounds is uttered. In this *acoustic sequence*, the last level of the table, one can see acoustic segments of the kind visible on a spectrogram. Notice that one acoustic segment does not necessarily correspond to a single phoneme. The phoneme /p/ is associated with at least three acoustic segments: a silent period corresponding to the bilabial closure, a noise burst produced as the lips are rapidly opened, and an aspiration interval related to a gradual closure of the vocal folds in preparation for voicing the following vowel.

Although Table 1–8 is fairly detailed, it represents only part of the complexity of speech. In the linguistic-phonetic organization of speech behavior, we need to consider three major components: the segmental (or phonetic) component, the suprasegmental *(prosodic)* component, and the *paralinguistic* component. The first two already have been discussed in this chapter. The paralinguistic component is similar to the prosodic component in that it might be called nonsegmental. This component includes those aspects of speech represented by terms such as *emotion* and *attitude*. A speaker who plans an utterance must decide not only about phonetic sequencing but also about prosodic structure and emotional and attitudinal content (that is, the "tone of voice"). The segmental component includes words, syllables, phonemes, and features. The suprasegmental or prosodic component includes stress, intonation, juncture, rate, loudness, and pitch level. The paralinguistic component is made up of tension, voice quality, and voice qualifications (Crystal, 1969).

The complexity of speech behavior can be illustrated by listing the various types of information represented in the speech signal. A *partial* listing (mostly from Branigan, 1979) is

1. A set of articulatory targets or goals corresponding to the intended phonetic sequence
2. Assignment of stress to the syllables that make up the sequence
3. Adjustments of syllable duration to stress, phonetic composition, and position of the syllable in the utterance
4. Specification of junctural features, including transitions between elements and terminal juncture at the end of the utterance
5. Internal ordering of words as it reflects syntactic form to convey semantic intentions (meaning)
6. Determination of other prosodic features such as speaking rate, pitch, level, and loudness
7. Use of paralinguistic features to convey emotion or attitude

It is important to remember that even an apparently simple aspect of speech behavior can be influenced by a host of variables. For example, the duration of a vowel is determined by tongue height, tenseness or laxness, consonant context, stress pattern, frequency of occurrence of the word in which the vowel occurs, syntactic ordering of the word in which the vowel appears, and rate of speaking (Klatt, 1976).

CONCLUDING NOTE ON IMPLICATIONS FOR SPEECH ACQUISITION

Speech articulation has its early roots in the vocalizations of infants. Just how the coos and babbles of the first year of life relate to the development of speech is not well understood, but there is growing evidence that early vocalizations prepare the child for acquisition of a phonetic system. The syllable appears to be an important unit in early sound patterns, and the development of syllabic organization of sounds may be a major framework of speech development. If so, it is of interest to chart the way in which syllabic structures develop during the first year of life. The following account is based on several chapters in a recently published book, *Precursors of Early Speech Development*, edited by Bjorn Lindblom and Rolf Zetterström.

The major phases in syllable development are as follows: (1) Continuous phonation in a respiratory cycle provides the basic phonatory pattern from which refinements in articulation can develop; (2) intermittent phonation within a respiratory cycle breaks the basic pattern of continuous phonation and, thus, is a

Normal Aspects of Articulation

precursor of syllable units; (3) articulatory (supraglottal) movements interrupting or combined with phonation provide early experience in the control of co-occurring phonation and articulation; (4) marginal syllables (in isolation or in sequence) are early syllabic forms that, while lacking the detailed structure of adult syllables, prefigure the basic syllable shape; (5) canonical syllables (in isolation or in sequence) anticipate important structural properties of adult speech and may be particularly important in relating an infant's perceptions of adult speech with his or her own productive patterns; and (6) reduplicated babble (repeated syllable patterns) gives the infant experience with both prosody (especially rhythm) and sequences of articulations. It is on this vocal bedrock that speech develops. For a time, babbling and early words coexist, sharing some phonetic properties but, perhaps, differing in others.

The CV syllable, occurring in virtually all of the world's languages, has long been recognized as a preferred basic unit of speech articulation. It appears to be an optimal unit for learning perceptual discriminations in infancy. Infants younger than four months can discriminate segments contained in sequences of the form CV, CVC, VCV, and CVCV (Bertoncini and Mehler, 1981; Jusczyk and Thompson, 1978; Trehub, 1973); and an alternating CV pattern seems to enhance the infant's ability to discriminate variations in place, manner and voicing. Since redundant syllable strings, such as [ba ba ba ba] (Goodsitt, Morse, and Ver Hoeve, 1984), further enhance this performance, we can conclude that the CV syllable train characterizing reduplicated babble is an excellent perceptual training ground for the infant.

The advantage of the CV syllable applies to production as well. This syllable form is one of the earliest syllables to be identified in infant vocalizations; the vocalizations of 1-year-olds are, predominantly, simple V or CV syllables and their elaborations, for example, VCV or CVCV (Kent and Bauer, 1985). Branigan (1976) regarded the CV syllable as a training ground for consonant formation. Most consonants are produced first in the initial position of CV syllables and then, later, in postvocalic (e.g., VC) position.

The importance of the canonical CV syllable as a unit for perceptuomotor integration is indicated by its long-delayed appearance in the vocal development of hearing-impaired infants (Kent, Osberger, Netsell, and Hustedde, 1987; Oller, 1986). There is also evidence that early CV syllable production is linked, in a developmental chain, to early word production and to the articulation of word-final consonants (Menyuk, Liebergott, and Schultz, 1986).

Speech acquisition is a complex process, one that involves learning a language (its syntax, semantics, and phonology)—a speech code that relates meaning to sound, and a motor skill by which the speech organs are controlled to produce rapid and overlapping movements. The layman often characterizes developing speech in the child by reference to frequently occurring substitutions (as when the child says *wabbit* for *rabbit* or *thee* for *see*) or other common misarticulations. But developing speech differs from adult speech in other ways.

First, children's speech generally is slower than adult speech. For example, McNeill (1974) reported speaking rates of slightly over 3 words per second for adults, about 2.5 words per second for 4- to 5-year-olds, and 1.6 words per second for children of about 2. Not surprisingly, then, the durations of individual segments are longer in children's speech (Naeser, 1970; Smith, 1978; Kent and Forner,

1980). Smith reported that the durations of nonsense utterances were 15 percent longer for 4-year-olds than for adults and 31 percent longer for 2-year-olds than for adults. Similarly, when Kent and Forner measured durations of phrases and short sentences, they found them to be 8 percent longer for 12-year-olds than for adults, 16 percent longer for 6-year-olds than for adults, and 33 percent longer for 4-year-olds than for adults. Some individual segments, such as the duration of stop closure, were observed by Kent and Forner to be twice as long in children's speech as in adult speech. The speaking rates of children have implications for both the production and perception of speech. It has been shown that children more successfully imitate sentences spoken at a rate nearer their own than at slower or faster rates (Bonvillian, Raeburn, and Horan, 1979).

Second, children's speech differs from adult speech in its variability. When children make the same utterance several times, the duration of individual segments varies more than for adults (Eguchi and Hirsh, 1969; Tingley and Allen, 1975; Kent and Forner, 1980). This difference in reliability of production may be an index of the child's linguistic and neuromotor immaturity. In general, a young child's speech patterns are less well controlled than an adult's, and there is evidence that the control continues to improve until the child reaches puberty (Kent, 1976).

A third difference between the speech of children and adults is in patterns of coarticulation. Data on this difference are not abundant, but Thompson and Hixon (1979) reported that with increasing age, a greater proportion of their subjects showed nasal air flow beginning at the midpoint of the first vowel in /ini/. They interpreted this to mean that anticipatory coarticulation occurred earlier for progressively older subjects. In other words, more mature speakers show increased anticipation in producing a phonetic sequence.

In summary, young children differ from adults not only in their obvious misarticulations, but also in their slower speaking rates, greater variability (error) in production, and reduced anticipation in articulatory sequencing.

REFERENCES

Adams, S.G., "Rate and clarity of speech: An x-ray microbeam study." Ph.D. dissertation, University of Wisconsin–Madison, 1990.

Beckman, M.E., "Stress and non-stress accent." *Netherlands Phonetic Archives 7*. Dordrecht: Foris, 1986.

Beckman, M.E., and J. Edwards, "Prosodic categories and duration control." *Journal of the Acoustical Society of America, 87*, Supplement 1 (1991): S65.

Behne, D., "Acoustic effects of focus and sentence position on stress in English and French." Ph.D. dissertation, University of Wisconsin–Madison, 1989.

Bernhardt, B., "Application of nonlinear phonology to intervention with six phonologically disordered children." Unpublished Ph.D. thesis, University of British Columbia, Vancouver, B.C., Canada, 1990.

Bernthal, J.E., and D.R. Beukelman, "Intraoral air pressures during the production of /p/ and /b/ by children, youths, and adults." *Journal of Speech and Hearing Research, 21* (1978): 361–371.

Bertoncini, J., and J. Mehler, "Syllables as units in infant speech perception." *Infant Behavior and Development, 4* (1981): 247–260.

Bock, J.K., "Toward a cognitive psychology of syntax: Information processing contributions to sentence formulation." *Psychological Review, 89* (1982): 1–47.

Bonvillian, J.D., V.P. Raeburn, and E.A. Horan, "Talking to children: The effects of rate, intonation, and length on children's sentence imitation." *Journal of Child Language, 6* (1979): 459–467.

Branigan, G., "Syllabic structure and the acquisition of consonants: The great conspiracy in word formation." *Journal of Psycholinguistic Research, 5* (1976): 117–133.

Branigan, G., "Some reasons why successive single word utterances are not." *Journal of Child Language, 6* (1979): 411–421.

Normal Aspects of Articulation

Cavagna, G.A., and R. Margaria, "Airflow rates and efficiency changes during phonation." *Sound Production in Man, Annals of the New York Academy of Sciences, 155* (1968): 152–164.

Chiat, S., "The relation between prosodic structure, syllabification and segmental realization: Evidence from a child with fricative stopping." *Clinical Linguistics and Phonetics, 3* (1989): 223–242.

Chin, S.B., and D.A. Dinnsen, "Feature geometry in disordered phonologies." *Clinical Linguistics and Phonetics*, in press.

Chomsky, N., and M. Halle, *The Sound Pattern of English.* New York: Harper & Row, 1968.

Clements, G.N., and S.J. Keyser, *CV Phonology.* Cambridge, Mass.: M.I.T. Press, 1983.

Cohen, A., R. Collier, and J. t'Hart, "Declination: Construct or intrinsic feature of speech pitch?" *Phonetica, 39* (1982): 254–273.

Crystal, D., *Prosodic Systems and Intonation in English.* Cambridge (U.K.): Cambridge University Press, 1969.

Crystal, D., "Non-segmental phonology in language acquisition: A review of the issues." *Lingua, 32* (1973): 1–45.

Daniloff, R.G., and K.L. Moll, "Coarticulation of lip rounding." *Journal of Speech and Hearing Research, 11* (1968): 707–721.

Dewey, G., *Relative Frequency of English Speech Sounds.* Cambridge: Harvard University Press, 1923.

Eguchi, S., and I.J. Hirsh, "Development of speech sounds in children." *Acta Orolaryngologica*, Supplement No. 257 (1969).

Fry, D., "Duration and intensity as physical correlates of linguistic stress." *Journal of the Acoustical Society of America, 27* (1955): 765–768.

Gandour, J., "The nondeviant nature of deviant phonological systems." *Journal of Communication Disorders, 14* (1981): 11–29.

Giles, S.B., "A study of articulatory characteristics of /l/ allophones in English." Ph.D. dissertation, University of Iowa, 1971.

Goldsmith, J., "Autosegmental phonology." Ph.D. dissertation, Massachusetts Institute of Technology, 1976 (published by Garland Press, 1979).

Goldsmith, J.A., *Autosegmental and Metrical Phonology.* Oxford: Basil Blackwell, 1990.

Goodsitt, J., P. Morse, and J. Ver Hoeve, "Infant speech recognition in multisyllabic contexts." *Child Development, 55* (1984): 903–910.

Hardcastle, W.J., *Physiology of Speech Production.* London: Academic Press, 1976.

Hayes, B., "Metrics and phonological theory." In F. Newmeyer (Ed.), *Linguistics: The Cambridge Survey. II. Linguistic Theory: Extensions and Implications.* Cambridge (U.K.): Cambridge University Press, 1988, pp. 220–249.

Hixon, T.J., "Mechanical aspects of speech production." Paper read at Annual Convention of the American Speech and Hearing Association, Chicago, November 17–20, 1971.

Hockett, C.F., "A manual of phonology." In *International Journal of American Linguistics* (*Memoir II*). Baltimore: Waverly Press, 1955.

Hyman, L.M., *Phonology: Theory and Analysis.* New York: Holt, Rinehart and Winston, 1975.

Ingram, D., *Phonological Disability in Children.* New York: Elsevier, 1976.

Jong, K.J. de, "The oral articulation of English stress accent." Ph.D. dissertation, Ohio State University, Columbus, Ohio, 1991.

Jusczyk, P., and E. Thompson, "Perception of phonetic contrasts in multisyllabic utterances by 2 month old infants." *Perception and Psychophysics, 23* (1978): 105–109.

Kantner, C.E., and R. West, *Phonetics.* New York: Harper & Row, 1960.

Kent, R.D., "Anatomical and neuromuscular maturation of the speech mechanism: Evidence from acoustic studies." *Journal of Speech and Hearing Research, 19* (1976): 421–447.

Kent, R.D., and H.R. Bauer, "Vocalizations of one year olds." *Journal of Child Language, 12* (1985): 491–526.

Kent, R.D., and L.L. Forner, "Speech segment durations in sentence recitations by children and adults." *Journal of Phonetics, 8* (1980): 157–168.

Kent, R.D., R.E. Martin, and R.L. Sufit, "Oral sensation: A review and clinical prospective." In H. Winitz (Ed.), *Human Communication and Its Disorders: A Review—1990.* Norwood, N.J.: Ablex, 1990, pp. 135–191.

Kent, R.D., and F.D. Minifie, "Coarticulation in recent speech production models." *Journal of Phonetics, 5* (1977); 115–133.

Kent, R.D., and K.L. Moll, "Vocal-tract characteristics of the stop cognates." *Journal of the Acoustical Society of America, 46* (1969): 1549–1555.

Kent, R.D., and K.L. Moll, "Cinefluorographic analyses of selected lingual consonants." *Journal of Speech and Hearing Research, 15* (1972): 453–473.

Kent, R.D., and K.L. Moll, "Articulatory timing in selected consonant sequences." *Brain and Language, 2* (1975): 304–323.

Kent, R.D., and R. Netsell, "Effects of stress contrasts on certain articulatory parameters." *Phonetica, 24* (1972): 23–44.

Kent, R.D., M.J. Osberger, R. Netsell, and C.G. Hustedde, "Phonetic development in identical twins differing in auditory function." *Journal of Speech and Hearing Disorders, 52* (1987): 64–75.

Klatt, D.H., "Linguistic uses of segmental duration in English: Acoustic and perceptual evidence." *Journal of the Acoustical Society of America, 59* (1976): 1208–1221.

Ladefoged, P., *Preliminaries to Linguistic Phonetics*. Chicago: University of Chicago Press, 1971.

Ladefoged, P., *A Course in Phonetics*. New York: Harcourt Brace Jovanovich, 1975.

Lehiste, I., *Suprasegmentals*. Cambridge, Mass.: M.I.T. Press, 1970.

Lieberman, P., *Intonation, Perception and Language*. Cambridge, Mass.: M.I.T. Press, 1967.

Lindblom, B.E.F., "Spectrographic study of vowel reduction." *Journal of the Acoustical Society of America, 35* (1963): 1773–1781.

Lindblom, B., "Explaining phonetic variation: A sketch of the H&H theory." In W.J. Hardcastle and A. Marchal (Eds.), *Speech Production and Speech Modelling*. Amsterdam, The Netherlands: Kluwer, 1990, pp. 403–439.

Lindblom, B., and R. Zetterström (Eds.), *Precursors of Early Speech Development*. New York: Stockton, 1986.

McCarthy, L., "Feature geometry and dependency: A review." *Journal of Phonetics, 43* (1988): 84–108.

MacNeilage, P.F., "Speech physiology." In H.H. Gilbert (Ed.), *Speech and Cortical Functioning*. New York: Academic Press, 1972, pp. 1–72.

McNeill, D., "The two-fold way for speech." In *Problèmes Actuels en Psycholinguistique*. Paris: Editions du Centre National de la Recherche Scientifique, 1974.

Menyuk, P., J. Liebergott, and M. Schultz, "Predicting phonological development." In B. Lindblom and R. Zetterström (Eds.), *Precursors of Early Speech*. Basingstoke, Hampshire (U.K.): MacMillan, 1986, pp. 79–93.

Moll, K.L., and R.G. Daniloff, "Investigation of the timing of velar movements during speech." *Journal of the Acoustical Society of America, 50* (1971): 678–684.

Moon, S.J., and B. Lindblom, "Formant undershoot in clear and citation-form speech: A second progress report." *Royal Institute of Technology (Stockholm, Sweden) Speech Transmission Laboratory, Quarterly Progress and Status Reports, 1* (1989): 121–123.

Naeser, M.A., "The American child's acquisition of differential vowel duration." Technical Report No. 144, Wisconsin Research and Development Center for Cognitive Learning, University of Wisconsin, Madison, 1970.

Oller, D.K., "Metaphonology of infant vocalizations." In B. Lindblom and R. Zetterström (Eds.), *Precursors of Early Speech*. Basingstoke, Hampshire (U.K.): MacMillan, 1986, pp. 21–35.

Parker, F., "Distinctive features in speech pathology: Phonology or phonemics?" *Journal of Speech and Hearing Disorders, 41* (1976): 23–39.

Perkell, J.S., *Physiology of Speech Production*. Cambridge, Mass.: M.I.T. Press, 1969.

Picheny, M.A., N.I. Durlach, and L.D. Braida, "Speaking clearly for the hard of hearing. II: Acoustic characteristics of clear and conversational speech." *Journal of Speech and Hearing Research, 29* (1986): 434–446.

Rabiner, L., H. Levitt, and A. Rosenberg, "Investigation of stress patterns for speech synthesis by rule." *Journal of the Acoustical Society of America, 45* (1969): 92–101.

Read, C., and P.A. Schreiber, "Why short subjects are harder to find than long ones." In E. Wanner and L. Gleitman (Eds.), *Language Acquisition: The State of the Art*. Cambridge (U.K.): Cambridge University Press, 1982.

Sagey, E., "The representation of features and relations in non-linear phonology." Unpublished Ph.D. thesis, Massachusetts Institute of Technology, Cambridge, Mass., 1986.

Schwartz, R.G., "Nonlinear phonology as a framework for phonological acquisition." In R.S. Chapman (Ed.), *Processes in Language Acquisition and Disorders*. Chicago: Mosby-Year Book, in press.

Sloat, C., S.H. Taylor, and J.E. Hoard, *Introduction to Phonology*. Englewood Cliffs, N.J.: Prentice Hall, 1978.

Smith, B.L., "Temporal aspects of English speech production: A developmental perspective." *Journal of Phonetics, 6* (1978): 37–68.

Spencer, A., "A nonlinear analysis of phonological disability." *Journal of Communication Disorders, 17* (1984): 325–348.

Spencer, A., "A phonological theory of phonological development." In M.J. Ball (Ed.), *Theoretical Linguistics and Disordered Language*. London: Croon Helm, 1988, pp. 115–151.

Stampe, D., "The acquisition of phonetic representation." In R.I. Binnick et al. (Eds.), *Papers from the Fifth Regional Meeting of the Chicago Linguistics Society*. Chicago: Chicago Linguistic Society, 1969, pp. 443–453.

Stampe, D., "A dissertation of natural phonology." Ph.D. dissertation, University of Chicago, 1972.

Subtelny, J., J. Worth, and M. Sakuda, "Intraoral pressure and rate of flow during speech." *Journal of Speech and Hearing Research, 9* (1966): 498–518.

Thompson, A.E., and T.J. Hixon, "Nasal air flow during speech production." *Cleft Palate Journal, 16* (1979): 412–420.

Tingley, B.M., and G.D. Allen, "Development of speech timing control in children." *Child Development, 46* (1975): 186–194.

Trehub, S., "Infants' sensitivity to vowel and tonal contrasts." *Developmental Psychology, 9* (1973): 91–96.

Walsh, H., "On certain practical inadequacies of distinctive feature systems." *Journal of Speech and Hearing Disorders, 39* (1974): 32–43.

Wise, C.M., *Introduction to Phonetics*. Englewood Cliffs, N.J.: Prentice Hall, 1957a.

Wise, C.M., *Applied Phonetics*. Englewood Cliffs, N.J.: Prentice Hall, 1957b.

chapter

2

Early Phonological Development

Marilyn May Vihman, Rutgers University

As a prelude to our discussion of normal phonological development, let us consider what a child accomplishes in a mere three or four years of exposure to language. At the outset of adult-like vocal production, sometimes called the babbling period, the vocalizations of children exposed to different languages are virtually indistinguishable (Atkinson, MacWhinney, and Stoel, 1968). Babies learning languages as different as English and Spanish (Thevenin, Eilers, Oller, and LaVoie, 1985) or French and Chinese (de Boysson-Bardies, Sagart, and Durand, 1984) cannot be reliably distinguished, based on tape recordings, by adult judges speaking one of these languages. Francescato suggested that "two hypotheses are possible: Either all children, of all languages, at the beginning of their linguistic activity share the 'same' language, or every child, of every language, speaks from the beginning its own language" (1968; 152f.). Today, the consensus seems to be that both hypotheses are true. Children in different language environments draw on the same "universal" repertoire of syllable shapes and sounds. At the same time, it seems that each child creates, out of these universal syllable shapes and sounds, a unique subset of sound preferences and patterns as he or she develops a phonological and communicative system of his or her own. Gradually, these unique or idiosyncratic patterns accommodate to and, finally, are replaced by the adult system to which the child is exposed.

In a remarkably short time most children develop intelligible speech. In fact, they even come to articulate well enough so that people outside the immediate family can understand what they are saying. At that point, the child can already be recognized as a member of a specific language community by his or her speech patterns; that is, he or she will have acquired the incidental phonetically distinguishing features as well as the system of contrasting sounds of the specific language spoken in his or her environment. In other words, in learning the phonology of, for example, American English, the infant also will have learned to pronounce like an American from Kansas or California or New Jersey. How do such profound changes take place in such a short time? The challenge of research in phonological development is to arrive at a better understanding of this process.

MODELS OF PHONOLOGICAL DEVELOPMENT: THE CHILD AS AN ACTIVE LEARNER

Linguists and psychologists have long sought to explain how children learn to distinguish and produce the sound patterns of the adult language. Not surprisingly, the earliest studies were largely *diary studies* or descriptions of the investigator's own child; several detailed studies of this sort were available by the 1940s. The first well-articulated model of phonological development—namely, Jakobson's structuralist model—was formulated at that time. Although it continues to be influential today, a number of other models, based on different perspectives and assumptions, have since been proposed (cf. Ferguson and Garnica, 1975; Ferguson, Menn, and Stoel-Gammon, 1992). In the past 20 years, there has been a notable increase in available data, due, in part, to the advent of tape recording as a common observational procedure, and, at the same time, there has been a shift in thinking about other areas of language acquisition. The earlier structuralist model presupposed little initiative on the part of the learner. Today, however, most investigators agree that the child, whose goal is to "sound like the adults around her" (Menn, 1981; 131), is an active participant in the learning process.

BEHAVIORIST MODEL

In the United States, the prevailing view from the 1950s to the early 1970s was the behaviorist model associated with Mowrer (1960) and Olmsted (1971). This model applied a psychological theory of learning to the human infant and emphasized the role of contingent reinforcement in speech acquisition. The child's babbling was held to be gradually "shaped," through classical conditioning principles, into forms appropriate for the adult speech community in question. Specifically, it was held that, in the course of the daily caretaking routines of feeding and changing, the infant comes to associate the vocalizations of the caretaker, usually the mother, with "primary reinforcement," such as food and comfort; thus, the adult's vocalizations acquire the value of "secondary reinforcement." The child's own vocalizations acquire secondary reinforcing value as well, by virtue of their similarity to the caretaker's vocalizations. The speech sound repertoire is further refined as the caretaker selectively reinforces sounds that resemble those used in the adult language and as the child is "self-reinforced" for producing sounds that match those in the environment.

STRUCTURALIST MODEL

In contrast to the behaviorists, who drew on psychological theory for their assumptions about learning, Jakobson (1941/68) drew on the linguists' structuralist theory of language to account for the observed phenomena of babbling and early speech. Jakobson postulated that phonological development follows a universal and innate order of acquisition. The distinctive features, arranged in a hierarchy, "unfold" in a predictable order as the child produces phonemic contrasts embodying them. The child was thought to start with two maximally contrasting sounds: a bilabial stop, /p/, and a low vowel, /a/. The child then begins to differentiate the consonant system by acquiring the contrast between nasal and oral: /p/ (oral) versus /m/ (nasal). The next feature contrast divides both oral and nasal consonants into a labial (/p/, /m/) and a dental pair (/t/, /n/). Jakobson proposed that the child's consonant and vowel systems continue to diversify and differentiate, step by step, as the child learns new feature contrasts. Features needed to differentiate stops, nasals, bilabials, and dentals were held to be acquired earlier than those needed to differentiate fricatives, affricates, and liquids. It should be pointed out that for Jakobson, babbling was a random activity which had little, if anything, to do with the development of the sound system of language.

Comment on the Behaviorist and Structuralist Models

Both the behaviorist and structuralist models concentrated on the relation between babbling and early speech. The behaviorists emphasized **continuity** between these two kinds of early vocalization. The structuralists, on the other hand, insisted on a **discontinuity** between the two, a view which followed from their conception of language as an autonomous structured system. The behaviorist paradigm is no longer widely accepted today as a model for language acquisition, primarily because it fails to account for the infinite capacity to produce *new patterns* that is the hallmark of human language (cf. Chomsky's [1959] critique of B.F. Skinner's *Verbal Behavior*): With specific reference to phonology, there is little evidence that caretakers selectively reward (or "shape") the child's sound productions in the prelinguistic period.

Though Jakobson's views provided a vital stimulus to research and are still widely cited, recent data have tended to weaken several aspects of his position. For one thing, the existence of regularities in prelinguistic (or babbling) vocal patterns has now been clearly demonstrated (cf., e.g., Ferguson and Macken, 1983) as has the gradual emergence of adult-based word shapes from the babble vocalizations (Vihman, Macken, Miller, Simmons, and Miller, 1985). Thus, the hypothesis of discontinuity between babble and speech appears to be unfounded.

A more basic difficulty is Jakobson's postulation of phonemic contrast as the basis of phonological development in the earliest stages. As Kiparsky and Menn (1977) pointed out, the corpus of words a child begins with is typically too small to provide clear evidence for or against the hypothesized sequence of **phonemic oppositions**. No set order of use of consonants is evident in the early words of the many different children whose data have been carefully recorded and analyzed. More importantly, the order of emergence of phonemic oppositions (nasal vs. oral, labial vs. dental) is extremely difficult to ascertain, as this requires an evaluation of the child's system based on the adult phonemes attempted as well as on the phonetic patterns used by the child. The undertaking is further complicated since many children seem to selectively **avoid** attempting words that include certain consonants. In fact, the child is now widely thought to be targeting *whole-word shapes* rather than individual segments or phonemes (Ferguson and Farwell, 1975). Furthermore, in light of the great *variability* found to be char-

Early Phonological Development

65

acteristic of early child forms, the issue of a universal order of acquisition of phonemes has lost much of its original interest.

NATURAL PHONOLOGY MODEL

The natural phonology model proposed by Stampe also emphasizes the universal and maturational aspect of phonological acquisition (Stampe, 1969; Donegan and Stampe, 1979). According to Stampe, the child comes innately equipped with a universal set of phonological processes—operations which change or delete phonological units—that reflect the natural limitations and capacities of human vocal production and perception. The innate processes correspond to the phonological regularities found in the languages of the world; the child's task is to suppress those processes which do not occur in the particular adult language to which he or she is exposed. For example, a child may be expected to devoice word-final obstruents (i.e., at first, the English-speaking child would pronounce *bad* as [bæt]), since this is a phonetically natural process found in many languages. In German, where *Hund* ('dog') is pronounced [hunt], the devoicing process accurately reflects adult phonology, and thus, the German-speaking child need not "suppress" it; however, the English-speaking child must suppress the process to match adult pronunciation (eventually producing *bad* as [bæd]).

GENERATIVE PHONOLOGY MODEL

Another influential model was developed in the 1970s by Smith (1973). Smith presented a lengthy formal description of the phonology of his son Amahl, from age 2 to 4. He described the child's phonology in terms of two distinct models: (1) a mapping of the adult forms into the child's, using "re-write rules" (e.g., "/f, v/ become [w] prevocalically," or in other words, "rewrite /f/ or /v/ as [w] . . ." to account for *feet* → [wi:t], *fork* → [wɔ:k], etc.); (2) an account of the child's system viewed in its own right, with the functional units and their interrelations defined and organized differently than in the adult system. Smith concluded that there is no psychological reality to the child's system; that is, he found no evidence that the system which seemed to underlie the child's forms, irrespective of the latter's relationship to the adult models, was productive. It did not bear upon the child's response to unfamiliar adult forms, his or her phonological treatment of new forms, or his or her reorganization of older forms under the influence of new patterns. Smith postulated a set of ordered universal tendencies, such as the use of consonant and vowel harmony and cluster reduction, that he considered to be either innate or learned very early.

COMMENT ON THE NATURAL PHONOLOGY AND GENERATIVE PHONOLOGY MODELS

In recent years, the natural phonology and generative phonology models have been influential in clinical practice with disordered speakers. The models of Stampe and Smith agree in several respects. Both reject the possibility of the child having a system of his or her own. Both insist on the "innate" or universal status of child phonological rules or processes—a position which remains highly controversial, though use of the term *process* and of the re-write or realization rule format has become general in the fields of normal and disordered child phonology (cf. Ingram, 1976; Grunwell, 1981; Edwards and Shriberg, 1983). Finally, both assume full, accurate perception from the earliest stages of speech production; that is, the child is assumed to perceive and store or *represent* speech forms correctly. According to this position, it is the innate constraints on the child's *production* that lead to simplification in the child's output forms.

PROSODIC MODEL

Waterson's (1971, 1981) prosodic model is rooted in the linguistic theory developed by J.R. Firth. Firth's prosodic linguistics differs sharply from traditional (especially American) linguistic practice, which has emphasized rules affecting individual segments. Waterson, like other Firthian linguists, focuses on the *word* rather than the segment as a basic unit of phonological structure. She describes groups of early words as schemata that share certain overall features derived from the adult form, such as intonation pattern, syllable structure, nasality, continuance (presence of fricatives), or voicing. In Waterson's view, the child's perception of the phonetic features of adult words is incomplete or partial at first. For Waterson and others (e.g., Braine, 1976; Maxwell, 1984), both child perception and production are likely to involve imperfect matches with the adult model at first, and therefore, both must undergo development and change before the child can arrive at an adult-like system.

COGNITIVE MODEL

Another widely adopted perspective is the "cognitive" or "problem-solving" model (Menn, 1983; Macken and Ferguson, 1983; Ferguson, 1978, 1986). In this view, the child encounters and eventually masters a series of challenges in acquiring the phonological system of the adult language. Individual strategies vary considerably across children, probably depending on their natural predispositions as well as on a number of external factors (such as the child's birth order and the interactional style of the primary caretakers).

Longitudinal studies have provided converging evidence for the view that active hypothesis testing and problem solving play an important role in phonological acquisition. Some of the major types of evidence follow.

Selectivity in Early Word Choice. In their earliest word productions, children have been found to begin by targeting adult words of certain shapes while avoiding sounds or sound patterns which are outside their repertoire. For example, one child initially used only two-syllable words with open syllables beginning with a stop or nasal (*daddy, mommy, doggy, patty(-cake)*, and *bye-bye*: Ferguson, Peizer, and Weeks, 1973). Different children begin by mastering different articulatory patterns and, accordingly, by attempting different (identifiable) adult words.

Unique Reduction Devices. Children use unique reduction devices to produce long words (Ferguson, 1978). For example, Priestly (1977) described the use by his son Christopher of the pattern [CVjVC] to produce a number of polysyllabic words—for example, *Panda* → [pajan], *berries* → [bɛjas], and *tiger* → [tajak]. Though these "exploratory forms" fail to match the adult forms in segmental terms, they accurately, if idiosyncratically, capture the correct syllable count.

"Phonological Idioms" and Regression. A child may first produce a complex adult word in a relatively advanced form (e.g., *pretty*, pronounced [prəti]) and

only later revert to a simplified form which conforms more closely to the other forms in his or her productive vocabulary (e.g., *pretty* → [bɪdi]; Leopold, 1947). In such cases, the child apparently takes a step backward or regresses since the new form is farther from the adult model. On the other hand, the new form fits into the child's own emerging **phonological system**. Thus, the **regression** seems to reflect systematization on the child's part, suggesting that the child's own system has psychological validity of some sort.

COMMENT ON THE PROSODIC AND COGNITIVE MODELS

Waterson's approach provides a useful complement to the phonological process–based (segmental) analysis, which was most widespread in the 1970s. In particular, Waterson is able to capture the "gestalt" or the "canonical form" underlying certain child productions that are highly irregular in terms of segment-by-segment comparison with the adult model. Waterson also differs with Stampe and Smith in her position regarding perception in the period of early words.

Like Waterson, the cognitive model focuses primarily on the earliest period of word production, when the child appears to be targeting whole words rather than segments (Ferguson and Farwell, 1975; Menyuk, Menn, and Silber, 1986). Although Waterson did not frame her findings in those terms, her prosodic analyses of child language data provide rich illustrations of the characteristic **individuality** of early phonological development later emphasized by the cognitive model. In fact, that model may be criticized for overemphasizing the individual creative aspects of phonological acquisition. Within the framework of the biologically possible, the child is seen as having considerable space for active exploration, hypothesis-formation, and systematization. Little attention is paid to the **constraints** on learning which may result from maturation, both physiological and psychological, or from the structure of language in general and also from the particular language of the child's environment.

BIOLOGICAL MODEL

Locke (1983, 1990; Locke and Pearson, 1992) has proposed a biological model of the origins of phonological system in the child (cf. also Kent, 1992). He suggests that innate perceptual biases and dispositions to certain motor action are at the root of phonological acquisition. In babbling, the child's phonetic repertoire is essentially universal, being constrained by biological factors such as the size and shape of the infant vocal tract and the relative complexity of neuromotor control required for various articulations. For example, simply raising and lowering the jaw can result in alveolar stop production at a time when independent manipulation of the tongue has not yet come under voluntary control. Babbling is critical in that it allows the child to construct auditory-kinesthetic links which can serve as a phonetic guidance system for acquiring language (Fry, 1966; Vihman, 1991).

Influence from the language of the child's environment is thought to emerge only with the production of first words, and is based on the storage and retrieval of some relatively stable perceived forms of the language. However, constraints on production remain basically unchanged until the child has a larger vocabulary (by about 18 months), and begins to deviate from the biologically given babbling production patterns to produce forms that reflect specific phonetic characteristics of the target adult language. At this point the child manifests the developmental

Early Phonological Development

mechanisms of **maintenance** (of babbling production patterns which occur in the adult language as well), **learning** (of patterns of the adult language not found in babbling), and **loss** (of patterns not found in the adult language).

SELF-ORGANIZING MODEL

Biological and linguistic approaches to vocal development have converged in the idea of self-organizing principles (Lindblom, 1992). According to this view, phonetic forms in all languages have evolved to meet the complementary needs of the two participants in vocal communication, the *listener* and the *speaker*. The needs of the listener are met when a language uses vowels such as /i/, /a/, and /u/, which are maximally distant from one another and thus *easy to discriminate*. On the other hand, the needs of the speaker are met when a language uses consonant-vowel sequences which require little tongue movement and are thus *easy to articulate*, such as apico-dental /t/ followed by a front (or "apical") vowel (/i/), or velar /k/ followed by a back vowel (/u/). The compromise between these two sets of **performance constraints** leads to phonetic universals, specifying "core" segments used in most languages and "exotic" segments which occur only in languages with large phonetic inventories.

In the case of the child learning to speak, a small number of articulatory gestures are used over and over in different combinations to produce word patterns, or articulatory **motor scores** corresponding to **unitary acoustic patterns**. The overlapping use of the same articulatory gestures to produce different word patterns or syllables (/ti/, /tu/, /ki/, /ku/) will eventually lead to the emergence of a network of phonologically contrastive segments (/t/, /k/, /i/, /u/) by "self-segmentation."

COMMENT ON THE BIOLOGICAL AND SELF-ORGANIZING MODELS

Despite the evidence that problem solving plays a role in phonology, as in other areas of learning, universal biologically or linguistically based constraints undoubtedly set the parameters within which acquisition must occur. Beyond this, both **maturation** (natural biological development and change) and **practice** may be said to influence learning. Both Locke's and Lindblom's models are similar to Jakobson's in their emphasis on the *universal* aspects of early speech. However, neither model accepts the notion of *discontinuity* between babbling and speech.

An apparent difficulty for Locke's view is the extent of **individual differences** that have been reported among children from a single language background in the babbling stage (Vihman, Ferguson, and Elbert, 1986). If the earliest period of linguistic development is under relatively strict biological or maturational control, one might expect greater uniformity across infants at this stage. However, genetic variation across individual members of a species is the rule in developmental biology and may account for the early differences in phonetic production (Locke, 1988). On the other hand, some global influence of the specific ambient language has been detected in infant vocalizations as early as 10 months (de Boysson-Bardies, Halle, Sagart and Durand, 1989; de Boysson-Bardies and Vihman, 1991), suggesting that phonetic "learning" must begin in the pre-lexical period.

The basis of the principle of self-organization is that neither genetic specification nor linguistic input is sufficient to account for the development of a phonological system, but that the *interaction* of the two promotes novelty and complexity in the child's emergent system.

SUMMARY

The earlier behaviorist and structuralist models developed out of the prevailing American and European linguistic schools of the mid-century and were, to a great extent, deductive rather than empirically based. Extensive analysis of the vocal productions of children in the past two decades has led to rejection, for the most part, of both these views. Currently, the remaining models are more controversial. Stampe and Smith emphasize universal constraints and a systematic, smooth progression toward the adult model; both explicitly deny any reality to the child's "own system," and both posit accurate perception of the adult forms from the start. Waterson, on the other hand, allows for individual or idiosyncratic child systems, based on imperfect perception of adult forms. Ferguson, Macken, and Menn emphasize the active role of the child, involving individual strategies, hypothesis-formation, and problem solving. The work of Locke, Kent, and Lindblom complements the prosodic and cognitive models and reflects current renewed interest in the biological roots of language in humankind as well as in the individual child.

INFANT PERCEPTION: BREAKING INTO THE CODE

Having reviewed the main theories of normal phonological development, we will now present a chronological account of infant perception and production. We begin with speech perception by infants, since perception of the sounds of the adult language would logically seem to precede adult-like sound production. Perception and production are thought to develop in parallel but to interact with each other. Perception and production are treated separately here for expository purposes only.

The study of infant perception is a relatively new field of inquiry, dating back to the early 1970s. Nevertheless, research findings in this area are abundant. The data base is sufficient to establish that very young infants are capable of differentiating most of the sounds used in speech. In attempting to construct a picture of the child's phonological acquisition, we start with these findings since they afford a clue to the perceptual capacities with which the infant first begins to attend to the "blooming buzzing confusion" around him.

PROBLEMS FACING THE CHILD

At the outset of our inquiry, we must ask how the child gets started on the difficult task of "learning to pronounce." To begin with, what do we know about how the child hears the sounds of language? The stream of speech is not naturally segmented into separate sounds, but rather consists of a continuous flow of overlapping sounds. This presents a **segmentation** problem for the infant. The adult listener applies his or her knowledge of the language to pick out contrasting syllables and segments as well as words and phrases. But what of the naive ear of the infant? How does the child pick out the sound units of language?

Equally problematic is the question of **perceptual constancy**. How does the child listening to speech decide what counts as the "same sound," despite differences in the physical features of the sound? The acoustic signals produced by males, females, and children are quite different due to significant differences in vocal tract size and configuration. Equally important acoustic differences result from differences in phonetic context (e.g., consonant before /i/ versus /u/), positional context (e.g., word-initial versus word-final), and rate (e.g., the rapid, fluent speech of "small talk" versus the slower, more hesitant production of carefully considered discourse). How does the child recognize as the "same sound" variations associated with different speakers, different contexts, and different rates of speech?

RESEARCH METHODOLOGY USED TO STUDY INFANT PERCEPTION

A considerable body of evidence concerning the perceptual abilities of infants is available as a result of the ingenious research methodologies developed in the past two decades. These methodologies are based on a simple observation: Infants, like older people, react to *changes* they perceive in their environment and become bored by ("habituate to") repetitions of the same event.

In 1971, Eimas, Siqueland, Jusczyk, and Vigorito reported a procedure known as the **high-amplitude sucking** paradigm to test infants' discrimination of voiced and voiceless and aspirated and unaspirated stops. This procedure has been used to obtain data on the discriminatory skills of infants from birth to 3 or 4 months of age. It allows the infant to control the presentation of a speech stimulus by the rate of sucking on a pacifier attached to a pressure transducer. Once the infant's baseline sucking rate has been established, a repeating speech stimulus such as [pa pa pa] is presented. The frequency of repetition of the sound is controlled by the infant's sucking rate. The presentation of the speech sound is presumed to serve as "contingent reinforcement" for the infant; increased sucking is interpreted as an expression of awareness of, and interest in, the sound stimulus. After several minutes, the infant's sucking rate typically levels off (reaches asymptote) and then decreases. Decreased sucking is taken to indicate that the infant has habituated and is no longer interested in the stimulus. The stimulus is then changed for the experimental group of infants, who hear a different repeated syllable (e.g., [ba ba ba]), while the infants in the control group continue to hear the sound stimulus first presented.

The sucking responses of the experimental group during this changed-stimulus condition are compared with those of the control group, which receives only a single stimulus throughout the experiment. If, following presentation of the second stimulus, the experimental group increases its sucking response while the control group maintains or slows its sucking rate, it is inferred that the experimental subjects perceive the difference between the two stimuli.

The other procedure most often used to test infant perception is the **visually reinforced head turn**, which is most appropriate for older infants (aged 6 to 12 months). Originally developed for assessing audiometric thresholds, this localization technique typically presents a repeated background sound for a time, follows it with a minimally different stimulus for a few seconds, and then repeats the original background stimulus. A head turn toward the sound source when the second sound is introduced is reinforced with the presentation of a lighted, animated toy that "rewards" the infant for discriminating the new sound from the old. If the infant turns his or her head during **change** trials (in which a new sound is introduced) but not during **control** trials (in which the same sound continues to be presented), it is concluded that the infant is able to discriminate the two contrasting sounds.

There are difficulties in the use of each of these procedures. In particular, since not all infants will habituate, large numbers of subjects must be tested to obtain statistically meaningful results. Nevertheless, several of the findings have been replicated many times over, in different laboratories by different investigators, so the results appear to be robust.

CATEGORICAL PERCEPTION

The acoustic cues relevant to speech sounds—such as the cues associated with voicing and aspiration or with place of articulation—may vary along a continuous parameter, but adults respond to these acoustic signals as if sharp boundaries were present at specific points along the continuum. For example, in producing the syllable /pa/ or /ba/, the speaker completely closes off the flow of air through the vocal tract (by bringing his or her lips together) and then releases the closure (by opening his or her mouth) in order to produce the following vowel. The difference between /p/ and /b/ is determined by the timing of the opening of the lips and the onset of vocal-cord vibration for vowel production. If the vocal cords begin to vibrate *before* the release of the oral closure, the stop is "pre-voiced," as in French word-initial /b/ or English intervocalic /b/. If the vocal cords begin to vibrate *at about the same time* that the lips are opened, an English (word-initial) /b/ is heard, but if the vibration of the vocal cords is *delayed*, English (word-initial) /p/ (aspirated [pʰ]) is heard. The parameter just described is referred to as *voice onset time*, or VOT.

A continuum of VOT possibilities exists beyond those associated with English "pre-voiced" (intervocalic) /b/, word-initial /b/, and word-initial /p/, although most languages seem to make use of one or more of these three in their phonemic system. Using **speech synthesis** (the artificial production of speech sounds), investigators have tested adult perception of the acoustic cues corresponding to the VOT continuum (Lisker and Abramson, 1964). Presented with a series of synthetic speech-like sounds resembling a range of different VOT values, adults generally perceive the stimuli as belonging to one of the phonemic categories distinguished in their own language. Thus, English-speakers hear virtually all stimuli as either /ba/ or /pa/, as if a sharp boundary divided the two; this is known as **categorical perception**. For some years, these findings were assumed to reflect adults' experience with the categories of their language. However, research with infants led to the surprising finding that 2- to 4-month-old babies also hear in terms of categories—despite their inexperience with the sounds of any language. The infants do not discriminate between acoustically different stimuli *within* the adult categories, but they are able to discriminate similar acoustic differences *between* categories.

English /b/ versus /p/ are discriminated by infants as if the two phonemic categories were known to them. This finding was initially attributed to an *innate mechanism* in humans for the recognition of speech categories. Later research has shown that not only human infants but also chinchillas and monkeys can distinguish this categorical boundary (Kuhl, 1987). So the argument for an innate human mechanism *specialized for speech perception* lacks strong supporting evidence. It is more likely that the phonetic boundary between the English language categories of voiceless and voiced stops happens to correspond to a *naturally salient physical boundary* distinguished by infants, whether or not they have been exposed to English, and also by certain mammals possessing auditory biases similar to those of humans.

The human auditory system seems to be especially attuned to **abrupt discontinuities,** or natural breaks, in the acoustic stream, like those created by stop consonants. Such a phonetic predisposition, together with the ability to discriminate continuous acoustic signals in a categorical way, may be crucial in enabling the child to solve the segmentation problem; that is, to break into a code based on overlapping sounds embedded in an ongoing speech stream.

UNIVERSAL PERCEPTION: EARLY ABILITIES

Using the various procedures described earlier, investigators have been able to demonstrate infant discrimination of a wide range of phonetic contrasts used in adult languages, regardless of the language of the child's environment (for overviews, see Eilers, 1980; Kuhl, 1987). Thus, children as young as 2 to 3 months of age can discriminate **place of articulation** in syllable-initial [b], [d], and [g]. Two-month-old infants can also discriminate [d] versus [g] in medial and final position. Only the distinction between contrasting unreleased (C)VC syllables (e.g., *bat* [bæt] and *back* [bæk]), which are not always easily identified by adults (Householder, 1956), were found to exceed infants' perceptual abilities. Investigation of **manner of articulation** contrasts has shown that infants can discriminate stops from nasals and glides and [ra] from [la].

Furthermore, 1- to 4-month-old infants have been found to discriminate the three vowels most commonly contrasted in languages ([a] vs. [i] and [i] vs. [u]). Embedding the vowels in a syllable ([pa] vs. [pi]) did not impede discrimination. In addition, infants of this age raised in an English-speaking environment were able to distinguish **oral** versus **nasal** vowels ([pa] vs. [pã]), even though the oral–nasal contrast is not used phonemically in English vowels (Trehub, 1976). (It does function phonemically in French and Hindi.) Finally, Kuhl (1987) reviews a number of studies in which she and her colleagues tested 1- to 4-month-old infants for perceptual constancy by presenting tokens of the vowels [a] and [i], each produced on monotone and rise-fall **pitches,** with the different pitch-tokens varied randomly. The children were able to discriminate the vowels and disregarded the differences in pitch. However, when the reverse situation was tested, contrasting the two pitch contours with random shifting between [a] and [i] as the vowel carrying the pitch, the infants failed to discriminate the pitch contrast. Thus, infants showed perceptual constancy with respect to the vowel-color dimension (i.e., [a] vs. [i]), which appeared to be more salient to them than the pitch-contour dimension (monotone vs. rise-fall). Similar testing of vowel contrasts produced by adult male versus female and child talkers showed that infants easily discriminate even the acoustically similar vowels /a/ and /ɔ/ regardless of changes in the speaker.

A few contrasts have been reported to resist discrimination in the early months and thus to require learning by the child. These include contrasts of voicing and place in fricatives, for example ([sa] vs. [za], [fa] vs. [θa], [fi] vs. [θi]: Eilers and Minifie (1975); Eilers, 1977). These results are interesting because the /f/

versus /θ/ distinction is a notoriously difficult one for children, even as late as age 3 or 4 (cf., e.g., Locke, 1980b); and, under less than ideal listening conditions, it can prove difficult for adults as well. However, other studies have shown that when computer-synthesized tokens are used instead of naturally produced syllables, 2- to 3-month-olds can discriminate [fa] versus [θa] (Jusczyk, Murray, and Bayly, 1979).

Another type of discrimination that may exceed infants' perceptual capacities is that between different stops embedded in multisyllabic vocalizations with relatively short syllables (less than 300 milliseconds: [ataba] vs. [atapa]: Trehub, 1973). This observation is interesting in light of children's use of syllable deletion and unique reduction devices well into the third year, which reflects the difficulty that the production of multisyllabic words poses for them. These production problems may result from perceptual as well as articulatory difficulties; that is, the relatively shorter syllables embedded in long words may continue to be difficult to perceive and store in sufficient segmental detail even when the child is successfully producing one- and two-syllable words. Later studies have shown that the difficulty of making discriminations within a "long word" context can be attenuated by adding exaggerated stress to the contrasting syllable, as caretakers typically do in speaking to children (Fernald and Simon, 1984; Karzon, 1985).

In summary, in the first few months of life, infants are capable of distinguishing between consonants that differ in place and manner of articulation, and also between some vowels. Distinguishing among certain fricatives and between stops embedded in longer, multisyllabic vocalizations is more problematic for young children.

THE ROLE OF LINGUISTIC EXPERIENCE

Some investigators have suggested that *linguistic experience* within the first six months of life may influence the child's perceptual capacities, particularly with respect to voicing and aspiration contrasts in stops. Children exposed to Spanish (Eilers, Gavin, and Wilson, 1979) or Kikuyu (Streeter, 1976) were found to discriminate pre-voiced from voiced (unaspirated) stops, whereas infants exposed only to English did not make this discrimination. Since the pre-voiced/voiced stop distinction is phonemic in Spanish and Kikuyu but not in English, it was inferred that the phonemic contrasts used in the adult language to which the child is exposed may affect the child's ability to discriminate phonetic categories within the first few months of life. Interpretation of the findings, however, has been criticized on both logical and methodological grounds. In particular, exposure to the speech of a given language does not ensure that a specific **phonemic category** or contrast will be perceived (MacKain, 1982). Recall that pre-voiced stops do occur in English, though only in intervocalic position. Thus, the child exposed to English does "experience" pre-voiced stops, though they are not contrastive. It is unclear how the young child's exposure to the phonetic realization of different phonemic categories in particular languages could lead to differential categorical perception of speech at this stage of development.

THE ROLE OF PROSODY

The most recent line of research on infant perceptual capacities has focused on larger speech units (sequences of sentences, clauses, and phrases rather than isolated syllables) and on other influences affecting infant attention to the speech

Early Phonological Development

signal (own mother or own language vs. other mother, other language; speech directed to infants, or "motherese", vs. speech directed to adults). Such studies have provided evidence that infants are strongly attracted to the sound of their own language, especially when spoken by the mother and especially when she uses the wide pitch contours characteristic of motherese. The attraction of prosodically varied speech is thought to be related to its emotional tone; it is part of the process of bonding between mother and infant. In addition, the infant's close attention to the caretaker's speech most likely plays an important facilitory role in beginning to identify the relevant **units** of the adult language. Specifically, infants appear to be sensitive to the perceptual unity of **clauses** by 6 months of age; **phrasal** units (subject noun, predicate verb) appear to be detectable by 9 months. It has been argued that the salience of prosodic cues reflects an **innately guided learning process,** like the tendency for goslings to follow the mother shortly after hatching or for the sparrow to attend to and learn the song typical of its species (Jusczyk and Bertoncini, 1988).

SUMMARY

What perceptual capabilities are infants born with? How do they break into the acoustic flow of speech? And which capabilities develop with age and exposure to the sounds of the language used around them? Researchers report that during the first months of life, infants respond differentially to different speech stimuli and treat some sounds varied along a continuum as if they belonged to categories of sounds used in the adult language. These discriminations probably reflect inherent biases in the auditory systems of mammals, including humans. Certain natural boundaries between sounds appear to be universally salient to infants, whether or not the natural boundary is matched by a phonemic contrast in the adult language to which the child is exposed. These built-in biases make it possible for the infant to begin finding recognizable patterns in the stream of overlapping sounds that constitute speech.

Many contrasts used in language are discriminable from an early age, including the differences among place of consonant articulation (labial/dental/velar) or manner of articulation (stops vs. nasals or glides, and /ra/ vs. /la/); other contrasts, especially distinctions among different fricatives, unreleased final stops, and those embedded in multisyllabic utterances, may be discriminated only later, as they require maturation and increased exposure to language. Attempts to demonstrate the effects of experience with different phonemic systems during the first few months of life remain controversial and the potential effects unclear.

Prosodic characteristics of speech play an important role in language acquisition, although only limited data are available at this time and the role of prosody is not yet well understood.

INFANT PRODUCTION: INTERACTION OF MATURATION AND EXPERIENCE

The problem facing the infant learning to produce speech sounds can be broken down into a series of increasingly complex tasks, ranging from vocal production per se to communicative use, in context, of adult-based sound patterns, or *words* (Menyuk, Menn, and Silber, 1986). These tasks include (1) learning to produce a variety of vocal sounds, (2) matching sound patterns produced by adults to some of the well-practiced vocal patterns already in the infant's repertoire, (3) associating certain adult sound patterns with situations where they are often produced (the basis for situation-bound word use), (4) achieving the understanding that sound-pattern production can be used as a means to share a focus of attention or to make a request, and (5) marshaling adult-based words to serve communicative goals in novel settings (the referential and symbolic use of words).

The task analysis outlined above identifies the cognitive challenges in learning to speak. Mastery of the articulatory gestures alone will take five years or more; perceptual development presumably plays a role in this process as well. When the process is barely underway, however, the child has already begun work on other aspects of communicative development, including the problem of apprehending the significance of regular and recurrent form-meaning correspondences (i.e., developing comprehension of words and of communicative gestures, such as pointing, clapping, or waving). As outlined above, the cognitive problems for the would-be language user involve matching his or her own productive capacities to the sound patterns of the adult language, developing the ability to access them at will, and developing the skills to use language to refer to events outside the immediate situational context. These tasks are largely encountered and mastered in the course of what is called "the transition period"; that is, the phase of development which reflects the transition from babbling to speech. We begin our account of vocal production with the first task—learning to produce a variety of vocal sounds.

LEARNING TO PRODUCE A VARIETY OF VOCAL SOUNDS

It is important to note that the infant's vocal tract is not simply a miniature or smaller version of the adult's (see Figure 2–1). Differences include: (1) a much shorter vocal tract; (2) a relatively shorter pharyngeal cavity; (3) a tongue mass placed relatively farther forward in the oral cavity; (4) a gradual, rather than a right-angle, bend in the oropharyngeal channel; (5) a high larynx; and (6) a close approximation of the velopharynx and epiglottis (Kent and Murray, 1982). The differences in anatomical structure affect the nature of infant vocal productions. For example, the close relationship of laryngeal and velopharyngeal cavities leads to nasal breathing and early nasal vocalizations by the infant; it is only after the velum and epiglottis grow farther apart, when the infant is about 4 to 6 months old, that nonnasal vocal sounds first appear in significant quantities.

EARLY STAGES OF PRODUCTION

Oller (1980) and Stark (1980) have provided compatible descriptions of vocal production over the first year of life (cf. also Roug, Landberg, and Lundberg, 1989, who offer a similar description for Swedish infants). "Reflexive" vocalizations (i.e., vocalizations arising as automatic responses to internal or external stimulation, such as hunger or discomfort) will not be discussed in this text. Rather, the presentation will focus on the nonreflexive prelinguistic vocalizations, which are assumed to be under voluntary control. Oller divides the first six months into three sequential stages, which he terms the *phonation stage*, the *cooing stage*, and the *expansion stage*. He also identifies two stages in the second half of the first year, *canonical* and *variegated babbling*. Considerable overlap exists be-

Early Phonological Development

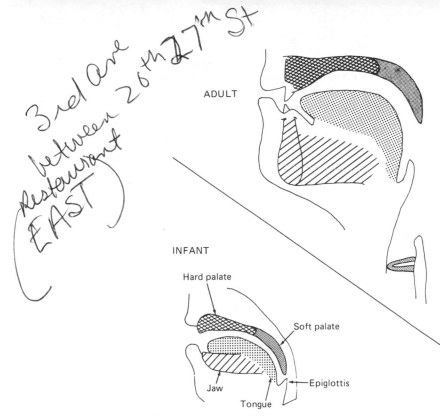

FIGURE 2–1. **Vocal tracts of adult and infant.** From R.D. Kent and A.D. Murray, "Acoustic Features of Infant Vocalic Utterances at 3, 6, and 9 Months." *JASA,* 72 (1982): 353–365. Used with permission.

tween stages, and the ages assigned to each stage are only approximations. Furthermore, although the appearance of canonical babbling is a landmark event, variegated babbling has been found to be difficult to distinguish as a chronologically separate "stage."

1. In the **phonation stage** (birth to 1 month), speech-like sounds are rare. The largest number of nonreflexive, nondistress sounds are the "quasi-resonant nuclei," which Oller characterizes as vocalizations with normal phonation but limited resonance, produced with a closed or nearly closed mouth. These elements give the auditory impression of a syllabic nasal.

2. In the "goo" or **cooing stage** (2 to 3 months), velar consonant-like sounds are produced with some frequency and "primitive syllabification" may be detected (Zlatin, 1975), but the rhythmic properties of adult syllables and the timing of the articulatory gestures for adult consonants have not yet been mastered. Acoustically, the cooing sounds are similar to rounded back vowels such as [u].

3. In the **expansion stage** (4 to 6 months), the child appears to gain increasing control of both laryngeal and oral articulatory mechanisms. He or she explores the vocal mechanism through the playful use of squealing, growling, yelling, and "raspberry" vocalizations (bilabial trills). "Fully resonant nuclei" (adult-like vowels) begin to be produced in this period, as does "marginal babbling," in which consonant-like and vowel-like features occur but lack the mature regular-syllable timing characteristics of canonical babbling.

Stark (1978) emphasized the interrelationship of earlier and later vocal behaviors in the first 6 months of life. The emergence of cooing is dependent on increased control over voicing, which is first found only in crying. The new co-occurrence of voicing, egressive breath direction, and consonant-like closures results from the overlap between the maturation in voluntary laryngeal control and continuing reflexive activity of the vocal tract. The acquisition of control over this new behavioral combination is probably derived from the interaction of maturation and the experience of exercising the new behavior. The modified combination is then ready to begin to form new combinations with other more primitive behaviors. Thus, cooing or comfort sounds are expanded through the use of vocal play, which allows the infant to gain greater control over the activity of the tongue, lips, and jaw.

BEGINNINGS OF ADULT-LIKE PRODUCTION: THE EMERGENCE OF CONSONANTS

The first probable evidence of adult language influence on production is manifested by the emergence of **canonical babbling** (Oller's Stage 4; also known as reduplicated babbling), typically at about 6 to 8 months. The sudden appearance of genuine syllabic production involving a true consonant and a "fully resonant nucleus" or vowel, often (though not exclusively) chained in repeated sequences such as [bababa], [dadada], or [mamama], constitutes the chief production milestone in the first year. The onset of this stage is easily recognized by parents, who report the child to be babbling or even "talking," although few if any consistent sound-meaning relations are likely to be observed.

Canonical babbling has been viewed primarily as the outgrowth of physiological maturation, uninfluenced by exposure to the adult language. However, Oller and his colleagues have reported that deaf children do not produce canonical babbling within the first year (Oller and Eilers, 1988; cf. also Stoel-Gammon and Otomo, 1986), whereas such babbling typically occurs in hearing babies by 10 months at the latest. These recent findings suggest that canonical babbling depends on auditory exposure and, thus, may reflect the influence of the adult language as well as physiological maturation.

The onset of canonical babbling may be viewed as a production discontinuity since it represents the first use of true consonantal articulation. The fact that stops (and nasals, or stops articulated with a lowered velum) are the earliest true consonants to be produced may be related to the natural perceptual salience of syllables with a stop onset. Stops present the sharpest possible contrast with vowels and provide the most obtrusive break in the acoustic stream of speech sounds. On the other hand, stop production is also relatively undemanding: Syllables such as [ba], [da], and [na] may be articulated through mandibular action alone (Kent, 1992). It is likely that this production milestone represents an advance in: (1) motoric control, which is **maturational**, or tied to natural physiological development in the first year; (2) the **experience-based** integration of visual and auditory perception of adult sequences of open–closed mouth and voice–silence alternation, and (3) the **expression** of the percept of adult vocalization through global imitation. In other words, children *see* as well as *hear* stop consonants in adult speech, produce such sounds themselves, and engage in repetitive vocal production or sound play, re-creating their impression of adult speech.

Variegated Babbling and Universal Production Patterns. The last babbling stage (Oller's Stage 5) is **variegated babbling**, in which continued use of adult-like syllables is supplemented by the use of increasingly varied consonants and vowels within a single vocalization (e.g., from the babbling of a 9-month-old girl, [ʔəmæːʰ], [wətʌ], [teːkæ], [hətapa]: Vihman, Ferguson, and Elbert, 1986). Elbers (1982) has traced the development from reduplicated to variegated babbling in the speech of one child, between 6 and 12 months of age. Elbers views babbling in this period as "a systematic, continuous and largely self-directed process of exploration," in which the child constructs a phonetic "spring-board" to speech (1982: 45). Variegated babbling may emerge very soon after the onset of canonical babbling, and because of the difficulty of distinguishing between these two types of babbling, some have suggested that variegated and canonical babbling be considered a single stage of development (Smith, Brown-Sweeney, and Stoel-Gammon, 1989; Mitchell and Kent, 1990).

A number of studies have looked at the sound **repertoire** found in the variegated babbling of children learning different languages. These segmental repertoires are virtually indistinguishable. Locke (1983) cited the babbling repertoires for infants (aged 9 to 15 months) acquiring one of 15 languages each. He found that stops and nasals formed the core of each inventory, with relatively low incidence for most other sounds. However, direct cross-linguistic comparisons of sound production **frequencies** in babbling vocalizations, examined through both instrumental analysis (of vowels) and phonetic transcription (of consonants), have revealed the first language-specific differences at 10 months, when word production is barely underway or has not yet begun (de Boysson-Bardies et al., 1989; de Boysson-Bardies and Vihman, 1991).

Vowel Production in the First Year

Up until now, we have concentrated mainly on the early development of consonants since the onset of true consonant use seems to mark the beginning of adult-like vocal production. However, vowel production dominates infant vocalization throughout the first year. Vowels have been less extensively investigated, primarily because they are particularly difficult to transcribe reliably and, thus, difficult to characterize. For example, Lieberman (1980) reported inter-transcriber reliability of 73 percent for the vowels produced by children aged about 3 to 14 months. He reported frequencies only for vowels identified as belonging to the English repertoire. Lieberman's findings for a single child are summarized below, but the relatively low reliability figure should be kept in mind.

Lieberman used spectrographic analysis as a supplement to phonetic transcription and reported little change in average formant frequency values over the period investigated. However, the various vowels transcribed for four months showed considerable acoustic overlap in formant frequencies. A month later, spectrographic analysis yielded identification of a rudimentary vowel triangle. The gradual differentiation in the acoustic vowel space could be seen to continue (based on data from other subjects) until age 3.

The vowels most often perceived over the entire period were lax—[ɛ, ɪ, æ, ʌ, u]—and were already present at the earliest session. [ɛ] was heard most frequently (33 percent of all the vowels transcribed), and the remaining lax vowels each accounted for 11 percent–17 percent of the data. The remaining (tense)

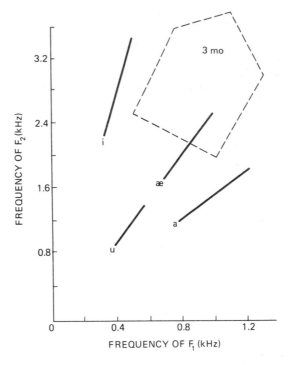

FIGURE 2–2. **F₁–F₂ region for 3-month-olds (area bounded by broken line) compared to isovowel lines for /i æ o u/.** From R.D. Kent and A.D. Murray, "Acoustic Features of Infant Vocalic Utterances at 3, 6, and 9 months." *JASA, 72 (1982): 353–365. Used with permission.*

vowels each accounted for no more than 5 percent, with the back-rounded [o] and [u] least frequent (1 percent each).

Kent and Murray (1982) investigated the acoustic features of vocalic utterances at 3, 6, and 9 months (seven infants at each age). Their findings were similar to those reported by Lieberman. The range of F1 and F2 frequencies increased somewhat across each age interval, but the majority of the vowels used by the 9-month-old infants showed roughly the same formant pattern as did the vowels of the younger subjects. Given the anatomical differences between adults and infants, it is not surprising that the range of possible infant vowel productions should be more restricted than those of adults. The formant patterns of infant vowels fit within the range of mid-front or central adult vowels (Figure 2–2).

In a study of 10-month-old infants' vowel productions drawn from four linguistic communities—Arabic, Chinese, English, and French—de Boysson-Bardies and her colleagues (1989) found that the categories of *front-low* and *mid-central* vowels accounted for the vast majority of vowels from all four groups. Acoustic analysis revealed characteristic patterns of vowel production for each group within those limits, however, with more high-front vowels for English, for example, and more low-back vowels for Chinese. The investigators interpreted these differences in vowel production to show that infants begin to position their lips and tongue in a manner specific to the language of their environment even before they produce word-forms modeled on adult speech.

Early Phonological Development

Languages differ not only in segmental patterns but also in terms of nonsegmental aspects of sound production, such as pitch, loudness, voice quality, and timing. de Boysson-Bardies and her colleagues (1984) presented comparative data from 6- and 8-month-old infants exposed to French and Arabic and suggested that the very earliest language-specific differences in vocal production reflect nonsegmental or prosodic characteristics. Specifically, the infants differed in phonation types (rapidly alternated sequences of inspiratory and expiratory phonation characterized the Arabic babbling, whereas the direction of air flow was always expiratory in the French samples) and in the organization of pitch and intensity contours (rhythmical weak–strong contrasts were prominent only in the babbling of Arabic infants).

The development of the intonational patterns of language has received considerably less attention than has the development of segments and segmental contrasts. This reflects, in part, the fact that the prosodic properties of adult languages are also less well understood. Nevertheless, the literature points to a few conclusions. Acoustic analysis of infant vocalizations across the first year of life shows that falling pitch is the most common contour during this period (Delack and Fowlow, 1978; Kent and Murray, 1982). Kent and Murray offer a physiological explanation, suggesting that a falling fundamental frequency, or pitch contour, is the natural result of a decline in subglottal pressure in the course of a vocalization. A reduction of vocal fold length and tension as the muscles of the larynx relax at the end of a vocalization could also lead to a falling pitch contour. A rising pitch contour requires an increase in vocal fold length or tension at the end of the vocalization or an increase in subglottal pressure or both. It seems natural, then, that the development of contrastive, rising pitch contours should develop later than falling pitch contours. It appears that this sequence is a general one, regardless of the language being acquired.

Once the variegated babbling stage has been reached, the child may also produce jargon. This phenomenon, which Oller (1980) calls "gibberish," results when adult-like pitch movement and rhythm are imposed on rapidly produced multisyllabic strings of variegated babble. In children acquiring English, multisyllabic jargon strings of this kind typically end with a relatively low pitch on the next-to-last syllable followed by a shift to a mid or mid-falling pitch on the last syllable. Notice that a phrase-final shift in pitch is a characteristic adult English intonation pattern. Jargon seems to represent the child's attempts to "reproduce the surface impression of longer strings of speech, that is, of phrases or sentences instead of isolated words" (Vihman, 1986); the result often impresses the adult listener as conversation without words (cf. Menn, 1976; de Boysson-Bardies, Bacri, Sagart, and Poizat, 1981).

Summary

Young children face a series of production tasks on their way to learning the language of their environment. To begin with, they must gain control of laryngeal and articulatory gestures to develop the precision necessary to produce the sounds of language at will. Developing such control involves both maturation of the laryngeal, articulatory, and perceptual mechanisms and accommodation to the sound patterns of the specific language spoken to the child. Thus, phonological development in the young child involves the interaction of physical maturation and social experience.

During the first six months of life, three stages of voluntary vocal behavior can be distinguished: the phonation stage, the cooing stage, and the expansion stage. Acquisition of control over each new behavioral combination is the result of the interaction of maturation and experience or practice in using the new motor behavior.

Between age 6 and 10 months, canonical babbling begins to be produced. This constitutes the main discontinuity, or sharp qualitative change, in infant production in the first year and provides the first concrete evidence of the influence of auditory experience with an adult language. In the last babbling stage, variegated babbling, the child prepares the phonetic ground for his or her first attempts at adult words. At this stage, infant consonantal repertoires are largely indistinguishable across languages, but consonant and vowel production frequencies begin to reflect differences in the child's linguistic experience.

During the first year, infant vowel production shows little change. Adult transcribers typically perceive the primitive vowels as mid-front or central.

The influence of the specific language environment is manifested at its earliest in nonsegmental parameters of speech, such as phonation type and rhythmical organization. Falling pitch contours predominate in the children's productions in the first year, perhaps for (universal) physiological reasons. Once the child has begun producing variegated babble, adult-like stress patterns and intonation contours may also be used, giving the surface effect of adult language, but without content or meaning.

THE TRANSITION PERIOD: FROM BABBLE TO SPEECH

We have reviewed the infant's perception and production of speech during the first year of life. The infant manifests impressive discriminatory abilities for speech sounds at a very early age. However, we have not yet considered how these abilities serve the child in linguistic perception nor in identifying and remembering meaningful sound patterns of the adult language. The child also faces a series of tasks in learning to produce meaningful speech. So far, we have discussed only the first of these tasks—learning to produce a variety of vocal sounds. By the end of the first year, the child is babbling or, in other words, producing adult-like sequences of syllables that include a range of different consonants (primarily stops and nasals) and vowels. Furthermore, the child is no longer restricted to a single consonant or vowel type per vocalization. Some use of rising pitch contours may occur alongside the more common falling pitch.

Having surveyed the infant's perceptual and productive abilities, we turn now to the transition period when the babbler becomes a talker. The critical development in this period is the linking of sound patterns with meaning, first in comprehension, then in word production. Sporadic signs of understanding may occur in the middle of the first year, so we will have to backtrack slightly in our chronological account to pick up the trail of the child's first steps in the use of meaning and communication.

The transition period is best defined by certain developmental events. It

Early Phonological Development

begins with the onset of comprehension of the adult language, and it closes when word use begins to dominate babble, typically when the child is using about 50 different words spontaneously. The age range in which these developments occur is extremely variable. Some normally developing children fail to produce many recognizable words before the age of 2, although they will show evidence of good language comprehension long before this time. For many, and perhaps most, children, the transition to speech will occur during the period from about 9 to 18 months.

RELATING SOUND PATTERNS TO MEANINGS

When the child first begins to respond differentially to particular words or phrases of the adult language, that is, begins to show comprehension, he or she has begun to match discriminable differences in sound patterns with differences in the use or function of those patterns. The first reports of language comprehension, found in the diary records kept by linguist parents, noted earliest signs of comprehension at age 4 or 5 months. At 20 weeks, Hans Lindner responded to *tick-tack* (German for 'tick-tock') by looking toward the large, loudly ticking wall clock that had often been pointed out to him (Lindner, 1898, reported in Ferguson, 1978). At 6 months, Deville's daughter responded to *bravo* by clapping her hands, and at 7 months she would respond to French *chut* ('quiet!') by refraining from touching an item of interest (Deville, 1890, 1891, reported in Lewis, 1936). Lewis observed his child's first responses to words at 8 or 9 months: a smile for *cuckoo!* "uttered in a special tone of voice," recoil from a movement for *no!*, and a wave for *say goodbye!* (Lewis, 1936; 107). In each case, the child had heard the word repeatedly in context, and the expected behavior (e.g., the appropriate gesture for routines involving clapping or waving) had been made clear on numerous occasions. The earliest signs of word recognition may be isolated occurrences. By 10 or 11 months, there is generally considerable language comprehension although it is difficult to determine precisely how much the child understands.

PERCEPTION IN THE TRANSITION PERIOD: ENTRY INTO THE NATIVE LANGUAGE

The beginnings of comprehension of the adult language, combined with production of the first learned gestures (e.g., clapping, waving), mark a significant new step in the child's development. We assume that at this point children have begun to develop a store of familiar phonetic patterns drawn from the adult language and linked with specific meanings. Unfortunately, little direct testing has been done on perception of word-patterns or phonemic contrasts (linguistic perception) by children in the transition period. It would be of great interest to know whether certain meaningful sound patterns are more easily distinguished than others. For example, do children distinguish between words or phrases on the basis of pitch or rhythm before they make a distinction between words differing only in their segmental properties, as anecdotal accounts suggest (Lewis, 1936)? Are differences carried by syllable shape (e.g., presence or absence of a final consonant) easier to recognize than differences carried by specific segments, or do children vary in this regard? Is there a relationship between the patterns most consistently recognized by a given child and the patterns in that child's babbling? Reliable experimental results regarding the relationship between perception and production would be helpful in deciding between the views espoused, on the one hand, by Smith and Stampe, who posit complete, accurate representation of the adult language from the earliest period of word production and, on the other hand, by Waterson, who presupposes imperfect perception as the source of production constraints on early words (cf. also Schwartz and Leonard, 1982; Menn, 1983).

Recent investigations of infant perception at the end of the first year have revealed an important shift whose timing coincides with the beginnings of word recognition—or at least with early comprehension of language in well-established contexts. Werker and her colleagues (Werker, Gilbert, Humphrey, and Tees, 1981; Werker and Tees, 1983) set out to discover the point at which the infant's broad capacities for discrimination of phonemic contrasts are replaced by the adult's language-specific responses to speech sounds (see Trehub, 1976). They tested adults and 4-, 8- and 12-year-old children on two contrasts which are phonemic in Hindi but unfamiliar to English-speakers: place of articulation (dental /t/ vs. retroflex /ṭ/) and voice-onset time (voiceless aspirated /tʰ/ vs. breathy voiced /dʰ/). In addition, they tested a contrast used in an Interior Salish Northwest Indian language, glottalized velar /kʔ/ versus glottalized uvular /qʔ/. Less than half of the adults and children aged 4 or over were able to discriminate these foreign contrasts, whereas most of the 6- to 8-month-old infants tested showed evidence of discrimination. In a critical study, Werker and Tees (1984) tested infants in age groups spanning the last half of the first year (6 to 8, 8 to 10, and 10 to 12 months) on the Hindi and Salishan place of articulation contrasts. The youngest group again showed discrimination, while the oldest group did not. The 8- to 10-month-olds were relatively successful with the Hindi contrast, but most of them did not discriminate the Salishan contrast.

The apparent decline in "universal" perceptual capacity at the end of the first year is intriguing and has aroused a good deal of controversy. Have infants "entered into" the phonemic system of the language to which they are exposed at this time (Werker, 1991), when they are just beginning to attend to language with some sign of understanding of the (arbitrary) association of verbal sounds and (situation-based) meanings? It is difficult to see how the child could have structured perceptual information to that extent at this early stage. Furthermore, the earliest word *production* by the child appears to reveal a broad or holistic phonological base rather than a full-blown set of phonemic (segmental) contrasts. One hypothesis for the apparent reorganization of perception at the onset to speech is that it is mediated by the child's emerging productive (articulatory) abilities (Locke, 1990; Vihman, 1991). As the child develops articulatory control and familiarity, through self-monitoring, with the *sound* as well as the *feel* of a few well-practiced articulatory gestures, we may suppose that certain salient sound patterns of the adult language begin to "stand out" perceptually, since they appear to *match* those familiar vocal patterns that the child has been repeatedly producing. Since influence from the particular language of the child's environment has just begun to affect the child's babbling at this age, it is possible that such an articulatory filter may serve to alter the child's initial "unbiased" response to speech sounds, replacing the "universal" readiness for any language by a more finely tuned readiness for the language of the child's caretakers (Werker and Pegg, 1992).

Early Phonological Development

The time at which the first word appears has long been of interest to individuals concerned with language development, yet the notion that the first word is in itself a significant milestone is problematic for at least two reasons. First, communicative gestures, or gestures used with meaning such as pointing, waving, or signaling *all gone* with outspread, upturned palms, typically begin to be used somewhat earlier than forms of oral language (Bates, Bretherton, Shore, and McNew, 1983). This may be due to the fact that motor control of the hands matures earlier than does comparable motor control of the vocal tract. Second, children often develop their own idiosyncratic sound-meaning pairings during this period, inventing "words" derived from their own babble. This occurs both before and after their first use of adult-based words (Ferguson, 1978). In other words, the child is developing intentional communication at the same time he or she is improving articulatory control and increasing the capacity to store and retrieve adult sound patterns. Thus, a child may communicate meaning with gestures and invented words before doing so consistently with adult-like words.

A child may rely on gestures or invented words for some weeks or even months before he or she embarks on adult-based word use (cf., e.g., Halliday, 1975). On the other hand, a child may imitate sound patterns without much regard for meaning or function, so the same form that appears to be a word in some well-structured interactions is also widely used in apparent sound play or babble (Vihman and Miller, 1988). Before a child can be confidently credited with adult-like word use, we must find evidence for the integration of all of these strands: **communicative intent, articulatory control**, and the capacity for **internal representation**, or memory for adult forms and their associated functions (McCune, 1992).

Identification of early words is difficult (Vihman and McCune, in submission). First of all, the criteria used to identify words must be established. We might decide to count as a word only the spontaneous, productive pairing of form and meaning. In other words, an acceptable word candidate cannot immediately follow an adult use of the word (i.e., it must represent spontaneous as opposed to imitative use by the child), and the same form or pattern must occur more than once in the same situational context or function (i.e., it must be used "productively"). Beyond the definitional issues, the most important source of difficulty in identifying early words is the continuity of phonetic form in the shift from babbling to speech; that is, a child's early word vocalizations come from the same phonetic pool as that child's contemporaneous babbling. Specifically, any child's phonetic preferences will be reflected in both that child's early word forms and his or her babbling (Vihman et al., 1985). When we consider that the child's forms (e.g., [baba], [dat]) are typically schematic approximations of the adult target (e.g., *bottle, light*), it is clear that recognition of adult-based word use will present a challenge.

In summary, many difficulties affect the identification of early words, chief of which is the similarity between babble and word-forms during this period. A number of criteria may be used to determine which vocal productions are best interpreted as words. Most commonly used are the functional criterion of repeated use in a plausible context and the formal requirements of recognizable similarity to an adult model and relative stability of the sound pattern across different instances of use.

INVENTED WORDS

Sometimes a child appears to invent words. The child will use a vocal pattern consistently although there may be no apparent adult counterpart to the child's pairing of sound and meaning (cf. Dore, Franklin, Miller, and Ramer, 1976; Ferguson, 1978). Typically, these idiosyncratic forms express broad meanings or rather general communicative functions.

A child may consistently use a particular form when her attention is focused. Such a form may be used not to communicate—a function which develops somewhat later, but rather to mark for the child herself an object or event of interest. For example, from 9 to 11 months, one child produced the vocalization [pwi] quietly, often in a whisper, in moments of focused attention. Idiosyncratic forms may be nonverbal rather than verbal. One 11-month-old child who observed adults blowing gently on the mobile above his crib apparently associated that gesture with the affective meaning "delight" or "wonder" and began using it to express that meaning; for example, he began blowing softly as he approached a Christmas tree.

Another broad meaning or function often expressed through idiosyncratic forms is "request." The use of a consistent form for requesting involves several notions. It presupposes the intent to communicate, memory for a consistent form, and the more complex idea that it is possible to make use of others to achieve a goal (cf. Bates, 1979). The more complex meaning is unlikely to emerge before the second year of life. Even children who already have a sizable conventional vocabulary may use invented or idiosyncratically generalized words or gestures, frequently together with pointing. It should also be noted that some children have been observed to develop idiosyncratic uses of intonation to express certain functions (cf. Halliday, 1975; Menn, 1976).

PHONETIC CHARACTERISTICS OF LATE BABBLING AND EARLY WORDS

Vocalization at the end of the first year has just begun to be affected by the phonetic makeup of the specific language of the child's environment and is not markedly different when an adult word is intended. What phonetic characteristics of the vocalizations are typically used in the period when word use is first being established? How similar are these vocalizations across infants learning the same language?

Several detailed reports are available on the phonetic characteristics of vocalizations during this period. Kent and Bauer (1985) described the syllable structures, vowel- and consonant-like segments, and intonation contours used by five 13-month-old children. Vihman et al. (1986) focused on vocalization length, syllable shape, and consonants in a longitudinal study of 10 children, aged 9 to 17 months. Davis and MacNeilage (1990) described vowel production for one child learning English (14 to 20 months). These studies addressed the same phenomena for children of approximately the same age and reported similar findings. de Boysson-Bardies, Vihman, Roug-Hellichius, Durand, Landberg, and Arao (1992) extended the Vihman et al. study to three more languages—French, Japanese, and Swedish (five subjects each)—and reported both similarities and differences across the four languages. For English-learners, monosyllabic (one-syllable) vocalizations were the most common form of vocalization, followed by disyllables (or two-syllable productions), while disyllables predominated in the other three language groups studied. Of the consonants used, stops were by far the most common for all the infants, followed by nasals and fricatives.

Kent and Bauer (1985) noted a difference in consonant use in vocalizations of different structures. Although stops dominated consonant use in CV vocalizations, they made up less than half of the consonants in VCV vocalizations and were greatly exceeded by fricatives and nasals in VC vocalizations. Bilabial and apical consonants were used the most often. Consonant clusters were very rare. Kent and Bauer found that the basic consonant-vowel contrast was primarily learned within the framework of the CV syllable, and concluded that such a syllable, which is found in all languages, may be viewed as "a simplest form . . . or a kind of atom in the formulation of speech" (1985: 517).

Kent and Bauer (1985) found that the most common vowels used were central, mid-front, and low-front ([ʌ, ɛ, æ]), while high vowels ([i, u]) were rare. Of the various intonation contours used, the fall and rise-fall accounted for over 75 percent of all vocalizations; a simple rising contour accounted for 10 percent more. Kent and Bauer stressed the fact that in all respects, the vocalizations of 13-month-olds were continuous with the vocalizations of both younger children and children in the second year of life.

Davis and MacNeilage (1990) were less impressed than Kent and Bauer by the evidence of continuity between babbling and early words. Although they found the expected predominance of relatively low, lax vowels, especially in babbling production, they also found high use of [i], especially in the second syllable of word productions. Finally, they noted that the vowels of babbling were not produced more *correctly* in speech but did tend to be used as *substitutions* for other vowels. In other words, the well-established vowels of babbling were overused in speech production, but a vowel less often used in babbling—[i]—appeared frequently in the child's words, reflecting the influence of the adult language.

Another major finding of the Davis and MacNeilage study (1990) was the interaction of consonant and vowel productions. High-front vowels were found to occur most frequently following alveolars, high-back vowels (when used at all) after velars, and central vowels after labials. In a replication of this analysis based on 23 subjects learning four languages—English, French, Japanese and Swedish—Vihman (1992) reported some of the same associations. Both velars and back vowels were rare, but they tended to be produced together when they did occur. Labials were typically followed by central vowels in the vocalizations of several children. Alveolars were not significantly associated with front vowels. Davis and MacNeilage suggested that the alveolars and velars may each tend to be followed by the high vowel closest in articulatory space for *mechanical* reasons, reflecting a lack of differentiation of articulatory gestures. However, Vihman reports a tendency for these CV associations to reflect the influence of different adult languages (e.g., /(alveolar) Ci/ is a common sequence in English—*daddy, pretty, lady, dolly*—while /ko/ occurs in many Japanese words used by the children), and suggests that reliance on such sequences may be a strategy particular to word production. Only the labial–central vowel association appears to reflect an early physiological basis, in which the tongue remains in a neutral, resting position while the lip gesture is actively recruited for articulation.

Vihman and her colleagues have investigated the extent of common tendencies versus individual differences in early vocalizations, both across children learning the same language and across different languages (1986, 1991, 1992). In order to assess variability across subjects at comparable stages of development, they defined sampling points on the basis of lexical use. Two early points reflected the beginnings of word use (ages ranged from 8 to 15 months), and two later points were taken from half-hour sessions in which 15 or more different words were used spontaneously (in this later period, the children had cumulative vocabularies, as reported by their mothers, of about 30 to 50 words; ages ranged from 12 to 23 months).

These studies found that variability in the phonetic categories analyzed was greatest at the earlier stages; a trend toward uniformity across subjects learning the same language was detected as the children's productive vocabularies increased. The strongest finding for the early lexical period was the considerable differences across subjects learning the same language, both in specific phonetic choices and in the degree of stability of phonetic preferences over time. This finding is discussed later in this chapter when individual learning styles are considered.

We can see the growing influence of the adult language in various ways during the transition period. A trend toward increased use of consonants begins for all infants with the onset of canonical babbling (Kent and Murray, 1982), although this trend levels off toward the end of the first year if lexical acquisition is proceeding slowly. Once lexical acquisition is underway, early words are considerably more likely to include a true consonant (stop, nasal, fricative, or liquid) than are babble vocalizations. This finding suggests that increasing knowledge of the adult language plays a significant role in the continued shift toward the use of consonants in this period.

The use of labials is highly variable in the earlier lexical stages, when the children had 10-word vocabularies at most. In the later stages, however, when the children had 30 to 50 words, labials accounted for over a third of all consonant productions for the English-learning subjects and for over half for the French-learning subjects (infants acquiring Swedish and Japanese used fewer labials). Labial use is more characteristic of words than of babble in all four languages. In fact, labial consonants accounted for nearly a third of the consonants in words attempted by the children overall. (The French "target words," or adult models attempted by the children, had over 50 percent labials, while Japanese and Swedish target words had fewer labials, especially in word-initial position, which appears to be particularly salient to the children.)

The disproportionate production of labials in words might be ascribed, in part, to the visibility of labial articulation. Since one can see the articulatory movement involved in producing the *b* of words like *baby* or *bottle*, it may well be easier for the child to gain control of the production of labials than of other consonants. Interestingly, this "overuse" of labials is not found in the early lexicon of blind children (Mulford, 1988), but is particularly characteristic of the vocalizations of the deaf (Stoel-Gammon and Otomo, 1986). We can expect the sighted and normally hearing child's preference for labials to gradually diminish as he or she gains greater control over articulatory production.

In summary, then, by the end of the transition period, when the child has a cumulative vocabulary of about 50 words, several signs exist for the influence of the adult language on the segmental shape of the child's vocalizations. Some of the characteristics of the child's vocal patterns reflect characteristics of all adult language, such as the dominance of true consonants. The preference for producing words with labials is also detectible in a range of languages, but it probably reflects characteristics of the **learning process**—mastering an articulation for which visible as well as auditory cues are available—rather than the form of adult languages. On the other hand, some early signs of the influence of the specific language environment are also evident by this point. For example, some children learning English, a language particularly rich in word-final consonants, begin to make use of final consonants in babble and especially in words by the end of the transition period, whereas children learning languages with fewer final consonants make negligible use of them.

PROSODIC ADVANCES

Cross-linguistic study has shown that prosodic organization begins in the transition period. Whalen, Levitt, and Wang (1991) analyzed pitch contours in the multisyllabic reduplicative babbling of five children each learning French and English, from 5 to 13 months. Whereas the children learning English produced mainly falling contours, the French infants produced roughly equal numbers of falling and rising contours. In a study of four children each learning French and Japanese, aged about 17 or 18 months, Hallé, de Boysson-Bardies and Vihman (in press) compared disyllabic vocalizations (both words and babble) for both pitch and final syllable lengthening, which is a near-universal in the world's languages (Cruttenden, 1986). They too found that the French children produced a predominance of rising pitch contours, while Japanese infants used more falling pitch. Furthermore, the French showed the expected lengthening of final syllables, while Japanese infants typically terminated their vocalizations abruptly with a glottal stop and thus showed no final syllable lengthening. These findings were interpreted as supporting the idea of a physiological basis to final lengthening (Robb and Saxman, 1990), with a learned suppression of natural lengthening in the case of children learning the abrupt glottal offset of Japanese.

The changes that occur in infant perception and production during the transition from babbling to speech have been reviewed. By the beginning of the transition period (from about age 9 to 18 months), the child has begun to demonstrate understanding of a variety of words, even if only in narrow or routine contexts. A shift in perception has been identified as occurring at about this time: "exotic" sounds, those not used in the language to which the child is exposed, are no longer discriminated. This may reflect the fact that children at this age have begun listening to speech as a meaningful model, potentially matching their own vocalizations. At this time children also express their growing interest in communication through the use of idiosyncratic word forms, gestures, or intonational patterns to express broad meanings such as "focus," "affect," and "request." By the end of the transition period the child's experience with a particular language is reflected in both production and perception. Once the child has begun to relate particular adult sound patterns (form) to particular situations (meaning), phonological organization has begun.

The sounds which occur most commonly in a child's babbling are likely to be the sounds the child uses in early words. Both words and babble are characterized at this time by a high proportion of mono- and disyllabic forms, stops, and open syllables. Use of consonants increases with knowledge of the adult language, and relatively extensive use of labials is particularly characteristic of early words. Language-specific phonotactic features, such as final consonants in English, and prosodic features, such as rising pitch for French and abrupt offset for Japanese also emerge over this period.

The bulk of phonological development takes place over the age range 1 to 3 years, at a time when the child is also experiencing an extraordinary growth of word knowledge and embarking on the acquisition of syntax. Yet it seems fair to say that the biggest hurdle of all—that of "getting the idea" of what language is all about, apprehending form-meaning correspondences, and learning to match, store, and reproduce them at will—has already been surmounted.

INDIVIDUAL DIFFERENCES: PROFILE OF TWO ONE-YEAR-OLD GIRLS

Although a general sequence of vocal development can be identified for the first year and a half of life, the extent of individual variability is striking. For one thing, children differ greatly in amount of vocalization during this period. In one study, for example, the average number of vocalizations produced by nine infants ranged from 97 to 265 per half-hour session (the children's interaction with their mothers was sampled at monthly intervals: Vihman et al., 1985).

Individual differences are also apparent in other aspects of phonological development. Infants vary in the sounds they produce (phonetic preferences) and in the stability of these sound preferences. Finally, infants may differ in the organization of their phonological systems and in their approaches to learning phonology. These differences can be identified as early as the period of transition from babbling to speech. We will illustrate differences in phonetic preferences and in phonological organization in this period by describing the development of two girls.

PHONETIC PREFERENCES AND WORD SELECTION

Molly and Deborah are both firstborn daughters of well-educated parents with a strong interest in their children's development. Both girls are naturally "talkative" (in fact, they ranked first and third in amount of vocalization among the nine children studied by Vihman et al., 1985), and both developed large vocabularies by the end of the study (50 words or more at 16 months).

Although Molly and Deborah were similar in many respects, they differed substantially in their phonetic preferences, their word selection, and the stability of their word shapes (Vihman, Ferguson, and Elbert, 1986). In the early lexical period, Molly showed a striking preference for labials (66 percent: mean use for the group, 44 percent) and nasals (41 percent: group mean, 16 percent), while Deborah more closely resembled the other nine children sampled. In the later period, Molly developed a strong focus on final consonants (23 percent: mean use for the group, 12 percent), while Deborah began using an unexpectedly large proportion of fricatives (26 percent against a mean of 10 percent).

Children select their early words at least partly on phonetic grounds (Ferguson and Farwell, 1975; Schwartz and Leonard, 1982). The word-initial consonant is most likely to be the child's target in deciding to attempt a word (cf. Shibamoto and Olmsted, 1978), although overall word shape, prosody, and vowel pattern undoubtedly play some role in the selection of early words (cf. Stoel-Gammon and Cooper, 1984; Davis and MacNeilage, 1990). Deborah's preference for fricatives is reflected in the words she attempts, which tends to include the sounds [s] and [tʃ]: *scratchy* [tʃi:tʃi], *Sesame Street* [si:si] (14 months), while Molly selects an unusually large number of words with final nasals (*bang, down, name, around*: Vihman and Velleman, 1989).

The two girls also differed in phonological organization. Although Molly gradually increased the number of different consonants she would attempt, she largely restricted herself to stops and nasals throughout this period of early word use. Even in a session in which she used over 20 different words (at 15 months), she still did not attempt words with sibilants or liquids. Deborah, on the other hand, used a broad array of consonants from the beginning. By the end of this period she had greatly expanded her repertoire by attempting words with interdentals as well as sibilants. In general, Deborah seemed to advance in an exploratory way, whereas Molly's progress was more systematic.

Finally, the two girls differed in the extent of variability in their productions of different tokens of a single word. Table 2–1 presents the different phonetic shapes used for four words that both girls happened to produce in recorded sessions which included over 30 different spontaneous words. Molly's word production was highly repetitive (i.e., she produced many tokens of a single-word type), with remarkably little variation across the different tokens or productions of a single word. In contrast, Deborah produced a different shape for almost every token of a given word. This appeared to be due, in part, to her inclusion of extra syllables at the beginning of a word, perhaps as a tentative effort to reproduce the sound of the English articles *a* and *the* and the possessive pronoun *my* (*a baby, my baby, the glasses*: cf. Ramer's [1976] discussion of *presyntactic forms*). Here again, Molly's highly stable word production seems to reflect a systematic approach to the learning of phonology, whereas Deborah appears to be exploring new forms before she has a good grasp of their function. The difference between the two girls appears to illustrate Ferguson's (1979) distinction between an unanalytic, risk-taking (exploratory) style and a cautious, analytic (systematic) style.

In summary, these two children differed widely in the phonetic preferences they displayed during babbling although they were matched for sex, socioeconomic status, amount of vocalization, and relative rate of lexical development. These same individual phonetic preferences appeared to carry over to the children's choices of early words. We see the beginnings of phonological structure as each child gradually expanded her range of phonetic segments and attempted increasingly complex syllable shapes.

SUMMARY

We have suggested that differences in approach to learning can be discerned among children early in their language acquisition. We provided evidence of individual differences in phonetic preferences, word selection, and stability or variability of word shapes. One child showed a cautious, systematic approach, while

TABLE 2-1. **Variability in Word Shapes.**

A. MOLLY (16 MONTHS; 39 SPONTANEOUS WORDS USED)

No. Shapes	Word Type	Phonetic Shapes	No. Tokens of Same Shape
1	*baby*	[pebi]	2
1	*down*	[ta^{n}nə]	9
		[dæ^{n}nə]	4
	cf. also *bang*	[pa^{n}nə]	2
	green	[kɔ:ni]	1
		[gə^{n}ni]	1
5	*glasses*	[kak^{h}i̥]	4
		[ta͜k k^{h}I]	5
		[tak]	1
		[kak]	8
		[kat]	3
		[kɛt]	1
4	*mama*	[əmæ]	1
		[mama]	4
		[jɛma^m ma:mi]	1
		[ʔe:mæmi]	1
13 shapes	**4 types**		

B. DEBORAH (17 MONTHS; 34 SPONTANEOUS WORDS USED)

No. Shapes	Word Type	Phonetic Shapes	No. Tokens of Same Shape
13	*baby*	[pep]	7
		[pepe]	2
		[pipi]	3
		[mibi]	1
		[miʔpe]	1
		[gəpe:b]	1
		[mipebi]	1
		[mapɛpi]	1
		[həpepi]	1
		[hipepi]	1
		[pipipi]	1
		[pepepe]	1
		[hənœpebi]	1
2	*down*	[tæ]	1
		[te]	1
7	*glasses*	[t^{h}æ]	1
		[k^{h}æ]	3
		[uk^{h}a]	1
		[ŋkæ]	1
		[hŋk'æ]	1
		[nœt^{h}æ]	2
		[hŋgxk^{h}æ]	1
2	*mommy*	[mami]	7
		[ʔama]	1
22 shapes	**4 types**		

the other made bold leaps from one point to another in word selection, with exploration of a wide range of sounds in both babble and first words. In both cases, the child's phonetic preferences were found to influence her choice of early words.

Early Phonological Development

LINGUISTIC PERCEPTION: REPRESENTING SPEECH SOUNDS

We began our account of the origins of phonological development by asking what perceptual abilities or natural biases the infant brings to the task of learning to pronounce. Before reviewing phonological development beyond the transition period, we will consider what is known about perceptual development during the period of rapid phonological advancement, from the transition to speech through the mastery of the sound system. Current theories of phonological development differ crucially on the issue of the timing of perceptual development. Some scholars view linguistic perception, or the ability to identify and represent or store the sound patterns of lexical items, as essentially complete even before the child has acquired a small lexicon of 50 words or so. From this perspective, the child's production errors may be largely ascribed to difficulties in motor control and phonological organization. Other scholars believe linguistic perception continues to develop during the preschool period and even beyond, and thus, some production errors may be due to perception-based differences between the adult word and the sound pattern the child is targeting—that is, to inaccuracies and gaps in the child's perception and consequent internal representation of the adult word.

It is important to note that the term *linguistic perception* refers not only to the auditory perception or identification of contrasts between different sounds but also to the *storing and accessing for recognition* of the particular sound patterns that constitute words and phrases in the language being acquired. Previously, we dealt with the child's auditory capacities. Here, we are concerned with the child's use of those capacities in constructing a repertoire of word forms and extrapolating from them a store of phonological knowledge—knowledge of the sound system of his or her language.

In our account of infant perception, we stressed that infants in the first few months of life seem to respond to graduated differences in the acoustic signal in a categorical way and, furthermore, that these categorical responses resemble adult responses, which are based on knowledge of phonemic (meaning-bearing) contrasts in the language. We ascribed the infants' surprising discriminatory ability to natural biases in the auditory structure of humans (and other mammals). Given the wide range of phonemic differences to which infants have been found to be sensitive, it is easy to see why some scholars have concluded that perception of speech patterns can be assumed to be completely accurate by the time children begin to produce lexical items on their own. It is important, however, to bear in mind the distinction between the nonlinguistic sensory *capacity* (the ability to make same–different distinctions) tested in studies of infant perception and the *use* of that discriminatory capacity to distinguish different meaningful lexical items, as well as to store or remember them (**internal representation**). Infant perception tasks used in research investigations involve an essentially **passive response** to change in the signal, which indicates auditory sensitivity to the change. But perception of sound patterns as a basis for language use involves **active attention** to contrasting speech sounds and sequences in order to identify, store, and recognize distinct lexical items (Ferguson, 1975). Furthermore, discrimination between phonemes involves a learned response to a range of different and variable acoustic signals in terms of a single (abstract) linguistic category. With respect to the child who is beginning to speak, we shift our focus from the perception of differences between sounds per se to the perception of phonemic contrasts and the use of that perception to recognize different words and, thus, to understand language. This shift in focus naturally leads to a shift in the methods used to investigate linguistic perception.

We cannot directly observe a child's perception of speech sounds. Instead, tasks must be devised requiring the child to respond in a way that reveals something about his or her perceptions. As Locke (1980a) has pointed out, this is a formidable challenge since both linguistic perception itself and the required behavioral responses are complex processes involving several steps. First, the salient features of the speech sound stimuli must be *heard* ("go in the ear of the subject") and then *registered* and *interpreted* by the child ("reach and reside briefly in the brain": Locke, 1980a; 433). In other words, the child's perception of a speech sound involves receiving the auditory stimulus and identifying the auditory cues in terms of the phonemic system, or the speech sound categories, of the adult language. Secondly, in order for the observer to judge the "accuracy" of the child's perception, or the extent to which it agrees with that of adults from the child's linguistic community, the perception must be *translated* into an interpretable behavioral response. Considerable ingenuity is required to devise satisfactory tasks since they not only must be within the child's conceptual capacities and repertoire of behavioral responses but also require the child to make a comparison of an adult surface form with his or her own internal representation. Additional ingenuity is needed to determine the critical acoustic cues leading to the child's response.

The difference between two speech sounds may depend on any combination of multiple acoustic cues (cf., e.g., Lisker, 1978). This built-in redundancy helps to make speech intelligible even in noisy or otherwise distracting surroundings. For example, the difference between voiced and voiceless final stops in English is cued by the length of a preceding vowel (which is greater before voiced consonants), by the voicing of the voiced stop, and by differences in the release, if any, of the voiced versus the voiceless stop. The discrimination of contrasting sounds, then, involves *knowledge of a particular phonemic system* as well as discrimination per se. Fluent users of a language disregard some sound-differences that are irrelevant to the phonemic categories of their language (recall the earlier discussion of categorical perception). In the case of children, auditory discrimination is subject to multiple interpretations; we do not necessarily know which cues the child is attending to; for example, vowel lengthening or voicing or release burst in the discrimination of the voicing contrast (cf. Greenlee, 1978).

METHODOLOGICAL CONSIDERATIONS

Over the past quarter century, many experiments have been conducted to test the speech sound discrimination abilities of children. The experiments have originated in such diverse fields as speech perception, child development, linguistics, and speech-language pathology, and their specific goals have ranged from the establishment of a universal order of acquisition for the perception of phonemic contrasts to the establishment of norms for preschool- or school-age children. Subjects have ranged in age from under one to adolescence. Methods have been accordingly diverse; both live or recorded real speech and synthetic stimuli have been used, and tasks have included naming nonsense objects after extensive training as well as picture-naming. We will review here some of the major methodological factors that may affect the interpretation of findings and thus, our conception of perceptual development. We will then describe a few selected studies.

Natural versus Synthetic Stimuli. In general, two conflicting demands must be weighed in making methodological choices. On the one hand, we are usually interested in "real world" behavior, or speech discrimination under everyday circumstances. From this point of view, live presentation of real speech has an obvious advantage. On the other hand, we must be concerned to carefully control the experiment to be sure that we are actually testing the ability of interest. As regards presentation, a live speech test is much more difficult to control than a recorded one. The experimenter may inadvertently cue the child by emphasizing a contrasting sound, looking toward the object the child is expected to choose, or simply allowing the child to see the experimenter's face as he or she pronounces a labial versus a dental, so it becomes unclear whether the task is testing visual or auditory discrimination or both. The greatest control is achieved in the use of synthetic stimuli designed to differ along a particular criterial acoustic dimension. Compared with real-life discrimination tasks this method is unnaturally simplified. Specifically, the child is not required to selectively attend to the criterial dimensions while ignoring irrelevant variations as is necessary in the case of natural speech. Furthermore, the perceptual weighting of the various cues may differ markedly from live speech.

Meaningful versus Nonsense Stimuli. There are advantages and disadvantages to both real and nonsense words as stimuli. Setting out to determine the age at which children can discriminate the phonemic contrasts of English, one soon discovers that some contrasts are relatively rare, and the minimal pairs that do occur may be difficult to illustrate clearly or are likely to be unfamiliar to young children. For example, the contrast between /f/ and /θ/ minimally distinguishes relatively few common word-pairs (such as *fin–thin*). Thus, there is an advantage in inventing (nonsense) speech sound sequences that are ideally suited for testing the contrasts of interest.

The use of nonsense words, however, gives rise to other difficulties, in particular, the problem of assuring that the child's internal representation of speech sounds is consulted. If we are interested in the child's knowledge of speech sounds and mental representation of the forms of words, as well as in the purely auditory ability to distinguish sounds, we must somehow contrive to tap his or her internal lexicon. When nonsense syllables are used, the child is often asked to decide whether two stimuli are the same or different. A purely auditory comparison of the two stimuli, without reference to any internal representation, is therefore possible; *linguistic* perception is not necessarily involved at all. On the other hand, when real words are used, the child is typically asked to look at two pictures representing similar sounding words while one of the words is named (e.g., *rake* vs. *lake*). In order to decide which of the two pictures goes best with the sound pattern just heard, the child must refer to some internal representation of the relevant words.

But words unfamiliar to the child are, in effect, no different from nonsense words. If the child is unfamiliar with a word, he or she may develop a strategy, for example, of always responding with the familiar picture, thereby avoiding entirely the intended discrimination task (Clumeck, 1982). When word familiarity has been controlled, error scores have been found to be higher for contrasts involving a relatively unfamiliar word (Barton, 1976; Clumeck, 1982; Smit and Bernthal, 1983).

RESEARCH WITH YOUNG CHILDREN

Methodological difficulties are the most acute with younger children. By the age of 10 or 12 months, children are beginning to understand and produce language and, thus, have already internalized a certain number of meaningful sound patterns. It would be of great interest to determine if children's internal representations of words conform more completely with adult models than do the word patterns they are able to produce. At this age, however, the child's cognitive capacities (e.g., attention span) and repertoire of behavioral responses are limited, and it is difficult to obtain on command consistent responses, such as pointing to a named picture or fetching a named object, from a child under the age of 2 or 3. Considerable ingenuity has gone into the development of experiments usable with children under 3, but the results remain disappointingly ambiguous.

Order of Acquisition. The classic study of phonological perception in very young children is that of the Russian linguist, Shvachkin (1948/73). In Shvachkin's procedure, 19 Russian children (10 to 24 months old) were painstakingly taught nonsense CVC names for objects. For each phonemic contrast of interest, three object names were taught. Two were minimally contrastive (e.g., /mak/, /bak/), and the third differed in all three segments (/zub/). Once a child could identify the objects by name, he or she was presented with all three and asked to carry out some task involving one of the two objects with minimally contrasting names. Shvachkin was primarily interested in determining an order of acquisition for the distinctive features used in the minimal contrasts (recall Jakobson's interest in the order of acquisition of distinctive features in early production).

Based on studies with Russian children, Shvachkin suggested a universal sequence of phonemic perception, beginning with the discrimination of different vowels, the presence versus absence of consonants, and the discrimination of sonorants from stops, and then proceeding to discrimination among sonorants, continuants, and obstruents. The last discrimination was that of voiced from voiceless obstruents. Shvachkin reported that all of the children were able to make all the tested phonemic discriminations tested before the age of 2.

Unfortunately, Shvachkin gave little detail regarding his methods or analysis (e.g., number of trials per child for each opposition, criterion used to judge successful discrimination). His methods were adapted for use with English-speaking children by Garnica (1973). Although she essentially replicated Shvachkin's results, Garnica found greater variability and suggested that Shvachkin's order of acquisition be considered only a general outline for perceptual development. In contrast to Shvachkin, she reported that perception of certain consonant distinctions was not acquired by age 2. Edwards (1974) used Shvachkin's method to examine differences between liquids and glides and between voiced and voiceless fricative pairs, with respect to the production of contrasts. She found that her 3-year-old subjects had not mastered all the phonemic contrasts tested.

Barton (1975) criticized the methods and statistical treatment of both Garnica and Edwards and questioned the acquisition orders they reported. Barton (1976) attempted to verify Shvachkin's order (postulated for Russian phonemic contrasts)

Early Phonological Development

by comparing it with his reanalysis of the data reported in several English studies on the difficulty of various contrasts. He found little relationship between Shvachkin's order and the level of difficulty reflected in the English data. The question of an order of acquisition remains moot.

Other studies of children's perception have established that pairs of sounds that differ from each other in more than one feature are easier to discriminate than pairs that contrast in only one feature (Tikofsky and McInish, 1968; Graham and House, 1971). Features have differential value, however, depending on their context of use. The contrast in voicing is generally reported to be the most difficult, for example, but voicing errors in these studies typically affect contrasts involving fricatives. Just as the acquisition of fricative production differs from one segment to the next, with no automatic "learning transfer" or "spread" from one contrasting pair (e.g., /f/–/v/) to another (e.g., /s/–/z/), the ability to detect voicing in one pair does not necessarily imply the ability to detect voicing in another pair. Therefore, it may not be sensible to refer to certain *features* as being "difficult to discriminate" without specifying the particular pair of contrasting sounds involved (Barton, 1980).

The search for a universal order of acquisition for the perception of distinctive features, like the search for a universal order of emergence of distinctive features in production, now generally arouses little interest. Although the concept of the distinctive feature, or the minimal phonetic difference between two speech sounds, is theoretically justifiable, it has, on the whole, failed to fulfill early expectations that it would yield significant insight into children's phonological development. Current research has largely abandoned the assumption that the distinctive feature and the minimally contrasting pair of segments are the primary functional units in perceptual acquisition. Instead, investigators are now looking for evidence to establish the syllable or the word as the earliest contrasting unit (cf. Menyuk, Menn, and Silber, 1986) in perception as well as in production.

Full versus Partial Linguistic Perception. In an effort to test the idea that full perception is achieved very early, Barton (1976) developed two procedures, one for use with children aged 2;3 to 2;11, the second adapted for use with younger children. In the first case, after assessing each child's ability to identify a given set of pictures and training them on unfamiliar labels, Barton repeatedly presented two cards at a time—each pair representing a minimal contrast, while a recorded voice instructed the child to point to one of the pictures. A wide range of contrasts was tested, including differences in voicing, nasality, and place of articulation, as well as /l/ versus /r/, /w/ versus /r/, and /tr/ versus /tʃ/. Overall discrimination was 80 percent; errors primarily occurred when one of the pictures was initially unfamiliar to the child.

In his second study, Barton used just two minimal pairs (*pear–bear* and *coat–goat*), focusing on the contrast in voicing, which Shvachkin and Garnica had reported to be a late or difficult discrimination. He began with teaching sessions in which the children played various games with small objects that represented each of the words but with no need to discriminate the minimal contrasts. After checking familiarity with the object names at least a day later, he tested the children on the minimal contrasts by repeatedly asking them to take different objects out of a bag or to place them back in it. Eight out of 10 subjects (aged 1;8 to 2;0) succeeded in making one or both discriminations. Failures of discrimination due to task difficulty could not be clearly differentiated from failures due to difficulty with the linguistic discrimination of interest. Despite the methodological difficulties, Barton (1976) interpreted his data as evidence for the position that full perception occurs at an early age. He concluded that discrimination was less difficult for 2-year-olds than had been reported in some earlier work.

The significance of the effect of word familiarity on the child's discrimination should not be overlooked. If children make more errors in discriminating contrasts in *new words*, then it may be wrong to assume that they are typically able to draw on accurate internal representations of surface forms when they produce words. Instead, it seems likely that children's internal representations continue to change for some years. When first attempting a word, the child may be operating with a partially correct internal representation. In time, this representation becomes more accurate as the child profits from additional exposure to the adult form. But the child may fail to notice the discrepancy between his or her initial internal representation and the adult surface form and could then persist in the perception-based error for some time.

Examples of such changing internal representations are difficult to obtain in any systematic or experimental way but may be revealed by careful analysis of longitudinal data (cf. Macken, 1980). Specifically, when a child begins to produce a new adult sound (such as /θ/) for which he or she formerly produced a substitute sound (such as /f/), we can look to see if the change seems to occur "across the board" (Smith, 1973), in all and only the words containing the relevant phoneme. If so, we can assume that the words were correctly represented although they were not yet correctly produced. On the other hand, if the child begins to use the new sound (/θ/) in words that were formerly correctly produced with the substituting sound (*wife, frosty* as /waiθ/, /θrɔsti/), we conclude that /θ/ words had formerly been mistakenly represented with /f/, and the child is now faced with the problem of sorting out which are actually /θ/ words and which are /f/ words. This process may take a matter of months or even years (cf. Vihman, 1982, for a fuller account of just such an error).

Interaction of Perception and Production. What is needed to resolve the question as to whether or not internal representations may be assumed to reflect adult surface forms accurately from the earliest stages of lexical acquisition is data on both production and perception from the same subjects. Several studies of this kind have been reported for normal children.

Eilers and Oller (1976) specifically expected to find a relation between ease of perception of a contrast and frequency of production errors involving the contrast. They adapted a technique of Vincent-Smith, Bricker, and Bricker (1974), using both real and nonsense words, to test 14 two-year-old children. Eilers and Oller combined familiar objects, such as fish, with nonsense toys given minimally contrasting names, such as /θiʃ/. To test discrimination, the child was told to choose a specific toy; a reward was hidden under the object named. The pairs were of three types: (1) pairs in which the second element typically substitutes for the first in child production of the pairs: [kʰ]–[k], [pl]–[p], [θ]–[f], [Vŋk]–[Vk], and [r]–[w]; (2) pairs of elements not typically involved in such a substitution relationship: [pʰ]–[tʰ] and [pl]–[pʰ]; and (3) non-minimal pairs. Eilers and Oller reasoned that if the substitutions were motivated by perceptual confusions, type (1) pairs should prove more difficult for children to discriminate than type (2) or

(3) pairs. The hypothesis was partially confirmed. Some of the type (1) pairs were not discriminated by any of the children ([θ]–[f], [V̄ŋk]–[Vk]), but one was unexpectedly discriminated by most of the children ([kʰ]–[k]). The type (3) pair was the easiest, as predicted. Transcription of the children's productions of each of the test pairs showed that the type (1) pairs were the least well distinguished, as predicted. In short, Eilers and Oller showed that some production errors may derive from perceptual difficulties although others (e.g., the contrast in voicing or aspiration) are more likely to relate to motor constraints.

Strange and Broen (1980) conducted a careful test of both the production and the perception of word-initial /w/, /r/, and /l/ by 21 children aged 2;11 to 3;5. Production was examined through the use of an imitation task and transcription of the child's forms; each phoneme was scored for each child as a "correct" production, a distortion, a substitution by another approximant, or a substitution by a segment outside the class of approximants. The children made virtually no errors on /w/; responses with /r/ and /l/ fell into three groups: (1) mastery, (2) few errors, and (3) many errors. Perception was tested through the use of live voice, recorded, and synthetic stimuli for the pairs *rake–lake, wake–rake*, and (as a control), *wake–bake*. The acoustic stimuli were designed to differ in not just one, but several, of the criterial dimensions that distinguish the target phonemes, but they had identical rhyming portions (*-ake*). The children were asked to point to one of two pictures. They proceeded from live voice to recorded to synthetic tests.

Overall accuracy was over 90 percent; /w/–/r/ was the most difficult contrast, /w/–/b/ the easiest. The synthetic stimuli gave rise to more errors for some pairs, but there was no consistent overall pattern of errors in relation to type of stimulus. Identification accuracy was clearly related to /r/ and /l/ production ability, with far more errors made by the eight children in group (3), who had made the most production errors. However, there was a great deal of variability in performance among those subjects, and all showed better than chance identification of all three contrasts on one or more tests. Strange and Broen tentatively concluded that both perception and production of phoneme contrasts develop gradually and that perception of a contrast normally precedes its production. However, they emphasized that their test situation was highly constrained; it involved only two response alternatives and a long series of tests using the same stimuli, which could serve as training on the contrast. Thus, the study does not reflect "intentional, coordinated perception," such as ordinary life requires, in which the child-listener is actively involved in extracting the relevant phonetic cues from a complex set of stimuli in order to determine which words were intended by the speaker.

Locke (1980b) has argued that evaluation of a child's perception of speech sounds should be based on the child's patterns of sound substitutions, with attention paid to the **particular phonetic contexts** that give rise to the child's production errors. He developed a *speech production-perception task* in which the perceptual stimuli used are based on a preliminary test of the child's productions. The child is tested on the sounds he or she misarticulated (the *stimulus phoneme*), on the substituting sound (the *response phoneme*), and on a perceptually similar control sound. The different stimulus types are presented six times each in a live-voice object or picture identification task ("Is this X?"), with the tester seated beside the child. For more detail and a copy of the test form, see Chapter 6.

Locke reported that of 131 children tested, ranging in age from 3 to 9 (mean age 5.3), most had speech substitutions, but they did not necessarily have speech disorders. About one third of the contrasts misproduced were also misperceived. However, misperception was not equally likely to be involved in all production errors. Specifically, only 49 percent of those errors consisted in the substitution of one voiceless fricative for another, yet this type of substitution accounted for fully 89 percent of the misperceived contrasts. The pair that accounted for the largest number of perception errors was /f/–/θ/ (67 percent incidence of misperception). Of 52 children who substituted /f/ for /θ/ in production, the 26 younger subjects (mean age 3.7) were much more likely also to misperceive the contrast than were the older subjects (mean age 6.2).

Finally, Velleman (1988) designed a study to test the hypothesis that some English phonemes typically involved in production errors (e.g., /s/) are easy to perceive, so late acquisition is likely to be due to articulatory difficulty. She predicted that in the case of /s/, poor production would occur in the *absence* of poor perception. For other phonemes, the production problem might be related to a perceptual problem; specifically, the articulation of /θ/ and /f/ yields signals that are relatively weak and can be confused with one another. Velleman predicted that in this case, production would be dependent on perception: "Only children with high perception scores would also have high production scores" (223).

Velleman tested 12 English-speaking children aged 3 to 5. She sampled production in free speech as well as in picture- and toy-naming and imitation of nonsense syllables. Initial fricatives were judged on the basis of three independent transcriptions and were then subjected to detailed acoustic analysis. To test perception, Velleman first assessed word familiarity and then used a live-voice, real-word picture-identification task. The pairs of interest were *thumb–some, thumb–fum* (as in *fee, fi, fo,* _____), and *some–fum*.

Velleman's results confirmed her hypotheses. Perception and production of /s/ showed no correlation. Some children with poor /s/ production had good perception of contrasts involving /s/, and in general, perception errors with /s/ were rare. In contrast, perception and production of /θ/ were highly correlated, with production of /θ/ better for children with perception scores of over 80 percent. More errors were made in both perception and production in the case of /θ/ than in the case of /s/.

In summary, the results of the few studies examining production and perception in the same children all point to an identical conclusion: Some phonemic contrasts remain difficult to discriminate perceptually as late as age 3 or older (e.g., /θ/–/f/, /r/–/w/), and production errors involving these pairs typically continue to occur in the later preschool period. It should be mentioned that the /f/–/θ/ contrast in particular is notoriously difficult for adults as well. Other production errors show no evident relation to perception (voicing in stops at age 2, /s/ at age 3 to 5).

Internal Representations. We can now reconsider the question raised earlier regarding internal representations. Note, first of all, that linguistic perception has not yet been successfully tested in the earliest period of lexical production (age 12 to 18 months). Anecdotal data are available from diary studies, but they are sparse, often based on once-only occurrences, and difficult to evaluate in the absence of transcriber reliability or other statistical procedures. Based on production data from this period, a bias toward perception and/or storage in terms of the favored shapes of the babbling period (e.g., CV syllables) seems likely (Locke, 1983; Vihman, 1991). By about age 2, when the child has a sizable lexicon but many production errors, we can assume that the child is perceiving words in a shape that closely resembles the adult surface forms. For some elements (e.g., fricatives, clusters, and /r/), however, non–adult-like perception may still be the rule, and it is precisely those sound classes that continue to give rise to production difficulties for many children into the later preschool and early school years. It is possible, then, that some children persist in misproducing a few sounds because they are inaccurately storing the adult form. Such errors may arise in an early period, when the child is unable to either produce the relevant articulatory gestures or *represent* (store) the relevant distinction. The production error may persist long after the child's motoric or articulatory difficulty has been resolved, due to the child's lack of self-monitoring or lack of attention to the difference between his or her inaccurately stored form and the adult form.

The possible effect on the child's phonology of the child's perception of his or her *own* output forms has received little attention. Straight (1980), who insists on a sharp dichotomy between auditory and articulatory processes, suggested that, in some cases, the child's own simplified or otherwise distorted output may lead to a radically inaccurate internal representation that then underlies the child's subsequent spontaneous productions. Vihman (1982) offered two possible illustrations of such "feedback" from the child's own productions to his or her internal representations. For a discussion of the complex interrelation between children's perceptions, misarticulations, and self-monitoring on the phonetic and phonemic level, see Locke, 1979.

Summary

Infants have been found to respond differentially to a wide range of contrasting speech sounds. Linguistic perception, however, requires active attention to speech sound contrasts, in order to identify, store, and recognize distinct lexical items. Given a variety of potential acoustic cues to speech sound contrasts, the child must be able to select and integrate the relevant cues while disregarding those that play no contrastive role in the phonemic system of the language in question.

Testing linguistic perception in children presents many methodological challenges. For example, the investigator must balance the need for *control* to ensure a valid test against the need for *naturalistic* data. As a result, studies of young children have used both real and nonsense words, live-voice, recorded, and synthesized stimuli. It has also proven important to test children on words that are familiar to them since more errors are made in the identification of relatively unfamiliar words.

Children aged 1 to 3 were taught to associate nonsense words with novel objects and then tested on a variety of tasks involving manipulation of these objects. This painstaking procedure led to a hypothesized universal sequence of phonemic perception, based on data from Russian children. Attempts to replicate the procedure with English-speaking children have met with methodological and statistical difficulties, however, so that no clear order of acquisition of distinctive features has emerged.

The question of whether or not a child's perception of lexical items is fully accurate from the beginning of speech production is currently of considerable theoretical interest. Attempts to test children younger than age 2 have been limited and not entirely successful. Nevertheless, the role of word familiarity has proven to be highly significant, suggesting that some production errors may derive from perceptual misinterpretations, that is, internal representations that fail to match the adult model, since initial attempts at a new word inevitably reflect an internal representation based on perception of a relatively unfamiliar word. The results of studies of production and perception in the same children support the idea that imperfect perception is involved in production errors with respect to certain contrasts, such as /f/ versus /θ/ and /w/ versus /r/. The production errors that appear to be related to perceptual difficulties are errors that typically persist into the later preschool or even early school-age years.

SYSTEMATIZATION AND REORGANIZATION: FROM WORD TO SEGMENT

It has been suggested that the earliest units the child targets for production are whole-word patterns rather than segments or even syllables (cf. Ferguson and Farwell, 1975). At least three different kinds of evidence have been adduced to support this view. The first kind involves variation in the child's production across different target words, the second, the relation of particular child word shapes to their adult models, and the third, the interrelation of child forms at a given point in time.

Lexical Idiosyncrasy. Individual segments vary across words, even in similar phonetic contexts. For example, *baby* may be realized with initial [d], while *bye-bye* has initial [b] in the child's forms. Similarly, some words are relatively stable in form from the beginning (e.g., Hildegard Leopold's *papa*: [papa~baba]), while others vary widely from one attempt to another (e.g., Hildegard's *mama*: [mama-ma~bama~maba]). Data of this sort suggest that the child does not target word-initial /b/ or /m/ in isolation from the particular adult word patterns in which the consonants occur.

Prosodic Phenomena. In some cases, the child's form seems to match the adult word as a whole, but with no evident sequential segment-to-segment correspondence. Ferguson and Farwell provide two examples: *shoe*: [gutçi], [gutʃidi]; *feet* ['fiʔ] (cf. also, e.g., Waterson, 1971). This strongly suggests that the child is targeting a whole gestalt, not a sequence of individual segments.

Phonological Idioms. It has been noted (cf. especially Moskowitz, 1973) that some early words may occur in surprisingly advanced form, for example, with consonant clusters produced as in the adult model. The best-known instance is Hildegard's first permanent word, *pretty* pronounced [prəti], at 10 months. This represents a relatively rare case of an unusually good reproduction of a difficult adult form, but it is unlikely to have been planned and produced segment by segment. Several months later, Hildegard simplified the form to [piti] and [bidi], structures that conformed more closely with her other word forms. These later productions seem to be integrated into Hildegard's phonological system at that stage of development and may be viewed as at least partially analyzed (into two syllables, say) prior to production. The more complex early form seems to be

Early Phonological Development

extra-systemic or "pre-systemic," since it is unrelated to other sound patterns in Hildegard's own repertoire.

As the child begins to acquire new vocabulary at an accelerated pace, typically after accumulating 50 words or more, there is pressure to "systematize" the phonological representations and production routines to allow smoother functioning of word production (cf. Chiat, 1979; Menn, 1983). The changes that occur at this time reflect a process of internal reorganization, like that shown to occur in other domains of language acquisition, such as syntax and semantics (cf., e.g., Slobin, 1973; Bowerman, 1982). The classic examples come from English morphology. Although the child at first produces apparently correct (irregular as well as regular) plural and past tense forms (*shoes, feet, walked, broke*), at a later point, he or she will begin to apply the regular inflectional endings to words that happen to have irregular plural or past tense forms in English (*foots, breaked*). This is generally taken as evidence that the child has "analyzed out" or "discovered" the productive inflectional suffixes marking regular plural and past tense forms. The "overregularized" forms thus reflect new knowledge and reorganization. Only much later will the child again begin to use the correct irregular forms, which, at that point, have a new status as known exceptions to the general morphological rule.

Evidence for phonological reorganization is indirect and thus difficult to trace in terms of specific stages. Nevertheless, there are data from a range of children learning different languages that suggest that such reorganization, based on internal analysis and systematization, does occur. This reorganization will affect the basic unit of the child's phonological system. While the primary unit at the earliest stage appears to be the word, re-analysis will allow the child to operate with a more efficient, segment-based system. We will consider three characteristics of the process of reorganization and, at the same time, illustrate different children's responses to phonological challenges.

Apparent Regression

Hildegard Leopold's production of *pretty*, first in a more complex, adult-like form and only later in a simplified form, is a good example of apparent regression; that is, a step backward for an individual lexical form in the service of greater progress or coherence for the child's phonological system as a whole. The extensive data available on the phonological development of Hildegard, who was raised as a bilingual speaker of English and German, provides a fuller illustration of this process as it pertains to the acquisition of /l/ (Leopold, 1947; our account is based on the analysis in Ferguson and Farwell, 1975). The word *hello* appeared in the form [ʔəlɔ] at 1;5 and showed no change until 1;10, when Hildegard began to produce it as [jojo], a superficially more primitive form. The substitution of the palatal glide [j] for /l/ affected some, but not all, of the /l/ words Hildegard attempted (see Table 2–2). In its original form, *hello* could be considered a phonological idiom. It showed no evidence of analysis below the word level, whereas [jojo] appears to reflect the "discovery" of the medial *l*, a troublesome segment for Hildegard, and the consequent application of the gliding rule, which began to play a role in Hildegard's phonology only after the time of her first use of *hello*. This is a classic example of "regression," or "non-linear progression," in which early attempts at systematization—themselves a sign of progress toward a more

TABLE 2–2. Development of the Lateral /l/ in H's Speech during the Second Year.

	hello	alle "all"	bottle	lie	Loch "hole"	Löscher "eraser"
1;5	ʔəlo					
1;6			ba:ɪ			
1;7		ʔatə	ba:ɪ			
1;8		ʔajə	baɪu			
1;9			balu			
1;10	jojo	ʔalə	baju		lok'/jok'	
1;11	jojo		balu	jal		loko/joke

Source: From Vihman, M. M., C. A. Ferguson, and M. Elbert, "Phonological Development from Babbling to Speech: Common Tendencies and Individual Differences." *Applied Psycholinguistics,* Vol. 7 (1986), 3–40, © Cambridge University Press. Used with permission.

sophisticated phonology—result in a more primitive child form of a word formerly pronounced in an adult-like way.

CREATIVE STRATEGIES

Virve Vihman acquired Estonian as her first language although she was exposed to some English as well (see Vihman, 1978). Multisyllabic forms were difficult for her. Among her first 50 words, only two had adult models longer than two syllables. At 17 months, her first trisyllabic form appeared: /ˈapːelsin/ → [ˈapːəsi] 'orange'. Within the same month, the child began to make use of an idiosyncratic long-word production strategy. Starting from a three-syllable adult model, she would produce a three-syllable form in which the last two (unstressed) syllables were always identical. She maintained the syllable count and overall syllabic structure of the adult word, but she abandoned any attempt at segmental fidelity for all three syllables. Instead, her choice of segments seemed to reflect a prosodic approach, in which certain features of the adult word were adopted and spread over more than one syllable, while other segments or features were disregarded. For example:

/ˈtakasi/ → [ˈtasisi] "(to go, take) back" (1;5)
/ˈlenːukːitː/ → [ˈnanunu] "airplane (obj.)" (1;6)
/ˈporkantitː/ → [ˈpɔnini] "carrot (obj.)" (1;6)
/ˈraːmatːutː/ → [ˈmaːnunu] "book (obj.)" (1;6)

Virve continued to produce new long words according to her invented pattern for five months. Ferguson (1978) has used the term *unique reduction device* to describe such creative strategies for coping with words of greater complexity than the child's production system can handle. Here again, the use of an adult-like form ([ˈapːəsi]) was followed by a more primitive type of production (e.g., [ˈtasisi]); the latter, however, reflects hypothesis-formation or system-building and, therefore, can be viewed as a step toward a more complex phonology.

CHANGING HYPOTHESES

Macken's (1979) description of the phonology of a Spanish-speaking child, Si, demonstrates the development from a word-based to a segment-based system. The child was recorded weekly from 1;7 to 2;5. For the first six months of the study, Si had a strong preference for a CVCV word pattern consisting of an initial labial consonant followed by a medial dental. Subpatterns developed during this

Early Phonological Development

period through the expansion of earlier patterns; as a new word pattern became dominant, some words would change patterns. Most strikingly, in order to achieve an output form which agreed with the preferred pattern "labial–dental," the child would restructure different adult models in different ways, selectively deleting the initial syllable(s) of *Ramon* and *elefante* ("elephant"), for example, but the medial syllable of *manzana* ("apple") and *Fernando*.

> *manzana* → [mən‿na] ("apple") (1;7)
>
> *Fernando* → [man‿nə - wan‿no - nan‿no] (1;8)
>
> *Ramon* → [mən] (1;8)
>
> *elefante* → [bat‿te] ("elephant") (1;9)

Si gradually increased her repertoire of sounds and syllable shapes over a six-month period while maintaining some control over the range of complexity she had to handle in terms of contrasting consonants in a single word. Any attempt to match Si's forms segment-for-segment to the adult model, as in a strict phonemic analysis like the one Smith (1973) provides to account for his son's development, would prove extremely difficult since Si's output depended heavily on her own current repertoire of word patterns. In the last four months of data collection, Si's phonemic system quickly grew to include most of the phonemes of adult Spanish, and the unusual substitution patterns of the earlier period disappeared, along with the constraints on co-occurrence of consonants that had motivated those patterns.

SUMMARY

The first units targeted in the earliest period of adult-based word production appear to be whole-word patterns rather than segments. This is suggested by the variation typically found in the treatment of individual segments across different words, by the gestalt-like match of early child forms to adult models, and by the occasional occurrence of extra-systemic forms or phonological idioms. After this early period, the pressure of a rapidly growing lexicon leads to gradual reorganization. Indirect evidence of this process may be found in the phenomenon of non-linear progression, in which superficially more advanced forms are later produced in a less adult-like form—but one that is integrated into the child's repertoire of phonological forms and appears to reflect the operation of regular phonological processes.

REFERENCES

Atkinson, K., B. MacWhinney, and C. Stoel, "An experiment on the recognition of babbling." *Language Behavior Research Laboratory Working Paper, 14.* Berkeley: University of California, 1968.

Barton, D., "Statistical significance in phonemic perception experiments." *Journal of Child Language, 2* (1975): 297–298.

Barton, D., "The role of perception in the acquisition of phonology." Ph.D. thesis, University of London, 1976. (Reprinted by the Indiana University Linguistics Club, 1978.)

Barton, D., "Phonemic perception in children." In G. Yeni-Komshian, J. Kavanagh, and C.A. Ferguson (Eds.), *Child Phonology*, Vol. 2. *Perception.* New York: Academic Press, 1980.

Bates, E., *The Emergence of Symbols: Cognition and Communication in Infancy.* New York: Academic Press, 1979.

Bates, E., I. Bretherton, C. Shore, and S. McNew, "Names, gestures, and other objects." In K.E. Nelson (Ed.), *Children's Language*, Vol. 4. New York: Academic Press, 1983.

Bowerman, M., "Reorganizational processes in lexical and syntactic development." In E. Wanner and L.R. Gleitman (Eds.), *Language Acquisition: The State of the Art.* Cambridge (U.K.): Cambridge University Press, 1982.

de Boysson-Bardies, B., N. Bacri, L. Sagart, and M. Poizat, "Timing in late babbling." *Journal of Child Language,* *8* (1981): 525–539.

de Boysson-Bardies, B., P. Hallé, L. Sagart, and C. Durand, "A crosslinguistic investigation of vowel formants in babbling." *Journal of Child Language, 16* (1989): 1–17.

de Boysson-Bardies, B., L. Sagart, and C. Durand, "Discernible differences in the babbling of infants according to target language." *Journal of Child Language, 11* (1984): 1–15.

de Boysson-Bardies, B., and M.M. Vihman, "Adaptation to language." *Language, 61* (1991): 297–319.

de Boysson-Bardies, B., M.M. Vihman, L. Roug-Hellichius, C. Durand, I. Landberg, and F. Arao, "Material evidence of infant selection from the target language: A crosslinguistic phonetic study." In C.A. Ferguson, L. Menn, and C. Stoel-Gammon (Eds.), *Phonological Development: Models, Research, Implications.* Parkton, Md.: York Press, 1992.

Braine, M.D.S., "Review of N.V. Smith, *The Acquisition of Phonology: A Case Study." Language, 52* (1976): 489–498.

Chiat, S., "The role of the word in phonological development." *Linguistics, 17* (1979): 591–610.

Chomsky, N., "A review of B.F. Skinner's *Verbal Behavior*" (New York: Appleton-Century-Crofts, 1957). *Language, 35* (1959): 26–58.

Clumeck, H., "The effects of word-familiarity on phonemic recognition in children aged 3 to 5 years." In C.E. Johnson and C.L. Thew (Eds.), *Proceedings of the Second International Congress for the Study of Child Language,* Vol. 1. Lanham, Md.: University Press of America, 1982.

Cruttenden, A., *Intonation.* Cambridge: Cambridge University Press, 1986.

Davis, B.L., and P.F. MacNeilage, "Acquisition of correct vowel production: A quantitative case study." *Journal of Speech and Hearing Research, 33* (1990): 16–27.

Delack, J.B., and P.J. Fowlow, "The ontogenesis of differential vocalization: Development of prosodic contrastivity during the first year of life." In N. Waterson and C. Snow (Eds.), *The Development of Communication.* New York: John Wiley, 1978.

Deville, G., "Notes sur le développement de l'enfant." *Revue de Linguistique, 23* (1890): 330–343; *24* (1891): 10–42, 128–143, 242–257, 300–320.

Donegan, P., and D. Stampe, "The study of natural phonology." In D. Dinnsen (Ed.), *Current Approaches to Phonological Theory.* Bloomington: Indiana University Press, 1979.

Dore, J., M.B. Franklin, R.T. Miller, and A.L.H. Ramer, "Transitional phenomena in early language acquisition." *Journal of Child Language, 3* (1976): 13–28.

Edwards, M.L., "Perception and production in child phonology: The testing of four hypotheses." *Journal of Child Language, 1* (1974): 205–219.

Edwards, M.L., and L.D. Shriberg, *Phonology: Applications in Communicative Disorders.* San Diego, Calif.: College-Hill, 1983.

Eilers, R.E., "Context-sensitive perception of naturally produced stop and fricative consonants by infants." *Journal of the Acoustical Society of America, 61* (1977): 1321–1336.

Eilers, R.E., "Infant speech perception: History and mystery." In G. Yeni-Komshian, J. Kavanagh, and C.A. Ferguson (Eds.), *Child Phonology,* Vol. 2. *Perception.* New York: Academic Press, 1980.

Eilers, R.E., W. Gavin, and W.R. Wilson, "Linguistic experience and phonemic perception in infancy: A cross-linguistic study." *Child Development, 50* (1979): 14–18.

Eilers, R.E., and F.D. Minifie, "Fricative discrimination in early infancy." *Journal of Speech and Hearing Research, 18* (1975): 158–167.

Eilers, R.E., and D.K. Oller, "The role of speech discrimination in developmental sound substitutions." *Journal of Child Language, 3* (1976): 319–329.

Eimas, P., E. Siqueland, P. Jusczyk, and J. Vigorito, "Speech perception in infants." *Science, 171* (1971): 303–306.

Elbers, L., "Operating principles in repetitive babbling: A cognitive continuity approach." *Cognition, 12* (1982): 45–63.

Ferguson, C.A., "Sound patterns in language acquisition." In D.P. Dato (Ed.), *Developmental Psycholinguistics: Theory and Application.* Georgetown University Roundtable, 1–16. Washington, D.C.: Georgetown University Press, 1975.

Ferguson, C.A., "Learning to pronounce: The earliest stages of phonological development in the child." In F.D. Minifie and L.L. Lloyd (Eds.), *Communicative and Cognitive Abilities—Early Behavioral Assessment.* Baltimore: University Park Press, 1978.

Ferguson, C.A., "Phonology as an individual access system: Some data from language acquisition." In C.J. Fillmore, D. Kempler, and W. S-Y. Wang (Eds.), *Individual Differences in Language Ability and Language Behavior.* New York: Academic Press, 1979.

Ferguson, C.A., "Discovering sound units and constructing sound systems: It's child's play." In J.S. Perkell and D.H. Klatt (Eds.), *Invariance and Variability of Speech Processes.* Hillsdale, N.J.: Lawrence Erlbaum, 1986.

Ferguson, C.A., and C.B. Farwell, "Words and sounds in early language acquisition." *Language, 51* (1975): 419–439.

Ferguson, C.A., and O.K. Garnica, "Theories of phonological development." In E.H. Lenneberg and E. Lenneberg (Eds.), *Foundations of Language Development*. New York: Academic Press, 1975.

Ferguson, C.A., and M.A. Macken, "The role of play in phonological development." In K.E. Nelson (Ed.), *Children's Language*, Vol. 4. Hillsdale, N.J.: Lawrence Erlbaum, 1983.

Ferguson, C.A., L. Menn, and C. Stoel-Gammon, *Phonological Development: Models, Research, Implications*. Parkton, Md.: York Press, 1992.

Ferguson, C.A., D.B. Peizer, and T.A. Weeks, "Model-and-replica phonological grammar of a child's first words." *Lingua, 3* (1973): 35–65.

Fernald, A., and T. Simon, "Expanded intonation contours in mothers' speech to newborns." *Developmental Psychology, 20* (1984): 104–113.

Francescato, G., "On the role of the word in first language acquisition." *Lingua, 21* (1968): 144–153.

Fry, D.B., "The development of the phonological system in the normal and the deaf child." In F. Smith and G. Miller (Eds.), *The Genesis of Language: A Psycholinguistic Approach*. Cambridge, Mass.: M.I.T. Press, 1966.

Garnica, O.K., "The development of phonemic speech perception." In T. Moore (Ed.), *Cognitive Development and the Acquisition of Language*. New York: Academic Press, 1973.

Graham, L.W., and A.S. House, "Phonological oppositions in children: A perceptual study." *Journal of the Acoustical Society of America, 49* (1971): 559–566.

Greenlee, M., "Learning the phonetic cues to the voiced-voiceless distinction: An exploration of parallel processes in phonological change." Ph.D. thesis, University of California, Berkeley, 1978.

Grunwell, P., "The development of phonology." *First Language, 2* (1981): 161–191.

Hallé, P.A., B. de Boysson-Bardies, and M.M. Vihman, "Beginnings of prosodic organization: Intonation and duration patterns of disyllables produced by French and Japanese infants." *Language and Speech*, in press.

Halliday, M.A.K., *Learning How to Mean—Explorations in the Development of Language*. London: Edward Arnold, 1975.

Householder, F.W., "Unreleased PTK in American English." In M. Halle (Ed.), *For Roman Jakobson*. The Hague: Mouton, 1956.

Ingram, D., *Phonological Disability in Children*. London: Edward Arnold, 1976.

Jakobson, R., *Child Language, Aphasia and Phonological Universals*, A.R. Keiler (Tr.). The Hague: Mouton, 1968. (Original title *Kindersprache, Aphasie und allgemeine Lautgesetze*. Uppsala: Almqvist and Wiksell, 1941.)

Jusczyk, P.W., and J. Bertoncini, "Viewing the development of speech perception as an innately guided learning process." *Language and Speech, 31* (1988): 217–238.

Jusczyk, P.W., J. Murray, and J. Bayly, "Perception of place of articulation in fricatives and stops by infants." Paper presented at Biennial Meeting of Society for Research in Child Development, San Francisco, 1979.

Karzon, R.B., "Discrimination of polysyllabic sequences by one- to four-month-old infants." *Perception and Psychophysics, 39* (1985): 105–109.

Kent, R.D., "The biology of phonological development." In C.A. Ferguson, L. Menn, and C. Stoel-Gammon (Eds.), *Phonological Development: Models, Research, Implications*. Parkton, Md.: York Press, 1992.

Kent, R.D., and H.R. Bauer, "Vocalizations of one-year-olds." *Journal of Child Language, 13* (1985): 491–526.

Kent, R.D., and A.D. Murray, "Acoustic features of infant vocalic utterances at 3, 6, and 9 months." *Journal of the Acoustical Society of America, 72* (1982): 353–365.

Kiparsky, P., and L. Menn, "On the acquisition of phonology." In J. Macnamara (Ed.), *Language Learning and Thought*. New York: Academic Press, 1977.

Kuhl, P.K., "Perception of speech and sound in early infancy." In P. Salapatek and L. Cohen (Eds.), *Handbook of Infant Perception*, Vol. 2. *From Perception to Cognition*. New York: Academic Press, 1987.

Leopold, W.F., *Speech Development of a Bilingual Child*, Vol. 2. *Sound-Learning in the First Two Years*. Evanston, Ill.: Northwestern University Press, 1947.

Lewis, M.M., *Infant Speech: A Study of the Beginnings of Language*. New York: Harcourt Brace, 1936.

Lieberman, P., "On the development of vowel production in young children." In G. Yeni-Komshian, J. Kavanagh, and C.A. Ferguson (Eds.), *Child Phonology*, Vol. 1. *Production*. New York: Academic Press, 1980.

Lindblom, B., "Phonological units as adaptive emergents of lexical development." In C.A. Ferguson, L. Menn, and C. Stoel-Gammon (Eds.), *Phonological Development: Models, Research, Implications*. Parkton, Md.: York Press, 1992.

Lindner, G., *Aus dem Naturgarten der Kindersprache*. Leipzig: Th. Grieben's Verlag, 1898.

Lisker, L., "Rabid vs. rapid: A catalogue of acoustic features that may cue the distinction." Haskins Laboratories Status Report on Speech Research (SR-54). New Haven, Conn., 1978.

Lisker, L., and A.S. Abramson, "A cross-language study of voicing in initial stops: Acoustical measurements." *Word, 20* (1964): 384–422.

Locke, J.L., "The child's processing of phonology." In W.A. Collins (Ed.), *Minnesota Symposium on Child Psychology*, Vol. 12. Hillsdale, N.J.: Lawrence Erlbaum, 1979.

Locke, J.L., "The inference of speech perception in the phonologically disordered child, Part I: A rationale, some criteria, the conventional tests." *Journal of Speech and Hearing Disorders, 4* (1980a): 431–444.

Locke, J.L., "The inference of speech perception in the phonologically disordered child, Part II: Some clinically novel procedures, their use, some findings." *Journal of Speech and Hearing Disorders, 4* (1980b): 445–468.

Locke, J.L., *Phonological Acquisition and Change.* New York: Academic Press, 1983.

Locke, J.L., "Variation in human biology and child phonology: A response to Goad and Ingram." *Journal of Child Language, 15* (1988): 663–668.

Locke, J.L., "Structure and stimulation in the ontogeny of spoken language." *Developmental Psychobiology, 23* (1990): 621–643.

Locke, J.L., and D. Pearson, "Vocal learning and the emergence of phonological capacity: A neurobiological approach." In C.A. Ferguson, L. Menn, and C. Stoel-Gammon (Eds.), *Phonological Development: Models, Research, Implications.* Parkton, Md.: York Press, 1992.

McCune, L., "First words: A dynamic systems view." In C.A. Ferguson, L. Menn, and C. Stoel-Gammon (Eds.), *Phonological Development: Models, Research, Implications.* Parkton, Md.: York Press, 1992.

MacKain, K.S., "Assessing the role of experience on infants' speech discrimination." *Journal of Child Language, 9* (1982): 527–542.

Macken, M.A., "Developmental reorganization of phonology: A hierarchy of basic units of acquisition." *Lingua, 49* (1979): 11–49.

Macken, M.A., "The child's lexical representation: The '*puzzle-puddle-pickle*' evidence." *Journal of Linguistics, 16* (1980): 1–17.

Macken, M.A., and C.A. Ferguson, "Cognitive aspects of phonological development: Model, evidence and issues." In K.E. Nelson (Ed.), *Children's Language,* Vol. 4. Hillsdale, N.J.: Lawrence Erlbaum, 1983.

Maxwell, E.M., "On determining underlying phonological representations of children: A critique of the current theories." In M. Elbert, D.A. Dinnsen, and G. Weismer (Eds.), *Phonological Theory and the Misarticulating Child.* ASHA Monographs, 22. Rockville, Md.: ASHA, 1984.

Menn, L., "Pattern, control, and contrast in beginning speech: A case study in the development of word form and word function." Ph.D. thesis, University of Illinois, 1976. (Reprinted by the Indiana University Linguistics Club, 1978.)

Menn, L., "Theories of phonological development." In H. Winitz (Ed.), *Native Language and Foreign Language Acquisition.* New York: Academy of Sciences, 1981.

Menn, L., "Development of articulatory, phonetic, and phonological capabilities." In B. Butterworth (Ed.), *Language Production,* Vol. 2. London: Academic Press, 1983.

Menyuk, P., L. Menn, and R. Silber, "Early strategies for the perception and production of words and sounds." In P. Fletcher and M. Garman (Eds.), *Language Acquisition: Studies in First Language Development,* 2nd ed. Cambridge (U.K.): Cambridge University Press, 1986.

Mitchell, P.R., and R.D. Kent, "Phonetic variation in multisyllable babbling." *Journal of Child Language, 17* (1990): 247–265.

Moskowitz, A.I., "The acquisition of phonology and syntax: A preliminary study." In K.J.J. Hintikka, J.M.E. Moravcsik, and P. Suppes (Eds.), *Approaches to Natural Language.* Dordrecht: Reidel, 1973.

Mowrer, O., *Learning Theory and Symbolic Processes.* New York: John Wiley, 1960.

Mulford, R., "First words of the blind child." In M.D. Smith and J.L. Locke (Eds.), *The Emergent Lexicon: The Child's Development of a Linguistic Vocabulary.* New York: Academic Press, 1988.

Oller, D.K., "The emergence of the sounds of speech in infancy." In G. Yeni-Komshian, J. Kavanagh, and C.A. Ferguson (Eds.), *Child Phonology,* Vol. 1. *Production.* New York: Academic Press, 1980.

Oller, D.K., and R.E. Eilers, "The role of audition in infant babbling." *Child Development, 59* (1988): 441–449.

Olmsted, D., *Out of the Mouth of Babes.* The Hague: Mouton, 1971.

Piaget, J., *The Origins of Intelligence in Children.* M. Cook, tr. New York: W.W. Norton & Co., 1963. (First published, 1952.)

Priestly, T.M.S., "One idiosyncratic strategy in the acquisition of phonology." *Journal of Child Language, 4* (1977): 45–65.

Ramer, A.L.H., "Syntactic styles in emerging language." *Journal of Child Language, 3* (1976): 49–62.

Robb, M.P., and J.H. Saxman, "Syllable durations of preword and early word vocalizations." *Journal of Speech and Hearing Research, 33* (1990): 583–593.

Roug, L., I. Landberg, and L.J. Lundberg, "Phonetic development in early infancy: A study of four Swedish children during the first eighteen months of life." *Journal of Child Language, 16* (1989): 19–40.

Schwartz, R., and L.B. Leonard, "Do children pick and choose? An examination of phonological selection and avoidance in early lexical acquisition." *Journal of Child Language, 9* (1982): 319–336.

Shibamoto, J.S., and D.L. Olmsted, "Lexical and syllabic patterns in phonological acquisition." *Journal of Child Language, 5* (1978): 417–456.

Shvachkin, N.KH., "The development of phonemic speech perception in early childhood." In C.A. Ferguson and D.I. Slobin (Eds.), *Studies of Child Language Development.* New York: Holt, Rinehart & Winston, 1973.

(Original title "Razvitiye fonematicheskogo vospriyatiya rechi v rannem vozraste." *Izvestiya Akademii Pedagogicheskikh Nauk RSFSR, 13* [1948]: 101–132.)

Slobin, D.I., "Cognitive prerequisites for the development of grammar." In C.A. Ferguson and D.I. Slobin (Eds.), *Studies of Child Language Development.* New York: Holt, Rinehart & Winston, 1973.

Smit, A.B., and **J. Bernthal,** "Performance of articulation-disordered children on language and perception measures." *Journal of Speech and Hearing Research, 26* (1983): 124–136.

Smith, B.L., S. Brown-Sweeney, and **C. Stoel-Gammon,** "Reduplicated and variegated babbling." *First Language, 9* (1989): 175–189.

Smith, N.V., *The Acquisition of Phonology: A Case Study.* Cambridge (U.K.): Cambridge University Press, 1973.

Stampe, D., "The acquisition of phonetic representation." Paper presented at the Fifth Regional Meeting of the Chicago Linguistic Society, Chicago, Illinois, 1969.

Stark, R.E., "Features of infant sounds: The emergence of cooing." *Journal of Child Language, 5* (1978): 379–390.

Stark, R.E., "Stages of speech development in the first year of life." In G. Yeni-Komshian, J. Kavanagh, and C.A. Ferguson (Eds.), *Child Phonology,* Vol. 1. *Production.* New York: Academic Press, 1980.

Stoel-Gammon, C., and **J.A. Cooper,** "Patterns of early lexical and phonological development." *Journal of Child Language, 11* (1984): 247–271.

Stoel-Gammon, C., and **K. Otomo.** "Babbling development of hearing-impaired and normally hearing subjects." *Journal of Speech and Hearing Disorders, 51* (1986): 33–41.

Straight, H.S., "Auditory versus articulatory phonological processes and their development in children." In G. Yeni-Komshian, J. Kavanagh, and C.A. Ferguson (Eds.), *Child Phonology,* Vol. 1. *Production.* New York: Academic Press, 1980.

Strange, W., and **Broen, P.A.,** "Perception and production of approximate consonants by 3-year-olds: A first study." In G. Yeni-Komshian, J. Kavanagh, and C.A. Ferguson (Eds.), *Child Phonology,* Vol. 2. *Perception.* New York: Academic Press, 1980.

Streeter, L.A., "Language perception of 2-month-old infants shows effects of both innate mechanisms and experience." *Nature, 259* (1976): 39–41.

Thevenin, D.M., R.E. Eilers, D.K. Oller, and **L. La Voie,** "Where's the drift in babbling drift? A cross-linguistic study." *Applied Psycholinguistics, 6* (1985): 3–15.

Tikofsky, R.S., and **J.R. McInish,** "Consonant discrimination by seven-year-olds." *Psychonomic Science, 10* (1968): 61–62.

Trehub, S.E., "Auditory-linguistic sensitivity in infants." Ph.D. thesis, McGill University, Montreal, 1973.

Trehub, S.E., "The discrimination of foreign speech contrasts by infants and adults." *Child Development, 44* (1976): 466–472.

Velleman, S.L., "The role of linguistic perception in later phonological development." *Applied Psycholinguistics, 9* (1988): 221–236.

Vihman, M.M., "Consonant harmony: Its scope and function in child language." In J.H. Greenberg (Ed.), *Universals of Human Language,* Vol. 2. *Phonology.* Stanford, Calif.: Stanford University Press, 1978.

Vihman, M.M., "A note on children's lexical representations." *Journal of Child Language, 9* (1982): 249–253.

Vihman, M.M., "Individual differences in babbling and early speech: Predicting to age three." In B. Lindblom and R. Zetterstrom (Eds.), *Precursors of Early Speech.* Basingstroke, Hampshire (U.K.): MacMillan, 1986.

Vihman, M.M., "Ontogeny of phonetic gestures: Speech production." In I.G. Mattingly and M. Studdert-Kennedy (Eds.), *Modularity and the Motor Theory of Speech Perception.* Hillsdale, N.J.: Lawrence Erlbaum, 1991.

Vihman, M.M., "Early syllables and the construction of phonology." In C.A. Ferguson, L. Menn, and C. Stoel-Gammon (Eds.), *Phonological Development: Models, Research, Implications.* Parkton, Md.: York Press, 1992.

Vihman, M.M., C.A. Ferguson, and **M. Elbert,** "Phonological development from babbling to speech: Common tendencies and individual differences." *Applied Psycholinguistics, 7* (1986): 3–40.

Vihman, M.M., and **L. McCune,** "When is a word a word?" In submission.

Vihman, M.M., M.A. Macken, R. Miller, H. Simmons, and **J. Miller,** "From babbling to speech: A reassessment of the continuity issue." *Language, 61* (1985): 395–443.

Vihman, M.M., and **R. Miller,** "Words and babble at the threshold of lexical acquisition." In M.D. Smith and J.L. Locke (Eds.), *The Emergent Lexicon: The Child's Development of a Linguistic Vocabulary.* New York: Academic Press, 1988.

Vihman, M.M., and **S. Velleman,** "Phonological reorganization: A case study." *Language and Speech, 32* (1989): 149–170.

Vincent-Smith, L., D. Bricker, and **W. Bricker,** "Acquisition of receptive vocabulary in the toddler-age child." *Child Development, 45* (1974): 189–193.

Waterson, N., "Child phonology: A prosodic view." *Journal of Linguistics, 7* (1971): 179–211.

Waterson, N., "A tentative developmental model of phonological representation." In T. Myers, J. Laver, and J. Anderson (Eds.), *The Cognitive Representation of Speech.* Amsterdam: North-Holland, 1981.

Werker, J.F., "Ontogeny of speech perception." In I.G. Mattingly and M. Studdert-Kennedy (Eds.), *Modularity and the Motor Theory of Speech Perception.* Hillsdale, N.J.: Lawrence Erlbaum, 1991.

Werker, J.F., J.H.V. Gilbert, K. Humphrey, and R.C. Tees, "Developmental aspects of cross-language speech perception." *Child Development, 52* (1981): 349–353.

Werker, J.F., and J.E. Pegg, "Infant speech perception and phonological acquisition." In C.A. Ferguson, L. Menn, and C. Stoel-Gammon (Eds.), *Phonological Development: Models, Research, Implications.* Parkton, Md.: York Press, 1992.

Werker, J.F., and R.C. Tees, "Developmental changes across childhood in the perception of non-native speech sounds." *Canadian Journal of Psychology, 37* (1983): 278–286.

Werker, J.F., and R.C. Tees, "Cross-language speech perception: Evidence for perceptual reorganization during the first year of life." *Infant Behaviour and Development, 7* (1984): 49–63.

Whalen, D.H., A.G. Levitt, and Q. Wang, "Intonational differences between the reduplicative babbling of French- and English-learning infants." *Journal of Child Language, 18* (1991): 501–516.

Zlatin, M., "Explorative mapping of the vocal tract and primitive syllabification in infancy: The first six months." *Purdue University Contributed Papers, 5* (1975): 58–73.

chapter
3

Later Phonological Development

Marilyn May Vihman, Rutgers University

The two different research strategies most commonly used in the study of later phonological development lead to somewhat different pictures of that process. In the **longitudinal** studies of individual children, extensive data are collected from different points in a particular child's development. This strategy, typically used by linguists, highlights the variability in any one child's production at one point and over time, and across different children. Close analysis of individual differences can provide insight into the learning process. But such intensive data analyses are available for only a relatively small number of children, and therefore the validity of any generalizations about the time-course for acquisition of specific speech sounds is uncertain. Child development specialists and speech-language pathologists interested in the study of normal phonological development for the purpose of comparison with disordered speakers most often use a different strategy—a **cross-sectional** research design. In this approach, no single child is followed over time; rather, different children at different age levels are tested at a single point in time on their ability to produce speech sounds, and a composite profile is extrapolated from the data.

We will begin our discussion of later phonological development by reviewing some of the best-known large-scale studies. This will set the stage for a closer look at the particular paths followed by a smaller number of individual children. We will also consider issues relating to the perception of running speech by older children in comparison with adults. Finally, we will review ways in which phonetic and phonological variation and change continue beyond the early childhood years.

Long before the field of child language acquisition began to burgeon in the 1960s, there was considerable practical interest in determining the age at which most children are able to correctly produce each of the phonemes of their language; that is, there was a need to establish developmental norms. Such an enterprise, however, has inherent methodological and theoretical problems. In order to establish production norms, one must test large numbers of children, but fully adequate evaluation of any one child's ability to produce contrasts between speech sounds requires both time and patience. Use of imitation may yield different results than spontaneous speech, and speech sound production in single words may differ from that in running conversation, as it does in adults. The many recent intensive studies of small groups (e.g., Ingram, Christensen, Veach, and Webster, 1980) have confirmed what a careful reading of earlier diary data suggested: Individual differences across children are so great in some areas—in the acquisition of fricatives, for example—that it may be impossible to establish meaningful age norms. Nevertheless, the need for such normative information is undeniable. Furthermore, developmental norm studies are based on the testing of children covering a broad age range (2 to 10 years) and, thus, can provide a useful overview of development beyond the earliest period of lexical acquisition.

Table 3–1 lists salient characteristics of the major cross-sectional studies undertaken in the United States in this century. These large-sample studies generally follow the same model, which may be described as follows.

Subject Selection. First of all, an effort is made to ensure that the sample reflects the socioeconomic distribution of the population as a whole; Templin (1957), who reported the parameters of her study in full, weighted her sample toward the lower end of the scale (70 percent of the children, based on father's occupation) and included only urban children. Second, audiometric screening and parental report are typically used to exclude children with hearing losses or delayed language development.

Obtaining the Sample. Children are asked to name a picture representing a target word, usually only once; if the child does not produce the word spontaneously, an imitation is elicited. Consonants and clusters are tested in initial,

TABLE 3–1. **Major Cross-Sectional Production Studies in the United States. (I = initial, M = medial, F = final; Sp = spontaneous, Im = imitated)**

DATE	AUTHOR(S)	NO.Ss	AGE RANGE	WORD POSITION	SP/IM	CRITERION
1931	Wellman et al.	204	2;0–4;0	I, M, F	Sp, Im	75%
1934	Poole	140	2;5–8;5	I, M, F	Sp	100%
1957	Templin	480	3;0–8;0	I, M, F	Sp, Im	75%
1963	Snow	438	6;5–8;7	I, M, F		
1967	Bricker	90	3;0–5;0	I	Im	
1971	Olmsted	100	1;3–4;6	I, M, F	Sp	
1972	Sax	535	5;0–10;0	I, M, F	Sp	93%
1975	Prather et al.	147	2;0–4;0	I, F	Sp, Im	75%
1976	Arlt and Goodban	240	3;0–5;6	I, M, F	Im	75%
1990	Smit et al.	997	3;0–9;0	I, F	Sp, Im	75%

Later Phonological Development

medial, and final position, or a subset of those; vowels and diphthongs are also tested in some studies.

Analysis. A criterion is set to determine "age of acquisition" *for the group as a whole.* For Templin, this criterion was correct production in each of three word positions by 75 percent of the children. For Prather, Hedrick, and Kern (1975), it was correct production in two positions, again by 75 percent of the children, and scores were averaged over the two positions. Vowels and diphthongs were generally found to be acquired by age three, and will not be further considered here.

In these studies, only group data are used. No results are given regarding individual responses, so there is no information regarding either individual differences between children of the same age or actual errors made for a given sound. The basic goal is to establish the age at which parents, teachers, and clinicians may reasonably expect a child's production of a given sound to match the adult standard.

Sander (1972) pointed out that the widely quoted ages of acquisition for speech sounds, based on the earlier studies cited in Table 3–1, are misleading if taken to reflect "average" performance, given the strict criteria used. Instead, they must be understood to represent upper age limits for acquisition. In an effort to derive a more representative profile, Sander reanalyzed the Wellman, Case, Mengert and Bradbury (1931) data (for age 2: 15 subjects) and the Templin data. He established a range between "customary production" (correct production in two out of three word positions by 50 percent of the children) and "mastery" (correct production in all three word positions by 90 percent of the children). Prather et al. (1975) also utilized this strategy; they presented their normative data in a similar manner, and then compared it with Sander's reanalysis (see Chapter 7, Figure 7–1).

Figure 7–1 vividly illustrates the difference between customary production and mastery, given data based on group behavior. Acquisition of /k/, for example, ranges from customary production (i.e., use by half the children sampled) at age 2 to correct production by virtually all the children at nearly age 4. The data regarding correct production of /t/ are strikingly discrepant in the two studies. Whereas Prather et al. find a range from under 24 months to 32 months, Sander's reanalysis of the data from Wellman et al. and from Templin shows a range from 24 months to over 48 months. However, Sander points out that the late age of acquisition cited for /t/ in Templin (age 6) is entirely due to the younger children's failure to produce a voiceless [t] in medial position. In fact, in American English /t/ is normally produced as a (voiced) flap in medial position following a stressed vowel (as in *skating*). The coding of an error here reflects an unrealistic, idealized standard.

Relatively small differences in methodology may greatly affect the age of acquisition reported. Smit (1986) analyzed the differences between Templin's study, which appears to be the one most frequently consulted by clinicians, and the more recent studies by Prather et al. (1975) and Arlt and Goodban (1976). The latter studies reported younger ages of acquisition for most sounds, as is evident for Prather et al. Arlt and Goodban suggested that children were learning speech sounds at younger ages at the time of their study than 20 years earlier. Use of this more recent standard, then, would entail concern about children at an earlier age if their production of some sounds (most likely fricatives or liquids) failed to meet expectations based on the reported data.

Smit noted several methodological reasons for the discrepancy, particularly differences in analysis, like the decision to use two positions instead of three and to *average* scores across word-positions rather than require that 75 percent of the children produce a sound correctly in *each* position. Furthermore, Templin reported data only for children who attempted all sounds, whereas Prather et al. reported *partial* data, especially at the younger ages. Since missing data likely reflects an unwillingness to make errors in producing a difficult sound, this difference alone can have a significant effect on the results.

Given their cursory sampling (one production per segment in each word-position) and the differences in methods of analysis of these large-scale studies, it would clearly be a mistake to place a great deal of faith in an exact age at which a given phoneme can be expected to be produced correctly. Nevertheless, the results of the studies do agree sufficiently to provide a general picture of the order of acquisition of English consonants up to the point of mastery of the system as a whole. Nasals, stops, and glides are acquired relatively early; fricatives and affricates are mastered relatively late. Consonant clusters are also acquired late, with two-consonant clusters (for example, /kl/ and /st/) preceding the three-consonant clusters (for example, /str/ and /spl/). Most single consonants and consonant clusters are apparently mastered by age 7 or 8. As Locke (1983) has pointed out, the consonants acquired early are, generally speaking, those which occur most frequently in the languages of the world.

Three other large-scale studies carried out in the United States provided more qualitative data than those described so far. Snow (1963) tested 438 first-grade children, using two test words per consonant for each of three word-positions. Unlike Templin, Snow reported in some detail the particular errors made on each sound. Bricker (1967) tested imitation of word-initial consonants in nonsense syllables by 90 children aged 3 to 5, and reported substitutions for the 10 consonants which elicited the most errors. Finally, Olmsted (1971) collected spontaneous speech samples of varying lengths from 100 children aged 1;3 to 4;6. He, too, reported substitutions for the 10 consonants most "prone to error."

Noting that these three studies are "more sophisticated in methodology and interpretation" than the earlier large-scale studies, Ferguson (1975) provided a thorough review and comparison of their data on fricatives, which account for the largest proportion of errors in all three. Despite differences in testing procedure, analysis, and the reporting of results, Ferguson found that the order of acquisition of the eight English fricatives across all three studies could be summarized in terms of three (internally unordered) groups: first /f, s, ʃ/, then /v, z/, and finally /θ, ð, ʒ/—an ordering which is largely consistent with the predictions of Jakobson (1941/68). On the other hand, the specific substitutions reported for these fricatives are not typically stops, as Jakobson predicted, except for /v/ (> /b/) and sometimes /ð/ (> /d/). Instead, /s/ substitutes for several other fricatives, /f/ substitutes for /θ/, and the affricate /dʒ/ is the most common substitute for /ʒ/, which has marginal status in English and is often replaced by /dʒ/ word-finally, even by adults. Linguists have yet to provide a plausible or widely accepted explanation for the occurring pattern of fricative to stop and fricative to fricative substitutions, whether based on the physiology of the speech tract, the nature of mental processes, the structure of English phonology, or the phonological usage of different members of society in the English-speaking world.

Smit, Hand, Freilinger, Bernthal, and Bird (1990) reported on a study conducted in Iowa and Nebraska which was larger in scale than anything undertaken previously. The study excluded data from 2-year-olds because of the large number who either failed to complete the test or refused to produce some of the test words. For the remaining children, Smit et al. reported a significant gender difference for children at ages 4;0, 4;6, and 6;0. Comparing their overall results with Templin's, they reported a plateau in the *boys'* developmental speech sound curve, between ages 3;6 and 4;0 or 4;6. A comparable plateau appears in the Templin data for boys beginning six months later. Close analysis of the various speech sounds tested reveals that the gender difference can be traced back to consonant cluster development, with either a plateau or a drop in performance for most clusters for boys, beginning at age 3;6. No explanation for this developmental difference is apparent at this time.

SUMMARY

Despite methodological difficulties, investigators have attempted to establish age norms based on the testing of large numbers of children at different age levels. Several cross-sectional studies of 100 or more English-speaking children have been conducted. Most report group data in terms of a set criterion, such as the age at which three quarters of the children correctly produce each consonant in three word-positions. It is important to bear in mind that there is often a long temporal gap between average age of customary production of a sound (correct use by 51 percent of the children in two out of three positions), and mastery of the sound (correct use in all positions by 90 percent of the children). Analysis in terms of customary production yields lower ages of acquisition. Other methodological variables—such as inclusion versus exclusion of data from subjects who fail to attempt some of the target sounds—also strongly affect the resultant chronology.

Large-scale studies do agree on certain general points. Nasals, stops, and glides are acquired early; fricatives, affricates, and consonant clusters are acquired later. Reporting of qualitative results (e.g., specification of the errors made for each sound) greatly enhances the value of a cross-sectional study. Developmental norm studies are designed to provide information about a large number of children and thus afford an overview of phonological development. Their limitation in principle is their inability to reveal the particular course of development of any one child. In providing a broad range of data, such studies can serve as a useful complement to the more narrowly based diaries and longitudinal studies of small groups of children.

PHONOLOGICAL PROCESSES: SYSTEMATICITY IN PRODUCTION ERRORS

One fact about phonological development on which linguists of virtually all theoretical persuasions can agree is the systematic nature of the child's simplifications and restructuring of adult words (Macken and Ferguson, 1981). As Oller (1975) explicitly puts it, "the sorts of substitutions, deletions and additions which occur in child language are not merely random errors on the child's part, but are rather the result of a set of systematic tendencies" (299). It is the systematic relationship between the adult target and the child's reproduction of that target that is expressed by the linguist's "rewrite" or "realization rule":

$$X \rightarrow Y/Z$$

or "X 'goes to' [is substituted by or realized as] Y in the environment Z." For example, when a 3-year-old produces a series of words like [tænt] for *can't*, [tɔz] for *'cause*, [taᵘ] for *cow*, and [oᵘt'e¹] for *okay*, the linguist formulates a rule to express the observed regularity: [k] → [t]; in this case no "conditioning environment" or context is given since the substitution appears to occur in a wide range of contexts. In fact, when we notice that the child also says [dɛt] for *get*, [doᵘ] for *go*, ['doᵘfɚs] for *gophers*, and [di:n] for *green*, we can express the rule more generally as "a velar stop is realized as a dental (or alveolar) stop."

Phonological substitutions typically show great regularity in the language of children past the earliest stage of lexical acquisition. Linguists express that regularity by using phonological rules, or what have come to be known in the child language literature as "phonological processes." The theoretical status—and the psychological reality—of these processes remains highly controversial. If perception of phonological contrasts continues to develop over the preschool years, the phonological processes that the child appears to operate with may not be strictly production rules; rather they may be perception or "interpretation" rules, meaning that the error underlying the mismatch between child form and adult form is actually present in the child's internal representation of the target word. Most likely, distortions of different kinds occur in both perception and production and may be due to a variety of factors including such idiosyncrasies as affective peculiarities of certain words and interrelationships between lexical items which the child associates. In any case, our understanding of phonological development has undoubtedly benefited from the extensive cataloging of common processes used by different children learning different languages. At our present stage of knowledge regarding the child's actual processing of language, references to phonological processes are generally a descriptive convenience rather than an attempt to directly reflect the child's mental activity.

Let us now take a closer look at the most common phonological processes that children have been found to apply to adult words. In general, these processes appear to be used regardless of the particular language the child is learning, although the structure of the adult language may affect the frequency with which a given process is used (Ingram, 1986; Vihman, 1978, 1980). The processes are used to some extent by virtually all children in the earlier stages of word acquisition, but a given child will quickly master certain difficulties (e.g., the production of velars or fricatives or closed syllables, depending on his or her phonetic preferences and the words he or she has been attempting) and thereby obviate the need for the corresponding processes (velar fronting, stopping, final consonant deletion) while continuing to make use of other processes. Finally, more than one process may be implicated in a child's production of a single word (e.g., cluster simplification as well as velar fronting must be posited to account for the realization of *green* as [di:n], cited above).

Phonological processes may be grouped into two functionally distinct categories: **whole-word processes,** which simplify word or syllable structure and segmental contrast within a word (generally through reduction or assimilation), and **segment change processes,** which involve (context-free) changes in specific segments or segment types, regardless of syllable- or word-position. We will briefly characterize a few of the most common processes representing each of these types; further discussion, using examples taken from the extensive literature on normal phonological acquisition, follows. For a fuller list of common phonological processes, see Chapter 7.

WHOLE-WORD PROCESSES

Unstressed syllable deletion: omission of an unstressed syllable of the target word

Ramon → [mən]   (Si: Macken, 1979)

Final consonant deletion: omission of a final consonant of the target word

because → [pi′kʌ]
thought → [fɔ]   (Vihman and Greenlee, 1987)

Reduplication: production of two identical syllables, based on one or more of the syllables of the target word

Sesame Street → [si:si]   (Deborah: Vihman et al., 1986)
hello → [jojo]   (Hildegard: Leopold, 1947)

Consonant harmony: one of the contrasting consonants of the target word takes on features of another consonant in the same word

duck → [gʌk]
tub → [bʌb]   (Daniel: Menn, 1971)

Consonant cluster simplification: a consonant cluster is simplified in some manner

cracker → [kæk]   (Molly: Vihman et al., 1986)

Assimilatory processes (like consonant harmony) take the whole word as their domain, whereas reduction processes (involving consonant or syllable deletion) alter the phonotactic or syntagmatic structure of the adult model, reducing the number of syllables or simplifying the shape of syllables. The two types of reduction processes are often treated together and have variously been referred to as "phonotactic rules" (Ingram, 1974), "syllable structure processes" (Ingram, 1986: see also Ch. 7), "structural simplifying processes" (Grunwell, 1981), "syntagmatic processes" (Nettelbladt, 1983), or "processes affecting sequential structure" (Magnusson, 1983). Following the order of processes given above, we will first consider two of the most common reduction processes, syllable deletion and consonant deletion, and then two assimilatory processes, reduplication and consonant harmony; finally, we will illustrate consonant cluster simplification, which is closely related to the segment change processes.

Reduction Processes. Vihman (1980) examined "long word reduction" in 11 children (aged 1;0 to 2;9) acquiring five languages. She restricted analysis to words of three syllables or more in the adult model. She found a strict language-based order for the proportion of long words attempted: Frequencies ranged from about 25 percent for two Spanish-speaking children to about 3 percent for three English-speaking children. Use of syllable deletion to handle the long words varied independently of the particular language spoken, and ranged from 90 percent for Hildegard Leopold (German- and English-speaking) to 26 percent for Jiri, a Czech-speaking child.

Syllable deletion most often affects an unstressed syllable. Even a stressed syllable may be omitted, especially if it is the first of three or more syllables. There is a strong tendency for children to preserve a final syllable, whether it is stressed or not, presumably because final position is perceptually salient. Klein (1981) provides a great many examples of syllable deletion. The following instances were produced by Jason, a child who made moderate use of the process of deletion.

> *alligator* → ['ægejʌ]
> *banana* → ['nǽnæ̃]
> *butterfly* → ['bʌfaɪ]
> *watermelon* → ['mõmīn]   (omitting the stressed initial syllable)

One of the 3-year-olds included in the study reported in Vihman and Greenlee (1987) was continuing to apply syllable deletion to many words:

> *animals* → ['æml̩z]
> *ambulance* → ['æmʌns]
> *dessert* → [ɝt]

Consonant deletion most often affects final consonants, though initial and medial consonants may also be omitted. Berman (1977) reported that her daughter Shelli (age 18 to 23 months, acquiring both Hebrew and English) frequently used consonant deletion, particularly to avoid producing word-forms with both initial and final consonants. Difficulty with individual segments appears to have dictated the choice of segment to omit: Stops and nasals were retained, with preference for stops; fricatives and liquids were omitted. The chief mark of phonological advance in the period under study was the production of formerly omitted consonants and the admission of new CVC words without reduction. Some examples of consonant deletion (from Berman, 1977):

1. Word-initial

> /'ruti/ → ['uti] "Ruthie" (mother's name)
> /ʃa'lom/ → ['alom] "hello"
> /xam/ → [am] "hot"

2. Word-final

> *peach* → [pi]
> *spoon* → [pu]
> /tov/ → [to] "good"

Deletion of a medial consonant is cited for one 3-year-old in Vihman and Greenlee (1987):

> *mommy* → [mãi]

Later Phonological Development

Assimilatory Processes. Although some writers view use of **reduplication** as the mark of a developmental stage that all children pass through (Moskowitz, 1973; Fee and Ingram, 1982), others maintain that reduplication, like other phonological processes, represents an individual strategy characterizing the speech of some but not all children at the same developmental point (Schwartz, Leonard, Wilcox, and Folger, 1980; cf. also Schwartz and Leonard, 1983). The function of reduplication is also a subject of controversy. It may serve as a strategy for producing multisyllabic adult words—retaining the syllable count while reducing the number of contrasting elements, or as a way to avoid final consonant production.

Schwartz et al. collected spontaneous speech data from 12 (English-speaking) children aged 1;3 to 2;0, half of whom proved to be "reduplicators," using full or partial reduplication in 20 percent or more of their recorded lexicon. Fee and Ingram drew on 24 heterogeneous data sets (mostly parental diaries) for children aged 1;1 to 2;6. Some examples of reduplication provided by Schwartz et al. (1980):

> *Christmas* → [dzɪdzɪ]
> *kitten* → [kɪkɪ]
> *water* → [wɔwɔ]

Whereas Schwartz et al. found no correlation between age or linguistic stage and relative use of reduplication for their narrower age range, Fee and Ingram found that the reduplicators in their sample were younger than the non-reduplicators (they did not assess stage of linguistic development). Both studies found that reduplication is primarily used to reduce the complexity of multisyllabic words. (Application of the process to monosyllables—e.g., *ball* → [bʌbə]—proved rare.) The relation between reduplication and final consonants remains unclear. Moreover, the suggestion that heavy use of reduplication may characterize slower learners (Ferguson, Peizer, and Weeks, 1973) has yet to be tested on a large scale.

Ferguson (1983) pointed out that reduplication has also been found to serve a "play" or "practice" function, not only in babbling but also in the sound-play of 2- to 5-year-olds (cf. Ferguson and Macken, 1983). Furthermore, reduplication may help the child to identify and learn to produce phonologically distinctive syllables and segments; production of a reduplicative pattern reflecting the shape of one of the syllables of the adult model seems to provide the child with a well-controlled way to move from a whole-word to a segment-based phonology (cf. Macken, 1978; Lleo, 1990).

Consonant harmony, or the assimilation of non-contiguous consonants, is essentially the same as "partial reduplication" (vowel harmony is a parallel process but is less frequently noted in child language data). Unfortunately, neither Schwartz et al. nor Fee and Ingram specified the proportion of full versus partial reduplication (i.e., assimilation) in their data. In a study of relatively large data sets from 13 children (aged 1;0 to 2;9) acquiring six languages, Vihman (1978) found a range from 1 percent to 32 percent in the use of consonant harmony (for words containing different consonants in the adult model); mean use was 14 percent. Differences in frequency of harmony use did not appear to be tied to differences in target language.

Smith suggested that consonant harmony is "part of a universal template which the child has to escape from in order to learn his language'' (1973; 206). In some children, however, it is rare, and when it is used, it often enters the child's lexicon as a simplification of words produced earlier in a form closer to the adult model. The use of consonant harmony can be taken to reflect the child's effort to systematize his or her word production. More specifically, consonant harmony often provides a way of avoiding difficult segments (such as liquids and fricatives) or of allowing the child to produce new segments or longer words by reducing overall complexity.

Consonant harmony may also be described as "full" or "partial," depending on the resultant child form. In full harmony, the consonants of a word, which contrasted in the adult model, are identical in the child form; in partial harmony, the consonants of the child form are more similar than in the adult model but are not identical. Some examples (from Vihman, 1978):

1. Full

     Amahl Smith   *tiger* → [gaigə]
     Virve Vihman   *tuppa* → [pup:a] "into the room"

2. Partial

     Virve Vihman   *suppi* → [fup:i] "some soup"

Notice that the differences reflected here between adult and child forms could all be described in terms of a single distinctive feature: alveolar to velar (plus automatic word-initial voicing) for *tiger*, alveolar to labial or labiodental for *tuppa* and *suppi*. Full versus partial harmony describes only the resultant form, not the extent of the difference between adult and child form.

Grunwell's chronology (1981) showed that neither reduplication nor consonant harmony is normally used by age 3. Full reduplication did not occur in the 3-year-old samples in Vihman and Greenlee (1987), and consonant harmony occurred only sporadically (a few instances in a three-hour sample) and only for a few of the children.

1. Full

    yellow → ['lɛloʊ]
    mailboxes → ['meɪlmaksɪz]

2. Partial

    slimy → ['snaɪmi]

Consonant Cluster Simplification. Like the reduction processes, cluster simplification alters syllable structure, but it is also closely related to the segment change processes in that the specific consonants omitted or changed are typically those difficult to produce as singleton consonants. Cluster simplification is virtually always present in the first year of language use, and it is one of the longest lasting processes. At age 3, cluster simplification still accounted for a substantial proportion of the phonological errors made by the 10 children followed in Vihman and Greenlee (1987), and it still accounts for over 10 percent of the errors of 5-

year-olds responding to standardized test items (Haelsig and Madison, 1986; Roberts, Burchinal, and Footo, 1990).

Among the 11 younger subjects of Vihman (1980), cluster simplification affected from 52 percent to 100 percent (mean 80 percent) of all target words with clusters (which themselves made up nearly a third of the children's words, on average; the three children learning Slavic languages averaged 38 percent words with clusters). Several general relationships emerged in this study. In clusters made up of liquid plus another consonant, the liquid was typically omitted, and when stop and fricative were combined, the stop was the more likely to be preserved. Nasal plus stop clusters were more likely to be maintained as clusters, but when such a cluster was reduced, the nasal was likely to be retained before a voiced stop and omitted before a voiceless stop. Perceptual rather than articulatory factors may be at work here (Braine, 1976) since nasals, like vowels, are longer before voiced obstruents and, thus, may be more easily perceived in that context.

In a study of the acquisition of stop-plus-liquid clusters Greenlee (1974) found the course of development to be very similar in all six of the languages investigated. She identified three stages: (1) omission of the liquid, (2) substitution for the liquid (usually by a glide), and (3) correct production. Some examples (from Greenlee, 1974):

Amahl Smith: *bread* → [bɛd], [blɛd]

Edmond Grégoire (a Belgian child acquiring French):

bras → [bwa] "arm"
croute → [tut] "crust"
grillé → [dije] "toasted"
tram → [kam], [tʃam] "streetcar"

From English-speaking 3-year-olds (Vihman and Greenlee, 1987):

flower → ['fawr̩]
monster → ['māt̩r̩]
stinker → ['sɪɔkr̩]
thread → [sɛd]

SEGMENT CHANGE PROCESSES

Velar fronting: a velar is replaced by an alveolar or a dental

/kikeriki:/ → [titi:]   (Virve: Vihman, 1976)

Stopping: a fricative is replaced by a stop

sea → [ti:]
say → [tʰei]   (Amahl: Smith, 1973)

Gliding: a liquid is replaced by a glide

lie → [jaɪ]   (Hildegard: Leopold, 1947)

Of the commonly found changes, **velar fronting** is the only one to affect stops, and it is, no doubt, the first common change process to be outgrown (Preisser, Hodson, and Paden, 1988). Of the ten 3-year-olds described in Vihman and Greenlee, only one exhibited consistent velar fronting. Regular use of velar fronting contributed significantly to the relative unintelligibility of the speech of that child, who was very advanced syntactically and, thus, often produced long, complex sentences. For example:

> *called* → [tald]
> *cow* → [tau]
> *gophers* → ['doufɚs]

The process of **gliding,** which also plays a role in the acquisition of stop + liquid clusters, persists considerably longer. Examples can be found in many languages, but Ingram (1986) claimed that this process does not appear in French acquisition data. Adult French lacks /w/, and /j/ does not occur word-initially. Ingram cited French examples in which word-initial liquids are simply omitted:

> *lampe* → [ãp] "lamp"
> *lapin* → [apē] "rabbit" (used by two children)
> *laver* → [ave] "to wash"

Examples of gliding from English-speaking 3-year-olds (Vihman and Greenlee, 1987):

> *love* → [jʌv]
> *red* → [wɛd]

Thus, the changes used in phonological processes appear to be influenced by the particular phonological system the child is acquiring.

Mastering Fricatives

The most common process affecting fricatives is **stopping,** but replacement by a stop is not the only error type found. In particular, the interdentals—the most difficult segments for English-speaking children to acquire (comparable to r-trills in languages which have them)—are frequently substituted by other fricatives (/f/ or /s/ for /θ/, somewhat less commonly /v/, /z/, or even /l/ for /ð/). As mentioned earlier, perceptual difficulties have been implicated in production errors involving both fricatives and liquids, although the low incidence of fricatives in babbling suggests that these sounds present articulatory problems for many children. Some examples of stopping from English-speaking 3-year-olds (Vihman and Greenlee, 1987):

> *move* → [mu:b]
> *shoes* → [ʃu:t]
> *some* → [tʌm]

Perhaps the most important lesson to be learned from the rather extensive literature on the acquisition of fricatives (e.g., Moskowitz, 1975; Edwards, 1979; Ingram, Christensen, Veach, and Webster, 1980) is that each fricative is acquired by its own individual path of development. There is no rapid spread of a feature of "frication" or "continuancy" to relevant segments (Ferguson, 1975). Other points of particular interest raised by Ferguson include the following: (1) Fricatives may be acquired in postvocalic, final position or intervocalically before initial position, and may precede the acquisition of stops in these word-positions, and (2) language-specific constraints on the frequency and freedom of occurrence of particular fricatives may affect the order of acquisition (e.g., English /ʒ/ is rare and largely limited to word-medial position, and it consequently tends to be a late acquisition).

THE ACQUISITION OF VOICING

Ingram (1986) noted that the voicing of prevocalic consonants has been reported primarily for English. This raises a question as to whether English-speaking transcribers may be mishearing **lack of aspiration** as "voicing." Acoustic studies of voice onset time in children's productions suggest that both aspiration, or "long lag," and pre-voicing, or "voicing lead," are relatively difficult for children to master (Gilbert, 1977; Barton and Macken, 1980; Macken and Barton, 1980a, b; Clumeck, Barton, Macken, and Huntington, 1981; Eilers, Oller, and Benito-Garcia, 1984; Allen, 1985). Children first produce only voiceless unaspirated stops (regardless of the language being learned); any contrasting stop classes will be acquired later (Macken, 1980).

Smit and Bernthal (1983) found that their 11 normally developing (English-speaking) 4-year-old subjects tended to use fewer fully voiced stops in initial position than adults. But these children did maintain a phonological voicing contrast in initial position: They used disproportionately long voice onset times (or heavy aspiration) in producing (word-) initial voiceless stops (all productions were embedded in a carrier phrase, "the _____ away").

In a study of consonantal devoicing in **final position** in English, Smith (1979) found that both 2- and 4-year-old subjects used substantially fewer voiced stops in all contexts than adults. He reported as much as 50 percent (partial) devoicing in final position by adults, but over 90 percent partial devoicing by both 2- and 4-year-olds. Smith attributed these results to the difficulty children have in controlling the physiological mechanisms needed to sustain voicing during stop closure.

The evidence from careful acoustic analyses, then, suggests that the observed contrast between early word-initial voicing of stops and word-final "devoicing" derives from adult (mis)interpretation of a single child phonetic type— voiceless unaspirated stop—used in both positions. Because final stops are not necessarily aspirated (or even released) in English, the voiceless unaspirated phone (used to realize final voiced as well as voiceless stops in target words) is perceived by observers as devoicing, whereas in initial position, where aspiration is an important cue to the English phonemic voicing contrast, the same child phone (again used to realize voiced as well as voiceless stop targets) is heard as voicing. For illustration of the unusual strategies children may resort to in the effort to produce an acceptable voiced stop word-finally, see Fey and Gandour (1982) and Clark and Bowerman (1986).

SUMMARY

The regularity found in phonological substitutions after the earliest stage of lexical acquisition can be conveniently formulated in terms of phonological rules or processes. Two types of processes are usually distinguished on functional grounds.

Whole-word processes simplify word or syllable structure and segmental contrast within a word, and segment change processes account for errors involving difficulty with specific segments. Whole-word processes are generally typical of the earlier stages of phonological development. They include assimilatory processes (reduplication and consonant harmony) and consonant cluster simplification. The most common segment changes are velar fronting, gliding, and various substitutions affecting fricatives. Only voiceless unaspirated stops are used in the earliest stage of phonological development, regardless of the language being learned; later, any contrasting classes of stops found in the adult language will gradually be added.

PROFILING THE PRESCHOOL CHILD: INDIVIDUAL DIFFERENCES REVISITED

We have reviewed both the findings of large-scale studies aimed at establishing norms for the acquisition of particular phonemes of the adult language and the phonological processes found to apply most often in intensive studies of small groups of children (or even just one child). In both cases, the analyses involved may be termed *relational*; that is, they are concerned with the relationship between the child's productions and the adult forms (Stoel-Gammon and Dunn, 1985). "Independent" analyses, on the other hand, describe the sounds and syllable structures of the child's productions in their own right, without reference to the adult forms. In order to form an idea of the kind of phonological production that we can expect to characterize a normally developing 2- or 3-year-old child, we will consider the results of two studies reporting phonological analyses of data drawn from naturally occurring conversation. The first is a study of 2-year-olds and makes use of both relational and independent analyses; the second is an intensive examination of the kinds of errors made by a smaller group of 3-year-olds. In addition, we will consider the results of two longitudinal studies, one comparing the phonological status at age 3 of the two 1-year-old girls profiled in Chapter 2, the other comparing phonological process use in two boys at ages 2, 3, and 6.

Phonetic Tendencies of Two-Year-Olds

Stoel-Gammon (1987) characterized the "phonological skills" of thirty-three 2-year-old children acquiring English. Subjects were recruited through a mailing to parents of newborn children in the Seattle area and observed from the age of 9 to 24 months on a trimonthly basis (cf. also Stoel-Gammon, 1985). The data were derived from two half-hour play sessions involving conversational interaction between child and observer rather than from attempts to elicit pre-selected target words. Stoel-Gammon pointed out that the "large-scale" studies of Wellman et al. (1931), Sander (1972), and Prather et al. (1975) were, in fact, based on a rather small number of 2-year-old subjects (no more than 10 or 20), since a large number of children failed to produce many of the target words. She argued that a better assessment of a 2-year-old's phonological skills can be attained through the recording of naturally occurring conversational data.

Stoel-Gammon established the use of at least 10 different adult-based words in the course of one hour of recording as a base criterion for including a speech

Later Phonological Development

sample in the 2-year-old analyses. She then developed a corpus of up to 50 words for each subject, taken from the first 100 fully or partially intelligible utterances in each sample. No one word *type* was represented by more than two variable *tokens* or productions of the same word (e.g., [su] and [du] for *shoe*). The number of words analyzed ranged from 20 to 50 per child (mean 36). Three different analyses were carried out.

Word and Syllable Shapes, Based on the Co-Occurrence of Consonants and Vowels. All the children produced at least two different open monosyllables (CV), and only one child failed to produce two different closed monosyllables (CVC). Disyllabic word shapes (CVCV[C]) occurred in over half the samples, as did word-initial clusters. Word-final clusters were produced by 48 percent of the children and medial clusters by only 30 percent.

Phonetic Inventories. Word-initial consonant inventories typically included stops at all three places of articulation ([t, k, b, d, g] occurred in at least 50 percent of the samples). In addition, nasals ([m, n]), fricatives ([f, s, h]), and a glide ([w]) typically occurred in initial position. In final position, three voiceless stops, one nasal ([n]), one fricative ([s]), and one liquid ([r]) were typically used. There was a strong tendency for children with large inventories in initial position to have a large inventory in final position as well. No one cluster (such as [sp-, pl-]) was used by more than half the children in either initial or final position.

Accuracy of Consonant Production. The mean percentage of correct consonants, based on a procedure developed by Shriberg and Kwiatkowski (1982), was 70 percent (range 43 percent to 91 percent). There was a tendency for the children with larger inventories to achieve greater accuracy with respect to the adult form than those with smaller inventories. Stoel-Gammon pointed out that the difference in inventory size between adult English and the "typical" 2-year-old in her study is considerable, and thus, the 70 percent accuracy level achieved by the children suggests that 2-year-olds attempt mainly words with consonants that fall within their productive range. The relationship between the number of different consonants produced and the appropriate use of consonant phones to match segments in the model further suggests that phonetic and phonological abilities are developing parallel to one another.

PHONOLOGICAL PROCESS USE AT AGE THREE

After age 3, the majority of simplifying phonological processes no longer apply regularly in most cases. The data we will describe here derive from three hours of recorded natural interaction between each of ten 36-month-old children and the child's mother (30 minutes), a familiar peer (30 minutes) and the observer (including phonological, grammatical, and cognitive probes: Vihman and Greenlee, 1987). The children were drawn from a middle-class population in California and were the same children observed weekly for seven months in the period of transition to speech (Vihman et al., 1985). Despite the socioeconomic homogeneity of the sample, wide differences were found in intelligibility, specific processes used, and phonological organization.

Intelligibility. All of the children could be clearly understood more than half the time; on average, 73 percent of their utterances were judged intelligible by three raters unfamiliar with the children, but the range was broad: 54 percent to 80 percent. As might be expected, the children judged most intelligible were generally those who made the fewest phonetic or phonological errors. Yet misarticulation and phonological process use were not the only factors contributing to unintelligible speech at this age. The children who used the highest proportion of complex sentences tended to be relatively difficult to understand. Some examples of complex sentences produced by these children:

> It's sort of necklace, but it's a string where you put beads on.
> It hurts when I crash into something.
> I can buckle 'em when people say that's alright, and then when they say that's not alright, I don't do it.

Most of the 3-year-olds were apparently unable to produce complex sentences and still speak clearly enough to be easily understood by unfamiliar adults.

Specific Processes Used. In addition to the common processes discussed earlier, the following additional processes were used by these children:

Epenthesis: addition of a consonant not present in the target word

save → [steɪv]
popsicles → ['patstɪpr̩z]

Metathesis: reordering of the consonants or syllables of the target word

xylophone → ['zaɪʌfloʊn]

Contiguous assimilation: a consonant takes on the place and/or manner of articulation of an adjacent consonant

Oscar → ['astʌ]

Reduction of variation: a gestalt-like restructuring of the syllables of a polysyllabic word or phrase: cf. Magnusson, 1983

let's don't → [ʃlɛ'lɔʔ]

Palatal fronting: a palatal is replaced by an alveolar

shy → [saɪ]

Flap deletion: a medial alveolar flap /D/ is omitted

putting → ['puɪn]
not a → ['naʌ]

Deaffrication: substitution of a stop for the affricates /tʃ/ and /dʒ/

cheese → [tiːz]
orange → ['ər̩nd]

Lateralization: flap /D/ is replaced by lateral [l]

water → ['waːli]
got it → ['gaːlɪt]

Only the substitution of interdental fricatives by other consonants (stops or other fricatives) was regularly used by all subjects. Two other processes—gliding and palatal fronting—were regularly used by over half the subjects. The remaining processes were used by no more than one to three subjects. Of the processes

Later Phonological Development

affecting sequential structure, cluster simplification was regularly used by three subjects, but the prosodic processes typical of 1-year-olds were each regularly used by only one or (in the case of consonant and syllable deletion) two of these 3-year-old subjects.

Phonological Organization: Profile of Two Three-Year-Old Girls. Earlier, we described two talkative firstborn girls, Deborah and Molly. Both had developed large vocabularies by the time they were 16 months old, but they showed different phonetic preferences and differences in phonological organization; we characterized Deborah's style as exploratory and Molly's as systematic. To what extent were the differences between the two girls present at age 3?

Both the girls were still quite talkative. Molly ranked first and Deborah fourth in average length of conversational turn at age 3 (based on interaction with their mothers). Both were also still lexically advanced, with Deborah ranking first and Molly second on a scale of lexical diversity (reflecting the number of different words used in the course of interaction with their mothers). And, with respect to phonology, they continued to diverge. Deborah was judged the most intelligible of the 10 children in the study and was found to make the next-to-least use of phonological processes (i.e., had the next-to-fewest phonological errors). Molly was third from last of the 10 children on both the intelligibility ranking and the phonological error score.

Deborah and Molly continued to differ in their respective error patterns. Deborah's errors were fairly evenly balanced between whole-word and segment change processes. She was the only 3-year-old who made relatively high use of **metathesis,** the reordering of segments. She made regular use of the segment change processes typical of the majority of the 3-year-olds (**palatal fronting, interdental fricative substitution**), and she was one of four children who did not replace liquids with glides. All of Molly's whole-word errors were sporadic or rare, as was true of the group as a whole, but she had a great many more cluster and segment errors than Deborah had. She was one of the three children who often, although inconsistently, reduced Cl-clusters.

What kind of comparison can be made with the specific phonetic preferences exhibited by these children at age 1 (see Chapter 2)? Several of the phonetic preferences seen at age 1 are no longer present at age 3. For example, place of articulation errors were rare at this age and were not made by Deborah or Molly. At age 1, Deborah made unusually extensive use of fricatives, yet at age 3, it was Molly, not Deborah, who showed relatively high accuracy in fricative use. On the other hand, Molly was exceptional at age 1 in her high use of final consonants, yet it was Deborah, not Molly, who showed no tendency to delete final consonants at age 3. In general, the specific phonetic tendencies found at age 1 seemed to be unrelated to the phonological errors made at age 3 (Vihman and Greenlee, 1987).

Turning to the question of phonological organization, the chief difference between Deborah and Molly at age 3 was Deborah's willingness to abbreviate words and to slur or scramble segments (e.g., ['dalfoz]~[du'ralfoz] for *Rudolfo's*), despite her relatively accurate production of individual consonants. Molly made relatively few errors affecting the structure of the word as a whole, yet she was unintelligible some of the time because of her difficulty with a number of individual consonants (especially /l/, /r/, and /ʃ/). Recall that Molly's systematic approach to phonological learning was expressed in (1) her highly constrained choice of words—rarely attempting fricatives, in particular (whereas Deborah attempted a wider range of sound patterns), and (2) the unusually low degree of variability across different tokens of the same word. In general, the children who, like Molly, were relatively more constrained in their word selection patterns at age 1 were very likely to make little use of whole-word processes at age 3; and those who, like Deborah, explored a wide range of sounds at age 1 were also more likely to delete consonants and syllables, assimilate consonants, and change the order of segments in a word at age 3. Furthermore, there was a tendency for children whose word shapes were more variable at age 1 to make more *inconsistent* use of phonological processes at age 3 (Vihman and Greenlee, 1987). In summary, Deborah's phonological style at both ages was typical of more *exploratory* children, those with a high "tolerance for variability" (Kamhi, Catts, and Davis, 1984), and Molly's was typical of children with a lower tolerance for variability and hence, a more systematic approach.

PROFILE OF TWO BOYS: AGES TWO, THREE, AND SIX YEARS

Klein (1985) reported the results of a longitudinal study of phonological process usage of two boys, Jason and Joshua. The boys were first recorded at ages 1;8 and 2;0, during a four-hour naturalistic play session with the investigator (see also Klein, 1981). Analyses focused on a comparison of monosyllabic versus polysyllabic productions. The boys proved similar in many ways, each attempting polysyllabic words in a little over half of their single-word productions (Jason 60 percent, Joshua 51 percent), and each matching the syllable count of the adult model in the majority of their productions. However, they differed in their more specific production strategies. Joshua tended to use consonant harmony and reduplication, while Jason typically replaced the consonants in unstressed syllables with either glottals or glides. In addition, Jason made greater use of syllable deletion than Joshua, and was thus more variable in his approach to the production of polysyllabic words. These are some examples of words produced by both boys in the course of the first recording:

Adult model	Joshua	Jason
bunny	[babi]	[bʌi]
tiger	[tada]	[daɪja]
pocketbook	[bababuk]	[paʔəwu]
motorcycle	[mumulalak]	[modaɪʔu]

At ages 3 and 6 the boys were recorded for about one hour each, including both **continuous speech,** produced during play with the same materials provided at age 2, and **single words,** produced in response to the *Photo Articulation Test* (Pendergast, Dickey, Selmar, and Soder, 1969). Analysis of these data focused on comparison of phonological process use (instances of use relative to opportunities for use in the child's productions) in single-word versus continuous speech. A "whole word accuracy" score was derived by comparing the number of error-free words with the total number of intelligible productions. Based on norms reported by Schmitt, Howard, and Schmitt (1983), Joshua was found to fall one standard deviation above the mean for his age at both ages 3 and 6, while

Later Phonological Development

Jason fell slightly more than one standard deviation below the mean for his age. At both ages the boys made many more errors in continuous speech than on single-word productions; in fact, at age 6 Joshua failed to make any errors on the articulation test, while Jason evidenced only **stopping** and **deaffrication**. In continuous speech both children sometimes deleted final consonants, stopped /ð/, and simplified consonant clusters.

The relationship between use of supraglottal consonants at age 2 and relative accuracy in phonological production at ages 3 and 6 is striking. Klein (1985) suggested that an **articulatory timing factor** may explain Jason's difficulty with the production of both affricates (or consonant clusters which pattern as **segmental units** in English) and consonant clusters in general, particularly in the flow of running speech (see Gilbert and Purves, 1977, discussed below). As Klein pointed out, the same difficulty with articulatory timing may account for Jason's earlier overuse of glottals and glides, which require less precise articulatory control than other consonants. Interestingly, Vihman and Greenlee found low use of "true consonants" (or overuse of glottals and glides) to be the best phonetic indicator at age 1 of slower phonological advance at age 3 (1987).

PHONOLOGY AND COGNITIVE STYLE

Individual differences identified in the lexical and syntactic domain are undoubtedly related to phonological strategies as well. In particular, the use of phrases rather than isolated words in the earliest stages of lexical acquisition may reflect a language-learning strategy that differs from the analytic style typically described for the firstborn children of well-educated parents. The mothers of some of the 18 children in Nelson's (1973) study of lexical acquisition reported, among the first 50 words, short phrases or formulas that appeared to be unanalyzed words for the children (e.g., *stop-it!, go-away*). Bretherton, McNew, Snyder, and Bates (1983) related the tendency to make use of such unanalyzed or partially analyzed wholes in early word combination to the acquisition of prosodic sentence contours and the imitation of whole phrases. Both Peters (1977) and Landahl (1982), who traced the transition into syntax of three children aged 12 to 24 months, picked out the early use of long, relatively unintelligible utterances as one strategy in early language acquisition, which they termed a "gestalt" (or unanalytic, holistic) approach. According to Peters (1983), the child who begins with such long phrases is focusing on the phrase or sentence, rather than the word, as an initial unit of acquisition. In such cases, the child is generally more successful at reproducing the overall intonation of the adult form than the individual segments. Instead of building up longer phrases from a growing repertoire of words, the child may gradually begin to control and produce intelligibly more and more words or syllables embedded in the longer phrasal units he or she is producing.

Attempts have been made to relate reports of the use of a "gestalt" strategy to early use of more pronouns than nouns (cf. Bloom, Lightbown, and Hood, 1975), more social or interactional words (such as *bye-bye, please*) than object words (Nelson, 1973), and more context-bound than flexible nouns (Bretherton et al., 1983). Nevertheless our understanding of the relationship between patterns of individual differences in different domains of language acquisition remains primitive. It is clear that normally developing children advance along different routes, at different rates, and with different degrees of success in different domains of language (e.g., advanced use of complex syntax along with relatively slow progress in the articulation of particular segments, such as velars or consonant clusters: cf. Vihman and Carpenter, 1984). Some of the differences reported appear to reflect such uneven development at early stages and can be expected to disappear entirely as the child masters his or her language. Other differences may reflect a preferred approach to problem solving in general and, thus, may prove to be early indicators of an individual's broad and long-lasting cognitive or learning style.

SUMMARY

Analysis of the naturally occurring conversation of 2-year-old English-speaking children revealed that open monosyllables were still the dominant production shape at this time, followed by closed monosyllables, and open or closed disyllables. Word-initial consonant clusters were used frequently as well. Stops and nasals continued to be the most common consonants; word-initial inventories were richer than word-final inventories in every consonant category except liquids. The children were more accurate in consonant production than might be expected, given their relatively incomplete inventories.

Analysis of ten 3-year-old English-speaking children engaged in natural conversation revealed that over half their speech was intelligible to outsiders. Both specific phonological errors and high use of complex sentences appeared to contribute to unintelligibility. All the children made errors involving interdental fricatives; gliding and palatal fronting were also common.

Comparison of the phonological error patterns of two 3-year-old children whose phonological development at age 1 was described earlier showed that the specific phonetic strengths they had exhibited at age 1 bore no relationship to the errors made at age 3. On the other hand, their differing approaches to phonological learning—systematic versus exploratory—manifested themselves at both ages.

Comparison of two boys across three time points, ages 2, 3 and 6 years, suggested that difficulty with articulatory timing may underlie relatively slow phonological development, and may be identifiable as early as age 1 or 2 years in the relatively high use of glottals and glides, or relatively slow mastery of supraglottal articulation.

Early use of formulas or of long, unintelligible utterances has been identified as a gestalt strategy in phonological learning. Efforts to relate this strategy to learning patterns or cognitive styles reflected in the acquisition of syntax or the lexicon remain speculative.

DEVELOPMENT OF PERCEPTION BEYOND EARLY CHILDHOOD: UNDERSTANDING RUNNING SPEECH

Perceptual issues relevant to the time when the child must construct both a repertoire of lexical forms and a store of knowledge about the sound system of the language were discussed previously. As the child becomes a more fluent speaker and enters the world of discourse with unfamiliar adults as well as peers, one challenge is to master the complex task of understanding continuous or running speech. What factors enter into that task? Do children process spoken language differently than adults?

Under ordinary circumstances, listeners do not identify isolated words but rather retrieve a message from the flow of speech. Recently, investigators have begun to study the factors affecting the perception of continuous speech, by children as well as adults. A variety of research methods have been designed to investigate the complex process by which listeners interpret speech "on-line," without taking the time to make sure of what was heard, consult a lexicon of possible words, and compare the plausibility of one word or interpretation against another.

Studies addressing the comprehension of natural, continuous speech have exploited one of two research methods: (1) **fast reaction time** tasks, in which the listener is required to shadow the input speech (Marslen-Wilson, 1985) or to monitor the speech for occurrences of particular words (identical monitoring) or of word categories (Tyler and Marslen-Wilson, 1981), or of mispronunciations deliberately included in ongoing sentences or stories (Cole, 1981), and (2) the **gating** task, developed by Grosjean (1980), in which listeners are presented with successively longer fragments of a word (either isolated or in sentential context), and are required to respond at each new increment with a guess as to what word they are hearing.

Recognizing spoken words is thought to involve integrating two different sources of information (Tyler and Frauenfelder, 1987): (1) **sensory input,** or "bottom-up" (phonetic) information, deriving from the speech signal itself; and (2) **contextual constraints,** or "top-down" information, deriving from the speaker's knowledge of what has already been said, what might plausibly follow, what semantic and syntactic structures the language allows, and what words the language makes available, given the unfolding message.

Experimental evidence suggests that words are typically (though not always) identified *before* sufficient acoustic-phonetic information has become available to allow all words but one to be eliminated on the basis of the sound pattern alone (Marslen-Wilson, 1987). Such "early selection" means that word recognition is based on informed guessing as well as perception. That is, the listener is continually engaged in constructing an interpretation of the incoming message, so that the more predictable a particular word is, given the conversation up to that point, the preceding sentence, or the phrase in which the word is located, the more rapidly a listener can guess or "recognize" it from a brief phonetic clue—such as the first sound or the first syllable.

In addition to the important role of context in word recognition, word frequency must also be taken into account: Experimental manipulations have shown that high-frequency words are recognized more rapidly than low-frequency words, when both provide equally good matches to the initial phonetic shape of the input and each are plausible in context.

To what extent do children resemble adults in the recognition of words in running speech? Each of the factors that enter into adult word recognition— ongoing analysis of the acoustic-phonetic signal, expectations based on the semantic, syntactic, and pragmatic context, and relative lexical familiarity—may potentially reflect a long period of development. Both increasing *experience with language* and possible changes in *processing abilities* may affect the child's capacity to carry out the complex task of interpreting running speech.

Analysis of the Phonetic Signal. Elliott, Hammer, and Evan (1987) used a **forward gating procedure** to test children, teenagers, and adults aged 70 to 85 on their recognition of highly familiar spoken monosyllabic nouns under conditions of **limited acoustic information**. The subjects were required to make a response (i.e., to guess, if the word had not yet been recognized) to each successive stimulus. The teenagers performed more successfully on this task than either the children or adults. They recognized more words and did so more rapidly. Their guesses were usually real words which were phonetically compatible with the sounds heard, whereas the children's responses sometimes failed to match the phonetic stimuli. These results are consistent with the hypothesis, advanced by Walley (1984), that children require more acoustic information to identify stimuli than do teenagers or adults.

Cole and his colleagues (Cole and Jakimik, 1980; Cole and Perfetti, 1980) used a mispronunciation task to compare the processing of continuous speech by children and adults. The subjects' reaction times are assumed to reflect the time it takes to (1) identify the intended or target word (e.g., *pajamas*), and (2) note the acoustic mismatch (e.g., /pədaməz/ or "padamas"). By manipulating both the words and their sentence context, Cole has tested several hypotheses about the process of word recognition in context. Cole's work supports three major theoretical assumptions regarding the process of decoding or recognizing words in running speech.

1. Words are recognized through the *interaction* of sound perception and linguistic and pragmatic knowledge.

2. Words are typically recognized *in order*. As each word is recognized, it allows the listener to establish word boundaries. In addition, each decoded word imposes syntactic and semantic constraints on the following words, which enables the listener to progressively narrow the field of possible interpretations.

For example, after decoding the word *picnic*, the listener is well prepared for a word like *basket*. When the phonetic pattern [pʰæskət] is heard instead, a mispronunciation is quickly identified. When [pʰæskət] follows a word with which *basket* is less likely to be combined—such as *plastic*—the mispronunciation is detected less rapidly.

3. Words are decoded sequentially, using earlier-occurring sounds to narrow the range of possible candidates. Adults have been found to detect errors in second syllables more rapidly than in first syllables, presumably because the target word has already been identified when the mispronounced second-syllable error is heard. Similarly, mispronunciations in the second syllable of words beginning with relatively unusual first syllables (e.g., *sham-*) are recognized more rapidly than those in words with common first syllables (*com-*), presumably because the set of possible lexical matches can more quickly be narrowed to one. On the other hand, mispronounced word-final consonants are less likely to be detected than mispronounced word-initial consonants. This likely reflects the limited attention paid to the end of a word, even under the special circumstances of a mispronunciation-detecting task.

In three experiments with 4- and 5-year-old children and adults, Cole (1981) investigated the effects of word-position, consonant substituted, and phonotactic structure, or permissible versus impermissible consonant clusters, on the detection of mispronunciations in running speech. The children were tested on familiar songs and nursery rhymes. The main results were:

1. The children averaged about 50 percent detection in word-initial position; in medial position, detection fell to 25 percent, and in final position, to 12 percent. Adult detection frequencies were 95 percent, 86 percent, and 71 percent, respectively, in the three word-positions. Thus, the children, like the adults, paid most attention to initial position and least to final position.

2. In word-initial position, children were most sensitive to changes in place of articulation of stops and to changes of stop to nasal and of voiced to voiceless stop. Interchanges among nasals, fricatives, or liquids were less often detected. Most easily detected were common articulatory substitutions of a stop for a fricative. In a follow-up study, Bernthal, Greenlee, Eblen, and Marking (1987) also found that **developmental substitutions** were more easily detected than nondevelopmental substitutions by normally developing and misarticulating 4- to 6-year-old children as well as by adults.

Cole and Perfetti (1980) reported one important difference between children and adults: Though the children, like adults, detected errors more readily in words predictable from the context (an advantage of about 14 percent, across all ages), they failed to identify second-syllable errors more readily than first-syllable errors. This difference may mean that, unlike adults, children put off deciding which word was intended until they have heard several syllables. Such a strategy seems reasonable for listeners who, to some extent, lack confidence in their ability to recognize words. In other words, if a great many words in adult conversation are still unfamiliar, it is easy to see why children would be slower to settle on a lexical interpretation.

Contextual Effects. Tyler and Marslen-Wilson (1981) investigated the role of discourse and of syntactic context alone on the comprehension of running speech by children aged 5, 7, and 10 years. Children were tested on two tasks, **identical monitoring,** in which the occurrence of a particular word is to be noted as soon as it is spoken, and **category monitoring,** in which a word belonging to a particular category (body part, fruit, furniture) is to be identified when heard. The target words fell toward the end of the second of a pair of sentences of one of three kinds: normal prose, in which the first sentence provides a normal discourse context for the second; syntactic prose, in which the sentences are anomalous in meaning but syntactically correct; and random word order, which violates both semantic and syntactic structure and thus provides no contextual support for word recognition. Examples (with the target word in boldface):

> John had to go back home. He had fallen out of the swing and had hurt his **hand** on the ground. (normal)
>
> John had to sit on the shop. He had lived out of the kitchen and had enjoyed his **hand** in the mud. (syntactic)
>
> The on sit shop to had John. He lived had and kitchen the out his of had enjoyed **hand** mud in the. (random)

The results suggested that children as young as age 5 are able to make good use of discourse and even of syntactic context: Mean reaction times decreased significantly with age, but all three groups showed a marked facilitatory effect from the normal discourse, and a lesser effect from normal syntax only. The category monitoring task was considerably more difficult for the children than the identical monitoring task. The normal discourse context again aided recognition, but the semantically anomalous "syntactic" sentence sequences gave no significant advantage in this case.

Another study suggested that children's ability to make use of **semantic knowledge** continues to improve up to as late as age 15. Elliott (1979) tested 24 children at each of four age levels (11, 13, 15, and 17 years) on their understanding of sentences against a background of multitalker babble. The test sentences were designed to fall into two groups: **high predictability** and **low predictability**—a function of the presence or absence of two or three semantically related "pointer" words that could help cue the listener as to the identity of the final (target) word, always a monosyllabic noun. The test consisted of 25 sentences of each type; none was longer than 8 syllables. The subject's task was to repeat back the last word of the sentence.

Under just one set of conditions, when the target sentence was presented at the same intensity as the noise, a significant age trend was found, with the 11- and 13-year-olds performing less well on high-predictability sentences than the 15- and 17-year-olds, who did about as well as young adults tested earlier with written responses. No age differences were found in quiet or in comprehension of the low-predictability sentences. A later test of 9-year-old children showed significantly poorer performance than that of the 11-year-olds. The age-related differences are not a direct auditory effect since only the high-predictability sentences proved easier for older subjects. Rather, the difference appears to reflect the extent to which children of different ages were able to use the semantic information in the pointer syllables to guess at the final, difficult-to-hear, target noun.

Lexical Familiarity. Cole and Perfetti (1980) reported a significant difference between children and adults in the detection of mispronunciations in a simple, clearly articulated story: On average, preschool children (ages 4 to 5) detected about 50 percent of the mispronounced words, children kindergarten through fifth grade about 60 percent, and adults 95 percent. Cole and Perfetti suggested that children probably treat mispronunciations as unfamiliar words: "It seems likely that children learn to tolerate (or actively ignore) unfamiliar words, so that each occurrence of an unfamiliar word does not result in a breakdown of the comprehension process" (313).

It is important to note that the children detected mispronunciations in isolated words (95 percent) far more readily than in fluent speech. The high detection rate for isolated words is due in part to their slower articulation, and also to the cues provided by pictures that accompanied the test words. This procedure is commonly used in clinical tests of phonetic discrimination, and therefore, the tests may overestimate children's ability to perceive phonetic differences in the course of conversational speech (Cole, 1981).

The issue of **word familiarity** itself has also received attention. Walley and Metsala (1990) used mispronunciation tasks to test children aged 5 and 8. Subjective age-of-acquisition ratings were used to categorize test words as "early," "current," and "late." The familiarity factor proved to be important: Young children were more likely to detect mispronunciations in early and current words.

Furthermore, the children were biased toward identifying late (or for age 5, both late and current) words as mispronounced—including words which were correctly pronounced ("intact" words). Thus, whereas the subjects in Cole and Perfetti (1980) were found to treat mispronounced words as unfamiliar, Walley and Metsala showed through analysis of "false alarms" that their subjects were reluctant to treat unfamiliar words as intact, and preferred to label them mispronounced. These results call to mind the biasing role of familiarity in early tests of linguistic perception, mentioned in Chapter 2 (Barton, 1976; Clumeck, 1982). They are reminiscent also of several anecdotes reported in Vihman (1981: 248), in which preschool children misperceived unfamiliar words as relatively more familiar ones, disregarding the fact that their interpretation was at odds with the ongoing discourse context.

SUMMARY

Word recognition is a complex process, involving the integration of both the sensory input, or acoustic–phonetic signal, and contextual information, including both pragmatic and general knowledge-based inferences regarding the gist of the incoming message and specific structural effects relating to the phonotactic, syntactic, and semantic restrictions characteristic of the language code. The listener's lexical expectations are also influenced by word frequency.

On the whole, school-age children process continuous speech in an adult-like way, making use of context to aid in the interpretation of the acoustic signal. Also, developmental mispronunciations are more salient than other consonant substitutions to children as young as age 4 as well as to adults. In several respects children are different from adults, however. They appear to need more acoustic information before they commit themselves to a decision as to word identity, perhaps because so many words continue to be unfamiliar, at least up to the teens. Furthermore, their use of semantic knowledge as a clue to the unfolding message is not fully developed until the teen years. Finally, school-age children, like younger children, perceive familiar words more accurately than unfamiliar words, and take a cautious approach to apparent mispronunciations in running speech.

PRODUCTION IN THE SCHOOL-AGE CHILD: CONTINUING CHANGE

In characterizing the phonological production of 3-year-olds, we noted that the majority of simplifying phonological processes no longer apply at that age although consonant clusters are still frequently reduced and certain segment types (especially fricatives and liquids) continue to be substituted by other segments. According to the normative articulation data presented in Figure 7–1, half of the children tested had succeeded in using all of the relevant sounds correctly by age 4, but for fricatives and liquids, correct production by 90 percent of the children was achieved only later. Hodson and Paden (1981) reported that articulation by the 60 normally developing 4-year-old children they tested closely resembled that of adults.

It is reasonable, then, to ask whether phonetic and phonological acquisition can be said to be complete for most normally developing children by the time they reach school age. With respect to basic articulatory mastery and intelligibility outside the family, the answer is probably yes. It is important to note, however, that both phonetic and phonological variation and change continue in a number of respects, not only beyond early childhood but also throughout a person's life span. We will illustrate this point by briefly discussing three areas of continuing change: (1) temporal coordination of speech production, (2) phonological reorganization under the influence of literacy, and (3) phonetic and phonological influence from the peer group.

TEMPORAL COORDINATION OF SPEECH PRODUCTION

Smith (1978) inferred from durational measurements that segment and word production by 2- and 4-year-old children was consistently slower than adult productions of the same forms. However, the proportional relationships between segments were much like those of adults: For example, final syllables and stressed syllables tended to be longer than non-final and unstressed syllables; voiceless stops were longer than voiced stops while vowels were shorter before the (longer) voiceless stops. Smith concluded that children possess quite sophisticated timing-control systems, despite their still immature neuromuscular control capacities (as reported for other aspects of motor performance, such as reaction time in general, maximum rate of syllable repetition, and maximum finger-tapping rate).

A gradual increase in rate of articulation with age was reported by Hulme, Thomson, Muir, and Lawrence (1984). They tested children aged 3 to 4, 7 to 8, and 10 to 11 as well as adults on their maximum rate of repetition of one-, two-, and three- or four-syllable words. They found an increase in speech rate with age, as well as a tendency for subjects to repeat short words more quickly than long ones, but with less difference in rate for different word lengths in the younger subjects. Hulme et al. were not primarily interested in speech rate per se, however, but in the possible relationship between speech rate—and, hence, maximum potential rate for verbal *rehearsal*—and short-term memory. Their results showed a close connection between increases in verbal short-term memory and speech rate. They viewed this finding as strong support for the hypothesis that verbal short-term memory "is a time-based system limited by the amount of speech which it can store" (251): See Baddeley, Thomson, and Buchanan (1975); Baddeley (1986).

A number of studies of children's speech production have addressed the question of the timing of individual segments embedded in clusters, syllables, and words. There is evidence that word-initial clusters may first be represented as single consonants combining features of both the consonants in the cluster (cf., e.g., Menyuk, 1972). Only later is the cluster "unpacked" into its separate component segments. Gilbert and Purves (1977) pointed out that the level at which the child represents the cluster as a single segment—in perception, in the production plan, or only in the execution of the plan—is not clear. If, for example, the child perceives the cluster but cannot produce the segments sequentially, the problem could be purely articulatory (difficulty with the timing and/or motor control of the separate articulatory gestures), or it could reflect difficulty in applying the appropriate "segmentalization rules," that is, in sorting out the (overlapping) articulatory gestures (at the planning level) to achieve the proper sequential output. It has been hypothesized that the child may be constrained at first by a **timing-dominant system,** in which a rigid time schedule governs the execution of artic-

Later Phonological Development

ulatory gestures (cf. Ohala, 1970; Hawkins, 1973). As the timing-dominant system is gradually replaced by an **articulation-dominant** system, the limited time constraints are relaxed, leading to slower but more accurate speech production.

Results from detailed analyses of children's productions tend to support such a developmental sequence. Hawkins (1973) measured consonant durations based on production by seven children aged 4 to 7. Comparing her findings with results reported for adults, Hawkins found that in clusters, /l/ tended to be longer in the children's speech. There was, however, no apparent age trend in her data. Hawkins suggested that once the child is able to produce "acceptable but not necessarily mature forms" of particular sounds or sequences of sounds, speech production may remain essentially unchanged for several years (perhaps until puberty) (204).

Gilbert and Purves (1977) tested four groups of five children, one group each at age 5, 7, 9, and 11, and five adults on the production of closed monosyllables, beginning with /s/, /f/, /l/, /w/, /sl/, /fl/, and /sw/, to determine the relative duration of the fricatives, liquids, and glides as singletons and as part of a cluster. They found greater variation in duration values in the younger children's productions. Like Hawkins (1973), they also found that the only significant timing differences across age groups involved clusters with /l/. In adult production, consonants are shorter when combined in a cluster. Five-year-olds failed to shorten /l/ appropriately; they produced a longer /l/ after fricatives. For the remaining age groups, there was a progressive decrease in the duration of /l/ in clusters, as compared with singleton /l/, up to age 11, when the relative durations were about the same as those for adults. The positional differences in duration, however, were not significant.

In the view of Gilbert and Purves, these results reflected a late stage in the acquisition of consonant clusters. At first, /l/ is likely to be omitted. Later, some children "split" the cluster, producing *blue* (/blu/) as [belu]. This may reflect the child's attempt to circumvent the constraints of a timing-dominant system: Since the child lacks the articulatory control needed to produce the cluster within a single syllabic unit, an additional syllable is produced. Gilbert and Purves' data suggest that the elongation of the /l/ may represent a further stage in the splitting process. As the child's timing control improves, the lengthening of /l/ is no longer needed.

In another study involving timing, Gilbert and Johnson (1978) tested eleven 6-year-old children on the (imitative) production of 73 polysyllabic words containing the syllable C/jul/ (as in *ambulance, ridiculous*). Since most of the words were unfamiliar to the children, they could be considered the equivalent of nonsense words.

Correct production of the C/jul/ segment (in *folliculous*, for example) characterized only 14 percent of the tokens. The remaining tokens generally displayed one of four (cumulative) error patterns: (1) unrounding (sometimes with reduction) of the vowel, to [ɪ] or [ə] (13 percent), (2) with glide deletion ([kɪ], [kəɪ]: 24 percent), (3) with methathesis ([klɪ]: 23 percent), and (4) with vowel deletion ([kl]: 7 percent). In adult production, the duration of the first two syllables is slightly less than that of the last two (43 percent : 57 percent of total duration). This ratio typically was maintained in the children's productions as well, despite a tendency toward greater shortening of the last two syllables with each cumulative error type. In the case of the last error type, the ratio is reversed (54 percent : 46 percent).

Although all of the subjects tested could produce the component segments of the C/jul/ sequence in isolation, production of these segments within the sequence and time constraints posed by a long word proved difficult. Gilbert and Johnson contend that it is the relation between syllable durations that must be modified as the child learns the articulatory program for a new polysyllabic word.

In summary, studies of timing problems posed by the production of consonants in clusters and in long words have shown that school-age children, although able to produce acceptably adult-like speech, are continuing to develop fluency in the planning and production of complex sequences of sounds.

PHONOLOGICAL REORGANIZATION: THE INFLUENCE OF LITERACY

Linguistic theory in this century has strongly emphasized the primacy of oral as opposed to written language. As a corollary, it is typically assumed that the unconscious systemic knowledge which underlies productive language use derives solely from the learning of oral language in early childhood. Yet in a literate society, individuals spend many of their formative years learning to read, to write, to spell, and to alphabetize. Indeed, as Ferguson (1968) has pointed out, spoken language changes in subtle ways as a society becomes literate, as indicated, for example, by the sporadic occurrence of spelling pronunciations (such as /'fɔr'hɛd/ in lieu of /'fɔrɪd/ for *forehead*; /'ɔftən/ in lieu of /'ɔfən/ for *often*). It is likely that what children are taught in school "reshapes the psychological structures . . . built up previously, so that what is psychologically real for literate speakers includes at least some of what they have been taught about their language" (Jaeger, 1984; 22). Three types of studies have investigated the role of literacy in forcing a restructuring of phonological knowledge. These studies have focused on (1) knowledge of the vowel alternations partially reflected in the English spelling system, (2) the influence of spelling on perception and production, and (3) differences in lexical organization between children and adults.

Knowledge of Vowel Alternations. In their highly influential work *The Sound Pattern of English*, Chomsky and Halle (1968) posited a set of phonological rules to capture the systematic relationship between different vowels that is reflected in such word-pairs as *divine–divinity* (/ai:ɪ/), *serene–serenity* (/i:ɛ/), *profane–profanity* (/ey:æ/), *cone–conical* (/ow:a/), *lose–lost* (/u:ɔ,a/), *profound–profundity* (/aw:ʌ/). These and other phonological rules in Chomsky and Halle's account have been said to reflect psychologically real patterns of alternation; that is, it is assumed that speakers will unconsciously apply these rules to new words fitting into the same pattern. But this particular set of rules, which reflects a historical sound change known as the Great English Vowel Shift (fourteenth to seventeenth century), is no longer productive or transparent in present-day English, since many words entered the lexicon *after* the shift took place and now participate in other alternations (e.g., *retain–retention* (/e:ɛ/), *genteel–gentility* (/i:ɪ/). Jaeger (1984) reviewed a series of psycholinguistic tests carried out on adults and children in an effort to probe the psychological reality of the vowel shift rule for English speakers.

Moskowitz (1973) obtained positive results on a concept formation task used in testing children aged 9 to 12 on knowledge of the vowel shift alternations. She concluded, however, that these results were based on the children's knowledge of *spelling rules* rather than of the phonological rules underlying derived words that were still largely unfamiliar to them. Jaeger (1984) followed up on Moskowitz's suggestion with a concept formation task carefully designed to distinguish between responses based on the vowel shift alternations and responses based on spelling rules. The crucial patterns involved the pair /aw/–/ʌ/, in which the alternations are not spelled with the same letter, and /u/–/ʌ/, in which the alternations are spelled with *u* (as in *reduce–reduction*) but are not part of the vowel shift rule. Jaeger trained 15 adults to respond positively to English words reflecting the vowel shift alternations and negatively to other derivationally related word-pairs exhibiting other phonological relationships, such as tense–lax (*retain–retention, peace–pacify*), or the same vowel (*promise–promissory*). She then tested subjects with new word-pairs exhibiting these two types of relationships as well as pairs belonging to the two critical categories (/aw/–/ʌ/ or /u/–/ʌ/). The results were clear. Pairs containing the critical spelling-based pair /u/–/ʌ/ were generally accepted, while pairs containing the irregular vowel shift pair /aw/–/ʌ/ were generally rejected. Later interviews with the subjects further confirmed a tendency to rely on the spelling rule, as when the training category was described by one subject as "a long and a short version of the same vowel." Jaeger concluded that "certain entities can be psychologically real either because they have been brought to speakers' conscious attention as part of their education or because they have been intuited from the orthographic system of their language" (34).

Influence of Spelling on Perception and Production. Ehri (1984) reviewed the various ways in which learning to read and spell have been found to affect children's competence in the production and perception of speech. In Ehri's view, "the full representational system offered by printed language is acquired and stored in memory during acquisition" (123), including both the whole-word ("lexical") gestalt and the segmental ("phonetic") letter-sound correspondences that characterize each word. Specifically, Ehri maintains that in the course of learning to read, the "alphabetic" or "orthographic" image of a word is *added* to the store of information associated with each item in the mental lexicon. The orthographic image is integrated with other information about a word as printed words are read and understood in context. Gradually, orthographic representations come to stand for a word's meaning as well as its form and to be as intimately associated with the word as are the phonological, semantic, and syntactic aspects of its identity. (For words acquired later, through reading, the orthographic image may even be established *before* the actual oral pronunciation is known.)

Ehri's experimental investigations on the effect of orthography on perception and production have led to a number of interesting results. She found that knowledge of spelling helps children to detect and accurately segment out the sounds embedded in words. For example, through spelling children become aware of extra syllabic segments (e.g., in words like *different, comfortable, decimal*). On the other hand, knowledge of spelling may also misleadingly influence perception, as in the case of the English alveolar flap /D/ (as in *latter* or *ladder*), which children typically hear as /d/ until they learn that many words containing the flap are spelled with *t*. Surprisingly, knowledge of related words in which the flap is realized as /t/ or /d/ (*sit–sitting, ride–riding*) was not found to affect perception.

In a series of studies of older children, Templeton (1979, 1983; Templeton and Scarborough-Franks, 1985) established that knowledge of the complex phonological alternations between derivationally related English words, such as those investigated by Moskowitz and Jaeger, continues to increase at least through grade 10 and is typically acquired through *prior* learning of the more transparent orthographic relationship between these words. Templeton and Scarborough-Franks pointed out that it is easier to relate complex derived English words through spelling than through verbal production for two reasons: The derivational stem is more stable in orthography than in surface phonetics, and the processes which must be applied to relate the base and derived forms of the word are also less complex (compare the spelling and pronunciation shifts needed to relate *incline* and *inclination*, for example). These authors concluded that the subjects in their study (both "good" and "poor" spellers, in grades 6 and 10) had abstracted the orthographic patterns associated with such words by the end of elementary school, but in grade 10 they were still in the process of abstracting the patterns in pronunciation (so that they could be automatically applied to the production of novel forms, for example: see also Jaeger, 1986).

Differences in Lexical Organization. The study of malapropisms (e.g., *ornaments* or *monuments* in lieu of *condiments*), or the mistaken production of one word in lieu of another, can shed light on the organization of the mental lexicon. Aitchison and Straf (1981) analyzed 680 malapropisms, almost a third of which were produced by children (aged 12 or under). Separate analysis of the adult and child malapropisms in comparison with their target words was carried out with respect to number of syllables, stress pattern, initial and final consonant, and identity of the stressed vowel. The results for adults and children were then compared. The child malapropisms were found to be as close to the targets as those produced by adults. For both adults and children, the number of syllables, initial consonant, and stressed vowel all were likely to match the target. Where all three were not retained, adults were most likely to produce the same initial consonant (e.g., *acapulco* in place of *acupuncture:* 77 percent), whereas children were more likely to retain the number of syllables (e.g., *naughty story* in place of *multi-story* [*car-park*]: 84 percent, vs. 68 percent for adults) and least likely to retain the initial consonant (57 percent). Stress pattern largely correlated with number of syllables for both adults and children. Although final consonants were retained more or less equally often by adults (e.g., *jungle* for *conjugal:* 72 percent) and children (e.g., *faint* for *fête:* 68 percent), the initial consonant was more often retained than the final consonant in the adult data; children retained the final consonant (marginally) more often than the initial consonant. In longer words, the final consonant was especially likely to be preserved by both children and adults, perhaps because of the derivational suffixes in which target and malapropism often matched (especially in the adult data where about 50 percent of the malapropisms included a suffix: Recall the errors for *condiments*).

Aitchison and Straf (1981) suggested five interacting factors to account for the differences between adult and child lexical retrieval and storage:

1. Children may pay more attention to perceptually salient aspects of words, such as rhythm (i.e., *giggle* for *wriggle, fascination* for *vaccination*).
2. Children appear to pay more attention to word endings (cf. Slobin, 1973) and, perhaps consequently, less attention to initial consonants.
3. Consonant harmony, a preference for open syllables, and a tendency to alter unstressed syllables appear to affect older children's memory for unfamiliar words, just as they affect word production in younger children and perhaps for

the same reasons (cf. Aitchison and Chiat, 1981, who implicate "faulty perception," or incomplete representation, together with memory overload to account for the role of phonological processes in both younger and older children).

4. Literacy and experience with dictionaries may enhance the importance of initial consonants for adults.

5. Growth in importance of word beginnings may accompany growth in vocabulary since the high frequency of derivational affixes in more sophisticated English vocabulary renders attention to word endings relatively inefficient as a way of differentiating between words.

In summary, the analysis of adult and child malapropisms reveals some of the salient features that must characterize words in the mental lexicon since these features influence word retrieval. Rhythmic structure and word endings are salient from early childhood (cf. Vihman, 1981); with schooling, experience with dictionary and library work, and the growth of a more abstract, derived lexicon, the importance of the initial consonant increases. An experimental study of ninety 5- to 9-year-olds showed that, at those ages, the consonants of the stressed syllable were still more likely to be recalled than the initial consonant (Aitchison and Chiat, 1981). It is not clear at what age the shift to a preferential reliance on initial consonants begins to affect lexical retrieval.

INFLUENCE FROM THE PEER GROUP

In the introduction to Chapter 2, we mentioned that by the time children are speaking clearly enough to be understood outside the family, their speech patterns will have been stamped with the phonetically distinguishing features of the language of their home community. Yet phonetic and phonological development do not come to an end at this point. An extensive sociolinguistic study by Payne (1975, 1980) demonstrated the influence of the peer group on both the phonetic and the phonological levels after the period of early childhood.

In order to investigate ongoing linguistic change, Payne designed a study to observe the speech patterns of a large number of children who had moved from one dialect area to another. By noting the age at which the children moved to the new community as well as their length of stay there, she was able to roughly distinguish between parental and peer influence.

Payne carried out her investigation in King of Prussia, a small middle-class community on the outskirts of Philadelphia that had become a thriving industrial center attracting a large number of recent arrivals. She interviewed some 200 families, making contact through children playing on the block and through church leaders, and finally, extended her investigation to the school where some 50 groups of children were interviewed, including 10 of the children originally approached in the family context. Payne (1975) presented in detail the acquisition of the Philadelphia dialect by one family of four children that had moved to the area from New York five years earlier; the children were aged 8, 10, 11, and 13 at the time of the study.

Payne concentrated her analysis on seven specific vowel patterns that characterize the "stable, central core" of the Philadelphia dialect; these patterns include three phonological differences with other dialects of English (splitting or merger of classes of phonemically distinct vowels; for example, the stressed vowels of *merry–Murray* and *ferry–furry* are merged) and four phonetic differences,

FIGURE 3–1. **Peer group influence. Number of years the Morgan children have spent under King of Prussia peer-group influence versus New York City and parental influence.** From A. Payne, "The Reorganization of Linguistic Rules: A Preliminary Report." *Pennsylvania Working Papers on Linguistic Change and Variation, 2*, 1975. Used with permission.

in which the phonemic structure is not affected (e.g., the nucleus of /oy/ is raised to [u]).

Payne found that the phonetic variables had all been acquired by all of the children, whereas the phonological variables were only incompletely acquired. Furthermore, she found a correlation for the three older children between degree of acquisition of the Philadelphia dialect and number of years spent under the influence of the King of Prussia peer group. The youngest child, Mike, aged 3 on arrival in the new area, showed about the same degree of influence as the oldest child, Richard (aged 8 on arrival). Liz (aged 6 on arrival) showed more influence and Dan (aged 5 on arrival) showed full acquisition of the phonological and phonetic variables. Payne explained this pattern of dialect change in terms of the proportion of a child's peer-influence years (from about 4 to 14) spent in the new dialect area (see Figure 3–1). Liz and Dan had spent a larger proportion of their peer-influence years in King of Prussia than had Richard, and they showed it by sounding more like Philadelphians; Mike was presumably too young to be influenced by peers for two of the five years he had spent in the area at the time of the study.

Although Payne (1975) reported results for only a single family, she noted that observation of the community as a whole supports the generality and consistency of the pattern of findings reported. Payne's study suggests that the dialect a child learns from his or her parents can change almost completely in later years under the influence of peers (but see Deser, 1991).

SUMMARY

Phonetic and phonological variation and change continue at least into the school-age years. Difficulties with the precise timing of sequential articulatory gestures continue to be smoothed out over a period of several years. The learning of a written language supplies a visual-spatial model for speech that is internalized as a representational system in memory (Ehri, 1984). Once children begin learning to read and spell, they acquire an important added dimension of language that subtly affects many aspects of language processing and use. Lexical organization, as revealed by lexical selection errors, is also influenced by literacy skills and by the growth, associated with advancing education, of the derived-word vocabulary. Finally, language in the school-age years comes under strong peer influence. Where parental and peer dialects differ in this period the peer norm is likely to triumph.

Later Phonological Development

REFERENCES

NOTE: References cited in both Chapter 2 and Chapter 3 are listed only in Chapter 2.

Aitchison, J., and S. Chiat, "Natural phonology or natural memory? The interaction between phonological processes and recall mechanisms." *Language and Speech, 24* (1981): 311–326.

Aitchison, J., and M. Straf, "Lexical storage and retrieval: A developing skill?" In A. Cutler (Ed.), *Slips of the Tongue and Language Production*. Amsterdam, The Netherlands: Mouton, 1981.

Allen, G.D., "How the young French child avoids the pre-voicing problem for word-initial voiced stops." *Journal of Child Language, 12* (1985): 37–46.

Arlt, P.B., and M.J. Goodban, "A comparative study of articulation acquisition as based on a study of 240 normals, aged three to six." *Language, Speech, and Hearing Services in Schools, 7* (1976): 173–180.

Baddeley, A., *Working Memory*. Oxford: Clarendon Press, 1986.

Baddeley, A.D., N. Thomson, and M. Buchanan, "Word length and the structure of short-term memory." *Journal of Verbal Learning and Verbal Behavior, 14* (1975): 575–589.

Barton, D., and M.A. Macken, "An instrumental analysis of the voicing contrast in word-initial stops in the speech of four-year-old English-speaking children." *Language and Speech, 23* (1980): 159–169.

Berman, R.A., "Natural phonological processes at the one-word stage." *Lingua, 43* (1977): 1–21.

Bernthal, J.E., M. Greenlee, R. Eblen, and K. Marking, "Detection of mispronunciations: A comparison of adults, normal speaking children and children with articulation errors." *Applied Psycholinguistics, 8* (1987): 209–222.

Bloom, L., P. Lightbown, and L. Hood, *Structure and variation in child language*. Monograph of the Society for Research in Child Development, 160. Chicago: University of Chicago Press, 1975.

Bretherton, I., S. McNew, L. Snyder, and E. Bates, "Individual differences at 20 months: Analytic and holistic strategies in language acquisition." *Journal of Child Language, 10* (1983): 293–320.

Bricker, W.A., "Errors in the echoic behavior of preschool children." *Journal of Speech and Hearing Research, 10* (1967): 67–76.

Chomsky, N., and M. Halle, *The Sound Pattern of English*. New York: Harper & Row, 1968.

Clark, E.V., and M. Bowerman, "On the acquisition of final voiced stops." In J.A. Fishman, A. Tabouret-Keller, M. Clyne, Bh. Krishnamurti, and M. Abdulaziz (Eds.), *The Fergusonian Impact*, Vol 1. *From Phonology to Society*. Berlin: Mouton de Gruyter, 1986.

Clumeck, H., D. Barton, M.A. Macken, and D.A. Huntington, "The aspiration contrast in Cantonese word-initial stops: Data from children and adults." *Journal of Chinese Linguistics, 9* (1981): 210–224.

Cole, R.A., "Perception of fluent speech by children and adults." In H.B. Winitz (Ed.), *Native Language and Foreign Language Acquisition*. New York: New York Academy of Sciences, 1981.

Cole, R.A., and J. Jakimik, "A model of speech perception." In R.A. Cole (Ed.), *Perception and Production of Fluent Speech*. Hillsdale, N.J.: Lawrence Erlbaum, 1980.

Cole, R.A., and C.A. Perfetti, "Listening for mispronunciations in a children's story: The use of context by children and adults." *Journal of Verbal Learning and Verbal Behavior, 19* (1980): 297–315.

Deser, T., "Dialect transmission and variation: An acoustic analysis of vowels in six urban Detroit families." Ph.D. thesis, Boston University, 1990. (Reprinted by the Indiana University Linguistics Club, 1991.)

Edwards, M.L., "Patterns and processes in fricative acquisition: Longitudinal evidence from six English-learning children." Ph.D. thesis, Stanford University, 1979.

Ehri, L.C., "How orthography alters spoken language competencies in children learning to read and spell." In J. Downing and R. Valtin (Eds.), *Language Awareness and Learning to Read*. New York: Springer-Verlag, 1984.

Eilers, R.E., D.K. Oller, and C.R. Benito-Garcia, "The acquisition of voicing contrasts in Spanish and English learning infants and children: A longitudinal study." *Journal of Child Language, 11* (1984): 313–336.

Elliott, L.L., "Performance of children aged 9–17 years on a test of speech intelligibility in noise using sentence material with controlled word predictability." *Journal of the Acoustic Society of America, 66* (1979): 651–653.

Elliott, L.L., M.A. Hammer, and K.E. Evan, "Perception of gated, highly familiar spoken monosyllabic nouns by children, teenagers, and older adults." *Perception and Psychophysics, 42* (1987): 150–157.

Fee, J., and D. Ingram, "Reduplication as a strategy of phonological development." *Journal of Child Language, 9* (1982): 41–54.

Ferguson, C.A., "Language development." In J.A. Fishman, J. Das Gupta, and C.A. Ferguson (Eds.), *Language Problems of Developing Nations*. New York: John Wiley, 1968.

Ferguson, C.A., "Fricatives in child language acquisition." In L. Hellman (Ed.), *Proceedings of the Eleventh International Congress of Linguists*. Bologna: Mulino, 1975. (Also in V. Honsa and M.H. Hardman-Bautista (Eds.), *Papers on Linguistics and Child Language*. The Hague: Mouton, 1978.)

Ferguson, C.A., "Reduplication in child phonology." *Journal of Child Language, 10* (1983): 239–243.

Ferguson, C.A., D.B. Peizer, and T.A. Weeks, "Model-and-replica phonological grammar of a child's first words." *Lingua, 3* (1973): 35–65.

Fey, M.E., and J. Gandour, "The pig dialogue: Phonological systems in transition." *Journal of Child Language, 9* (1982): 517–519.

Gilbert, J.H.V., "A voice onset time analysis of apical stop production in 3-year-olds." *Journal of Child Language, 4* (1977): 103–110.

Gilbert, J.H.V., and C.E. Johnson, "Temporal and sequential constraints on six-year-olds' phonological productions: Some observations on the 'ambliance' phenomenon." *Journal of Child Language, 5* (1978): 101–112.

Gilbert, J.H.V., and B.A. Purves, "Temporal constraints on consonant clusters in child speech production." *Journal of Child Language, 4* (1977): 417–432.

Greenlee, M., "Interacting processes in the child's acquisition of stop-liquid clusters." *Papers and Reports on Child Language Development, 7* (1974): 85–100.

Grosjean, F., "Spoken word recognition and the gating paradigm." *Perception and Psychophysics, 28* (1980): 267–283.

Haelsig, P.C., and C.L. Madison, "A study of phonological processes exhibited by 3-, 4-, and 5-year-old children." *Language, Speech, and Hearing Services in Schools, 17* (1986): 107–114.

Hawkins, S., "Temporal coordination of consonants in the speech of children: Preliminary data." *Journal of Phonetics, 1* (1973): 181–217.

Hodson, B.W., and E.P. Paden, "Phonological processes which characterize unintelligible and intelligible speech in early childhood." *Journal of Speech and Hearing Disorders, 46* (1981): 369–373.

Hulme, C., N. Thomson, C. Muir, and A. Lawrence, "Speech rate and the development of short-term memory span." *Journal of Experimental Child Psychology, 38* (1984): 241–253.

Ingram, D., "Phonological rules in young children." *Journal of Child Language, 1* (1974): 49–64.

Ingram, D., "Phonological development: Production." In P. Fletcher and M. Garman (Eds.), *Language Acquisition: Studies in First Language Development*, 2nd ed. Cambridge (U.K.): Cambridge University Press, 1986.

Ingram, D., L. Christensen, S. Veach, and B. Webster, "The acquisition of word-initial fricatives and affricates in English by children between 2 and 6 years." In G. Yeni-Komshian, J. Kavanagh, and C.A. Ferguson (Eds.), *Child Phonology*, Vol. 2. *Production*. New York: Academic Press, 1980.

Jaeger, J.J., "Assessing the psychological status of the vowel shift rule." *Journal of Psycholinguistic Research, 13* (1984): 13–36.

Jaeger, J.J., "On the acquisition of abstract representations for English vowels." *Phonology Yearbook, 3* (1986): 71–97.

Kamhi, A.G., H.W. Catts, and M.K. Davis, "Management of sentence production demands." *Journal of Speech and Hearing Research, 27* (1984): 329–338.

Klein, H., "Productive strategies for the pronunciation of early polysyllabic lexical items." *Journal of Speech and Hearing Research, 24* (1981): 389–405.

Klein, H., "Relationship between early pronunciation processes and later pronunciation skill." *Journal of Speech and Hearing Disorders, 50* (1985): 156–165.

Landahl, K., "The onset of structured discourse: A developmental study of the acquisition of language." Ph.D. thesis, Brown University, 1982.

Lleo, C., "Homonymy and reduplication: On the extended availability of two strategies in phonological acquisition." *Journal of Child Language, 17* (1990): 267–278.

Macken, M.A., "Permitted complexity in phonological development: One child's acquisition of Spanish consonants." *Lingua, 44* (1978): 219–253.

Macken, M.A., "Aspects of the acquisition of stop systems: A cross-linguistic perspective." In G. Yeni-Komshian, J. Kavanagh, and C.A. Ferguson (Eds.), *Child Phonology*, Vol. 1. *Production*. New York: Academic Press, 1980.

Macken, M.A., and D. Barton, "The acquisition of the voicing contrast in English: A study of voice onset time in word-initial stop consonants." *Journal of Child Language, 7* (1980a): 41–74.

Macken, M.A., and D. Barton, "The acquisition of the voicing contrast in Spanish: A phonetic and phonological study of word-initial stop consonants." *Journal of Child Language, 7* (1980b): 433–458.

Macken, M.A., and C.A. Ferguson, "Phonological universals of language acquisition." In H.B. Winitz (Ed.), *Native Language and Foreign Language Acquisition*. New York: New York Academy of Sciences, 1981.

Magnusson, E., *The Phonology of Language Disordered Children: Production, Perception, and Awareness*. Travaux de l'Institut de Linguistique de Lund, 17. Lund: CWK Gleerup, 1983.

Marslen-Wilson, W.D., "Speech shadowing and speech comprehension." *Speech Communication, 4* (1985): 55–73.

Marslen-Wilson, W.D., "Functional parallelism in spoken word-recognition." In U.H. Frauenfelder and L.K. Tyler (Eds.), *Spoken Word Recognition*. Amsterdam, The Netherlands: Elsevier-Science Publishers, 1987.

Menn, L., "Phonotactic rules in beginning speech." *Lingua, 26* (1971): 225–251.

Menyuk, P., "Clusters as single underlying consonants: Evidence from children's production." *Proceedings of the Seventh International Congress of Phonetic Science, Montreal, 1971*. The Hague: Mouton, 1972.

Moskowitz, A.I., "The acquisition of fricatives: A study in phonetics and phonology." *Journal of Phonetics, 3* (1975): 141–150.

Nelson, K., *Structure and Strategy in Learning to Talk.* Monographs of the Society for Research in Child Development, 38. Chicago: University of Chicago Press, 1973.

Nettelbladt, U., *Developmental Studies of Dysphonology in Children.* Travaux de l'Institut de Linguistique de Lund, 19. Lund: CWK Gleerup, 1983.

Ohala, J.J., "Aspects of the control and production of speech." *U.C.L.A. Working Papers in Phonetics, 15,* 1970.

Oller, D.K., "Simplification as the goal of phonological processes in child speech." *Language Learning, 24* (1975): 299–303.

Payne, A., "The reorganization of linguistic rules: A preliminary report." *Pennsylvania Working Papers on Linguistic Change and Variation, 2* (1975).

Payne, A.C., "Factors controlling the acquisition of the Philadelphia dialect by out-of-state children." In W. Labov (Ed.), *Locating Language in Time and Space.* New York: Academic Press, 1980.

Pendergast, K., S. Dickey, J. Selmar, and A.L. Soder, *Photo Articulation Test.* Danville, Ill.: Interstate, 1969.

Peters, A., "Language learning strategies: Does the whole equal the sum of the parts?" *Language, 53* (1977): 560–573.

Peters, A., *The Units of Language Acquisition.* Cambridge (U.K.): Cambridge University Press, 1983.

Poole, E., "Genetic development of articulation of consonant sounds in speech." *Elementary English Review, 11* (1934): 159–161.

Prather, E., D. Hedrick, and C. Kern, "Articulation development in children aged two to four years." *Journal of Speech and Hearing Disorders, 40* (1975): 179–191.

Preisser, D.A., B.W. Hodson, and E.P. Paden, "Developmental phonology: 18–29 months." *Journal of Speech and Hearing Disorders, 53* (1988): 125–130.

Roberts, J.E., M. Burchinal, and M.M. Footo, "Phonological process decline from 2 ½ to 8 years." *Journal of Communication Disorders, 23* (1990): 205–217.

Sander, E., "When are speech sounds learned?" *Journal of Speech and Hearing Disorders, 37* (1972): 55–63.

Sax, M., "A longitudinal study of articulation change." *Language, Speech, and Hearing Services in the Schools, 3* (1972): 41–48.

Schmitt, L.S., B.H. Howard, and J.F. Schmitt, "Conversational speech sampling in the assessment of articulatory proficiency." *Language, Speech, and Hearing Services in Schools, 14* (1983): 210–222.

Schwartz, R., and L.B. Leonard, "Some further comments on reduplication in child phonology." *Journal of Child Language, 10* (1983): 441–448.

Schwartz, R., L.B. Leonard, M.J. Wilcox, and K. Folger, "Again and again: Reduplication in child phonology." *Journal of Child Language, 7* (1980): 75–88.

Shriberg, L., and Kwiatkowski, J., "Phonological disorders III: A procedure for assessing severity of involvement." *Journal of Speech and Hearing Disorders, 47* (1982): 256–270.

Smit, A.B., "Ages of speech sound acquisition: Comparisons of several normative studies." *Language, Speech, and Hearing Services in Schools, 17* (1986): 175–186.

Smit, A.B., and J. Bernthal, "Voicing contrasts and their phonological implications in the speech of articulation-disordered children." *Journal of Speech and Hearing Research, 26* (1983): 486–500.

Smit, A.B., L. Hand, J.J. Freilinger, J.E. Bernthal, and A. Bird, "The Iowa articulation norms project and its Nebraska replication." *Journal of Speech and Hearing Disorders, 55* (1990): 779–798.

Smith, B.L., "Temporal aspects of English speech production: A developmental perspective." *Journal of Phonetics, 6* (1978): 37–67.

Smith, B.L., "A phonetic analysis of consonantal devoicing in childen's speech." *Journal of Child Language, 6* (1979): 19–28.

Smith, B.L., "The emergent lexicon from a phonetic perspective." In M.D. Smith and J.L. Locke (Eds.), *The Emergent Lexicon: The Child's Development of a Linguistic Vocabulary.* New York: Academic Press, 1988.

Snow, K., "A detailed analysis of articulation responses of 'normal' first grade children." *Journal of Speech and Hearing Research, 6* (1963): 277–290.

Stoel-Gammon, C., "Phonetic inventories, 15–24 months: A longitudinal study." *Journal of Speech and Hearing Research, 28* (1985): 505–512.

Stoel-Gammon, C., "The phonological skills of two-year-olds." *Language, Speech, and Hearing Services in Schools, 18* (1987): 323–329.

Stoel-Gammon, C., and C. Dunn, *Normal and Disordered Phonology in Children.* Baltimore: University Park Press, 1985.

Templeton, S., "Spelling first, sound later: The relationship between orthography and higher order phonological knowledge in older students." *Research in the Teaching of English, 13* (1979): 255–264.

Templeton, S., "The spelling–meaning connection and the development of word knowledge in older students." *Journal of Reading, 27* (1983): 8–14.

Templeton, S., and L. Scarborough-Franks, "The spelling's the thing: Knowledge of derivational morphology in orthography and phonology among older students." *Applied Psycholinguistics, 6* (1985): 371–390.

Templin, M.C., *Certain Language Skills in Children*. Minneapolis: University of Minnesota Press, 1957.

Tyler, L.K., and U.H. Frauenfelder, "The process of spoken word recognition: An introduction." In U.H. Frauenfelder and L.K. Tyler (Eds.), *Spoken Word Recognition*. Amsterdam, The Netherlands: Elsevier-Science Publishers, 1987.

Tyler, L.K., and W.D. Marslen-Wilson, "Children's processing of spoken language." *Journal of Verbal Learning and Verbal Behavior, 20* (1981): 400–416.

Vihman, M.M., "From pre-speech to speech: On early phonology." *Papers and Reports on Child Language Development, 3* (1976): 51–94.

Vihman, M.M., "Sound change and child language." In E.C. Traugott, R. Labrum, and S. Shepherd (Eds.), *Papers from the Fourth International Conference on Historial Linguistics*. Amsterdam, The Netherlands: John Benjamins B.V., 1980.

Vihman, M.M., "Phonology and the development of the lexicon: Evidence from children's errors." *Journal of Child Language, 8* (1981): 239–264.

Vihman, M.M., and K. Carpenter, "Linguistic advance and cognitive style in language acquisition." In C. Brugman and M. Macaulay (Eds.), *Proceedings of the Tenth Annual Meeting of the Berkeley Linguistic Society*, 1984.

Vihman, M.M., and M. Greenlee, "Individual differences in phonological development: Ages one and three years." *Journal of Speech and Hearing Research, 30* (1987): 503–521.

Walley, A.C., "Developmental differences in spoken word identification." Ph.D. thesis, Indiana University, 1984.

Walley, A.C., and J.L. Metsala, "The growth of lexical constraints on spoken word recognition." *Perception and Psychophysics, 47* (1990): 267–280.

Wellman, B.L., I.M. Case, E.G. Mengert, and D.E. Bradbury, *Speech Sounds of Young Children*. University of Iowa Studies in Child Welfare, 5, Iowa City: University of Iowa Press, 1931.

chapter

4

Dialectal Variations

Aquiles Iglesias, Temple University

Noma Anderson, Howard University

INTRODUCTION

The speech patterns of the child's community are a very important consideration when assessing a child's phonological status. For example, if members of a child's speech community consist of individuals who are bilingual (Spanish and English) and the variety of English spoken in the child's community is Black English Vernacular (BEV), then the child will most likely speak a variety of English which will be influenced by BEV and Spanish. Phonological assessment of such a child must take into consideration the influence which BEV and Spanish might have on the child's phonological patterns.

Information on the characteristics of particular languages and dialects, together with information on normal phonological development can provide information for nonbiased phonological assessments, and for differentiating children with dialectal differences from those with phonological disorders. Clinicians must develop an intervention program for children that reflects the social situations in which a child interacts and the linguistic characteristics of his or her speech community. This sensitivity and knowledge are required for a child with a phonological disorder as well as for the client who elects intervention to modify or reduce this cultural dialect.

LANGUAGE VARIETIES

Several varieties of American English are spoken in the United States. Some of these depend on context and interlocutors (register), while others depend on the social, ethnic, and geographical characteristics of the speaker (dialect). **Registral**

varieties are dependent on the participants, setting, and topic. For example, one usually uses one register when talking to friends about an awesome weekend and another when speaking to a police officer about a speeding violation. **Dialects** are mutually intelligible forms of a language associated with a particular region, social class, or ethnic group. Southern White Standard, Appalachian English, Caribbean English, Black English Vernacular, Standard American English, Mexican American Spanish, Puerto Rican Spanish, and Cuban Spanish are all examples of dialects spoken in the United States.

No dialect of any language is considered linguistically superior to any other since particular thoughts can be expressed using any of the dialects of a language. This is not to say that all varieties of a language carry the same prestige. Some varieties of a language, specifically those used by the dominant groups in any socially stratified society, will be considered to have higher prestige (Wolfram, 1986), will be promulgated within the educational system (Adler, 1984), and will be valued by the private sector of the society (Shuy, 1972; Terrell and Terrell, 1983).

The promulgation of Standard American English, the prestige dialect in the United States, within the educational system has partially reduced dialectal diversity (**dialect leveling**). Contact through the broadcast media between members of different regional dialects has decreased the differences between dialects. At the same time, isolation of some groups such as lower socioeconomic African-Americans within our large urban centers has resulted in a communicative seclusion which has increased the distance between certain dialects. Greater immigration with subsequent ethnic isolation among some subgroups has also increased the number of ethnic dialects in our society. The "melting pot" hypothesis appears to be a myth, in terms of dialects, for certain segments of our society.

The courts have acknowledged the rights of linguistic minority populations, which has resulted in greater acceptance within the United States of dialects other than Standard American English. In addition, there has been a realization that, although English is the most common and dominant language spoken in the United States, other languages have a right to exist in our linguistically plural society.

Historically, the general pattern for most immigrants to this country was to adopt English as their native tongue. Some immigrant groups, however, maintained the use of their mother tongue (first language) from generation to generation with reinforcement from new immigrants and travel to their country of origin. One example of this phenomena is the Hispanic population in the United States. Over 20 percent of this population does not speak English "well or not at all" (U.S. Department of Commerce, 1983).

CHARACTERISTICS OF BLACK ENGLISH VERNACULAR

Black English Vernacular (BEV) is a dialect of American English that is spoken by many African-Americans. The most widely accepted explanation regarding the origin of BEV is that it began in West Africa when Europeans traveled to the African continent for trade and exploration. Initially, *lingua francas*, or trade languages, developed between European and African speakers as they intermingled and attempted to communicate verbally regarding business matters. As the slave trade evolved and Africans were brought from Africa to the Caribbean and the colonies in the southeastern United States, an African-European language combination evolved and developed from a lingua franca to a *pidgin* form. A pidgin is more developed than a lingua franca but is characterized by limited grammatical complexity and vocabulary and is not used as a person's native language (Dalby, 1971; Dillard, 1972).

As the African and European languages (especially English) became more intermingled in this country, the pidgin form of language evolved into a *creole*. Creole language, in contrast to pidgin, has an expanded grammar and a vocabulary sufficient for transmission as a native language to the next generation. Linguistic theory posits that BEV dialect represents a form of language that emerged from a lingua franca to a pidgin and then to a creole and represents a combination of European and African grammar, phonology, and vocabulary.

The great exodus of African-Americans from the southeast to the northeast and other parts of the United States in the early 1900s brought BEV to the urban areas of the North (Stewart, 1971a). In many cases, individuals from a particular state tended to migrate to particular cities (e.g., South Carolinians moving to Philadelphia). The restricted social environments in which many African-Americans lived, in addition to continued contact with their southern families and communities, reinforced the use of BEV.

Like all American English dialects, BEV is systematic with rule-governed phonological, semantic, syntactic, pragmatic, and proxemic features. BEV shares most of its linguistic features with Standard American English but also shares features of other dialects of English (Southern dialect, Cockney English), as well as features found in other languages such as French and Spanish (Stewart, 1971b). A number of linguistic features distinguish BEV from Standard American English (Williams and Wolfram, 1977). The eight major phonological features which distinguish these two dialects are reported in Table 4–1.

The above features are always optional, are not used in each possible phonetic context, and are not used by all BEV speakers. For example, the simplification of word-final clusters tends to occur when one of the consonants is an alveolar and the other (deleted consonant) a morphological marker. Hence, some BEV speakers may not differentiate between the present and past tense of the same verb (e.g., *miss* and *missed* pronounced as /mɪs/) but would retain the cluster in the word *mist*.

TABLE 4–1. **Major Phonological Features Which Distinguish Standard American English and Black English Vernacular.**

1. Word final consonant cluster simplification, particularly when one of the two consonants is an alveolar (e.g., *test* /tɛst/ → [tɛs])
2. Stopping of word-initial *they* (e.g., *they* /ðei/ → [dɛi]), *thought* /θɔt/ → /tɔt/)
3. Substitution of [f/θ] and [v/ð] in the intervocalic position (e.g., *nothing* /nʌθɪŋ/ → [nʌfɪŋ], *bathing* /beðɪŋ/ → [bevɪŋ])
4. Substitution of [f/θ] in word-final posittion (e.g., *south* /sauθ/ → [sauf])
5. Deletion of /r/ and /l/ (e.g., *sister* /sɪstə˞/ → [sɪstə], *help* /hɛlp/ → [hɛp], *Carol* /kæral/ → [kæal], *professor* /prəfɛsɚ/ → [pəfɛsə])
6. Devoicing of final stops (e.g., *pig* /pɪg/ → [pɪːk])
7. Substitution of I/E before nasals (e.g., "pin" /pɪn/ and *pen* /pɛn/ pronounced as [pɪn])
8. Nasalization of preceding vowel and deletion of nasal consonant in word-final position (e.g., *man* /man/ → [mæ̃])

The extent to which individuals use dialectal features often depends on socioeconomic status. For example, middle-class African-Americans use BEV features to a lesser extent than working-class African-Americans, especially in formal situations. Wolfram (1980, 1986) refers to this sociolinguistic phenomenon as the "social diagnosticity of linguistic structures." The term *social diagnosticity* refers to the observation that linguistic features lack similar patterns of usage across socioeconomic levels. Wolfram observed the frequency of occurrence of selected BEV features among the speech of individuals representing four socioeconomic groups: upper middle class, lower middle class, upper working class, and lower working class. His research revealed that certain BEV linguistic features show **gradient stratification** across the four groups. Gradient stratification is a progressive decrease in frequency of usage of a particular linguistic feature as one moves from lower to higher class groups. The lack of realization of postvocalic *r* (e.g., /sɪstɚ/ → [sɪstə]) is an example of gradient stratification since this BEV phonological feature is used by all four socioeconomic groups, albeit with different levels of frequency. On the other hand, certain BEV features show a pattern of usage referred to as **sharp stratification**. Sharp stratification refers to linguistic features that more clearly differentiate socioeconomic groups, based upon frequency of usage. An example of a BEV feature that presents sharp stratification is substitution of /f/ for /θ/ (e.g., /tuθ/ → [tuf]). The use of this BEV phonological characteristic contrasts middle-class with working-class groups, as working-class groups use the feature much more frequently than middle-class speakers. Wolfram indicated that features revealing sharp stratification are of greater social diagnosticity than those showing gradient stratification.

PHONOLOGICAL DEVELOPMENT OF BLACK ENGLISH VERNACULAR

Little information exists on the development of BEV phonology. Seymour and Seymour (1981) compared the performance on a standard articulation test of 4- and 5-year-old African-American children to a group of white children. They reported that both groups evidenced phonological variations characteristic of BEV (i.e., [f/θ] in medial and final positions: [d/ð] in initial and medial positions; devoicing of /b/, /d/, and /g/ in final word-positions; [b/v] in initial and medial positions); however, the BEV features occurred more frequently in the productions of the African-American children. Thus, both groups produced the same type of substitutions, but the frequency between the two groups differed. These results suggested that for the population they studied, the contrast between BEV and Standard American English dialects was *qualitatively* undifferentiated at this age.

Seymour and Seymour (1981) also reported considerable intersubject variability among the African-American subjects. Although the prevalence of BEV phonological features was higher among the African-American subjects than the white subjects, not all of the target features were present in each African-American speaker nor were the features equally distributed among speakers. They inferred that African-American children from BEV-speaking communities would likely show developmental variations similar to existing normative data.

Bleile and Wallach (1992) compared the articulation of non–speech-delayed and speech-delayed African-American children ranging in age from 3;6 to 5;5.

Head Start teachers who shared the same racial and linguistic background as the children differentiated the two groups of children. Data analysis was based on non-BEV phonological patterns exhibited by the children in a picture-identification, single-word test. The delayed and nondelayed groups reflected differences in the type and quantity of their speech errors. Speech-delayed children had a larger number of (1) stop errors (especially velars), (2) fricative errors in all positions (especially fricatives other than /θ/), and (3) affricate errors in all positions. Non–speech-delayed subjects reflected greater devoicing of final /d/, sonorant errors, and errors related to /r/. Both groups of children produced a large number of consonant cluster errors. Bleile and Wallach (1992) concluded that a combination of characteristics, rather than a single indicator, appears to be the most reliable index of speech delay in African-American speakers, just as it is with nonminority populations.

The acquisition of BEV features by English-speaking Puerto Rican children has also received attention. Wolfram (1974) studied the speech characteristics of Puerto Rican teenagers living in East Harlem, New York. His findings suggested that the degree of contact which his subjects had with BEV speakers influenced the number of BEV features in their speech. Those individuals with the greatest contact showed the largest number of features. Poplack (1978) examined BEV, Puerto Rican Spanish, and Philadelphia English variants in the speech of sixth-grade Puerto Rican children. She concluded that the specific variants used by the children were more related to "covert prestige" than to their linguistic environment, with the boys assigning more prestige to BEV speakers and the girls Philadelphia English. The results of both of these studies support the notion that speech patterns are greatly affected by peer interaction.

CHARACTERISTICS OF SPANISH AND SPANISH-INFLUENCED ENGLISH

Spanish has become the second most common language spoken in the United States with over 11 million individuals, or 5 percent of the U.S. population, speaking the language. Spanish dialects are largely determined by the country of origin. According to Dalbor (1980) there are six major dialects of American Spanish: Mexico and Southwest United States; Central America; Caribbean; Highlands; Chilean; and Southern Paraguayan, Uruguayan, and Argentinean. The principal differences among these dialects are in their vocabulary and phonology. Although all of these dialects are spoken in the mainland United States, the two more prevalent dialects are Southwestern United States Spanish and Caribbean Spanish. The prevalence of these two dialects is attributable to the large number of Mexican immigrants, the migration of large numbers of Puerto Ricans, and the immigration of political refugees from Cuba, El Salvador, and Nicaragua. The degree to which each of these groups speaks the "standard dialect" of the educated urbanites in their home country will largely depend on their prior socio-economic status.

The English dialect spoken in the geographical community of a Spanish speaker will influence both his or her Spanish and English dialects. Other influencing factors include the degree of contact with Spanish and English speakers; whether the speaker is learning both languages simultaneously or sequentially;

and the prestige attached to the various dialects with which the individual comes in contact. This multiplicity of factors affecting language usage results in multiple variations and accounts for considerable linguistic diversity within a population. It is important to have an understanding of the characteristics of Spanish in order to understand the influence that English and Spanish might have on each other.

SPANISH PHONOLOGY

Presented in the paragraphs that follow is a delineation of the segmental characteristics of Spanish phonology. There are 18 consonants in Spanish: the voiceless stops /p, t, k/, the voiced stops /b, d, g/, the voiceless fricatives /f, s, h/, the affricate /tʃ/, the glides /w, j/, the lateral /l/, the tap/trill /ɾ, r/, and nasals /m, n, ñ/. Each group is discussed separately by manner of articulation. Unless otherwise specified, the manner of production is identical to that of their English counterparts.

Stops. There are three voiceless stop consonants in Spanish: the bilabial /p/ (e.g., "papa" /papa/), the linguadental /t/ (e.g., "Tita" /tita/), and the linguavelar /k/ (e.g., "coco" /koko/). These phonemes occur in the initial and medial positions, and all three consonants are unaspirated. When either /p/ or /k/ occurs as the first element of a medial cluster, the phoneme tends to be assimilated to the following phoneme producing a lengthened consonant or a single consonant (e.g., "Septiembre" /septiembre/ → [settiembre] or [setiembre], "doctor" /doktor/ → [dottor] or [dotor]).

The three voiced stop consonants have a stop [b, d, g] (e.g., "beso" [beeso], "dama" [dama], "goma" [goma]) and a fricative allophone [β, ð and ɣ] (e.g., "nube" [nuβe], "radio" [raðɪo], "lago" [laɣo]). The stop and fricative allophones are in complementary distribution. The stop allophones occur in word-initial position or word-medial position if preceded by a nasal (e.g., "tengo" [tengo]) and, in some dialects, the word-final position (e.g., "sed" [sed]). The fricative allophones generally occur within the word or across-word intervocalic positions (e.g., [laɣo], [laɣata] but not [el ɣato]). The intervocalic /d/ is often deleted in conversational speech (e.g., "dedo" /deðo/ → [deðo] or [deo]).

Fricatives. There are three fricatives in Spanish: the labiodental /f/, the linguadental /s/, and the glottal /h/. The fricative /f/ occurs in the word-initial and word-medial positions (e.g., "feo" /feo/, "sofa" /sofa/). When /f/ occurs as part of an /nf/ cluster, the allophone [Φ] is often produced (e.g., "enfermo" [emΦermo]). The fricative /h/ occurs both in word-initial and word-medial positions (e.g., "jamón" /hamon/, "baja" /baha/). Some dialects of Spanish have the velar fricative phoneme /x/ instead of the phoneme /h/ (e.g., "hoja" /oha/ = /oxa/).

The fricative /s/ can occur in the word-initial position (e.g., "zapato" /sapato/), in the word-medial position as a singleton (e.g., "vaso" /baso/), as part of a consonant cluster (e.g., "esperar" /esperar/), and in word-final position (e.g., "dos" /dos/). Word-final /s/ can be a morphological marker, a noun plural marker, or a second-person verb marker (e.g., "gatos" /gatos/, "corres" /kores/). The /s/ has several allophones: [s], less strident [s], [ʰ], and [z]. The specific allophone used is determined by phonological environment, grammatical status, stress, register, speaker gender, and, in the case of the plural marker, other morphosyntactic information.

Deletion of /s/ is common in Caribbean Spanish and Spanish spoken in the coastal regions of Colombia, Mexico, and Venezuela (Dalbor, 1980; Terrell, 1983). Factors affecting word internal /s/ singletons are somewhat different than those affecting plural /s/ markers. Vernacular speech favors the deletion or reduction of word internal /s/, while formal speech favors its retention. The more formal registers require the use of the allophone [s], regardless of the dialect. In less formal dialects there is a tendency for females to aspirate (e.g., "este" [eʰte]) and for males to assimilate the following consonant (e.g., "este" [ette]), although both processes occur in both genders. In the Caribbean dialect of Spanish, male speakers also tend to produce a less strident /s/. An additional allophone of /s/, found only in the baby-talk register, is [tʃ] (e.g., "beso" /beso/ → [betʃo]).

The realization of plural /s/ is affected by the morphological, syntactic, and semantic constituents in which the plural /s/ marker appears. In Spanish, plurality is marked redundantly across the noun phrase by marking the determiner, the adjective, and the verb for number ("los platanos verdes estan aqui/the–plural green–plural bananas–plural be–plural here"). In addition, plurality of the noun can be marked by structures other than the s marker, including adding a quantifier (e.g., "mucha cosa/many thing"); adding [e] to words which normally form their plural by adding es (e.g., "árbol" + es /arboles/ → [arbole]); or using part of the masculine plural marker (e.g., "el muchacho/the–sing. boy" → "lo muchacho/ the–plural boy"). Any or all plural /s/ markers can be deleted as long as information on plurality is maintained in other constituents of the sentence. Dialects with high rate of plural s deletion have low plural verb marker (n) deletion (Poplack, 1979). Thus, an individual can delete the plural /s/ markers and still convey plurality by marking it in the verb.

Affricates. Spanish has only one affricate: /tʃ/ (e.g., "china" /tʃina/, "leche" /letʃe/). It occurs in the word-initial and intervocalic positions. As mentioned previously, [tʃ] is often used as an allophone of /s/ in the baby-talk register.

Glides. There are two glides in Spanish: /w/ and /j/. The allophones of /w/ are [w], [u], and [gw]. These allophones are in free variation (e.g., "hueso" [weso], [ueso], [gweso]). Because of the [gw] allophone, some linguists classify /w/ as an allophone of /g/. The allophones of /j/ are [j], [ɪ] and, in some dialects, [Y] (e.g., "yerba" or "hierba" [jerba], [ierba], or [Yerba]).

Liquids. There are three liquids: /l/, /ɾ/, and /r/. The /l/ can occur in word-initial, word-medial, and word-final positions (e.g., "lago" /laɣo/, "palo" /palo/, "sol" /sol/). The two other liquids, /ɾ/ and /r/, are produced by a rapid motion of the tongue tip on the alveolar ridge. The tap /ɾ/ is produced by a single rapid tapping motion. This allophone occurs in the word-medial and word-final positions (e.g., "caro" /kaɾo/, "mar" /maɾ/). In some dialects of Spanish, the allophone [l] occurs when the phoneme precedes a stop while in others the /ɾ/ is deleted (e.g., "carbon" /kaɾbon/ → [kalbon] or [kabon], "carta" /kaɾta/ → [kalta] or [kata], "barco" /baɾko/ → [balko] or [bako]). Poplack (1979) found that the lambdacization of /ɾ/ in informal speech marks social stratification and is affected by age, sex, educational level, and region of the speaker, with women favoring lambdacization. The trilled /r/ is also produced by rapid tapping motion, with the tongue tip striking the alveolar ridge at least twice in succession. The trilled /r/ occurs in the word-initial and word-medial positions (e.g., "roto" /roto/, "carro" /karo/). In the Puerto Rican dialect, the uvular trill, [R], is sometimes produced instead of the [r]. The usage of [R] shows social stratification in some speech communities but not in others.

Nasals. There are three nasals in Spanish: the bilabial /m/, the alveolar /n/, and the palatal /ñ/. The phonemes /m/ and /ñ/ occur in the word-initial and word-medial positions (e.g., "mapa" /mapa/, "cama" /kama/, "ñata" /ñata/, "niño" /niño/). The few words in Spanish which begin with "ñ" tend to be Caribbean or Central and South American in origin. The /n/ occurs in word-initial, word-medial, and word-final positions (e.g., "nariz" /naris/, "pino" /pino/, "con" /kon/). In word-final position regressive assimilation may accompany a vowel which precedes final consonant deletion of /n/ (e.g., "cajón" /kahon/ → [kahõ]. Word-final /n/ is also a morphological marker for the first- and third-person verbs. Deletion of this morphological marker without regressive assimilation is dependent on whether the dialect has a high or low rate of plural /s/ deletion, with greater deletion of /n/ found in dialects which maintain plurality by maintaining plural /s/ markers.

Table 4–2 provides a summary of all Spanish phonemes, their allophones, and their relative frequency. Although there are some minor differences in the relative frequency of consonants in English and Spanish, the rank order of consonants is similar between the two languages (Wilson, 1984). As in English, alveolar consonants are the most frequent and account for 52 percent of all consonants.

Differences between Spanish and English extend beyond the segmental level. As in English, monosyllabic words occur more frequently than multisyllabic words in spoken Spanish. However, unlike English in which nouns comprise a large proportion of one-syllable words, monosyllabic words in Spanish tend to be adjectives, adverbs, articles, and pronouns. The majority of nouns in Spanish are

TABLE 4–2. **Phonemes and Allophones of Spoken Spanish. (I = initial, M = medial, F = final)**

PHONEME	ALLOPHONES	POSITION	ORTHOGRAPHIC SYMBOL
p	p	I, M	p
b	b ß v	I, M	b or v
t	t	I, M	t
d	d ð	I, M, F	d
k	k	I, M	qu or k
g	g ɣ	I, M	g
f	f Φ	I, M	f
h	h	I, M	j
s	s	I, M, F	s or c
w	w u gw	I, M	hu, gu
j	j i ʤ	I, M	hi or y
t	t	I, M	ch
l	l	I, M, F	l
ɾ	ɾ	I, M, F	r
r	r R	I, M	rr r
m	m	I, M	m
n	n	I, M, F	n
ñ	ñ	I, M	ñ

Dialectal Variations

either two- or three-syllable words with the most frequent canonical form for nouns being CVC(C)V(C) and VC(C)V (Iglesias, Cohen, Gutierrez-Clellen, and Marcano, 1985).

One area in which the two languages differ significantly is in their vowel systems and the effect of speaking rate on vowels. Spanish includes five vowels, /a/, /e/, /i/, /o/, and /u/. Although vowel plus vowel combinations in Spanish are possible (e.g., "peine" /peine/), the vowels maintain their individual characteristics. The unique identity of each vowel is maintained even in rapid speech. As speaking rate increases, Spanish speakers tend to eliminate syllables (e.g., "para aqui y para alla" /para aki i para aia/ → [pakipaia]) or eliminate syllables and delete consonants (e.g., "dónde está Ana" /donde esta ana/ → [ontana]) rather than reducing vowel duration.

SPANISH-INFLUENCED ENGLISH

When there is contact between speakers representing each of two languages, a tendency exists for one language to influence the other. For example, English phonology can influence Spanish productions (e.g., "Cómo se llama su niño?" [koumou seɪ dʒama su ninou]) and Spanish phonology can influence the production of English (e.g., "Let me try to explain the theme" [le mi trai tu eʰple di tim]). Sounding like a native speaker is not a matter of just producing the correct phonemes, although this helps considerably, but also of appropriate application of phonological rules. For example, application of regressive assimilation of voicing in final clusters does not increase intelligibility as much as it increases one's ability to sound like a native English-speaker.

Several factors influence the extent to which one phonological system influences another. The influence may be due to the absence of phonemes or allophones in a language (e.g., [pʰ, tʰ] and [kʰ, θ, v, dʒ] do not occur in Spanish); differences in the distribution of sounds (in Spanish the only final consonants are /s, n, r, l, d/), or differences between the languages in place of articulation for consonants (Spanish /d/ and English /d/). Another influencing factor is when and how pronunciation is acquired. For some individuals learning English as a second language, their first exposure may be the written form. The lack of one-to-one correspondence between grapheme and phoneme in English necessitates explanations not usually part of learning a language orally.

PHONOLOGICAL DEVELOPMENT OF SPANISH

Most investigators of phonological development of Spanish have focused on the acquisition of phonetic rather than phonemic inventories. These data suggest that the phonetic system is largely developed by the age of 2;6 (Maez, 1981; Gonzalez, 1983). Maez (1981) studied the acquisition of Spanish in three children between the ages of 18 and 24 months. The children produced all the Spanish phonemes except [f, ɾ, and r] by 18 months. Jimenez (1987) examined the articulation skills of 120 Spanish-speaking Mexican-American children and reported that all consonants, except [s-, l-, x-, ɾ, -r-, ɾ- and r-], were produced by half of the subjects by age 3;3. The phone [r] was the latest to be acquired, with over 50 percent of the children producing [r] at the age of 4;7.

There is a paucity of data regarding the use of phonological patterns or

TABLE 4-3. Percentage of Occurrence of the Syllabic Processes of Final Consonant Deletion (FCD), Cluster Reduction (CR), and Weak Syllable Deletion (WSD) Based on the Standard Spanish Referent (StR) and the Puerto Rican Spanish Referent (PRR).

AGE	FCD		CR		WSD	
	StR	PRR	StR	PRR	StR	PRR
3;0–3;5	36.7	11.7	17.9	11.7	5.8	3.5
3;6–3;11	37.5	12.5	4.3	0.9	4.0	1.7
4;0–4;5	32.5	7.7	12.7	7.1	4.8	2.6
4;6–4;11	36.7	9.9	3.2	3.0	3.9	1.4

processes in Spanish-speaking children. Most investigators who have studied phonological acquisition in Spanish-speaking children have focused on phonetic forms; however, they have not taken into consideration the dialect spoken by the children's speech community. Gonzalez (1981) examined the phonetic development of 150 Puerto Rican children ages 2;6 to 5;0, and reported that final consonant deletion and cluster simplification were used by most children in over 50 percent of the instances in which they could occur. Anderson and Smith (1987) assessed six monolingual Puerto Rican Spanish-speaking children ranging in age from 2;4 to 2;10. Cluster reduction occurred in over 50 percent of the clusters. Initial-, medial-, and final-position consonant deletions occurred in 25 to 50 percent of potential instances of usage.

The most comprehensive analysis to date on the phonological development of Spanish-speaking children is that of Goldstein (1988). Thirty-nine Spanish-speaking Puerto Rican children, ages 3;0 to 4;11, were administered a 72-item, single-word articulation test. The data were analyzed for evidence of each of the following processes: final consonant deletion (FCD), cluster reduction (CR), weak syllable deletion (WSD), velar fronting (VF), stopping (ST), palatal fronting (PF), liquid simplification (LS), and assimilation (AS). Evidence of these processes was evaluated against two referents: Standard Spanish (StR) and the Puerto Rican dialect of Spanish (PRR). For example, if a child produced [koβa] for /eskoβa/ it would be marked as a WSD when the response was evaluated against Standard Spanish, but no process error was noted when the production was evaluated against the Puerto Rican dialect of Spanish. Data based on comparison of the children's productions to the Spanish Standard Referent (see Tables 4–3 and 4–4) show that among 3-year-olds, FCD, CR, and LS were evidenced in over 10 percent of the words in which they could occur. By the end of the fourth year,

TABLE 4-4. Percentage of Occurrence of the Substitution Processes of Velar Fronting (VF), Stopping (ST), Palatal Fronting (PF), Liquid Simplification (LS), and Assimilation (AS) Based on the Standard Spanish Referent (StR) and the Puerto Rican Spanish Referent (PRR).

AGE	VF		ST		PF		LS		AS	
	StR	PRR	StR	PRR	StR	PRR	StR	PRR	StR	PRR
3;0–3;5	*	*	*	*	*	*	17.5	3.9	7.4	3.6
3;6–3;11	*	*	*	*	*	*	17.3	5.1	7.6	2.9
4;0–4;5	*	*	*	*	*	*	13.2	2.6	7.2	2.2
4;6–4;11	*	*	*	*	*	*	12.1	1.3	3.2	1.3

* Less than 2 percent

FCD and LS still persisted beyond the 10 percent level. By contrast, when responses were compared to the Puerto Rican Spanish Referent, only FCD and CR occurred more than 10 percent of the time, at age 3, while by age 4 neither was evident 10 percent of the time. When data are contrasted for the two types of comparison, it is clear that a significantly greater percentage of processes occurred when the Standard Spanish Referent was used as the referent. Data in Tables 4–3 and 4–4 reflect the fact that the existence of a process varies as a function of the linguistic dialect against which it is compared. The results of this study support the notion that the dialect of the child's speech community must be taken into consideration when considering phonological differences.

Ramirez-Diaz (1988) evaluated the speech of 12 Puerto Rican children ranging in age from 2;0 to 2;11. Phonetic inventories of these subjects revealed that 75 percent of the children had acquired all phonemes except /r/ or its allophone [R]. The following syllabic processes were evident in the speech of these young children: final consonant deletion, syllable deletion, and cluster reduction. These findings generally support those of Goldstein (1988). Ramirez-Diaz's also reported that initial consonant deletion (/huɣo/ → [uɣo]) was common in some of the younger children. Additionally, Ramirez-Diaz's data indicated that the weak syllable deletion process varies as a function of the number of syllables in a word. For example, 7 out of 12 subjects showed evidence of this process in three-syllable words while 10 of the 12 subjects showed evidence of this process in four-syllable words. Cluster reduction was evident in all subjects.

In summary, available data suggest that Spanish-speaking children have acquired most of their phonetic inventory by the age of 3;0, which is similar to that reported for English-speaking children. Phonological process data also reflect patterns similar to those in children acquiring the English language. The data suggest the importance of evaluating the children's production against the standard used by their speech community.

IMPLICATIONS FOR ASSESSMENT

The assessment of phonological disorders requires a determination of whether the client's phonological system is within the norm of acceptable speech for his/ or her linguistic community. Thus, the assessment must be approached with an understanding of the social, cultural, and linguistic characteristics of that community. Such information must be obtained in order to guard against cultural stereotyping (Taylor, Payne, and Anderson, 1987). For example, it is inappropriate to assume that all African-Americans speak with BEV phonology. Members of the same race need not share the same speech community or culture. While one African-American's production of [t/d] in the word *bed* may be regarded as within acceptable norms for the BEV dialect, it would be inappropriate to make the same clinical judgment for another African-American who also produces [t/d]. While the first speaker may be a BEV dialect speaker, the second speaker may not be and, therefore, is reflecting a phonological error.

There are several issues which must be considered when assessing an individual whose language or dialect differs from that of the examiner. First, examiners must be aware of their own dialect and its effect on the assessment process. Seymour and Seymour (1977) noted that the client's perception of the formality of the situation affects linguistic phonological usage. Casual speaking settings may encourage the use of BEV, while a formal setting may inhibit and stigmatize speech forms other than Standard English. A similar issue may be encountered when a clinician uses Castillian Spanish (standard dialect of Spanish spoken in Spain and taught in most educational systems in the United States) when speaking to a speaker of any of the other major Spanish dialects. This is not to say that one should force her or himself to use the client's dialect. One must, however, realize the potential effect which one's particular dialect may have on a client.

Second, examiners must be aware of the limitations of existing assessment tools. Few test makers have specifically addressed the issue of linguistic diversity in the construction of phonological assessment instruments or procedures. It is imperative for speech-language pathologists to review items to determine which have the potential for eliciting nonstandard responses. With prior identification of such items, and with knowledge of the phonological features of both standard and nonstandard dialects, the clinician will be able to conduct culturally appropriate phonological assessments. Obviously, when a standardized test has been modified to accommodate dialectal variation, the norms for the test are no longer valid.

One approach suggested for determining acceptable responses is to ask a member of the client's speech community, preferably an adult family member, to say the word and then for the clinician to compare the adult's production with the client's production. However, as Eblen (1982) noted, children may use a casual speech form they have heard, while the adult in the interview setting would more likely use a formal variant. Another approach suggested by Hodson (1986) is to obtain normative data for clients in their respective communities by administering a test to normal peers in order to identify those dialectal patterns that may be unique for that particular speech community.

When conducting assessment, but especially when the child's language is other than the clinician's dominant language, care should be taken to familiarize oneself with possible alternative lexical responses. Lack of knowledge of these possibilities could result in an inappropriate analysis of the child's productions. For example, if a Spanish-speaking client is asked to label a picture of a turkey ("guajalote" in Mexican Spanish), a response of [paβo] is not incorrect and may be considered an acceptable alternative, while a response of [papalote] indicates that a child mistook the item to be a kite.

ASHA's position paper on social dialect (American Speech-Language-Hearing Association, 1983) officially acknowledges the distinction between a speech-language difference and a speech-language disorder. Appropriate differentiation between a difference and a disorder can be accomplished if one takes into consideration the assessment issues noted above.

IMPLICATIONS FOR INTERVENTION

Once the results of an assessment are obtained, clinicians must decide the next course of action. ASHA's position paper on social dialect referred to above provides guidelines to be followed if the client is a speaker of a dialect other than Standard English. As reflected in this paper, the traditional role of a speech-language pathologist is to provide clinical services for communication disorders but not to treat dialectal differences. The position paper, however, identifies the following expanded role for the speech-language pathologist (1983; 24):

> Aside from the traditionally recognized role, the speech-language pathologist may also be available to provide *elective* clinical services to nonstandard English speakers who do not present a disorder. The role of the speech-language pathologist for these individuals is to prepare the desired competency in Standard English without jeopardizing the integrity of the individual's first dialect. The approach must be functional and based on context-specific appropriateness of the given dialect.

Elective dialect therapy is not without its opponents. Adler (1984, 1987) supported the notion that "non-Standard" dialect reduction should not be elective but rather mandatory for "underclass and Appalachian English-speakers." Adler acknowledged the controversial nature of his proposal and cited literature to support the detrimental effects of speaking a "non-Standard" dialect on educational achievement and employability. He further argued that "if Standard English is the speech system used by members of the establishment, all members of our society should have the opportunity to learn this dialect system, thereby helping them to enter into the societal mainstream if they so desire" (1987; 43).

Regardless of whether therapy is elective or mandatory, the question of which characteristics should be targeted for intervention must be addressed. Wolfram (1980) suggested the following principles to guide linguistic features to be trained:

1. Sharply stratified phonological features should be taught before gradiently stratified features.
2. The more general the rule, the earlier it should be sequenced. Some BEV features reflect non-general rules and only affect a small subset of words, whereas others involve general rules which can operate on many words (i.e., [f/θ] can affect all words containing voiceless *th* while /ι/ for /e/ occurs only before nasal consonants, and therefore is not a general rule).
3. BEV features with general social significance should be addressed before features with regional social significance. This principle recognizes that some BEV features occur more frequently than others.
4. The more frequently occurring BEV features should be addressed before the less frequently occurring ones.

It is important to remember that elective therapy does not necessarily mean that the client wants to eliminate the first dialect (D_1). More often the client prefers to be bidialectal. Taylor (1986) proposed a series of steps which must be followed in order to maintain both dialects. First, a positive attitude toward D_1 must be established. Second, the client must learn to contrast the features of D_1 and D_2. Finally, the client uses D_2 in controlled, structured, and eventually spontaneous situations.

There is a paucity of guidelines for the clinical management of children with phonological problems in which English is not the first language or for whom the dialect spoken is very different from the standard dialect. There are, however, intervention questions which should be addressed. Such questions might include: Is the treatment objective for the client to use the appropriate speech sounds of his or her speech community? If so, then remediation should preferably be in the language(s) spoken in the child's environment. Such a decision requires the clinician to have a degree of competency in the client's first language–dialect. In spite of this, the decision is often made to provide remediation in English, a language which may not be spoken in the child's speech community. It is not uncommon for clinicians in this situation to suggest to parents that they speak English to their children; but they may later express concern that the English dialect spoken by the parents is not a "good model." While solutions to this problem are difficult to arrive at, it is clearly helpful if the clinician is bilingual.

SUMMARY

To provide adequate and appropriate speech and language services to linguistically diverse individuals, speech-language pathologists should be knowledgeable about the dialect of their clients. Furthermore, clinicians must be aware that not all speakers of a particular dialect will show or use every characteristic of it. It is common knowledge that the next 15 to 20 years will bring an increasing number of immigrants to the United States. Many of these immigrants will reflect either non- or limited-English proficiency. These immigrants will join the large number of Americans for whom English is not their first language. Members of this population will include individuals with a variety of languages and dialects. Regardless of whether services are provided in the individual speakers' first or second language, clinicians must know the phonological rules of the first language and its dialectal variations.

REFERENCES

Adler, S., *Cultural Language Differences: Their Educational and Clinical-Professional Implications*. Springfield, Ill.: Charles C Thomas, 1984.

Adler, S., "Bidialectism? Mandatory or elective." *Asha, 29* (1987): 41–44.

American Speech-Language-Hearing Association, "Social dialect position paper." *Asha, 25* (1983): 23–25.

Anderson, R., and B.L. Smith, "Phonological development of two-year-old monolingual Puerto Rican Spanish-speaking children." *Journal of Child Language, 14* (1987): 57–78.

Bleile, K.M., and H. Wallach, "A sociolinguistic investigation of the speech of African-American preschoolers." *American Journal of Speech-Language Pathology: A Journal of Clinical Practice, 1* (1992): 54–62.

Dalbor, J.B., *Spanish Pronunciation: Theory and Practice*, 2nd ed. New York: Holt, Rinehart and Winston, 1980.

Dalby, D., "Black through white: Patterns of communication in Africa and the New World." In W. Wolfram and N.H. Clarke (Eds.), *Black-White Speech Relationships*. Washington, D.C.: Center for Applied Linguistics, 1971.

Dillard, J.L., *Black English: Its History and Usage in the United States*. New York: Random House, 1972.

Eblen, R., "A study of the acquisition of fricatives by three-year-old children learning Mexican Spanish." *Language and Speech, 25* (1982): 201–220.

Goldstein, B., "The evidence of phonological processes of 3- and 4-year-old Spanish speakers." Unpublished master's thesis, Temple University, Philadelphia, Pa., 1988.

Gonzalez, A., "A descriptive study of phonological development in normal speaking Puerto Rican preschoolers." Unpublished doctoral dissertation, Pennsylvania State University, State College, Pa., 1981.

Gonzalez, G., "The acquisition of Spanish sounds in the speech of two-year-old Chicano children." In R.V. Padilla (Ed.), *Theory, Technology and Public Policy on Bilingual Education*. Rosslyn, Va.: National Clearinghouse for Bilingual Education, 1983.

Hodson, B., *Assessment of Phonological Process—Spanish*. San Diego, Calif.: Los Amigos Research Associates, 1986.

Iglesias, A., L. Cohen, V. Gutierrez-Clellen, and M. Marcano, "The phonological complexity of spoken Spanish." Paper presented at the American Speech-Language-Hearing Association Convention, Washington, D.C., November 1985.

Jimenez, B.C., "Acquisition of Spanish consonants in children aged 3–5 years, 7 months." *Language, Speech, and Hearing Services in Schools, 18* (1987): 357–363.

Maez, L.F., "Spanish as a first language: The early stages." Unpublished doctoral dissertation, University of California, Santa Barbara, Calif., 1981.

Poplack, S., "Dialect acquisition among Puerto Rican bilinguals." *Language in Society, 7* (1978): 89–103.

Poplack, S., "Function and process in a variable phonology." Unpublished doctoral dissertation, University of Pennsylvania, Philadelphia, Pa., 1979.

Ramirez-Diaz, M., "Phonological processes of two-year-old Spanish speakers." Unpublished manuscript, 1988.

Seymour, H.N., and C.M. Seymour, "A therapeutic model for communicative disorders among children who speak Black English Vernacular." *Journal of Speech and Hearing Disorders, 42* (1977): 247–256.

Seymour, H., and C. Seymour, "Black English and Standard American English contrasts in consonantal development of four- and five-year-old children." *Journal of Speech and Hearing Disorders, 46* (1981): 274–280.

Shuy, R.W., "Social dialect and employability: Some pitfalls of good intentions." In L.M. Davis (Ed.), *Studies in Linguistics*. Birmingham, Ala.: University of Alabama Press, 1972.

Stewart, W.A., "Continuity and change in American Negro dialects." In W. Wolfram and N.H. Clarke (Eds.), *Black-White Speech Relationships*. Washington, D.C.: Center for Applied Linguistics, 1971a.

Stewart, W.A., "Sociolinguistic factors in the history of American Negro dialects." In W. Wolfram and N.H. Clarke (Eds.), *Black-White Speech Relationships*. Washington, D.C.: Center for Applied Linguistics, 1971b.

Taylor, O.L., "Teaching standard English as a second dialect." In O.L. Taylor (Ed.), *Treatment of Communication Disorders in Culturally and Linguistically Diverse Populations*. San Diego, Calif.: College-Hill Press, 1986.

Taylor, O.L., K.T. Payne, and N.B. Anderson, "Distinguishing between communication disorders and communication differences." *Seminars in Speech and Language, 8* (1987): 415–427.

Terrell, S.L., and F. Terrell, "Effects of speaking Black English upon employment opportunities." *Asha, 25* (1983): 27–29.

Terrell, T.D., "Change: The explanatory value of the heterogeneity of variable rule application." In L. Elias-Olivares (Ed.), *Spanish in the U.S. Setting. Beyond the Southwest*. Rosslyn, Va.: National Clearinghouse for Bilingual Education, 1983.

U.S. Department of Commerce, Bureau of the Census, *National Data Books and Guides to Resources: Statistical Abstracts of the U.S.*, 104th ed. Washington, D.C.: U.S. Government Printing Office, 1983.

Williams, R.L., and W. Wolfram, "Social dialects: Differences versus disorders." In K. Jeter (Ed.), Bilingual Language Learning System. Rockville, Md.: American Speech-Language-Hearing Association, 1977.

Wilson, D., "Proportional occurrence of allophones in the Puerto Rican dialect of Spanish." Unpublished master's thesis, Temple University, Philadelphia, Pa., 1984.

Wolfram W., *Sociolinguistic Aspects of Assimilation: Puerto Rican English in New York City*. Arlington, Va.: Center for Applied Linguistics, 1974.

Wolfram, W., "Sociolinguistic implications for educational sequencing." In R.W. Fasold and R.W. Shuy (Eds.), *Teaching Standard English in the Inner City*. Washington, D.C.: Center for Applied Linguistics, 1980.

Wolfram, W., "Language variation in the United States." In O. Taylor (Ed.), *Nature of Communication Disorders in Culturally and Linguistically Diverse Populations*. San Diego, Calif.: College-Hill Press, 1986.

chapter

5

Factors Related
to Phonological Disorders

INTRODUCTION

In the study of phonological disorders, an abiding concern is the identification of variables that may relate to the presence of speech sound disorders. Various factors, such as cognitive-linguistic, psychosocial, speech mechanism, and hearing and auditory perception have been studied in an attempt to better understand phonological disorders.

For many children with phonological disorders it is difficult, if not impossible, to determine causal factors related to speech delay. For a small percentage of children, however, causal factors related to presence of a delay may be more readily identified. Since the medical model (i.e., determination of the cause of a disorder) is sometimes employed by speech-language pathologists during phonological evaluation, it is important that a book on phonological disorders include a discussion of current understandings of causality as it relates to the presence of phonological impairment.

As discussed in sections of this chapter, certain **causal factors** precipitate and may maintain the presence of phonological/articulatory disorders. For the most part, causal factors are related to impairments and/or interference with the structure and function of the speech and hearing mechanism. Since the percentage of clients in whom causal factors can be identified is relatively small, researchers have been interested in variables, called **causal correlates,** that may coexist with phonological impairments. From 1930 to around 1970 an extensive body of literature related to causal correlates was developed. A knowledge of these correlates is helpful in our understanding of causality as it relates to phonological impairment.

Correlational studies have been used to explore whether phonological proficiency and selected variables covary or coexist with each other. Stated more simply, such studies seek to determine whether one variable (such as status of articulation) is related to another variable (such as intelligence). A *high* correlation between two variables implies that such variables are related to each other. For example, a high correlation between a measure of articulation and a measure of intelligence would indicate that a high number of correct articulatory responses co-occur with a high score on a measure of intelligence, and a low number of correct articulatory responses co-occur with a low score on a measure of intelligence. A *low* correlation, on the other hand, would indicate that the score obtained on an articulatory measure and the score on an intelligence measure do not covary and are not systematically related to each other. When a correlation is high, the status of one variable can sometimes be predicted from knowledge of the status of the second variable. This does not mean, however, that a causal relationship exists between the two; it simply means that they are related to each other. The frequently cited warning, "Correlation does not imply causation," speaks to precisely this issue. Correlational studies of the relationship between a single variable and articulatory status have identified topics for further study, which may lead to identification of factors that affect phonological performance.

A second type of procedure used to examine factors potentially related to phonological impairment involves comparisons between normal children and children who are phonologically delayed. When reviewing studies of this type, several points should be kept in mind. First, a statistically significant difference between a group of normal persons and a group of phonologically impaired persons on a particular variable (for example, speech sound discrimination) does not imply a causal relationship between that variable and articulation. Other variables may account for the differences found between the articulatory-impaired and normal-speaking groups. Second, statistical significance does not imply clinical significance for two reasons: (1) group trends frequently do not reflect individual performance, and (2) relatively small quantitative differences resulting in statistically significant differences may have limited clinical utility. In a study reported by Dubois and Bernthal (1978), a small but statistically significant difference was found between two types of articulation measures (spontaneous picture-naming and a delayed imitation sentence production), and yet, the numerical difference in average performance, based on a 20-item task, was less than 2 items. Because of the small numerical difference, the clinical significance of such group findings might be questioned.

In studies of factors related to articulation, investigators typically have looked at only a single variable (for example, age or intelligence) as it relates to articulatory status. Several investigators have used **multivariate analysis** techniques to look at the relationship between articulation status and a number of variables simultaneously. Winitz (1969) thought it "quite possible that substantial relationships between articulation and other independent variables would be forthcoming if the independent variables were examined collectively rather than singularly" (216). Arndt, Shelton, Johnson, and Furr (1977) and Prins (1962a) used multivariate analysis to identify and describe homogeneous subgroups of misarticulating children. In both investigations, a subgroup was identified by the similarity of scores on variables potentially related to articulation.

Winitz (1969) has suggested that some variables that have been studied in relation to articulation disorders may best be viewed as **macrovariables** (variables formed from several other variables). The variable of age, for example, may be understood to comprise such components as physical maturation, motor coordination, and cognitive-linguistic maturity. As Winitz has pointed out, although a macrovariable may be found to correlate with articulation, the individual components accounting for the correlation may be difficult to identify.

In addition to examining status relationships between selected factors and phonology, investigators have explored changes that may simultaneously occur between certain variables and a phonological measure. Improvement relations are of two types: (1) changes in articulation as a function of a change in one or more other variables; and (2) changes in one or more other variables as a function of a change in articulation. For example, Williams and McReynolds (1975) reported that improvement in articulation had resulted in improved performance in speech sound discrimination. Correlational studies demonstrating that improvement in one or more variables results in improvement in articulation may have potential for clinical application.

The primary focus of this chapter is on correlational variables rather than causal variables. However, some variables have been identified as causal factors in phonological and articulatory disorders, and thus are discussed in this chapter. At the present time most of the identified causal factors are in the area of structure and function of the speech and hearing mechanism. Some of these causal factors call for surgical management; for example, a cleft in the palate. Such treatment may be a critical part of the remediation plan. In this first section, defects in structure and function of the speech and hearing mechanism that might interfere with the individual's phonological productions are reviewed; that is, hearing loss, certain structural anomalies, and certain neuromotor pathologies. The second section deals with cognitive-linguistic factors and the final section with psychosocial factors.

STRUCTURE AND FUNCTION OF THE SPEECH AND HEARING MECHANISMS

HEARING LOSS

Among the variables influencing articulation, perhaps none is as important as the ability to hear. Through this sensory channel, an individual is able to monitor his or her own productions as a speaker and receive incoming messages as a listener. The hearing-impaired person is unable to perceive certain sounds that are audible to others and, hence, may perceive the speech signal in a distorted fashion, if at all. The deaf child must learn how to produce speech by watching how sounds look on the face, how they feel through vibrations, what he or she is shown about them, and what he or she can perceive from a distorted auditory signal. A certain level of hearing is required to learn and maintain normal speech production. Ling (1989) summarized this relationship by noting that the more normal a person's hearing, the more natural his or her speech is likely to be.

Several aspects of hearing loss have been shown to affect speech perception

Factors Related to Phonological Disorders

and production; these include the level of hearing sensitivity, speech recognition ability, and configuration of the hearing loss. Individual hearing losses range from mild to severe or profound (greater than 70 dB HL). Labels such as *hard of hearing* and *deaf* are frequently applied to persons with varying degrees of hearing impairment.

Hearing sensitivity which is measured primarily through pure-tone audiometric testing typically varies somewhat from one frequency to another, with speech and language differentially influenced by the frequency configuration and severity of the hearing loss. Although information recorded on an audiogram is a useful prognostic indicator of speech reception ability, predictions based solely on pure-tone measurements are not always accurate. Thus, two children with similar audiograms may not perceive speech sounds in the same way. A pure-tone audiogram cannot measure a person's ability to distinguish one frequency from another or to track formant transitions (a skill critical to speech perception). For these and other reasons, individuals with similar pure-tone audiograms can differ greatly in their understanding of speech.

A second hearing-related factor important to phonological acquisition and maintenance is the age of onset of the hearing loss. If a severe loss has been present since birth, acquisition of language including phonologic, syntactic, and semantic aspects is difficult, and specialized instruction is necessary to develop speech and language. Such instruction may rely on visual, tactile, and kinesthetic cues as well as whatever residual auditory sensation the person possesses. Children and adults who suffer a serious loss of hearing after language has been acquired usually retain their articulation patterns for a time, but frequently, their articulatory skills deteriorate. Even individuals who can be assisted by amplification find it difficult to maintain their previous level of articulatory performance.

Influence on Speech. Investigators have explored the influence of hearing loss on speech sound productions. Levitt and Stromberg (1983) observed the following vowel patterns in individuals with hearing loss: (1) a number of vowel substitutions, (2) substitution of diphthongs for vowels (diphthongization) and vowels for diphthongs, (3) some omissions of the intended vowel or diphthong, and (4) schwa or schwa-like vowel substitutions (neutralization).

The most common consonant errors noted by Levitt and Stromberg (1983) were (1) omissions, especially in word-final position (final consonant deletions); (2) voiced and voiceless confusions (e.g., [t] for [d] or vice versa); (3) substitutions of stops for nasals (e.g., [b] for [m] caused by improper timing of velar closure due to lack of perception of auditory cues usually in conjunction with other articulatory events); (4) a tendency to over-constrict the vocal tract, resulting in the substitution of stops for fricatives and affricatives (e.g., [t] for [θ] or [tʃ]; (5) glottal substitutions, most frequently for stops and affricates; and (6) some place substitutions (e.g., [n] for [ŋ]) and some unidentifiable distortions. Regardless of the type of hearing loss, sibilant sounds have frequently been reported to be the most commonly affected sounds.

In addition to segmental characteristics, the suprasegmental patterns of hearing-impaired speakers differ from those seen in normal-hearing speakers. Hearing-impaired speakers generally speak at a slower rate than normal-hearing speakers due to longer duration of both consonants and vowels, and they also use more frequent pauses and slower articulatory transitions. Stress patterns tend to be inappropriate as many hearing-impaired speakers do not distinguish duration in stressed and unstressed syllables. Finally, hearing-impaired speakers frequently use too high or too low a pitch, use inappropriate inflectional patterns, use harsh or breathy voice quality, and are hypo- or hypernasal (Dunn and Newton, 1986).

There is a great deal of variation in speech patterns of individuals with hearing impairments. There still does not exist a comprehensive description of the speech and language of the hearing impaired, due to the complexity involved in analyzing their speech. Interestingly, there is less information available for individuals with mild to moderate hearing losses than for those with more severe losses.

Calvert (1982) reported that errors of articulation common to deaf children are not confined to productions of individual phonemes; errors also occur because of the phonetic context in which the phones are embedded. Calvert delineated the following common errors of articulation in the speech of the deaf (defined as those with hearing threshold levels for speech of greater than 92 dB) for whom everyday auditory communication is impossible or nearly so.

1. Errors of Omission
   a. Omission of /s/ in all contexts
   b. Omission of final consonants
   c. Omission of initial consonants
2. Errors of Substitution
   a. Voiced for voiceless consonants
   b. Nasal for oral consonants
   c. Low feedback substitutions (substitution of sounds with easily perceived tactile and kinesthetic feedback for those with less; e.g., /w/ for /r/ substitution)
   d. Substitution of one vowel for another
3. Errors of Distortion
   a. Degree of force (Stop and fricative consonants are frequently made with either too much or too little force.)
   b. Hypernasality associated with vowel productions
   c. Imprecision and indefiniteness in vowel articulation
   d. Duration of vowels (Deaf speakers tend to produce vowels with undifferentiated duration, usually in the direction of excess duration.)
   e. Temporal values in diphthongs (Deaf speakers may not produce the first or the second vowel in a diphthong for the appropriate duration of time.)
4. Errors of Addition
   a. Insertion of a superfluous vowel between consonants (e.g., /sʌnoʊ/ for /snoʊ/)
   b. Unnecessary release of final stop consonants (e.g., [stopʰ])
   c. Diphthongization of vowels (e.g., *mit* → [mɪʌt])
   d. Superfluous breath before vowels

Calvert reported that in those individuals who become deaf after acquiring speech and language, distortions and omissions occur for speech sounds characterized by low intensity and high frequency, such as /s/, /ʃ/, /tʃ/, /f/, and /θ/. In addition, such individuals may produce consonants in the final position of words with so little force that they are not heard by the listener.

Although there is no one-to-one correspondence between level and type of hearing loss and patterns of misarticulations, in general, the less severe the loss, the less articulation is affected. Since consonants, especially those with high-frequency energy (e.g., sibilants), have less inherent intensity in their production than vowels, consonants tend to be most frequently misarticulated.

Even relatively minor fluctuating hearing losses seen in children with recurrent middle-ear problems may affect those children's speech and language acquisition. Investigators have reported that children who are experiencing otitis media with effusion usually score poorer on articulation tests than those free of otitis media with effusion. Other researchers have reported that a delay in speech and language development at 3 years and older often follows with effusion, otitis media, and its accompanying fluctuating hearing loss. It has been reported that many children seen for phonological and articulation deficiencies have a history of middle-ear involvement, and children with a history of middle-ear involvement can be differentiated from those without such a history by the phonological patterns in their speech (Shriberg and Smith, 1983; Shriberg and Kwiatkowski, 1982). However, the existence of such a relationship between middle-ear involvement and later speech difficulties remains unclear due to conflicting results and methodological limitation of the investigations.

Shriberg and Kwiatkowski (1982) reported that up to one third of the children with moderate-to-severe phonological delays may have histories of middle-ear involvement. They inferred a possible relationship between a history of middle-ear problems and phonologic delay.

Shriberg and Smith (1983) reported that children with positive histories of middle-ear involvement made sound changes (errors) in nasals and word-initial consonants more frequently than phonologically delayed children without such histories. Initial consonants were deleted (e.g., *got* → [at]), or replaced by [h] (e.g., *tie* → [haɪ]) or glottal stop replacements (e.g., *to* → [ʔu]). The other changes noted were that nasal sounds were (1) replaced by another nasal or stop (e.g., *not* → [ma] or *my* → [baɪ]; (2) replaced by denasalization (e.g., *knee* → [n̆i:]); or that (3) nasals were preceded or followed by an epenthetic stop (e.g., *no* → [ᵈnoʊ]). Shriberg and Smith (1983) suggested that it may be possible to differentiate children who have a positive history of middle-ear involvement from those who do not on the basis of the phonological patterns in their speech. Churchill, Hodson, Jones, and Novak (1985) reported that deletion of the stridency feature was the distinguishing characteristic of children with middle-ear involvement.

Paden, Novak, and Beiter (1987) attempted to identify differences between children with frequent or persistent middle-ear problems who later required phonologic intervention from those who did not. They reported no distinguishing phonological patterns in their subjects with a history of middle-ear involvement. They concluded that children with similar hearing thresholds and length of middle-ear involvement differed widely in their mastery of phonologic skills. They also suggested that perhaps guidelines based on a number of variables—for example, the percentage of deviancy from age norms on velars, deletions of postvocalic obstruents, liquid durations, age of initial diagnosis of middle-ear problems, length of time the middle-ear problem persisted, and severity of the hearing impairment—could be developed to aid in the identification of 18- to 36-month-old children with a history of middle-ear involvement who are "at-risk" phonologically. In a subsequent study, Paden, Matthies, and Novak (1989) attempted to identify which young children, 19 to 35 months, who were below age level for phonology and had otitis media with effusion were at risk for continued phonologic delay even when pressure equalization tubes were inserted. They reported that of the original group they studied, 24 percent even with aggressive medical treatment did not attain normal phonologic development by age 4. It can be inferred from this finding that with aggressive medical treatment most children who are prone to have middle-ear problems will catch up with their peers without intervention but about 25 percent will not. A statistical procedure called discriminant analysis indicated that the best predictors between children who would likely achieve normal phonology by age 4 and those who would not were four variables:

1. Velar deviations
2. Cluster reduction
3. Score on the retest four months following insertion of tubes
4. A time lag between initial diagnosis of otitis media and age at first significant remission from otitis media of six months or more

On the basis of their findings, they recommended the following formula for identifying children for whom phonologic intervention is indicated:

Sum: Initial Adequacy Score × .045; Elapsed Time × −.087; Retest Adequacy × .050; a Constant 2.626.

Individuals who obtain negative scores with this formula are at risk for continued phonological delay at age 4.

Roberts, Burchinal, Koch, Footo, and Henderson (1988) studied 55 children in a longitudinal study and reported no significant relationship between otitis media during the first 3 years of life and the subsequent use of phonological processes and/or consonant errors during the preschool years. They concluded that "the magnitude of any adverse speech outcome associated with early childhood middle-ear problems is small and more likely to be evident when children are school age" (431). Although there is disagreement in the literature relative to the role early middle-ear involvement has on speech development, a history of middle-ear problems may be a contributing factor to later speech difficulties. Because middle-ear involvement has the potential to adversely affect speech development, the speech of children with reoccurring otitis media should be periodically monitored.

Intelligibility. Calvert (1982) argued that in evaluating the speech intelligibility of the hearing impaired, the listeners, the stimulus material, and the context for evaluation should be taken into account. He pointed out that as a listener becomes familiar with the speech of the hearing impaired, understanding improves and, furthermore, that most listeners develop this familiarity in a short time. Therefore, judgments of intelligibility cannot be made without knowing the listener's experience with speech of the hearing impaired as well as his or her personal familiarity with the subject's speech and language patterns.

Judgments of speech intelligibility have also been shown to vary with the materials on which they are based. For example, one-syllable words do not provide the linguistic redundancy available in sentence productions. Judgments based on material produced spontaneously may differ from judgments based on material that is read or elicited through questions just as judgments based on live speech reading may differ from those based on tape recordings. Familiarity with the subject matter may also influence judgments.

Monson (1983) studied 10 hearing-impaired adolescents and reported that:

1. Subjects used simple sentences with few consonant clusters, few polysyllabic words, and were more intelligible when using less complicated syntax than when using more complex sentences.
2. Experienced listeners understood more than inexperienced listeners.
3. Sentences presented within a verbal context were more intelligible than those presented out of context.
4. Sentences when the speaker was both seen and heard were better understood than those which were only heard.

Monson (1983) concluded that for the hearing-impaired speaker, speech intelligibility is influenced by ''the characteristics of the listener (listener experience), the articulatory and prosodic skill of the speaker, the phonology and grammar of the language, and the context or situation in which communication takes place'' (293).

Smith (1972) studied the speech intelligibility of 40 day and residential hearing-impaired pupils in two age groups—8 to 10 years and 13 to 15 years. All subjects had hearing losses greater than 80 dB at 1000 Hz. The percentage of intelligible words, as assessed by 120 listeners unfamiliar with the speech of hearing-impaired children, ranged from 76 percent to 0 percent, with a mean of 18.7 percent.

SPEECH SOUND PERCEPTION

Speech-language pathologists have long been interested in a possible relationship between the perception and production of speech sounds. Phonemic perception is a form of auditory perception in which the listener–speaker distinguishes among the sound contrasts in a language. Linguistic or phonemic perception also includes the storing and accessing of sounds for the recognition of words that are heard. From a clinical perspective, this skill includes the ability to detect differences between target sounds in the language and error productions that may be substituted for those sounds. Clinicians have been interested in determining whether or not production errors are related to errors in perception of speech sounds. Numerous investigations have been conducted to ascertain the relationship between production and perception in children with normal phonological development and children with delayed phonological development.

As was stated in our discussion of phonological acquisition (see Chapter 2), some investigators view phonemic perception as essentially completed by the time the normally developing child has acquired the first 50 words. If this assumption is correct, it follows that the child's speech sound production errors can be ascribed primarily to difficulties in motor (articulatory) control and/or phonological organization, rather than perception. If, however, the acquisition and development of speech sound perception continues at least into the preschool and even the early school years, as other investigators argue, then some production errors may be due to a mismatch between the adult form of the word and the child's perception and underlying representation (storage) of the word. In other words, some children's production errors may be related to phonemic perception. Finally, many treatment programs include auditory discrimination tasks on the assumption that such tasks help the child to learn the adult phonological system.

Before discussing studies concerned with the relationship between production and perception, it is useful to recall some of the previously reviewed data regarding auditory perception in normal infants and young children. In Chapter 2, evidence was presented that infants can perceive most contrasts used in the phonology of their language at the time they begin to speak. Indeed, experiments have shown that infants under 1 year of age are able to discriminate between speech sounds (Eimas, Siqueland, Jusczyk, and Vigorito, 1971; Butterfield and Cairns, 1974). Apparently, within the first few months of life, infants perceive differences in the acoustic signal as categorical differences similar to those serving as phonemic contrasts in adult languages. Speech sound perception experiments also suggest that as children begin to speak words, they do not perceive all of the relevant phonological contrasts. It is also important to remember that studies of infant perception require only that the subject note changes in the acoustic signal, whereas linguistic or phonemic perception involves an active attention to contrasting speech sounds and sequences in order to identify, store, and recognize distinct lexical items. The skills required for nonlinguistic discrimination (same–difference distinctions) tested in investigations of infant perception are very different from those required to distinguish and store lexical items.

Perceptual discrimination experiments with preschoolers, beginning with children at approximately age 2, have shown that young children can make most of the phonological distinctions in English. Barton (1976), who attempted to determine whether normal 2-year-olds had full or partial linguistic perception (see Chapter 2), reported that his subjects were not able to make all of the perceptions required on the experimental tasks but were able to perceive sounds they were not producing. He concluded that his subjects' perception was more advanced than their production and suggested that they may have had full or nearly full perception at this early age. He also pointed out that word familiarity influenced the children's performance on perceptual tasks: children made more errors on the perception of new or unfamiliar words than on words they knew well.

As was discussed in Chapter 3, perceptual errors may result from a partially correct internal representation that becomes more accurate with increased exposure to the adult form of the word. If a child fails to notice the discrepancy between his or her initial internal representation and the adult form, then a perceptually based error may exist.

The study of young children's perceptual skills has continued to be of interest to both clinicians and researchers. The extent to which the findings based on children with normal perceptual and production skills are applicable to the phonologically delayed population is unclear since it is not certain that inferences can be drawn from normal to phonologically delayed speakers. Locke (1980) has also suggested that a difference may exist between the role of perception in the acquisition of phonological errors and its role in the maintenance of a phonological disorder.

Clinical research on speech sound perception and its relationship to articulation disorders has sought to determine (1) if a relationship exists, (2) the relationship between general and phoneme-specific measures of discrimination and

Factors Related to Phonological Disorders

production, as well as that between external and internal monitoring, and (3) the relationship between perceptual training and production.

Relationship between Articulation and Speech Sound Discrimination. The possibility of a relationship between articulation disorders and speech sound (auditory) perception was first investigated in the 1930s. This early perceptual research, referred to as speech sound discrimination research, relied primarily on general measures of speech sound discrimination, which required the subject to judge whether word or nonsense pairs verbally presented by the examiner were the same or different. There was generally no attempt to compare the specific phoneme production errors with the specific perception errors the subject might have made.

Travis and Rasmus (1931) found that on a discrimination test of 366 paired nonsense-syllable items, groups of normal subjects performed significantly better than groups with mild articulation disorders. Other researchers comparing the discrimination skills of normal speakers and speakers with articulation errors (Kronvall and Diehl, 1954; Clark, 1959) reported similar findings; that is, that normal speakers had significantly better skills, and several investigators found a positive correlation between performance on an articulation test and performance on a test of speech sound discrimination (Reid, 1947b; Carrell and Pendergast, 1954).

A number of studies, however, found no relationship between discrimination and speech sound productions. In a study similar to that of Travis and Rasmus, Hall (1938) reported no significant differences in discrimination skill between normal speakers and two groups of defective speakers with mild and severe articulatory disorders. Hansen (1944), who studied discrimination and articulation in a college-age population, also reported little relationship between the two variables; and Mase (1946), Prins (1962b), Garrett (1969), and Veatch (1970) likewise found no significant differences in speech sound discrimination skills between children with articulation disorders and normal speakers.

Sherman and Geith (1967) suggested that one reason for the equivocal findings may have been that experimental groups were chosen on the basis of articulatory proficiency rather than speech sound discrimination performance, and consequently, etiologies associated with articulatory-impaired subjects may not have been limited to individuals with poor speech sound discrimination skills. In order to control for perceptual skill, Sherman and Geith administered a 50-item speech sound discrimination test to 529 kindergarten children and then selected from this group 18 children with high discrimination scores and 18 with low scores. These two groups were given a 176-item picture-articulation test. The authors reported that children with high speech sound discrimination scores obtained significantly higher articulation scores than the group with lower discrimination scores. They concluded that poor speech sound discrimination skill may be causally related to poor articulation performance.

Schwartz and Goldman (1974) investigated the possible effects on performance by young children of the type of discrimination task required and found that their subjects consistently made more errors when stimulus words were presented in a paired-comparison context (goat and *coat; coat* and boat) than when target words were included in carrier phrase and sentence contexts (as in, "The man brought a *coat*"). They also found that when background noise was present during stimulus presentation, performance was poorer, particularly for the paired-comparison words. The authors urged speech-language pathologists to test discrimination with tasks which are meaningful and familiar to children, and under the kind of listening conditions the child is likely to encounter in his or her environment.

After reviewing the articulation and discrimination literature, Weiner (1967) attributed the variations in findings to the fact that (1) different types of discrimination tasks were used; (2) subjects of different age levels were used; and (3) subjects reflected varying degrees of articulatory defectiveness from one study to another. He further concluded that speech sound discrimination is a developmental skill, which ceilings at about 8 years, and that a positive relationship exists between auditory discrimination problems and more severe articulation difficulties at age levels below 9 years. More recently, Winitz (1984) reported, after reviewing the studies on the relationship between auditory discrimination and articulation performance, that "With few exceptions, children with functional articulation disorders show lower discrimination scores relative to children who do not have articulation disorders" (22). He also identified a number of factors that may account for the absence of more consistent reports of a positive relationship between articulatory performance and speech sound discrimination measures: (1) a lack of relevance of the discrimination test items, (2) a lack of consideration of the child's specific articulation errors, and (3) a lack of consideration of phonetic context in which the production error occurs.

Relationship between General and Phoneme-Specific Measures; External and Internal Monitoring. In most of the investigations cited above, discrimination was tested through general speech sound discrimination measures; that is, tasks comprised of items sampling a wide variety of sound contrasts (e.g., *s*un–*b*un, *k*ey–*t*ea, *sh*oe–*z*oo) and designed to examine the subject's overall capacity to distinguish among a large number of speech sounds in a variety of phonetic contexts. Investigators (Spriestersbach and Curtis, 1951; Locke, 1980) have pointed out that in testing speech sound perception of articulatory-impaired clients, the critical issue is the clients' ability to discriminate the sound or segments that they misarticulate. Although clients may not have a general problem with speech sound discrimination, they may have phoneme-specific perceptual difficulties on sounds they misarticulate. Perceptual testing should involve stimuli that focus on the children's production errors. We see little value in administering general tests of discrimination that do not reflect the child's specific production errors when attempting to determine a relationship between articulation and speech sound discrimination.

Locke (1980) has gone a step further, urging that measures of sound perception should not only be phoneme-specific, but also context-specific. He argued that perceptual tasks should reflect the child's production errors and reflect those phonetic environments (words) in which error productions occur and include both the error productions and the target productions.

Locke studied children's ability to discriminate sounds they produced in error when those sounds were reproduced and contrasted with the correct sound by the adult examiner. Specifically, 131 children were tested on a perceptual task in which the examiner produced imitations of the subject's error productions, and the subjects were then required to judge whether the examiner's productions were

Factors Related to Phonological Disorders

correct productions of the target word. Locke reported that 70 percent of the children correctly perceived the correct and incorrect forms of the target words, thus indicating that many children could correctly discriminate sounds made by an adult, that they produced in error. About one third of the contrasts misproduced were also misperceived, but the misperceptions were not evenly distributed across all misproductions. Although the substitution of one voiceless fricative for another accounted for 49 percent of the production errors, these contrasts accounted for 89 percent of the misperceptions.

In a study of 14 two-year-old children, Eilers and Oller (1976) found some perceptual confusions in word and nonsense pairs where production of one segment was substituted for another. Yet other common production errors were discriminated by most of their subjects. They concluded that some production errors may be related to perceptual difficulties and others to motor constraints.

Strange and Broen (1980) compared 21 children between the ages of 2 and 11 and 3 and 5 with respect to their production and perception of word-initial /w/, /r/, and /l/. They concluded from their data that both perception and production of phonemic contrasts develop gradually and that perception of a contrast usually preceded its production.

Velleman (1983) collected data from children aged 3 to 5 on a production task that included naming of pictures and objects in a play situation and the imitation of nonsense syllables. She then tested the children's perception of /s/ and /θ/—/s/ because it is easy to perceive and /θ/ because it is not "acoustically salient" and is thus relatively difficult to perceive—and computed a correlation between the two tasks. The data confirmed her hypothesis that some frequently occurring production errors in children's speech are easier to perceive than others. Since contrasts involving /s/ were relatively easily perceived, Velleman inferred that the late acquisition of /s/ could be ascribed to motor constraints. In contrast, the /θ/ versus /f/ contrast is a difficult distinction to make and, as she predicted, only children with high perception scores (over 80 percent) obtained high production scores on these phonemes. More errors were made on both perception and production in the case of /s/, and there was no significant correlation between the two measures.

In summary, some speech sound contrasts remain difficult to discriminate as late as 3 years or older, even in normal developing children. There does not, however, appear to be a correlation between many of the production errors seen in children and measures of speech sound perception.

An additional testing variable frequently considered in phoneme-specific discrimination testing is the source of the speech production that the subject is required to judge. When the task involves discrimination of a stimulus presented from an external source, such as speech productions from another person or recorded stimuli, it is termed **external discrimination** or **monitoring**. External discrimination can also include **external self-discrimination**, of which listening to and making judgments of tape-recorded samples of one's own speech is an example.

When the discrimination or perceptual task involves a judgment of one's own live, ongoing speech sound productions, it is called **internal discrimination** or **internal monitoring**. During internal discrimination, the speaker has available both air- and bone-conducted auditory cues.

Studies of speech sound discrimination skills of young children with delayed phonological development have indicated that subjects frequently were able to make external judgments of sound contrasts involving their error sounds (Locke and Kutz, 1975; Chaney and Menyuk, 1975). In a study employing phoneme-specific discrimination tasks, Aungst and Frick (1964) utilized the *Deep Test of Articulation* (McDonald, 1964), in which the /r/ was tested in 58 productions, to study the relationship between /r/ production and four measures of speech sound discrimination. Three of the discrimination tasks were designed by the investigators to assess subjects' discrimination of their own /r/ productions as they occurred in a set of 30 words. These discrimination tasks required each subject to (1) make an immediate right–wrong judgment of his or her /r/ production after speaking each word, (2) make right–wrong judgments of his or her /r/ productions after such productions had been audio recorded and played back, and (3) make same–different judgments of his or her /r/ productions as they followed the examiner's correct productions presented via audio tape recording. The fourth discrimination task was the *Templin Test of Auditory Discrimination* (Templin, 1957), a general test of external discrimination. The subjects were children, 8 years or older, who made articulation errors only on /r/. The authors reported high correlations for relationships among their three discrimination tasks but low correlations between each of those tests and the Templin general discrimination measure. Moderate correlation coefficients of .69, .66, and .59 were obtained between each of the three phoneme-specific discrimination tasks and scores on the Deep Test for /f/. In contrast, the Templin discrimination test scores (a general discrimination measure) did not correlate well with the articulation measure. These findings indicate some relationship between performance on the Deep Test and the phoneme-specific discrimination measures but not between the Deep Test and the general test of discrimination.

Lapko and Bankson (1975) also compared external and internal monitoring with consistency of articulation, as measured by the Deep Test of Articulation, in a group of 25 kindergarten and first-grade children exhibiting misarticulations of /s/. All measures were phoneme-specific to /s/. They reported a significant correlation (r = .55) between the child's ability to discriminate his or her own productions of /s/ and the consistency of misarticulation of /s/. In other words, those subjects with the higher number of correct productions on the Deep Test of Articulation also had higher scores on the measure of internal discrimination. Such a correlation was not obtained between external monitoring tasks and articulation consistency as measured on the Deep Test of Articulation.

Wolfe and Irwin (1973) and Stelcik (1972) provided further evidence of a positive correlation between articulatory skill and self-monitoring (internal monitoring) of error sounds. But the results of other investigations (Woolf and Pilberg, 1971; Shelton, Johnson, and Arndt, 1977) have indicated that the findings in such studies may be influenced by such factors as the consistency of misarticulation, type of discrimination task used to test internal monitoring, and nature of the stimulus items.

After reviewing the findings of Aungst and Frick (1964) regarding the correlation between self-monitoring and production of /r/ and the findings of Lapko and Bankson (1975) regarding /s/, Shelton, Johnson, and Arndt (1977) concluded that "the self-discrimination testing procedures that are in use do not, by themselves, allow precise prediction of articulation behavior of individual subjects" (715). In other words, the finding that self-monitoring discrimination measures are significantly related to performance on the deep test does not necessarily imply that clinical instruction should focus on self-monitoring skills.

Some experimenters feel that more information about external monitoring is required before appropriate self-monitoring tasks can be developed. Hoffman, Stager, and Daniloff (1983) suggested that current phoneme-specific, external discrimination tasks may not be sensitive to allophonic variations that might be perceived by misarticulating children. For example, the prevocalic voicing contrast that a misarticulating child perceives and produces may not be within the perceptual boundary of an adult phoneme and, consequently, not perceived by the adult; what the child may perceive as a contrast between adult allophones of /z/ may not be perceived by the adult listener because both allophones are within the adult's perceptual boundary of /z/. Such sound variations may be used by some children to contrast forms that are not used in a contrastive manner by adults. It would follow that an adult examiner would evaluate such contrasts as a mismatch between the child's production and the adult standard. These authors have suggested that "meaningful subgroups of misarticulating children may be found to manipulate subphonemic, that is allophonic, acoustic cues in nonstandard manners and thus lead to their identification as misarticulations" (214). In order to understand the relationship between perception and production, we need to have a better understanding of the perceptual skills required for speech sound production.

Discrimination Improvement and Articulatory Productions. The influence of discrimination training on production has also been considered by investigators. Many clinicians routinely conduct some type of discrimination training, or "ear training," as a precursor to production training. Investigators have attempted to determine whether or not a functional relationship exists between articulation and discrimination and more specifically, whether or not discrimination training affects production.

Holland (1967) attempted to determine if programmed speech sound discrimination, focusing on a number of different sound contrasts, influenced speech sound discrimination and articulatory productions. She concluded that such training improved performance on general speech sound discrimination tasks, discrimination of the target phoneme, and articulation of the target sound and non-target sounds. Improvement in articulation, however, did not necessarily mean that speech sound errors were corrected; shifts from one type of error to another—such as omission to substitution or substitution to distortion—were regarded as evidence of improvement.

Sonderman (1971) reported an investigation designed to assess (1) the effect of speech sound discrimination training on articulation skills, and (2) the effect of articulation training on speech sound discrimination skill. Holland's speech sound discrimination program (1967) and the *S-Pack* (Mowrer, Baker, and Schutz, 1968) were administered in alternate sequence to two matched groups of 10 children between 6 and 8 years old, all of whom produced frontal lisps. Four measures were administered to obtain pre-training and post-training profiles for each child: (1) the *Wepman Test of Auditory Discrimination* (a general test of external monitoring skills), (2) an /s/ specific discrimination test, (3) an examiner-designed general articulation test, and (4) the criterion test from the S-Pack (a deep test of the /s/). Improvement in both discrimination and articulation scores was obtained from both discrimination training and articulation training, regardless of the sequence in which the two types of training were conducted. Again, these findings must be cautiously interpreted since articulatory improvement was based on the error improvement scale used by Holland (1967), rather than on right–wrong judgments.

Williams and McReynolds (1975) explored the same question as Sonderman. Two subjects were first given production training followed by a discrimination probe and then discrimination training followed by a production probe. Two additional subjects received the discrimination training first and the production training second. The probe measures, administered to determine if changes occurred in one modality after training in the other, indicated that production training was effective in changing both articulation and discrimination; in contrast to Sonderman (1971), however, Williams and McReynolds (1975) found that discrimination training was effective in changing only discrimination and did not generalize to production.

Shelton, Johnson, and Arndt (1977) also explored the influence of articulation training on discrimination performance. One group of subjects received articulation training on the /r/ and a second group on the /s/, and pre- and post-discrimination probes, consisting of 40 items specifically related to the error sound, were administered. Results indicated that both groups of subjects improved in articulation performance, but no improvement was noted in discrimination performance. The authors suggested that the variance between their results and those of other investigators presumably could be accounted for by one or more unidentified subjects or procedural variables.

Another group of investigators (Koegel, Koegel, and Ingham, 1986; Koegel, Koegel, Van Voy, and Ingham, 1988) has looked at a related topic and examined the relationship between self-monitoring skills and response generalization into the natural environment. School-age children were provided specific training in self-monitoring of the speech productions. These investigators reported that generalization of correct articulatory responses of the target sounds did not occur until a self-monitoring task was initiated in the treatment program. They concluded in the second study that such self-monitoring was required for generalization of the target sounds in the natural environment to occur. These studies will be discussed in more detail later in Chapter 9 (Remediation Concepts and Principles) in the discussion of generalization.

Summary. A relationship appears to exist between speech sound perception and articulation in subjects with impaired phonology although the precise nature of the relationship has not been determined. Self-monitoring of error productions would appear to be an important skill, but instruments to assess such a skill are lacking. Further data are needed to better understand the relationship between discrimination errors and articulation disorders. Although the efficacy of speech sound discrimination training as a predecessor to production training has yet to be established, when perceptual deficiencies are present, perceptual training would seem appropriate.

Speech clinicians are frequently required to make judgments about the structure and/or function of the lips, teeth, tongue, and palate. These oral structures can vary significantly among individuals. Investigators have attempted to identify relationships between articulatory status and structural variations of the oral mechanism, which can range from minor deviations to gross structural anomalies. Although a cause-and-effect relationship between articulation deviations and minor variations in oral structures has not been established, individuals with significant deformities of the orofacial region (such as patients who have undergone ablative surgery) may experience articulatory effects. Articulation deviations thought to be more directly associated with structural anomalies will be discussed later in this chapter.

Lips. Approximation of the lips is required for the formation of the bilabial phonemes /b/, /p/, and /m/; lip rounding is required for various vowels and the consonants /w/ and /hw/. An impairment that would inhibit lip approximation or rounding might result in misarticulation of these sounds.

Fairbanks and Green (1950) examined various dimensions of the lips in 30 adult speakers with superior consonant articulation and 30 with inferior consonant articulation and reported no differences on various lip measurements between the two groups.

Teeth. Several English consonants require intact dentition for correct production. Labiodental phonemes (/f/ and /v/) require contact between the teeth and lower lip for their production, and linguadental phonemes require interdental tongue placement for /ð/ and /θ/ productions. The tongue tip alveolars (/s/, /z/) require that the air stream pass over the cutting edge of the incisors.

Researchers investigating the relationship between deviant dentition and consonant production have examined the presence or absence of teeth, position of teeth, and dental occlusion. **Occlusion** refers to the alignment of the teeth when the jaws are closed, and **malocclusion** refers to the imperfect or irregular position of the teeth when jaws are closed. Lay terms to describe different types of occlusion include terms as *open bite* and *overjet*. Examples of different types of occlusion may be seen in Figure 5–1.

Bernstein (1954) identified malocclusions in children with normal and defective speech but did not find a higher incidence of malocclusion in children with articulation problems than in children with normal articulation skills. He found that articulation defects were generally not related to malocclusion, except in the case of the open bite (the bite is opened—that is, the teeth do not come together, from the first or second molar on one side to the same tooth on the opposite side). Fairbanks and Lintner (1951) examined molar occlusion, occlusion of the anterior teeth, and anterior spaces in 60 adults, 30 of whom were judged to have superior articulation skills and 30 with inferior articulatory skills. They found that neutrocclusion (normal jaw relationship with a slight malocclusion in the anterior segments) tended to predominate in the group of superior speakers, and distocclusion (malocclusion with retrusion of the mandible) and mesiocclusion (malocclusion with protrusion of the mandible) tended to occur more often in the group of speakers with production errors. When data on the subjects were divided according to (1) no marked dental deviation and (2) one or more marked dental

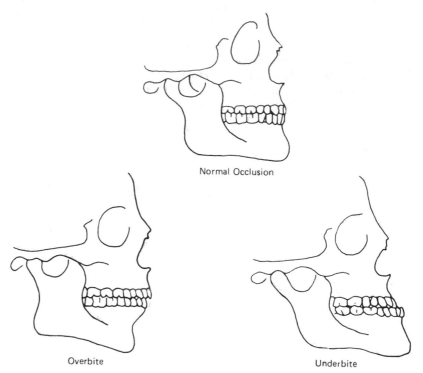

Normal Occlusion

Overbite

Underbite

FIGURE 5–1. **Examples of types of occlusions.**

deviations, the authors found that marked dental deviations occurred significantly more frequently in the inferior speakers than in the superior ones. Open bite was present in the inferior speaking group but not in the superior speaking group.

Although speakers with normal articulatory skills tend to have a lower incidence of malocclusion than speakers with articulatory errors, malocclusion itself does not preclude normal articulation. Subtelny, Mestre, and Subtelny (1964) found malocclusion to coexist with both normal and defective speech. They also noted that during /s/ production, normal speakers with malocclusion (distocclusion) tended to position the tongue tip slightly to the rear of the lower incisors when compared to normal speakers with normal occlusion.

Starr (1972) reported several clinical observations concerning dental arch relationships and speech production skills. He stated that an articulation problem is highly probable in individuals with a short or narrow maxillary (upper) arch and a normal mandibular (lower) arch. The consonants likely to be affected by such conditions are /s, z, ʃ, tʃ, f, v, t, and d/. He further noted that rotated teeth and supernumerary (extra) teeth do not generally present significant speech problems.

Another area of interest to investigators has been the influence of *missing teeth* on articulation. Bankson and Byrne (1962) examined the influence of missing teeth in kindergarten and first-grade children on the production of /s/, /ʃ/, and /f/ in the word-initial, -medial, and -final positions, and /z/ in the word-medial position. Initially, subjects were identified either as children who had correct

Factors Related to Phonological Disorders

articulation with their teeth intact or as children who had incorrect articulation with their teeth intact. After four months, articulation skills were reassessed and the number of missing central or lateral incisors tabulated. A significant relationship was found between presence or absence of teeth and correct production of /s/, but not of /f/, /ʃ/, or /z/. However, some children maintained correct production of /s/ despite the loss of incisors.

Snow (1961) examined the influence of missing teeth on consonant production in first-grade children. Subjects were divided into two groups: those with normal incisors and those with missing or grossly abnormal incisor teeth. The consonants examined were /f/, /v/, /θ/, /ð/, /s/, and /z/. Although Snow found that a significantly larger proportion of children with dental deviations misarticulated consonants, she also found that three quarters of the children with defective dentition did not misarticulate these sounds. In contrast to Bankson and Byrne, who noted significant differences only for /s/, Snow found significant differences for all phonemes. Snow suggested that although dental status may be a crucial factor in sound productions for some children, it does not appear to be significant for most.

Tongue. The tongue is generally considered the most important articulator for speech production. Tongue movements during speech production include tip elevation, grooving, and protrusion. The tongue is relatively short at birth, growing longer and thinner at the tip with age.

Fairbanks and Bebout (1950) investigated differences in tongue characteristics between 30 individuals with superior articulation and 30 with inferior articulation. They found no significant differences between the two groups on measurements of maximum length of protrusion, length of the tip, maximum amount of tongue face, or in the percentage of errors in duplicating tongue position.

Ankyloglossia, or "tongue-tied," are terms used to describe a restricted lingual frenum. At one time, it was commonly assumed that an infant or child with ankyloglossia should have his or her frenum clipped to allow greater freedom of tongue movement and better articulation of tongue tip sounds, and frenectomies (clipping of the frenum of the tongue) were performed relatively frequently. However, McEnery and Gaines (1941) examined 1,000 patients with speech disorders and identified only 4 individuals with abnormally short frenums. Their most extreme case of a short frenum was a 10-year-old boy, whose only articulation error was a /w/ for /r/ substitution; the error was corrected following speech instruction. The authors recommended against surgery for ankyloglossia because of the possibility of hemorrhages, infections, and scar tissue. It can be inferred from these data that a short frenum is only rarely the cause of an articulation problem.

Fletcher and Meldrum (1968) examined the relationship between length of the lingual frenum and articulation. They compared two groups of sixth-grade students, 20 with limited lingual movement and 20 with greater lingual movement, and reported that subjects with restricted lingual movement scored within normal limits on a measure of articulation but tended to have more articulation errors than the group with greater lingual movement.

Although too large a tongue (**macroglossia**) or too small a tongue (**microglossia**) might be expected to affect articulation skills, there appears to be little relationship between tongue size and articulation although these variables have not been adequately investigated. The tongue is a muscular structure capable of considerable change in length and width and thus, regardless of size, is generally capable of the mobility necessary for correct sound productions.

Hard Palate. The relationship between articulation disorders and variations in hard palate dimensions has received limited attention. Fairbanks and Lintner (1951) measured the hard palates of a group of young adults with superior consonant articulation and a group with inferior consonant articulation. They reported no significant differences in cuspid width, molar width, palatal height, and maximum mouth opening. Bloomer and Hawk (1973) pointed out that removal of any part of the maxilla, if not restored surgically or prosthetically, creates a serious problem for the speaker. Articulation problems related to structural anomalies of the palate will be discussed in this chapter under Major Structural Variations of the Speech Mechanism.

Facial Patterns. During the clinician's examination of the oral mechanism, the status and function of the facial and intraoral structures are evaluated. Although researchers have investigated the relationship between specific variations in such oral structures (e.g., teeth, lips, and tongue) and articulation skills, little has been written about the influence of minor variations of facial patterns on speech production skills.

An individual's facial pattern is determined by analyzing the relationship of the mandible and maxilla to the cranial base and to each other. Mason and Wickwire (1978) described the three types of facial patterns associated with orofacial variations as follows:

> The *Class One* facial pattern is considered normal, and refers to a good balance of skeletal and soft tissue components.
>
> The *Class Two* facial pattern shows midface protrusion. This may be due either to maxillary protrusion or mandibular retrusion or a combination of both. Such considerations relate to the denture bases or skeletal parts, not the teeth per se.
>
> The *Class Three* profile is characterized by procumbency of the lower face. Again, the relative position of the maxilla (deficient or retrusive) or mandible (protrusive), or a combination of each, may contribute to the Class Three pattern. It is interesting that although profiles may look alike, their etiology can be entirely different (8).

There is no indication in the literature that facial pattern variations affect articulation skills. Speech problems may or may not be present in individuals with different facial patterns. Clinicians have noted, however, that some individuals with Class Three facial patterns who demonstrated articulation errors and underwent surgery to correct the facial pattern variation, subsequently corrected their previously misarticulated speech sounds without intervention (Mason, 1979; Tabor, 1979).

MAJOR STRUCTURAL VARIATIONS OF THE SPEECH MECHANISM

Speech-language clinicians should recognize that significant anomalies of the oral structures are frequently associated with specific speech problems. Oral structural anomalies may be congenital or acquired. Cleft lip and/or palate is perhaps the most common congenital anomaly of the orofacial complex. Acquired structural deficits may result from trauma to the orofacial complex or surgical removal of oral structures secondary to oral cancers. For individuals with orofacial anomalies, the course of habilitation or rehabilitation often includes surgical and/or prosthetic management, and therefore, the speech clinician must work closely with various medical and dental specialists.

Lips. Surgical repair of clefts of the lip can result in a relatively short and immobile upper lip. Although this might be expected to adversely affect articulation skills, there is no evidence in the literature that this anomaly causes a significant problem for most speakers. Bloomer and Hawk (1973) reported the effects of ablative surgery on production of labial phonemes in a patient who underwent surgical removal of the external and internal nasal structures for treatment of cancer. Although surgery resulted in a relatively immobile and shortened upper lip, the patient maintained good overall speech intelligibility, producing labiodental approximations for all bilabial consonants. The development of compensatory articulatory gestures to achieve acoustically acceptable speech production is very common in many patients with structural anomalies.

Tongue. As we mentioned when addressing minor structural variations, the tongue is a muscular structure capable of considerable changes in length and width. Because the tongue is such an adaptable organ, speakers are frequently able to compensate for major lingual structural defects and still maintain intelligible speech. Clinical investigators have repeatedly reported intelligible speech production following partial glossectomies (surgical removal of the tongue). One such case study (Backus, 1940) recorded the speech pattern of a 10-year-old boy with an undersized tongue after excision of the tongue tip and the left half of the tongue. Initially, the child's articulation was characterized by numerous consonant substitutions, but after a period of treatment, he was able to produce all consonants with little identifiable deviation.

For many patients, however, speech production is affected in varying degrees when part of the tongue is excised. Skelly, Spector, Donaldson, Brodeur, and Paletta (1971) reported pre-treatment and post-treatment intelligibility scores for 25 glossectomy (14 total, 11 partial) patients. Intelligibility judgments were based on single-word productions audio tape-recorded and played back to listeners. Intelligibility scores for those who underwent partial glossectomy ranged from 6 to 24 percent on the pre-test and from 24 to 46 percent on the post-test. Intelligibility scores for those who underwent total glossectomy ranged from 0 to 8 percent prior to treatment and from 18 to 24 percent after treatment. The investigators noted that the compensatory articulatory patterns of the two groups differed. Partial glossectomy patients utilized the residual tongue stump to modify articulation; total glossectomy patients made mandibular, labial, buccal, and palatal adjustments. The compensatory behavior of the total glossectomy patients with the highest intelligibility were described by Skelly et al. (1971) following cinefluorographic analysis of articulatory patterns:

> . . . /z/ was produced by means of a bilabial tension obstruction of the airstream, with the lips in much closer approximation than usual for this phoneme; /n/ was produced by momentary velar contraction followed by a quick uvular relaxation, with the lips concurrently almost approaching true adduction . . . these patients appeared to differentiate /n/ from /m/ not only by degree of labial occlusion, but also by a shift in nasal resonance . . . /g/ was produced by a pharyngeal constriction, with slight bulging of the retrogrossal pharyngeal wall . . . /d/ was produced by utilizing the lower lip in contact with the upper teeth . . . (111).

Massengill, Maxwell, and Picknell (1970) reported that speech intelligibility in three patients decreased as the amount of tongue excised increased. The patients demonstrated minimal difficulty in verbal communication, though speech distortion was present. Skelly et al. (1971) reported that unilateral tongue excision required fewer speech adaptations than tongue tip excisions.

Weinberg, Christensen, Logan, Bosma, and Wornall (1969) reported on a 7-year-old girl with congenital hypoplasia of the tongue who acquired intelligible speech without instruction. They reported that unilateral labial speech movements were noted during speech and indicated that these movements were probably developed in order to produce normal sounding speech.

Hard Palate. Oral cancers often require surgical removal of the diseased tissues. Bloomer and Hawk (1973) stated that removal of any part of the maxilla, if not restored surgically or prosthetically, creates a serious problem for the speaker. Majid, Weinberg, and Chalin (1974) examined speech intelligibility following prosthetic obturation of surgically acquired maxillary defects. Six adults—three women and three men—recorded speech with and without maxillary prosthetic obturators. Without the dental prosthesis, average intelligibility scores ranged from 40 to 80 percent and with it from 92 to 98 percent. The authors concluded that normal intelligibility is a realistic treatment goal for patients with acquired maxillary defects.

Clefts of the hard palate are surgically repaired, typically within the first 12 to 24 months of life. Scarring associated with the surgery has not been found to interfere with articulatory production.

Soft Palate. The relationship of the soft palate (velum) to articulation has been a topic of considerable research, much of it focusing on the sphincteral closure of the velopharyngeal port and the effect of velopharyngeal competence on articulation. **Velopharyngeal competence** refers to the valving that takes place to separate the nasal cavity from the oral cavity during nonnasal speech production. Inadequate velopharyngeal closure is frequently associated with (1) hypernasal resonance of vowels, vocalic consonants, and glides and liquids; (2) reduced or diminished intraoral breath pressure during production of pressure consonants, i.e., fricatives, stops, and affricates; and (3) nasal air emission accompanying production of pressure consonants, e.g., substitutions of glottal stops for stop consonants and pharyngeal fricatives for sibilants. Although velopharyngeal incompetence is often associated with individuals with clefts of the soft palate, some speakers without clefting also demonstrate such incompetence—for example, individuals with dysarthria related to neurogenic paresis or paralysis of the velopharyngeal muscles (Johns and Salyer, 1978).

As stated above, the pharyngeal fricative and the glottal stop are two examples of compensatory articulatory gestures associated with velopharyngeal valving problems. The glottal stop is characterized by interruption of the airstream at the glottis, resulting in a glottal click, or cough-like sound. Glottal stops are generally substituted for stops, particularly velar stops, as well as fricatives and affricates. The pharyngeal fricative is produced with the source of friction in the pharyngeal area and is frequently substituted for fricatives and affricates. The presence of hypernasality, nasal emission of air, weak consonants, glottal stops, and pharyngeal fricatives are all signs of velopharyngeal valving difficulties.

When the oral cavity communicates in some way with the nasal cavity, for example, through palatal fistulae (openings), or following ablative surgery or velopharyngeal incompetence, varying degrees of hypernasality will usually result. On the other hand, hyponasality (denasality) may result when the nasopharynx or nasal cavity is obstructed during speech production. Inflammation of the mucous membranes of the nasal cavity or a deviated septum may also cause hyponasality.

Nasopharynx. The nasopharyngeal tonsils (adenoids) are located at the upper or superior pharyngeal area. Hyperthrophied (enlarged) adenoids may compensate for a short or partially immobile velum, by assisting in velopharyngeal closure. Thus, their removal may result in hypernasality. But the adenoids may become sufficiently enlarged as to constitute a major obstruction of the nasopharynx, resulting in hyponasal speech. Enlarged adenoids may also interfere with Eustachian tube function in some individuals.

Summary. Although individuals with oral structural deviations frequently experience articulation problems, the relationship between structural deficits and articulation skills is not very predictable. The literature cites many instances of individuals with structural anomalies who have developed appropriate compensatory gestures to produce acoustically acceptable speech. Why some individuals are able to compensate for relatively gross abnormalities and others are unable to compensate for lesser deficits has not been resolved. A speech-language clinician who evaluates or treats individuals with oral structural anomalies should work collaboratively with various medical and dental specialists during speech habilitation or rehabilitation.

ORAL SENSORY FUNCTION

Some treatment approaches include the practice of calling a client's attention to sensory cues. For example, McDonald's (1964) sensorimotor therapy includes having the client identify oral cavity contacts and movements that occur during speech. More recently, Bordon (1984) called for heightened awareness of kinesthesis (sense of movement and position) during therapy. Almost any phonetic placement technique used to teach speech sounds usually includes a description of articulatory contacts and movements necessary for the production of the target speech sound. If one assumes that since oral sensory and kinesthetic feedback play a role in the development and ongoing monitoring of articulatory gestures, the relationship between oral sensory function and speech sound production should be established and that such research would have potential clinical implications.

The investigation of somethesis (sense of movement, position, touch, and awareness of muscle tension) has focused on (1) temporary sensory deprivation during oral sensory anesthetization (nerve block anesthesia) to determine the effect of sensory deprivation on speech production and (2) the assessment of oral sensory perception; for example, two-point discrimination or oral form discrimination to see if such sensory perception was related to articulatory skill. Considerable research into oral sensory functioning was conducted in the 1960s using a variety of methods to assess oral tactile sensitivity in order to understand if a relationship existed between these sensory tasks and articulation performance. Later research examined articulation of individuals during periods of temporary sensory deprivation, sometimes referred to as **oral blockade.**

Netsell (1986) has suggested that it is likely that adults are not consciously aware of specific speech movements during running speech. He also speculates that children may not be aware of articulatory movements during the acquisition period. If Netsell is correct, the clinician who attempts to utilize somesthetic senses in monitoring running speech may be asking the client to respond to information that is not available at a conscious level without instruction.

Oral Tactile Sensitivity. Early investigators of oral sensory function attempted to explore the sensitivity or threshold of awareness of oral structures to various stimuli. Ringel and Ewanowski (1965) studied oral tactile sensitivity utilizing an esthesiometer, a device used in the measurement of two-point discrimination. This instrument allows one to vary the distance between two stimulus points and control the force of the points and determine how far apart the two points must be before the subject perceives two points rather than one. Ringel and Ewanowski examined discrimination sensitivity of various structures in a normal population and found that the maximal to minimal awareness hierarchy for two-point stimulation (awareness of two points rather than one) was tongue tip, finger tip, lip, soft palate, alveolar ridge, and that the midline of structures tended to be more sensitive than the lateral edges.

Fucci and associates (Arnst and Fucci, 1975; Fucci, 1972) have measured the threshold of vibrotactile stimulation of structures in the oral cavity in both normal and speech-disordered individuals. These investigators found that subjects with misarticulations tended to have poorer oral sensory abilities than normal speaking subjects.

Oral Form Recognition. Oral sensory function has also been investigated extensively through form recognition tasks. Ringel, Burk, and Scott (1970) speculated that form identification (**oral stereognosis**) may provide information concerning nervous system integrity since the recognition of forms placed in the mouth was assumed to require integrity of peripheral receptors for touch and kinesthesis as well as central integrating processes. Most form recognition tasks require the subject to match forms placed in the oral cavity with drawings of the forms, or to make same–different judgments. Stimuli for such testing are typically small, plastic, three-dimensional forms of varying degrees of similarity, such as triangles, rectangles, ovals, and circles. McDonald and Aungst (1970) reported that oral form recognition improves with age, through adolescence.

Investigators who have studied the relationship between oral form recognition and articulation performance have reported inconsistent results. Arndt, Elbert, and Shelton (1970) did not find a significant relationship between oral form recognition and articulation performance in a third-grade population. But Ringel, House, Burk, Dolinsky, and Scott (1970) reported significant differences on an oral form-matching task between normal-speaking elementary school children and children with articulation errors. In their study, children were required to make same–different judgments of various forms. They noted that errors tended to increase with the severity of the articulation disorders; that is, children with severe misarticulations made more form-recognition errors than children with mild articulation problems.

Some researchers have investigated the relationship between production of specific phonemes and oral sensory function. Weinberg, Liss, and Hillis (1970) studied a junior and senior high school population using visual, manual, and oral

Factors Related to Phonological Disorders

form-identification tasks. A group of normal speakers was compared with subjects in an experimental group who misarticulated /r/ and had received two or more years of speech instruction. Although no significant differences in visual and manual form tasks were noted, normal speakers performed significantly better than the experimental group on the oral form task. McNutt (1977) also found that children who misarticulated /r/ did not perform as well as the normal speakers on oral form perception tasks; there were, however, no significant differences between the normal speakers and the children who misarticulated /s/.

Bishop, Ringel, and House (1973) compared oral form-recognition skills in deaf high school students who were orally trained (taught to use speech) and in those who were manually trained (taught to use sign language). The authors noted skill differences that favored the orally trained students and postulated that ". . . while a failure in oroperceptual functioning may lead to disorders of articulation, a failure to use the oral mechanism for speech activities, even in persons with normal orosensory capabilities, may result in poor performance on oroperceptual tasks" (257).

Locke (1968) examined the relationship between articulation skills and oral form-recognition scores from a different perspective. Rather than comparing the performance of normal-speaking children with those of children who demonstrated articulation errors, he compared the performance on an articulation learning task of 10 normal children with high form-recognition scores with that of 10 normal children with low form-recognition scores. Each subject was required to imitate three German sounds heard on a tape recording of a native German speaker. Locke found that the group with high form-perception scores obtained significantly better production scores on two of the three consonant sounds than the group with low form-identification scores. It should be noted that because this task involved learning a nonphonemic sound, performance differences may have been related to factors other than those used in form perception.

McDonald and Aungst (1970) pointed out that an individual can have good articulation skills despite poor oral form-recognition scores. They cited the case of a 21-year-old neurologically impaired male who articulated normally yet demonstrated difficulty in oral form identification and in two-point discrimination on the tongue.

Oral Anesthetization. The relationship between speech sound productions and oral sensory functions has also been examined through sensory deprivation. In order to study the role of oral sensation during speech, researchers have induced temporary states of oral sensory deprivation through the use of oral nerve-block and topical anesthetization. They then compared speech under normal conditions with speech under anesthetization on a variety of dimensions, such as overall intelligibility, vowel and consonant articulation, rate, phoneme duration, and physiological and acoustic characteristics.

Gammon, Smith, Daniloff, and Kim (1971) examined the articulation skills of eight adult subjects reading 30 sentences under four conditions: (1) normal, (2) with masking noise present, (3) nerve-block anesthesia, and (4) nerve-block anesthesia with masking noise. They noted few vowel distortions under any of the conditions and a 20 percent rate of consonant misarticulation (especially fricatives and affricates) under anesthesia and under anesthesia with noise. Scott and Ringel (1971) studied the articulation of two adult males producing lists of 24 bisyllabic words under normal and anesthetized conditions. They noted that articulatory changes caused by sensory deprivation were largely nonphonemic in nature and included loss of retroflexion and lip-rounding gestures, less tight fricative constrictions, and retracted points of articulation contacts.

Prosek and House (1975) studied four adult speakers reading 20 bisyllabic words in isolation and in sentences under normal and anesthetized conditions. Although intelligibility was maintained in the anesthetized condition, speech rate was slowed and minor imprecisions of articulation were noted. The authors reported that, when anesthetized, speakers produced consonants with slightly greater intraoral air pressure and longer duration than under the normal non-anesthetized condition.

Horii, House, Li, and Ringel (1973) examined acoustic characteristics of speech produced during temporary loss of oral sensation. They noted a reduction and shift of high-frequency energy, prolongation of utterances, and higher and more variable fundamental frequencies. The authors suggested that the high intelligibility of speech produced by anesthetized speakers may be due, in part, to a selective effect of sensory deprivation on certain classes of speech sounds and to the human listener's adaptability to distortions of the speech signal.

In summary, studies involving anesthetization found that speech remained intelligible although subjects did not speak as accurately under anesthetization (deprived of certain sensory feedback) as they did under normal conditions. However, the subjects in these studies were adult speakers with normal articulation skills prior to the sensory deprivation. It is unclear if reduced oral sensory feedback might interfere with the acquisition of speech or effect remediation.

Oral Sensory Function and Articulation Learning. Jordan, Hardy, and Morris (1978) studied the influence of tactile sensation as a feedback mechanism in articulation learning. Their subjects were first-grade boys, nine with good articulation skills and nine with poor articulation skills. Subjects were fitted with palatal plates equipped with touch-sensitive electrodes and taught to replicate four positions of lingual-palatal contact, with and without topical anesthesia. Both groups learned the tongue placements, but children with poor articulation performed less well on tasks of precise tongue placement than children with good articulation. Since the subjects with poor articulation were able to improve their initially poor performance when given specific training on the tongue placement tasks, it appears that this group received the intraoral sensory feedback necessary to learn the tasks but needed more experience for the learning to occur. The type of feedback received was assumed to be from muscle spindles on deep receptors within the tongue, since touch-pressure receptors were thought to be anesthetized.

Wilhelm (1971) and Shelton, Willis, Johnson, and Arndt (1973) used oral form-recognition materials to teach form recognition to misarticulating children and reported inconsistent results. Wilhelm reported articulation improved as oral form recognition improved. Findings of Shelton et al. did not support that finding. Ruscello (1972) reported that form-recognition scores improved in children undergoing treatment for articulation.

Summary. The role of normal oral sensory function or somesthetic feedback in the development and maintenance of speech production is complex. Despite efforts to identify the relationship between oral sensory status and articulatory performance, conclusive findings are lacking. A review of the literature, however, has revealed the following:

1. Many methods have been used to measure oral sensory perception; that is form recognition, touch-pressure threshold, two-point discrimination, and oral vibro-tactile thresholds.

2. Oral form recognition improves with age, through adolescence.

3. The role of oral sensory information in the acquisition of phonology is unclear.

4. Individuals with poor articulation tend to achieve slightly lower scores on form-perception tasks than their normal-speaking peers. However, some individuals with poor form-identification skills have good articulation.

5. Investigators who have anesthetized oral structures reported that intelligibility is generally maintained during sensory deprivation but less accuracy in articulation was noted.

6. Although research has indicated that some individuals with articulation problems may also have oral sensory deficits, the neurological mechanisms underlying the use of sensory information during experimental conditions may differ from those operating in normal running speech.

7. Information concerning oral sensory function has not been shown to have clinical applicability or a place in treatment.

8. It would seem important to differentiate between the effects of sensory deprivation in individuals who have already developed good speech skills and the effects in individuals with defective articulation.

9. The effects of long-term sensory deprivation have yet to be explored.

MOTOR ABILITIES

Because speech is a motor act, researchers have explored the relationship between articulation skills and motor coordination, investigating performance on general motor tasks as well as oral and facial motor tasks.

General Motor Skills. Studies focusing on the relationship between general motor skills and articulatory abilities have yielded inconsistent and inconclusive results. Investigators have examined populations of different ages and with different speech disorders and have assessed different motor skills on both a formal and informal level (Bilto, 1941; Reid, 1947b; Prins, 1962b; Jenkins and Lohr, 1964). Because individuals with articulation problems have not been shown to have significant retardation in general motor development, little recent research on this topic has been reported.

Oral-Facial Motor Skills. Speech is a dynamic process that requires the precise coordination of the oral musculature. During ongoing speech production, fine muscle movements of the lips, tongue, palate, and jaw constantly alter the dimensions of the oral cavity. An assessment of the client's oral motor skills is typically a part of an articulatory evaluation. Tests of diadochokinetic rate or maximum repetition rate (rapid repetition of syllables) have been used most frequently to evaluate oral motor skills. Diadochokinetic rate is established either with a "count by time" procedure, in which the examiner counts the number of syllables spoken in a given interval of time, or a "time by count" measurement, in which the examiner notes the time required to produce a designated number of syllables. The advantage of the time by count measurement is that few operations are required since the examiner need only listen to the syllable count and turn off the timing device when the requisite number of syllables is produced. Performance is then compared to normative data. The syllables most frequently used to assess diadochokinetic rates are /pʌ/, /tʌ/, and /kʌ/ in isolation and the sequence /pʌtʌ/, /tʌkʌ/, /pʌkʌ/, /pʌtʌkʌ/. There is some evidence that diadochokinetic rates improve with age. Fletcher (1972) examined diadochokinetic rates in children aged 6 to 13 years using a count by time procedure. He reported that children increased the number of syllables produced in a given unit of time at each successive age from 7 to 13 years. Data reported by Canning and Rose (1974) indicated that adult values for maximum repetition rates were reached by 9- to 10-year-olds, whereas Fletcher's data show a convergence after age 15.

A better understanding of the relationship between oral motor skills and articulation skills in individuals without apparent neurological involvement is of interest to speech clinicians since individuals with speech problems who perform well on oral motor tasks are not uncommon.

McNutt (1977) and Dworkin (1978) examined diadochokinetic rates of children with specific misarticulations and of their normal-speaking peers. McNutt examined the rate of alternating syllable productions such as /dʌgə/ in children with normal articulation, children with /s/ misarticulation, and children with /r/ misarticulation. Both groups of children with misarticulations were noted to be slower than normal speakers in syllable production rates. Dworkin examined lingual diadochokinetic rates for the syllables /tʌ/, /dʌ/, /kʌ/, and /gʌ/, in normal speakers and frontal lisping speakers aged 7 to 12 years. The mean rate of utterances of the syllables tested was significantly lower in the disordered group.

Some researchers have questioned the usefulness of rapid syllable repetition tasks and their relationship to articulation skills. McDonald (1964) stated that diadochokinetic tasks have

> . . . only limited usefulness in assessing motor control of the articulatory mechanism because the movements of articulation are produced by the simultaneous contraction of different groups of muscles rather than the alternating contraction of opposed muscles. . . . Children are seen clinically who can skillfully produce diadochokinetic movements but who demonstrate considerable difficulty in producing patterns of overlapping movements (183).

Winitz (1969) also pointed out that because normal speakers have a history of success with speech sounds, they may have an advantage over subjects with misarticulations on diadochokinetic tasks. Tiffany (1980) pointed out that little is known concerning the significance of scores obtained on diadochokinetic tasks and, thus, "such measures appear to lack a substantial theoretical base" (895).

Summary. Individuals with articulation problems have not been shown to exhibit significantly depressed motor coordination on tasks of general motor performance. The relationship between oral motor skills and articulation skills in functional articulation disorders remains uncertain. Although individuals with defective articulation have been found to perform more poorly on diadochokinetic tasks than their normal-speaking peers, these results cannot be accurately interpreted until the relationship between diadochokinetic tasks and the ability to articulate sounds in context is clarified.

Factors Related to Phonological Disorders

Introduction. The term *tongue thrust* refers to excessive anterior tongue movement during swallowing or speech and the anterior placement of the tongue during resting posture (Christensen and Hanson, 1981). Proffit (1986) points out that tongue thrust is something of a misnomer since it implies that the tongue is thrust forward forcefully, when in reality such individuals do not seem to use more tongue force against the teeth than non-thrusters. Rather, tongue thrust swallow implies a directionality of tongue activity in swallowing. Other terms sometimes used to describe these behaviors include *reverse swallow, deviant swallow,* and *infantile swallow*. These terms should be avoided because of faulty implications inherent in them (Mason, 1988). The most salient features of a tongue thrust swallow pattern, according to Mason and Proffit (1974), include one or more of these conditions:

1. . . . during the initiation of a swallow, a forward gesture of the tongue between the anterior teeth so that the tongue tip contacts the lower lip;
2. During speech activities, fronting of the tongue between or against the anterior teeth with the mandible hinged open (in phonetic contexts not intended for such placements); and
3. At rest, the tongue carried forward in the oral cavity with the mandible hinged slightly open and the tongue tip against or between the anterior teeth'' (116).

Everyone starts out life as a tongue thruster because at birth the tongue fills the oral cavity and tongue fronting is obligatory. Sometime later, prior to about 5 years, most children replace an anterior tongue-gums/teeth seal during swallowing with a superior tongue-palate seal (Hanson, 1988b).

Tongue thrust during swallow and/or tongue fronting at rest can usually be identified by visual inspection. Mason (1988) has pointed out that two types of tongue fronting should be differentiated. The first is described as a *habit* and is seen in the absence of any morphological structural delimiting factors. The second is *obligatory* and may involve factors such as airway obstruction or enlarged tonsils with tongue thrusting being a necessary adaptation to maintain the size of the airway to pass food during swallow. Oral myofunction therapy for obligatory tongue fronting has been questioned by Shelton (1989) because of the poor prognosis for change, and thus it is important to differentiate between the two types of tongue thrust.

Hanson (1988a) suggested that a better description for these tongue position and movement behaviors would be "oral muscle pattern disorders." Orthodontists and speech-language pathologists have been interested in tongue thrusting and a forward tongue resting posture because of the perception that tongue function can cause certain types of (1) malocclusion problems, (2) altered patterns of facial development, and (3) articulation problems. The type of articulation disorder associated with tongue thrust and malocclusion is a frontal lisp characterized by anterior tongue placement for /s/ and /z/. Some children who evidence tongue thrusting also manifest articulatory errors. The number of children with lisps is higher in children who evidence tongue thrusting than for children who do not evidence such behavior. Sometimes tongue thrust is also associated with anterior placement for /ʃ/, /tʃ/, /dʒ/, /ʒ/, /t/, /d/, /l/, and /n/.

Although tongue thrusting has been a topic of interest to speech-language clinicians for some time, the validity of the label and the efficacy of treating the phenomenon are matters of controversy. In 1974, a *Position Statement on Tongue Thrust,* prepared by the Joint Committee on Dentistry and Speech Pathology and Audiology, was adopted by the American Speech and Hearing Association and by the House of Delegates of the American Association of Orthodontists. The position statement questioned the diagnostic label *tongue thrust,* expressed skepticism that myofunctional therapy produced significant changes in oral form or function, and called for research to establish the validity of tongue thrust as a clinical entity. This committee (*Asha,* 1975) went on to state that they "could not recommend that speech pathologists engage in clinical management procedures with the intent of altering function patterns of deglution" (331). In contrast, the statement adopted as an official statement by the ASHA Legislative Council in 1991 included the statement that abnormal fronting (tongue thrust) of the tongue can be identified reliably, that myofunctional therapy is effective in modifying disorders of tongue movement and lip posture, and that such treatment is within the purview of speech-language pathology.

Impact of Tongue Thrust on Dentition. The current view is that the resting posture of the tongue affects the position of the teeth and jaws more than does the tongue function during swallowing (tongue thrust) or speaking (Proffit, 1986). Tongue thrusting may play a role in maintaining or influencing an abnormal dental pattern when an anterior resting tongue position is present. If the position of the tongue is forward (forward resting position) and between the anterior teeth at rest, this condition can impede normal teeth eruption and can result in an anterior open bite. However, tongue thrusting patients, in the absence of an anterior tongue resting position, are not thought to develop malocclusions. The pressure or force on dentition associated with tongue thrust during speaking and swallowing are of short duration and do not exert enough force on the dentition to cause problems of dental occlusion. Mason (1988) pointed out that individuals who exhibit a tongue thrust pattern and forward tongue posture create morphological conditions that can potentially lead to dental occlusion problems and would be much more likely to develop a malocclusion than when only a tongue thrust is present.

Tongue Thrust and Presence of Articulation Errors. Investigators have reported that articulation errors, primarily sibilant distortions, occur more frequently in children who evidence tongue thrust than in those who do not. Fletcher, Casteel, and Bradley (1961) studied 1,615 school children aged 6 to 18 and found that children who demonstrated a tongue thrust swallow pattern were more likely to have associated sibilant distortions than children who did not. They also reported that subjects with normal swallow patterns demonstrated a significant decrease in sibilant distortion with age, whereas tongue thrusters did not.

Palmer (1962) found that clients referred for marked tongue thrusting nearly always demonstrated a sibilant "difference" but that the difference was perceived as only a slight lisp. He reported that such differences also occurred on /t/, /d/, and /n/.

Jann, Ward, and Jann (1964) examined the relationship between speech defects, tongue thrusting, and malocclusion in children in the early primary grades and reported a high incidence of /s/, /z/, and /l/ variations in children with tongue thrust swallow patterns.

Factors Related to Phonological Disorders

Subtelny, Mestre, and Subtelny (1964) used radiographic techniques to examine the relationship between normal and abnormal oral morphology and /s/ production. Their subjects, 81 adolescents and adults, were divided into three groups: (1) normal speakers with normal occlusion, (2) normal speakers with severe malocclusion, and (3) abnormal speakers with severe malocclusion. In contrast to earlier investigators, these authors found that the incidence of tongue thrusting and malocclusion in normal speakers was comparable to that in abnormal speakers. This finding is consistent with the reported developmental decrease in the reverse swallow pattern.

Dworkin and Culatta (1980) studied the relationships among protrusive tongue strength, open bite, and articulation in 141 children. They reported no significant difference among their group in tongue strength.

Treatment Issues. Hanson (1988a), in a review of the 11 studies which examined the effectiveness of tongue thrust therapy, reported that 10 of the investigators reported positive results concerning the efficacy of oral myofunctional therapy. Overstake (1976) studied 48 children aged 7 to 12 years who evidenced interdental /s/ defects, tongue thrusts, and open bite and/or overjet malocclusions. Half of the children received oral myofunctional therapy only, and the other half received oral myofunctional and speech services. Overstake reported that speech improved in both groups of subjects. Christensen and Hanson (1981) studied two groups of 6-year-old children, with five children in each group, all of whom exhibited tongue thrust and articulation errors (lisps). All subjects received 14 weeks of treatment, with half receiving treatment for articulation only and the other half receiving oral myofunctional services prior to and in conjunction with articulation instruction. Subjects in both groups made similar progress in correcting /s/, but only children who received oral myofunctional services modified their tongue thrust behaviors.

Other support for tongue thrust intervention has often come from clinical reports by clinicians who conduct oral myofunctional therapy. For example, Hilton (1984) stated "In my experience, many tongue-fronting children who begin speech articulation therapy without having had the early sensorimotor and stretching activities of myotherapy . . . begin with an unnecessary handicap . . . I provide every tongue-fronting speech articulation case these initial oral awareness, control, and flexibility exercises prior to initiation of the place-feature oriented therapy . . ." (51).

The official statement adopted by the ASHA Legislative Council (*Asha,* 1991) relative to the role of the speech-language pathologist in assessment and management of oral myofunctional disorders includes the statement that "Investigation, assessment, and treatment of oral myofunctional disorders are within the purview of speech-language pathology" (7). This statement, as well as others stated below, shows that ASHA's view of tongue thrust and oral myofunctional therapy has changed considerably from the skepticism about this group of disorders reflected in the 1974 joint statement and endorsement by the American Speech-Language-Hearing Association, the American Dental Association, and the American Association of Orthodontists.

1991 Position Statement. It is the position of the American Speech-Language-Hearing Association (ASHA) that:

1. Oral myofunctional phenomena, including abnormal fronting (tongue thrust) of the tongue at rest and during swallowing, lip incompetency, and sucking habits, can be identified reliably. These conditions co-occur with speech misarticulations in some patients.

2. Tongue fronting may reflect learned behaviors, physical variables, or both.

3. There is published research that indicates that oral myofunctional therapy is effective in modifying disorders of tongue and lip posture and movement.

4. Investigation, assessment, and treatment of oral myofunctional disorders are within the purview of speech-language pathology.

5. The speech-language pathologist who desires to perform oral myofunctional services must have the required knowledge and skills to provide a high quality of treatment. The provision of oral myofunctional therapy remains an option of individual speech-language pathologists whose interests and training qualify them.

6. Evaluation and treatment should be interdisciplinary and tailored to the individual. The speech-language pathologist performing oral myofunctional therapy should collaborate with an orthodontist, pediatric dentist, or other dentists, and with medical specialists such as an otolaryngologist, pediatrician, or allergist, as needed.

7. Appropriate goals of oral myofunctional therapy should include the retraining of labial and lingual resting and functional patterns (including speech). The speech-language pathologist's statements of treatment goals should avoid predictions of treatment outcome based on tooth position or dental occlusal changes.

8. Basic and applied research is needed regarding the nature and evaluation or oral myofunctions and the treatment of oral myofunctional disorders (7).

The ad hoc committee report (*Asha,* 1989) on labial-lingual posturing function developed the above statement based on the following concepts relative to oral myofunctional phenomena as they relate to communication disorders:

1. All infants exhibit a tongue thrust swallow as a normal performance.

2. This pattern changes with growth and maturation to the extent that many different swallow patterns can be identified from infancy to adulthood.

3. At some time in development, a tongue protrusion swallow is no longer the norm and can be considered undesirable or as a contributing and maintaining factor in malocclusion, lisping, or both.

4. A related condition that has a stronger link to malocclusion is a forward resting posture of the tongue. . . . This is consistent with orthodontic theory and research that long-acting forces against the teeth result in tooth movement whereas short-acting (intermittent) forces are not as likely to cause tooth movement.

5. There is descriptive evidence that during the course of oral myofunctional therapy, some individuals have corrected or controlled a tongue thrust swallow and an anterior resting posture.

6. Diagnostic attention should be directed toward determining whether a tongue thrust swallow and a forward tongue resting posture coexist in a given patient. When these conditions coexist, a greater link to malocclusion would be expected than from a tongue thrust swallow alone. However, there is insufficient evidence to show that a forward tongue posture and tongue thrust swallow are more detrimental than a tongue forward resting posture alone. There is also some evidence that a tongue forward resting posture or a tongue thrust swallow and lisping coexist in some persons. Correction of tongue function or posture may facilitate correction of the lisp, or the interdentalization of the /t/, /d/, /n/, and /l/ phonemes.

7. In normal development, slight separation of the lips at rest ("lip incompetence")

Factors Related to Phonological Disorders

is normal in children. With growth, the lips typically achieve contact at rest in the teenage years. Some individuals, however, persist in a lips-apart posture after development has advanced sufficiently to permit lip closure. Such individuals may be candidates for treatment.

8. There is some evidence that lip exercises can be successful in facilitating a closed-lip posture.

9. Sucking habits (e.g., finger, thumb, tongue, lips) can influence dental development. When tongue thrusting and thumb sucking coexist into mixed dentition, developmental correction of the tongue thrust would not be expected until the thumb, finger, or sucking habit ceases.

10. Variables in addition to learning influence tongue posture. They include posterior airway obstruction, which may involve tonsils, adenoids, nasal blockage, high posterior tongue position with a short mandibular ramus, or a long soft palate. Many morphologic features or combinations of features can reduce oral isthmus size and obligate the tongue to rest forward. Diagnostic procedures should distinguish such patients from those with other forward tongue postures or functions. The obligatory tongue forward posture group would seem unlikely candidates for myofunctional therapy in the absence of medical treatment. Any indicated remedial medical procedures are usually carried out prior to consideration of myofunctional therapy.

The *Asha* report strongly recommended an interdisciplinary approach to the planning, treatment, and further study of these disorders.

Summary

1. The current position of the American Speech-Language-Hearing Association as stated in the 1991 position statement relative to the clinical entity of tongue thrust as well as the management of oral myofunctional disorders was modified significantly from the 1974 statement.

2. Data are available which support the idea that abnormal labial-lingual posturing function can be identified, including abnormal fronting (tongue thrust) of the tongue at rest and during swallowing, lip incompetency, and sucking habits.

3. A forward tongue resting posture has the potential with or without a tongue thrust swallow to be associated with malocclusions.

4. There is some evidence that an anterior tongue resting posture or a tongue thrust swallow and lisping coexist in some persons.

5. Oral myofunctional therapy can be effective in modifying disorders of tongue and lip posture and movement.

6. Assessment and treatment of oral myofunctional disorders which may include some non-speech remediation are within the purview of speech-language pathology but should involve interdisciplinary collaboration.

7. Research is needed regarding the nature and evaluation of oral myofunctions and treatment of such disorders.

NEUROMOTOR DISORDERS

Speech production at a motor level requires muscle strength, speed of movement, appropriate range of excursion, accuracy of movement, coordination of multiple movements, motor steadiness, and muscle tone (Darley, Aronson, and Brown, 1975). Damage that impairs one or more of these neuromuscular functions may affect motor speech production. Motor speech disorders are not only disorders of articulation but also frequently involve other components of speech production, including phonation, respiration, or velopharyngeal function.

Neurologists and speech-language pathologists have sought to understand the possible relationship between the clinical (behavioral) responses associated with neurologically impaired individuals and the site and extent of the neurological lesions (brain damage). The reason for such inquiry is to identify some potential commonality across patients with respect to the specific brain damage and the concomitant cognitive language impairment.

Although entire books are devoted to motor speech disorders, the following offers a brief introduction to this topic.

Dysarthria. Dysarthria is a speech problem caused by neuromuscular impairment. It may result from a lesion of the central or peripheral nervous system that involves the pathways subserving the speech mechanism (Darley, Aronson, and Brown, 1969). Because this disorder has varying characteristics that can be caused by different types of lesions at different locations in the brain, the term *dysarthrias* is, perhaps, more accurate than *dysarthria.*

Dysarthrias are caused by a paralysis, weakness, or incoordination of the speech musculature, which may result from localized injuries to the nervous system, various inflammatory processes, toxic metabolic disorders, vascular lesions of the brain, degenerative disorders of the nervous system, or be associated with a brain tumor. The most significant characteristic of dysarthric speech is reduced intelligibility. Dysarthric speech can involve disturbances in respiration, phonation, articulation, resonance, and prosody. Phonemes misarticulated in spontaneous speech are also likely to be misarticulated in other situations, such as reading and imitation tasks.

Table 5–1 lists the five types of dysarthrias and the most prominent deviant speech characteristics associated with each. The most common of these characteristics is the production of imprecise consonants.

Apraxia. Apraxia is a motor speech disorder also caused by brain damage, but it is differentiated from the dysarthrias and described as a separate clinical entity. Apraxia of speech is characterized by an impairment of motor speech programming with no weakness, paralysis, or incoordination of the speech musculature. Whereas dysarthrias frequently affect all motor speech processes—respiration, phonation, articulation, resonance, and prosody—apraxia primarily affects articulatory abilities with secondary prosodic alterations.

A description of some of the clinical characteristics of this disorder has been provided by Darley, Aronson, and Brown (1975):

> Apraxia of speech is characterized by highly variable articulation errors embedded in a pattern of speech made slow and effortful by trial-and-error gropings for the desired articulatory postures. The off-target productions are usually complications of articulatory performance, that is, substitutions (many of them unrelated to the target phoneme), additions, repetitions, and prolongations. Less frequently, the errors are simplifications, that is, distortions and omissions. Errors are most often on consonants occurring initially in words, predominantly on those phonemes and clusters of phonemes requiring more complex muscular adjustment. Errors are exacerbated by increase in length of word and the linguistic and psychologic "weight" of a word in the sentence. They are not significantly influenced by auditory, visual, or instructional set variables. Islands of fluent, error-free speech highlight the marked discrepancy between efficient automatic-reactive productions and inefficient volitional-purposive productions (267).

Factors Related to Phonological Disorders

TABLE 5–1. **Dysarthrias and Associated Speech Deviations.**

TYPE	DISCRETE NEUROLOGICAL GROUP	RELATIVE PROMINENCE OF SPEECH DEVIATIONS
Flaccid Dysarthria—(Disorders of the Lower Motor Neuron)	Bulbar Palsy	1. hypernasality 2. imprecise consonants 3. breathiness (continuous)
Spastic Dysarthria—(Disorders of the Upper Motor Neuron)	Pseudobulbar Palsy	1. imprecise consonants 2. monopitch 3. reduced stress
Ataxic Dysarthria— (Disorders of the Cerebellar System)	Cerebellar lesions	1. imprecise consonants 2. excess and equal stress 3. irregular articulatory breakdown
Hypokinetic Dysarthria—(Disorders of the Extrapyramidal System	Parkinsonism	1. monopitch 2. reduced stress 3. monoloudness
Hyperkinetic Dysarthria—(Disorders of the Extrapyramidal System)	Chorea	1. imprecise consonants 2. prolonged intervals 3. variable rate
	Dystonia	1. imprecise consonants 2. distorted vowels 3. harsh voice quality
Mixed Dysarthrias—	Amyotrophic lateral sclerosis with relative prominence in pseudobulbar palsy and bulbar palsy	1. imprecise consonants 2. hypernasality 3. harsh voice quality

Source: Adapted from F. Darley, A. Aronson, and J. Brown, *Motor Speech Disorders* (Philadelphia: W. B. Saunders, 1975).

Some clients who demonstrate apraxia of speech (**verbal apraxia**) also demonstrate similar difficulty in volitional oral nonspeech tasks, a behavior described as **oral apraxia** (Darley, 1970; De Renzi, Pieczuro, and Vignolo, 1966). For example, an individual may protrude his or her tongue during eating but may be unable to perform this act voluntarily. Although oral apraxia often coexists with verbal apraxia, this is not always the case.

Johns and Darley (1970) compared apraxic and dysarthric speakers on tasks involving spontaneous speaking and reading at a "self-chosen rate" and at a rapid rate. They reported that (1) apraxic speakers were less consistent than dysarthric speakers in their articulatory errors; (2) apraxics made fewer articulation errors and were more intelligible when reading at rapid rates rather than slow rates; (3) apraxics performed better on the spontaneous speaking tasks than on the reading tasks; (4) dysarthrics made fewer errors and were more intelligible when speaking at slow rates rather than fast rates; and (5) distortions accounted for 65 percent of the errors made by dysarthrics but only 10 percent of the errors made by apraxic speakers; substitutions accounted for 50 percent of the errors made by apraxic speakers but only 10 percent of the errors made by dysarthric speakers.

Speech sound errors seen in apraxia have usually been identified as sound substitution errors and thereby differentiated from the speech sound distortions seen in dysarthrics. Itoh and Sasanuma (1984) have argued, however, that some of the substitutions seen in apraxia can better be described as distortions, and thus, apraxia may be characterized by both substitution and distortion errors. Lapointe and Wertz (1974) described patients who demonstrated a "mixed" articulation disorder consisting of a combination of apraxic and dysarthric speech characteristics.

Developmental Verbal Dyspraxia. Among the large number of children who evidence developmental phonological disorders is a relatively small group that has been identified as having an articulation disorder which may be associated with some type of congenital neuromotor impairment in the absence of dysarthria. The labels **developmental verbal dyspraxia** (DVD) and **developmental apraxia of speech** (DAS) are sometimes used to identify this subcategory of children. While the literature in this area is almost exclusively focused on children, Haynes, Johns, and May (1978) have suggested that the syndrome of conditions commonly associated with this disorder may persist to adulthood.

Descriptions of this unique subgroup of phonologically impaired children have existed for some time. In the late 1800s, Hadden (1891) described children who evidenced "defects of articulation in the presence of good mental capacity . . . associated neither with mechanical conditions in the mouth, nor with diseases of the auditory apparatus, but almost certainly dependent on some fault in the central nervous system." Morley (1957), along with other Europeans, was among the first in more recent times to call attention to this type of developmental speech disorder and to describe this subgroup of articulatory impaired youngsters. During the 1970s, the diagnostic label **developmental apraxia/dyspraxia** came into prominence in the United States to identify a particular subcategory of children who traditionally were identified as having "functional" articulation disorders (disorders of unknown etiology), but whom clinicians suspected as having a subtle motor or neurological basis to their phonological errors.

Apraxia in the adult population is viewed as a motor speech disorder associated with lesions of the nervous system and characterized by an impairment of motor speech programming with no weakness, paralysis, or incoordination of the speech musculature (Darley, 1970; Darley, Aronson, and Brown, 1975). The term *apraxia* has been borrowed from the adult literature to identify a somewhat behaviorally similar, but etiologically dissimilar (at least there is no evidence to substantiate similarity) phenomenon in children. Thus, the term *developmental verbal dyspraxia* or *developmental apraxia* has come to refer to children with articulation errors who also have difficulty with volitional or imitative production of speech sounds and sequences. These symptoms may or may not be accompanied by symptoms of oral apraxia.

Although DVD is widely discussed and a body of literature has developed that addresses the description, assessment, and treatment of the disorder, controversy persists over the existence of such a disorder. Of all the areas of controversy related to DVD, the issue of whether the disorder presents itself as an identifiable and consistent syndrome continues to be debated. Some have suggested that it is inappropriate to consider DVD as a "diagnostic entity" of phonologically impaired children since the symptoms attributed to the syndrome are not consistent enough in occurrence or unique enough to support such a designation.

Characteristics of DVD. Studies by Rosenbek and Wertz (1972) and Yoss and Darley (1974) are among the most frequently cited studies that have sought to document the characteristics of DVD. According to these studies and other references in the literature, behavioral symptoms commonly attributed to children reflecting developmental dyspraxia of speech include the following:

1. Delayed or deviant speech development
2. Language comprehension superior to language expression (lexical and syntactical formulation)
3. Oral apraxia frequently present
4. Difficulty sequencing articulatory movements; production poorer in connected speech than single words; metathetic errors (sound reversals)
5. Inconsistent error patterns; deletions more common than substitutions; errors most common on complex fricatives, affricates, and clusters; substitutions reflect two and three feature differences; errors with consonant voicing and devoicing; distortions; vowel errors
6. Slow improvement in treatment; lack of retention and generalization from one treatment session to the next
7. Fine and gross motor incoordination; high incidence of "soft" neurological signs
8. Family history of speech and language disorders

A replication of the Yoss and Darley (1974) study was conducted in Australia by Williams, Ingham, and Rosenthal (1981), using a non-hospital population. Their findings did not support those of Yoss and Darley relative to behavioral symptoms associated with DVD. It has been suggested (Guyette and Diedrich, 1981) that this discrepancy in findings may be related to the fact that Yoss and Darley selected apraxic subjects based on volitional oral movement skills, thus "building in" a subject selection characteristic that was to be studied, and secondly, that their subjects were selected from a hospital pediatric unit, which may have resulted in a biased sample of children with severe articulation problems.

Guyette and Diedrich (1981) presented an extensive review of the literature related to DVD and concluded that (1) there is little agreement on which symptoms or behaviors are important in diagnosis of the disorder; (2) there is a paucity of data to support agreed upon symptoms; and (3) even when data are available, there is no clear specification of how these data can be used in identifying children.

In spite of the arguments against the validity of the DVD syndrome, the diagnosis is supported by clinicians and researchers, including those with a primary concern for neurologically based communication impairments. For those clinicians working with children who are perceived to evidence dyspraxic characteristics, several concepts may be useful in guiding professional actions.

1. Jaffe (1986) has pointed out that DVD appears to be a syndrome in which all symptoms and signs need not be present to diagnose the disorder, nor must one typical sign or symptom be present to establish the diagnosis.
2. It has been suggested (Crary and Towne, 1984) that clinicians should work to better describe the basic motor properties of the deficits seen in dyspraxic children. In other words, keep better records of children's performances on both speech and non-speech tasks (for both those who are and are not perceived as evidencing motor articulation problems). In this way, we can refine our descriptions and make comparisons among clients.
3. One way to support the presence of a diagnostic category is to demonstrate that particular remediation procedures are effective in ameliorating symptoms. This may be accomplished by gathering data on how clients progress clinically in such areas as (a) contrast awareness, (b) acquisition of articulatory gestures, and (c)

phonological generalization patterns. Documenting progress (single subject research designs can be useful in this regard) in response to particular intervention procedures can be helpful in testing the viability of the DAS diagnosis.

4. Love (1992) suggested that

> . . . despite the serious questions raised about the etiology, pathology, and validity of the reported signs and symptoms of the DVD syndrome, it remains an appropriate and useful diagnostic category of childhood motor speech disability (95).

He further suggested that DVD

> . . . provides substantial assistance in the differential diagnosis of the most prevalent speech disorder encountered by the speech-language pathologist—a developmental phonologic disorder, or so called "functional articulation disorder." The appropriate identification of children with phonologic disorders whose etiology is likely neurogenic rather than learned or idiopathic provides added explanatory power to the understanding, assessing, and managing of a select group of children with severe and often unyielding articulation defects that make them special problem cases for the speech-language pathologist (98).

Based on the suggestions of Haynes (1985) and others who have identified modifications of traditional articulation treatment techniques that are helpful with the dyspraxic population, the following guidelines for treating developmental apraxia of speech are presented:

1. Employ imitation and verbal command drills focusing on non-speech tongue and lip movements.
2. Practice imitation of sustained vowels and consonants followed by production of simple syllable shapes (CV, VC, CVC).
3. Practice movement patterns and sequences in words, word-pairs, and phrases.
4. Emphasize slow rate and self monitoring of productions. Avoid traditional discrimination training.
5. Employ techniques designed to capitalize on orosensory perceptual awareness (tactile stimulation) and other special cueing techniques that can be associated with particular sounds and sound sequences (see Bashir, Grahamjones, and Bostwick, 1984).
6. Instruction needs to be frequent and employ systematic drills.
7. Teaching a core vocabulary may be helpful particularly with severe developmental apraxia.
8. If their speech remains so severely impaired that they cannot be understood, employ augmentative communication strategies to assist clients to meet their daily communication needs and develop their language systems.

COGNITIVE-LINGUISTIC FACTORS

INTELLIGENCE

When identifying factors related to the presence of phonological disorders, one might assume intelligence to be a relevant variable. The relationship between intelligence (as measured by IQ tests) and articulation disorders has been the subject of several investigations. Reid (1947a, 1947b) studied the intelligence level of 38 elementary and junior high school students identified as having disordered articulation. Mental ages were obtained from school records and the *California*

Test of Mental Maturity. The authors reported that articulation proficiency could not be predicted from intelligence scores when the IQ was 70 or above.

Winitz (1959a, 1959b), in his investigation of 150 children, reported similarly low positive correlations between scores obtained on the *Wechsler Intelligence Scale for Children* and the *Templin-Darley Articulation Screening Test.* Thus, in terms of the relationship between intelligence and articulation in children of normal intelligence, data indicated that one is not a good predictor of the other.

A second perspective on the relationship between intelligence and phonology may be gleaned from studies of the phonological status of mentally retarded individuals. Prior to 1970, a number of studies were conducted to explore the prevalence of articulation disorders in the mentally retarded population. Typical of these studies are those of Wilson (1966), Schlanger (1953), and Schlanger and Gottsleben (1957). Wilson used the *Hejina Articulation Test* in his study of 777 mentally retarded children whose chronological ages ranged from 6 to 16 years. He reported that 53.4 percent of the children evidenced articulation disorders. Errors of substitution, omission, and distortion tended to decrease as the mental ages of the children increased. Wilson (1966) concluded that "There is a high incidence of articulatory deviation in an educable mentally retarded population, and the incidence and degree of severity is closely related to mental-age levels" (432). Wilson's findings also indicated that articulatory skills which continue to improve until approximately age 8 in the normal population continue to show improvement well beyond that age in the retarded population.

Schlanger (1953) and Schlanger and Gottsleben (1957) reported similar findings to Wilson in their studies of articulation in the mentally retarded. Schlanger investigated 74 children in a residential school; the children's mean chronological age (C.A.) was 12;1, and their mean mental age (M.A.), 6;8. Of the 74 children, 56.7 percent were found to have articulation disorders. In their study of 400 randomly selected residents at a training school with a chronological age mean of 28.9 and a mean mental age of 7.8, Schlanger and Gottsleben reported that 78 percent presented articulation delays ranging from slight to severe. Individuals with Down's syndrome or whose etiologies were based upon central nervous system impairment demonstrated the most pronounced speech delay.

A review of specific phonologic errors (Bleile, 1982; Smith and Stoel-Gammon, 1983; Sommers, Reinhart, and Sistrunk, 1988) suggest that speech development and error patterns of persons with mental retardation are not qualitatively different from those of young normally developing children. Variability in phonological performance across test trials is, however, a characteristic of the mentally retarded, particularly those with Down's syndrome.

In a study of the phonology of 40 adults with mental retardation, Shriberg and Widder (1990) reported the following speech characteristics:

1. High rate of deletions (including final consonant deletions, cluster simplifications, and syllable deletions)
2. Overall inconsistency of token to token performance
3. Presence of vowel errors

These authors suggested that their findings reflect evidence that cognitive-linguistic deficits affect phonological acquisition and performance.

Shriberg and Widder (1990) indicated that findings from nearly four decades of speech research in mental retardation can be summarized as follows:

1. Persons with mental retardation are likely to have articulation errors.
2. The most frequent type of articulation error is likely to be deletions of consonants.
3. Articulation errors are likely to be inconsistent.
4. The pattern of articulation errors is likely to be similar to that of very young children or children with "functional" articulation delays.

Several investigators have explored the phonological characteristics of Down's syndrome (DS) individuals, a genetically controlled subset of the mentally retarded population. It is well established that DS children fail to develop normal communication, and a high percentage reflect articulatory errors resulting in reduced intelligibility (Schlanger and Gottsleben, 1957; Dodd, 1975). Research efforts in recent years have focused on more detailed descriptions of phonological productions of DS speakers.

Sommers, Reinhart, and Sistrunk (1988) reported that among the phonological errors evidenced by DS children ages 13 to 22 years, some were phonemes frequently seen in error in 5- and 6-year-olds (i.e., /r/, of normal intelligence /r/ clusters, /s/, /s/ clusters, /z/, /θ/, and /v/). The authors indicated that these errors would appear to support the assertion that the phonological development of children with DS follows the same general pattern as that of normal children. However, they also reported that DS children evidenced errors not typically seen in normal 5- and 6-year-olds (i.e., deletion of alveolar stops and nasals). They also reported that imitative and spontaneous single-word picture-naming responses of their subjects failed to identify many of the omission errors found in connected speech samples of their subjects.

Stoel-Gammon (1980, 1981) reported that DS children tended to reflect delay rather than deviancy in their use and elimination of certain phonological processes. While the pattern of usage appeared similar for both DS and younger normally developing children, the DS group evidenced a slower rate of elimination of processes.

Sommers, Patterson, and Wildgen (1988) reported that their DS subjects, ages 13 to 22, evidenced a combination of delayed and deviant phonology. Evidence of delayed phonology was reflected in final consonant deletions, cluster reductions, gliding of liquids, and vocalizations; simplification processes frequently observed in the speech of young children. However, the authors also reported that several of the subjects' speech characteristics might be interpreted as deviant, including (1) widespread usage of final consonant deletions by all subjects in connected speech, spontaneous picture-naming, and imitation; (2) the + vocalic feature (as reflected in /r/ and /l/) was the error feature maintained the longest by all subjects in terms of their distinctive feature profiles, followed by + nasal; and (3) a high percentage of errors on stop consonants (usually considered to be early developing).

Rosin, Swift, Bless, and Vetter (1988) studied the articulation of DS children as part of a study of overall communication profiles in this population. They compared a group of 10 DS male subjects ($\times$ C.A. = 14.7 years) with a control group of mentally retarded subjects, and two control groups of normals representing two age levels ($\times$ C.A. 6.1, 15.5). They reported that as M.A. increased across subjects, intelligibility on a language sample increased. The DS group was also significantly different from the mentally retarded and the younger age normal group (the older group was not compared) in terms of the percent of consonants correctly articulated on the *Goldman-Fristoe Test of Articulation.*

In addition to the speech measures mentioned above, Rosin et al. (1988) also included other language measures, an oral motor evaluation, and aerodynamic measures in their assessment. They reported that the DS group had more difficulty with production measures as demands for sequencing increased (e.g., consonant-vowel repetitions, length of words). The DS group needed significantly more cueing in order to articulate the target /pataka/, and had more variable intraoral pressure when producing /papapaps/. The mean length of utterance of the DS group was also significantly shorter. The authors indicated that these findings are in accord with observations of others and suggested that sequencing underlies both oral motor control and language problems evidenced in DS subjects.

Summary. Investigators concur that there is a low positive correlation between intelligence and articulatory function within the range of normal intelligence, and thus, it can be inferred that intellectual functioning is of limited importance as a contributing factor to articulatory skill, and can be viewed as a poor predictor of articulation. On the other hand, a much higher correlation has been found between intelligence and articulation in the mentally retarded population. The articulatory skills in individuals with Down's syndrome reflect error patterns similar to those seen in young normally developing children; however, they also evidence errors that are considered deviant or unusual.

LANGUAGE DEVELOPMENT

Because phonology is one component of a child's developing linguistic system, there has been a natural interest in the relationship between phonological development and development of other aspects of language (i.e., morphology/syntax, semantics, pragmatics). Of particular interest to clinical phonologists has been the extent to which delay or disorders in phonology may co-occur with delay or disorder in other aspects of language.

VanDemark and Mann (1965) compared the spontaneous utterances of 50 children with articulatory defects and 50 normal children ranging in age from 8 through 16 years. To be included in the articulatory impaired group, the children had to fall below the cutoff score for 8-year-olds on the Templin-Darley Articulation Screening Test. The investigators reported that the children with articulation disorders obtained lower scores than the normal group on grammatical completeness and complexity measures.

Whitaker, Luper, and Pollio (1970) reported that children with articulation defects were also impaired in language skills involving knowledge of phonological rules, form classes, and sentence structure. Subjects ranged in age from 6;1, to 7;7, and included both an articulation disorders group and a normal control group. All subjects in the disorders group failed to meet the cutoff score for 7-year-old children on the Templin-Darley Articulation Screening Test. The authors reported that the disordered group appeared to be developing language in the normal pattern but at a retarded rate.

Shriner, Holloway, and Daniloff (1969) compared the language skills of a normal control group with those of a group of 30 children between the ages of 5 and 8 who were considered to have severe articulation disorders (had at least seven articulatory errors and scored one standard deviation below the mean on the Templin-Darley Tests of Articulation). Subjects in the articulatory-defective group used significantly shorter and less complex utterances in their spontaneous conversation than members of the control group.

The relationship between articulation disorders and language comprehension was explored by Marquardt and Saxman (1972) using two groups of kindergarten children; one group performed one standard deviation or more below the norm for that age on the Templin-Darley Tests of Articulation, and the other (the control group) produced no more than one defective sound. The investigators administered the *Test of Auditory Comprehension of Language* and found that the impaired group made significantly more language comprehension errors than the control group. A correlation of scores obtained on both measures revealed that children who made the greatest number of articulation errors also made the greatest number of errors in language comprehension.

Gross, St. Louis, Ruscello, and Hull (1985) studied the language skills of three groups of school-age subjects: (1) a group with multiple articulation errors; defined as those with at least two errors in the final position, with /l/, /r/, and /s/ not included in this consideration; (2) a group with residual articulation errors; defined as two or more positional errors for at least one of the following phonemes: /l/, /r/, and /s/. Consonant cluster errors on these phonemes were allowed, but subjects could have no other phonemic errors; and (3) a normal control group. A total of 144 subjects from grades 1, 3, 5, and 7 were included in this retrospective study. The investigators reported that mean language structural scores for completeness and complexity were significantly lower for the multiple error group than the residual error and control groups. Scores for length of utterances were not significantly different among groups. The total number of language errors reduced progressively from multiple error to residual error to control groups.

Research investigations such as those cited above, which have attempted to explore the correlation between certain aspects of language and phonology, have generally reported a moderate correlation between phonologic and language disorders. After reviewing literature related to the language–phonology relationship, Tyler and Watterson (1991) indicated that one might expect to find disorders of language and of phonology co-occurring in 60 to 80 percent of the young children who have been identified as having a disorder of one type or the other.

Some investigators have attempted to further study and explain the interaction between phonology and other aspects of language, especially syntax. A common perception is that language is organized from the "top-down," or, in other words, a speaker goes from pragmatic intent, to semantic coding, to syntactic structure, to phonological productions. Thus, higher level linguistic formulations may ultimately be reflected in a child's phonological productions. If this theory is accurate, it might be expected that the more complex the syntax, the more likely a child is to evidence linguistic breakdown, which may then be evidenced in phonological productions. Schmauch, Panagos, and Klich (1978) conducted a study in which 5-year-old children with phonological and language problems were required to produce certain nouns (drawn from phonological inventories) in three syntactic contexts; that is, an isolated noun phrase, a declarative sentence, and a passive sentence. These investigators reported a 17 percent increase in articulatory errors between the noun phrase and each of the sentence contexts. They also reported that later developing consonants were those most influenced by syntactical complexity and that error productions reflected quantitative rather than qualitative changes.

A follow-up study of the "top-down" notion was conducted by Panagos, Quine, and Klich (1979). In this study, 5-year-old children were required to produce 15 target consonants in noun phrases, declarative sentences, and passive sentences; consonants appeared in the initial and final word-positions of one- and two-syllable words. Syntax was again found to significantly influence articulatory accuracy, as did number of syllables in target words. Word-position did not influence phonological accuracy. The authors further reported that two sources of complexity—phonological (including difficulty with later developing consonants as well as specific contexts) and syntax—combined addictively to increase the number of phonological errors. From the easiest context (final word-position, one-syllable word, noun phrase) to the hardest (final word-position, two-syllable word, passive sentence), there was a 36 percent increase in articulatory errors. The effects of grammatical complexity on articulatory accuracy were cumulative.

A second perspective on the language–phonology relationship suggests that linguistic influences operate from the "bottom-up." In this view, language expression is regulated by feedback (internal and external) from phonological performance. Feedback from phonological performance is needed to maintain syntactic processing and accuracy, especially when errors occur and must be corrected.

Panagos and Prelock (1982) conducted a study to test the hypothesis that phonological structure influences children's syntactic processing. Ten children with language disorders were required to produce sentences containing words with varying syllable complexity; that is, *simple:* "The (CV) kid (CVC) pushed (CVCC) the (CV) car (CVC) in (VC) the (CV) room (CVC)"; and *complex:* "The (CV) chocolate (CVCVCVC) is (VC) in (VC) the (CV) napkin (CVCCVC)." In addition, sentence complexity was varied from unembedded ("The girl washed the doll in the tub") to right embedded ("The cook washed the pot the guy dropped") to center embedded ("The lady the uncle liked sewed the coat"). The results of the study supported the hypothesis. When subjects repeated sentences containing words of greater syllable complexity, they made 27 percent more syntactic errors. In addition to this "bottom-up" influence, Panagos and Prelock (1982) also reported that syntactic complexity further compounded production difficulties. From the unembedded to the center embedded, there was a 57 percent increase in phonological errors. These findings support the view that a simultaneous "top-down"–"bottom-up" relationship exists between language and phonology. Another way of expressing this concept is to consider that children with disordered language–phonology have a limited encoding capacity; and the more this capacity is strained at one level or another, the greater the probability of delay in one component or more of language.

It should be pointed out that the study by Panagos and Prelock (1982), as well as others in a series of experimental studies, employed elicited imitation tasks, and thus complexity of utterances was controlled by the investigators. It can be argued that with this type of performance task, structural simplifications are expected outcomes. Elicited imitation tasks do not reflect the conditions present when a child is engaged in conversation, and thus we cannot assume that constraints of the nature demonstrated by Panagos and Prelock can predict behavior in a conversational context (Paul and Shriberg, 1984). In an investigation of Paul and Shriberg (1982) designed to study phonological productions as they relate to particular morphophonemic structures, continuous speech samples were obtained in 30 speech-delayed children. They found that in over half their subjects, general syntactic delays accompanied delayed phonological development. They also reported that certain of their subjects were able to produce complex morphosyntactic contexts spontaneously, which did not result in phonological simplifications. In other words, some of their subjects were able to maintain a similar level of phonological production in spite of producing more complex syntactic targets. They suggested (Paul and Shriberg, 1984) that children may "do things other than phonological simplification in an attempt to control complexity in spontaneous speech" (319). They summarized by indicating that some speech-delayed children are sometimes able to allocate their limited linguistic resources to realize phonological targets consistent with their linguistic knowledge in the context of free speech, even though at other times they may use avoidance strategies or other means of reducing the encoding load.

A "synergistic view" of language (Schwartz, Leonard, Folger, and Wilcox, 1980; Shriner, Holloway, and Daniloff, 1969) is a conception of the relationship between language and phonology that assumes a complex interaction and interdependency of various aspects of linguistic behaviors. Experimental evidence for this view was provided by Matheny and Panagos (1978), who looked at the effects of syntactic programming on phonological improvement and the effects of phonological programming on syntactic improvement in school-age children. Syntactic training resulted in both phonological and syntactic improvement, and phonological intervention resulted in significant gains in syntactic development as well as phonological performance. Similar findings were reported by Hoffman, Norris, and Monjure (1990). Based on a study of two siblings from a set of triplets, they reported that language-based therapy not only resulted in improvement in syntax–morphology but also in phonology. Phonological instruction, however, resulted only in improvement in phonology but not syntax morphology. These findings have not been supported in the research of Tyler and Watterson (1991) and Fey (1991), who reported that language-focused intervention did not impact phonological errors.

Results of the experimental treatment studies identified above reinforce the complexity of the language–phonology interaction. Tyler and Watterson (1991) hypothesized that the interactions among linguistic domains during treatment were influenced by both the type of treatment and the relationship between the subject's language and phonological disorders. They reported that subjects with a severe overall language and phonological disorder made improvements in language when presented with language therapy; however, gains were not made in phonology (they actually reported a tendency for performance to become worse). On the other hand, subjects with mild-moderate but unequal impairments in phonology and language, improved in both areas when presented with phonological therapy. The authors suggested that a language-based intervention program may not result in improvement in phonologic as well as other language skills for children whose disorders are severe and comparable in each domain. However, children with less severe problems in one or both domains may benefit from therapy with either

Factors Related to Phonological Disorders

a language or phonology focus. Clearly further developmental and clinical studies are needed to clarify the interactions between phonology and other aspects of language.

Summary. Research has shown that younger children with severe phonological disorders are more likely to evidence language problems than those with mild-moderate delay. Language and phonology may be related in what has been termed a synergistic relationship. Investigators face the challenge of further defining the intricacies of the relationship between phonology and other linguistic behaviors in terms of both development and clinical management of disorders.

ACADEMIC PERFORMANCE

The relationship between phonological disorders and educational problems is of interest to clinicians working with school-age children since oral language skills are fundamental to the development of many academic skills such as reading and spelling. Because the use of sounds in symbolic lexical units is a task common to learning to speak, read, and write, researchers have studied the co-occurrence of reading and articulation disorders, and have discussed possible common factors underlying the acquisition of literacy and other language-related skills.

Hall (1938) compared 21 children with functional articulation disorders with a normal control group on the *Gates Silent Reading Test* and the *Iowa Silent Reading Test* and reported no significant differences in silent reading achievement between the two groups. Everhart (1953) also used the Gates Reading Test in comparing the reading skills of children with articulation disorders and a control group of normal children. Everhart found no significant relationship between articulatory disorders and reading ability, although boys with normal articulation tended to obtain higher reading scores than the overall group of children with articulation disorders.

The relationship between reading readiness and articulation development in children with and without defective articulation was studied by Fitzsimons (1958) and Weaver, Furbee, and Everhart (1960). Fitzsimons used the *Metropolitan Reading Readiness Test* to determine the status of reading readiness and reported that below grade-level scores were more frequent among children with articulation disorders than among those with normally developing articulation. In a study of the relationship between parental occupational status and articulation defects, Weaver, Furbee, and Everhart (1960) also included a test of reading in their test protocol. Their findings indicated a significant relationship between articulatory performance and reading readiness as well as between articulatory performance and reading scores.

Sommers, Cockerille, Bowser, Fichter, Fenton, and Copetas (1961) studied the relationship between reading and articulation performance by examining the influence of clinical speech instruction and a speech improvement program (identification and discrimination of sounds) on reading scores of first-grade children. Reading was assessed before and after instruction using *The Primary Reading Profiles.* The authors reported no significant differences in reading improvement between normal speakers and children with articulation disorders who had been placed in the speech improvement program. Nor were significant differences in reading improvement found between those who received clinical speech instruction and a control group. However, significant differences in reading comprehension (but not other aspects of the reading test) were found between two groups of children with severe articulation disorders; the group receiving both speech instruction and speech improvement made greater gains than the group receiving only speech improvement.

Flynn and Byrne (1970) took a different approach to exploring the relationship between articulation disorders and reading. They compared articulatory performance of 52 advanced and 42 delayed third-grade readers on the Templin-Darley Tests of Articulation. Those who scored 4.2 or higher on the *Iowa Test of Basic Skills* were classified as advanced readers; those who scored 2.2 or lower as delayed readers. The authors reported no significant difference between the two groups in articulation test scores.

Lewis and Freebairn-Farr (1991) conducted a cross-sectional study designed to examine the performance of individuals with a history of a preschool phonological disorder on measures of phonology, reading, and spelling. Groups of subjects included at least 17 individuals from each of the following categories: preschool, school age, adolescence, and adulthood. Normal comparison groups at each age level were also tested. Significant differences between the disordered and normal groups were reported on the reading and spelling measures for the school-age group, and on the reading measure for the adult group. Although the reading and spelling measures for the adolescent group and the spelling measure for the adult group did not reach significance, the trend was for the individuals with histories of disorders to perform more poorly than normals. Data also indicated that subjects who evidenced a phonological disorder accompanied by additional language problems performed more poorly on measures of reading and spelling than subjects with phonological disorders only. The authors indicated that children evidencing phonological impairment are at risk for reading and spelling problems in school and may have special educational needs.

Interest has traditionally focused on the co-occurrence of reading–spelling and phonological disorders in children, but more recently there has also been interest in children's ability to process phonology as part of various reading tasks. More specifically, some reading disabled students may lack awareness of individual sounds, have difficulty dividing words into sounds, and recalling sound–symbol relationships. Catts (1986) found that reading-disabled children may have problems with these linguistically oriented tasks and yet not reflect phonological impairments.

Researchers have attempted to apply phonological concepts to aid in the understanding of reading and spelling disorders. This activity is based on the assumption that acquisition of speaking, reading, and writing skills involves the analysis of sounds in lexical units, which may be related to underlying cognitive-linguistic processes. In particular, the concepts of phonological processes and underlying internal knowledge of the sound system have been employed to aid in understanding the development of spelling and reading skills (Hoffman and Norris, 1989).

Liberman and Shankweiler (1985) in a discussion of the phonological basis of literacy indicated that reading success was related to the degree to which children were aware of "underlying phonological structure" and that poor readers often were unable to segment words into their phonological constituents. They

Factors Related to Phonological Disorders

suggested that a relationship exists between children's readiness for reading and spelling and their metalinguistic awareness of the internal structure of words.

Catts (1991) suggested that speech-language pathologists working in school systems should seek to develop programs designed to facilitate "phonological awareness" in children, particularly those at risk for reading disabilities. Catts suggested that "phonological awareness" activities might include activities designed to increase awareness of syllables, phonemes, manner of phoneme production, and sound positions in words. Activities to accomplish these goals could include sound play, rhyming, alliteration, and segmentation tasks.

Hoffman and Norris (1989) analyzed spelling errors of 45 elementary school children for evidence of phonological process patterns. They reported that many of the spelling errors involved both syllable reduction and feature changes similar to the sound simplifications seen in the speech of young children with normal speech development. They further indicated that even though children had acquired normal speech, they exhibited spelling errors similar to those seen in the speech simplifications of younger children. Hoffman (1990) related specific types of developmental spelling patterns to stages of normal phonological acquisition. For example, "precommunicative spellings" (seemingly random selection of letters of the alphabet to represent words), were described as parallel to the random sound productions of babbling. "Semiphonetic spellings" (letters used to represent sounds, but only some of the sounds are represented, e.g., *E* for *eagle*), were described as parallel to the stage where children delete syllables or segments and substitute sound classes for one another. He also indicated that because the speech-language pathologist is the school-based professional who has the most detailed knowledge of sound perception and production, phonological organization, stages of acquisition, and methods of phonological description, he or she is in a good position to serve as a resource to teachers regarding the application of phonological concepts to the understanding of spelling errors.

Summary. Research investigations that have focused on the co-occurrence of phonological and reading disorders are equivocal. These findings are perhaps partially related to the fact that children typically do not have severe phonological problems by the time they are learning to read (approximately age 6); and thus most investigators of these two behaviors have focused on children with milder phonological delays. Data indicate that young children with severe phonological and/or other language disorders are at risk for academic problems. More recently interest has focused on the role of "phonological awareness" in the development of reading and spelling skills. Parallels have been made between the use of phonological processes and stages in the acquisition of oral language and acquisition of reading and spelling skills. It has been suggested that speech-language pathologists are in a unique position to offer assistance to the classroom teacher in their efforts to assist children "at risk" for reading and/or spelling problems.

PSYCHOSOCIAL FACTORS

AGE

In Chapters 2 and 3 the literature concerning phonological acquisition was reviewed. Investigations of phonological development have revealed that children's articulatory skills continue to improve until approximately 8 years of age, by which time the normal child has acquired most aspects of the adult sound system.

Speech-language pathologists use normative information concerning phonological development as a guide in case selection and for determining treatment goals. Clinicians should keep in mind that the order in which sounds are incorporated into speech varies from child to child and does not necessarily follow a specific sequence. There is no indication that one sound is dependent on any other for its development.

Speech-language pathologists have shown a particular interest in the effect of maturation on children identified as having phonological disorders. Roe and Milisen (1942) sampled 1,989 children in grades 1 through 6 and found that the children's mean number of articulation errors decreased between grades 1 and 2, grades 2 and 3, and grades 3 and 4. In contrast, the difference in the mean number of errors between grades 4 and 5 and grades 5 and 6 was not significant. The authors concluded that maturation was responsible for improvement in articulation performance between grades 1 and 4 but was not an appreciable factor in articulation improvement in grades 5 and 6.

Sayler (1949) assessed articulation in 1,998 students in grades 7 through 12 as they read sentences orally. His findings indicated a slight decrease in the mean number of articulation errors at each subsequent grade level, but because the improvement in speech sound productions was so small, he concluded that maturation does not appear to be an appreciable factor in improvement in the secondary grades. Children in upper elementary and secondary grades appear to be more consistent in their phonological patterns than children in the lower elementary grades.

Summary. Acquisition by a child of the adult speech sound system has been shown to be related to maturation. There is a direct correlation between improvement in articulation skills and age through approximately age 8. In other words, the probability of a child outgrowing a phonological delay is much higher prior to than after age 9 in normally developing children.

Sex

Child development specialists have long been interested in contrasts between males and females in phonological acquisition, and, likewise, speech-language pathologists have investigated the relationship between gender and articulation status. Research in this area has focused on (1) a comparison of phoneme acquisition in males and females, and (2) a comparison of the incidence of phonological disorders in males and females.

Dawson (1929) examined the articulatory skills of 200 children from grades 1 through 12 on six measures of articulation. He reported that until approximately age 12, girls were slightly superior to boys in their articulatory skills. Templin (1963) reported similar findings: "In articulation development, girls consistently are found to be slightly accelerated . . . in all instances the differences are relatively small and often are not statistically significant" (13).

Smit, Hand, Freilinger, Bernthal, and Bird (1990) conducted a large-scale normative study of phonological development in children ages 3 through 9 from Iowa and Nebraska. They reported that the Iowa–Nebraska girls appeared to acquire sounds at somewhat earlier ages than boys, although this effect reached statistical significance only at age 6 and younger, and not in every preschool age group.

Speech surveys conducted by Hall (1938), Mills and Streit (1942), Morley (1952), Everhart (1960), and Hull, Mielke, Timmons, and Willeford (1971) indicated that the incidence of articulation disorders was higher in males than females, regardless of the age group studied. Smit et al. (1990) stated that "... it is a well-known fact that boys are at much greater risk than girls for delayed speech, and this propensity continues to be reported" (790). Kenney and Prather (1986), who elicited multiple productions of frequent error sounds, reported significant differences favoring girls in the age range 3 through 5. Contrary to the above findings, Roe and Milisen (1942) reported insignificant differences in the mean number of articulation errors between males and females from a sample of 1,998 children in grades 1 through 6. Likewise, Winitz (1959a) reported no significant differences between the articulatory skills of 75 males and 75 females entering kindergarten.

After a review of the literature concerning articulatory differences between the sexes, Perkins (1977) and Winitz (1969) both concluded that sex is a minor variable in the development of articulatory skill. Perkins (1977) stated: "The results . . . are conflicting, differences reported are small, and they are virtually non-existent in well-controlled studies" (257).

Summary. The sex of a child does not appear to be a significant factor in phonological acquisition, as is evidenced by the fact that most research concerning phonological disorders does not control for the sex of subjects. It should be recognized, however, that at certain ages, females tend to be slightly ahead of males in phonological acquisition, and more male than female children are identified as being phonologically delayed.

FAMILY BACKGROUND

Researchers have been interested in the influence of family background and how it may affect a child's speech and language development. In the paragraphs below we will review literature related to family background and phonology organized around three topics: (1) socioeconomic status, (2) family transmission, and (3) sibling influences.

Socioeconomic Status. The socioeconomic status of a child's parents, as measured by parents' educational background, parental occupation, income, and location of family residence, is a significant part of the child's environment. Since some behavioral deficiencies occur more frequently in lower socioeconomic environments, socioeconomic status has been of interest to speech-language clinicians as a possible factor in language development.

Everhart (1953, 1956) explored the variable of parental occupational status in an investigation of the relationship between articulation and other developmental factors in children. In speech surveys of children in grades 1 through 6, those classified as having articulation disorders were compared to children with normal articulation development with respect to parental occupation. No significant differences were found, and Everhart concluded that the occurrence of articulation disorders in children was not related to parental occupation. Winitz (1959a, 1959b) also reported no significant relationships between ratings of socioeconomic status and scores obtained from an articulation screening test on 150 kindergarten children.

Templin (1957) analyzed developmental language data from children aged 3 to 8 years in terms of parental occupation and reached a somewhat different conclusion. She used the *Minnesota Scale for Parental Occupations* to categorize parental occupation. At each age level, children whose parents were in the upper occupational group had fewer misarticulations than the children in the lower occupational group. In particular, 4-, 4½-, and 7-year-old children whose parents were in the lower occupational group had significantly more articulation errors than those whose parents were in the upper group. Templin concluded that parental occupation seemed to be a factor in children's articulation skill until about age 4 but that parental occupation no longer seemed to influence articulation development by the time children were 8 years old.

Weaver, Furbee, and Everhart (1960) also investigated the relationship between parental occupation and articulation proficiency in 592 first-grade children and found that a greater number of children with normal articulation skills came from homes in the upper occupational group, whereas more children with articulation errors came from homes in the lower occupational group. The poorest articulation proficiency, as judged by number of articulation errors, was found among children from the two lowest occupational classes.

Prins (1962a) found no significant correlation between articulation and socioeconomic level for 92 articulatory defective children between the ages of 2 and 6 years. Likewise, Smit et al. (1990) in the Iowa–Nebraska normative study reported that socioeconomic level did not have a significant relationship to articulatory performance. After an extensive review of the literature on the relationship between articulation and socioeconomic status, Winitz (1969) concluded that "more misarticulating children and more articulatory errors are found in the lower socioeconomic groups than in the upper socioeconomic groups. However, when a correlational index is used, the relationship is low or nonsignificant" (147).

Family Transmission. It is not uncommon for speech-language pathologists to observe a family history for developmental speech and language disorders. While information of this nature is often noted in diagnostic reports, until the 1980s few systematic attempts were made to study phonological disorders as they relate to family history. Neils and Aram (1986) obtained reports from the parents of 74 preschool language-disordered children and indicated that 46 percent reported that other family members had histories of speech and language disorders. Of this group, 55 percent were reported to have articulation disorders, the most prevalent type of familial disorder reported.

Two twin studies have been reported that contribute to our understanding of familial influences, including genetic factors that may relate to phonological disorders. Matheny and Bruggeman (1973) studied 101 same-sex twin sets, 22 opposite-sex twin sets, and 94 siblings between the ages of 3 and 8 years. An articulation screening test was administered to each child. Monozygotic twins' articulation screening correlated more closely with each other than did dizygotic twins' scores. The authors concluded that there is a strong hereditary influence on articulation status. In addition, sex differences were found to favor females. Locke and Mather (1987) examined speech sound productions in 13 monozygotic and 13 dizygotic twin sets. They reported more phonetic concordance in the monozygotic than the dizygotic twins.

Lewis, Ekelman, and Aram (1989) examined the familial basis of phonological disorders by comparing sibling articulation status for a group of children identified as evidencing a severe phonological disorder, and a group whose siblings

Factors Related to Phonological Disorders

reflected abnormal phonological development. Phonological measures included the *Natural Process Analysis*, repetition of 50 multisyllabic words, and the Screening Test for Developmental Verbal Apraxia. In addition, language, gross and fine motor skills, and reading were assessed. Family histories of communication disorders and/or learning disabilities were noted. Results revealed that the siblings of the disordered children performed more poorly than control siblings on phonology and reading measures. Disordered subjects' phonological skills correlated significantly and positively with those of their siblings, whereas controls' scores did not. Families of disordered children reported significantly more members with speech and language disorders and dyslexia than did families of controls. Sex differences were reflected in the incidence but not the severity or type of disorder present. The author concluded that their findings suggest a familial basis for at least some forms of severe phonological disorders.

It may be inferred from the studies reviewed above that genetic or biological inheritance factors may precipitate phonological impairment, yet it is often difficult to separate environmental from genetic/biological influences. A study that examined environmental influences was reported by Parlour and Broen (1991). Their research was predicated on the possibility that individuals who themselves experienced significant speech and language disorders as children are likely to become adults who will provide a less than optimal cultural or linguistic milieu for their own families.

Parlour and Broen collected follow-up family data of adults with and without a childhood history of delayed phonological development. Both groups of subjects were originally part of the large normative study that was conducted by Mildred Templin (1968), 28 years earlier. The group who had displayed a moderate to moderately severe phonological disorder in early elementary school was comprised of 24 individuals. The control group was comprised of 28 adults who had evidenced average or better articulation during the same time period.

Two environmental measures, the *Preschool HOME Scale* and the *Modified Templin Child-Rearing Questionnaire*, were employed to ascertain qualitative aspects of a child's environment including physical, emotional, and cognitive support available to preschool children, and child-rearing practices. These two measures included direct observation of the examiner, parental reports, and parental responses to a written questionnaire.

The two groups performed in a generally comparable manner for all of the environmental domains sampled, with one exception, *acceptance,* which assessed disciplinary practices. Parlour and Broen (1991) reported that families with a history of phonological disorders were more reliant on physical punishment than were control families. The authors suggested two possible interpretations of their findings: (1) adults with a history of moderately delayed phonological development are as likely as control adults to provide home environments which provide intellectual stimulation, warmth, and cohesiveness, or (2) true group differences may have existed but may not have been identified by the assessment instruments. In terms of future research efforts, the authors suggested that we keep in mind that although differences were generally not significant between the groups, the disordered group received lower mean scores than controls on each of the Home subscales, suggesting that some subtle differences may have been present, particularly for domains involving the use of punishment, learning, and language stimulation.

Sibling Influence. Another factor of interest to investigators of phonological acquisition has been sibling number and birth order. Since the amount of time that parents can spend with each child decreases with each child added to a family, some clinicians have questioned whether sibling status is related to articulatory development. Koch (1956) studied the relationships between certain speech and voice characteristics in young children and siblings in two-child families. In this study, 384 children between 5 and 6 years old were divided into 24 matched subgroups matched individual by individual on the basis of age, socioeconomic class, and residence. Data on speech and voice characteristics consisted of teacher's ratings on the *California Behavior Inventory for Nursery School Children.* Koch reported that firstborn children had better articulation than secondborn, and the wider the age difference between a child and his or her sibling, the better the child's articulation. Likewise, Davis (1937) reported that children without siblings demonstrated superior articulatory performance to children with siblings and to twins. On the other hand, Wellman, Case, Mengert, and Bradbury (1931) did not find a significant relationship between the number of siblings and level of articulation skill for 3-year-olds.

Twins have been reported to present unique patterns of speech sound acquisition (Perkins, 1977; Powers, 1971; Winitz, 1969). From birth, twins receive speech stimulation not only from others within their environment but also from each other. Powers (1971) indicated that the "emotional ties of twins, too, are likely to be closer than those of singled siblings, which further augments their interdependence in speech" (868). It is not uncommon for twins to reflect common phonological patterns and use similar phonological processes. Schwartz, Leonard, Folger, and Wilcox (1980) reported, however, that in the very early stages of phonological acquisition (the first 50 words), similarities in phonemes used, including phonological patterns and lexical items, were not present. Unique patterns of speech occasionally found in twins 2 years and older which have little resemblance to adult models and are meaningful only to the twins, are termed *idioglossia.*

Summary. Little relationship exists between socioeconomic and articulation status based on available reports. Although greater numbers of misarticulating children tend to be found in lower socioeconomic groups (especially children under 4 years), socioeconomic status does not appear to contribute to the presence of a phonological disorder.

Studies of phonological development in twins, as well as in families with a history of severe phonological impairment, suggest some sort of genetic or familial propensity toward the presence of such a disorder. While there is a paucity of data in this area, interest in the topic is growing.

Investigations examining phonological status and sibling relationships are limited, but findings have been fairly consistent. Firstborn and only children exhibit significantly better articulation performance than children with older siblings or twins. The age span between siblings also appears to affect phonological proficiency, with better articulation associated with wider age differences. One can speculate that the firstborn or only child receives better speech models and greater stimulation than the child who has older siblings. The possibility also exists that

Factors Related to Phonological Disorders

older siblings produce "normal" developmental phonological errors and, thus, at points in time present imperfect speech models to younger siblings. Unique patterns of sound productions have been found in twins; reasons for these patterns are speculative and tend to focus on the stimulation each twin receives from the other.

PERSONALITY

The relationship between personality characteristics and phonological behavior has been investigated to determine if particular personality patterns are likely to be associated with phonological disorders. Researchers have examined not only the child's personality traits but also those of the child's parents, using various assessment tools.

Lerea and Ward (1966), using spatial distance of human forms to infer a child's self-perception in his or her social milieu, found that personal relationships were more distant for 29 children with articulation disorders than for a control group of normal speakers. When the disordered group was instructed to place felt figures of themselves and family members on a board, the distance between the forms was significantly greater than for the 20 children in the control group.

Solomon (1961) used a questionnaire format to investigate the personality characteristics of children with phonological delay. Solomon interviewed the mothers of 49 children whose speech was characterized by misarticulations and the mothers of 49 normal-speaking children. Nine areas of child development and personality (including eating behavior, sleeping behavior, fears, and anxieties) were the focus of the interviews. The articulation-defective group was rated as being more poorly adjusted than the control group. Differences were noted in peer relationships, sleeping behaviors, fears, and anxieties. The children in the articulation disorder group were rated as being passive, submissive, timid, and exhibiting a high need for approval. Templin used the *Moore-Gilliland Test for Aggressiveness* to compare college students with and without articulation disorders and found that students with articulation problems scored lower in aggressiveness than those with normal speech.

Because of interactions between children and their parents, some investigators have explored the personality and adjustment characteristics of both phonologically impaired children and their parents. Wood (1946) studied 50 children between the ages of 5 and 14 who did not exhibit organic problems or intellectual deficiency. She administered a series of psychological tests and case history interviews to children and their parents and found that (1) the parents were separated in 24 cases, (2) severe discipline methods were practiced in 22 of the homes, and (3) parents reacted emotionally to the child's speech difficulty in 18 cases. Between one third and two thirds of the children showed withdrawing tendencies, a sense of frustration, a lack of affection, or manifestations of anxiety and insecurity. Wood concluded that a significant degree of emotional maladjustment occurs among parents, especially mothers, of children with functional articulatory disorders.

Using the *Parental Attitude Research Instrument* and *Wiley's Attitude Toward the Behavior of Children,* Moll and Darley (1960) studied the parents of articulatory defective children and the parents of children with normal articulation. They concluded that there were no clear differences between the two groups.

Dickson (1962) studied the parents of two groups of elementary school children originally identified as having phonological disorders. One group of children ultimately developed normal articulation; the other did not. The investigation explored emotional characteristics of the parents using the *Minnesota Multiphasic Personality Inventory*. Findings showed that the mothers of children who still had phonological errors showed a tendency toward neuroticism. No definite personality characteristics emerged for fathers from either group or for mothers from the control group.

Parlour and Broen (1991) studied environmental factors in the homes of 24 adults who as children evidenced moderate to moderately severe phonological disorders, and a control group of adults who as children evidenced average or better articulation. Two environmental measures, the *Preschool HOME Scale* and the *Modified Templin Child-Rearing Questionnaire,* were used to study and rate aspects of the home presumed to reflect the quality of physical, emotional, and cognitive support available to a preschool child. While the findings for the two groups were generally similar, mean scores for the group with a history of phonological disorders were lower than for the normal group. A significant difference between the two groups was found with regard to disciplinary practices, suggesting that "disorders" families were more reliant on physical punishment than were control families.

In a review of research in phonological disorders and personality, Spriestersbach (1956) criticized the term **personality** as vague and argued that numerous obstacles are confronted when trying to test a construct that has such divergent definitions. He concluded that "the contribution of research to an understanding of the relationship between articulatory defects and personality is largely negative" (334).

Bloch and Goodstein (1971) concluded, in a later review of similar literature spanning a 10-year period, that there is evidence of personality differences between parents of children who present articulatory deficits and parents of children with normal articulation. They noted that studies of the personality traits and emotional adjustment of individuals with articulatory disorders have shown contradictory findings, and attributed this to two major problems with the investigations: (1) the criteria for defining articulatory impaired has varied from one study to the next; and (2) the tools or instruments used to assess personality and adjustment have varied in their validity and reliability.

Summary. No cluster of personality characteristics has been identified that can be attributed to individuals with phonological disorders, nor is there any indication that individuals with phonological disorders or delays have severe emotional disorders that result from their speech problems. Although parents of children with articulation disorders may have a slight tendency toward maladjustment, experimental findings in this area are inconclusive and conflicting, and there is little evidence that personality characteristics of the parents are related to the presence of phonological disorders.

CONCLUSION

The speech-language pathologist must have a basic knowledge of factors related to phonological disorders in order to assess phonological status, plan remediation programs, and counsel clients and their parents. Despite the large body of literature reflecting investigations of variables potentially related to articulation impairments, many questions remain unanswered. One truth that emerges from the literature, however, is the absence of any one-to-one correspondence between the presence of a particular etiological factor and the nature of an individual's phonological status. Prediction of cause-effect relationships represents a scientific ideal, but determination of such relationships in the realm of human behavior, including communication disorders, is extremely difficult.

REFERENCES

American Speech and Hearing Association and American Association of Dental Schools, Joint Committee on Dentistry and Speech Pathology and Audiology. *Asha, 17* (1975): 331–337.

American Speech-Language-Hearing Association, "Report of ad hoc committee on labial-lingual posturing function." *Asha, 31* (1989): 92–94.

American Speech-Language-Hearing Association, "The role of the speech-language pathologist in management of oral myofunctional disorders." *Asha, 33* (Suppl. 5) (1991): 7.

Arndt, W., M. Elbert, and R. Shelton, "Standardization of a test of oral stereognosis." In J. Bosman (Ed.), *Second Symposium on Oral Sensation and Perception.* Springfield, Ill.: Charles C Thomas, 1970.

Arndt, W., R. Shelton, A. Johnson, and M. Furr, "Identification and description of homogeneous subgroups within a sample of misarticulating children." *Journal of Speech and Hearing Research, 20* (1977): 263–292.

Arnst, D., and D. Fucci, "Vibrotactile sensitivity of the tongue in hearing impaired subjects." *Journal of Auditory Research, 15* (1975): 115–118.

Aungst, L., and J. Frick, "Auditory discrimination ability and consistency of articulation of /r/." *Journal of Speech and Hearing Disorders, 29* (1964): 76–85.

Backus, O., "Speech rehabilitation following excision of tip of the tongue." *American Journal of the Disabled Child, 60* (1940): 368–370.

Bankson, N., and M. Byrne, "The relationship between missing teeth and selected consonant sounds." *Journal of Speech and Hearing Disorders, 24* (1962): 341–348.

Barton, D., "The role of perception in the acquisition of phonology." Ph.D. dissertation, University of London, 1976.

Bashir, A., F. Grahamjones, and R. Bostwick, "A touch-cue method of therapy for developmental verbal apraxia." *Seminars in Speech and Language, 5* (1984): 127–137.

Bernstein, M., "The relation of speech defects and malocclusion." *American Journal of Orthodontia, 40* (1954): 149–150.

Bilto, E., "A comparative study of certain physical abilities of children with speech defects and children with normal speech." *Journal of Speech and Hearing Disorders, 6* (1941): 187–203.

Bishop, M., R. Ringel, and H. House, "Orosensory perception, speech production and deafness." *Journal of Speech and Hearing Research, 16* (1973): 257–266.

Bleile, K., "Consonant ordering in Down's Syndrome." *Journal of Communicative Disorders, 15* (1982): 275–285.

Bloch, R., and L. Goodstein, "Functional speech disorders and personality: A decade of research." *Journal of Speech and Hearing Disorders, 36* (1971): 295–314.

Bloomer, H., and A. Hawk, "Speech considerations: Speech disorders associated with ablative surgery of the face, mouth and pharynx-ablative approaches to learning." In *ASHA Report #8: Orofacial Anomalies.* Washington, D.C.: ASHA, 1973.

Bordon, G., "Consideration of motor-sensory targets and a problem of perception." In H. Winitz (Ed.), *Treating Articulation Disorders: For Clinicians by Clinicians.* Austin, Tex.: Pro-Ed, 1984.

Butterfield, E., and G. Cairns, "Discussion-summary of infant reception research." In R. Schiefulbusch and L. Lloyd (Eds.), *Language Perspectives: Acquisition, Retardation and Intervention.* Baltimore: University Park Press, 1974

Calvert, D., "Articulation and hearing impairments." In L. Lass, L. Northern, D. Yoder, and L. McReynolds (Eds.), *Speech, Language and Hearing,* Vol. 2. Philadelphia: W.B. Saunders, 1982.

Canning, B., and M. Rose, "Clinical measurements of the speech, tongue and lip movements in British children with normal speech." *British Journal of Disorders of Communication, 9* (1974): 45–50.

Carrell, J., and K. Pendergast, "An experimental study of the possible relation between errors of speech and spelling." *Journal of Speech and Hearing Disorders, 19* (1954): 327–334.

Catts, H., "Facilitating phonological awareness: Role of speech-language pathologists." *Language, Speech, and Hearing Services in Schools, 22* (1991): 196–203.

Catts, H.W., "Speech, production/phonological deficits in reading-disordered children." *Learning Disabilities, 19* (1986): 504–508.

Chaney, C., and P. Menyuk, "Production and identification of /w, l, r/ in normal and articulation-impaired children." Paper presented at the convention of the American Speech and Hearing Association, Washington, D.C., 1975.

Christensen, M., and M. Hanson, "An investigation of the efficacy of oral myofunctional therapy as a precursor to articulation therapy for pre–first-grade children." *Journal of Speech and Hearing Disorders, 46* (1981): 160–167.

Churchill, J., B. Hodson, B. Jones, and R. Novak, "A preliminary investigation comparing phonological systems of speech disordered clients with and without histories of recurrent otitis media." Paper presented at the annual convention of the American Speech-Language-Hearing Association, Washington, D.C., 1985.

Clark, R., "Maturation and speech development." *Logos, 2* (1959): 49–54.

Crary, M., and R. Towne, "The asynergistic nature of developmental verbal dyspraxia." *Australian Journal of Human Communication Disorders, 12* (1984): 27–28.

Darley, F., "Apraxia of speech: Description, diagnosis and treatment." Paper presented at the annual convention of the American Speech and Hearing Association, New York, 1970.

Darley, F., A. Aronson, and J. Brown, "Differential diagnostic patterns of dysarthria." *Journal of Speech and Hearing Research, 12* (1969): 246–269.

Darley, F., A. Aronson, and J. Brown, *Motor Speech Disorders.* Philadelphia: W.B. Saunders, 1975.

Davis, E., "The development of linguistic skills in twins, singletons with siblings, and only children from age five to ten years." *Institute of Child Welfare Monograph Series, 14.* Minneapolis: University of Minnesota Press, 1937.

Dawson, L., "A study of the development of the rate of articulation." *Elementary School Journal, 29* (1929): 610–615.

De Renzi, E., A. Pieczuro, and L. Vignolo, "Oral apraxia and aphasia." *Cortex, 2* (1966): 50–73.

Dickson, S., "Differences between children who spontaneously outgrow and children who retain functional articulation errors." *Journal of Speech and Hearing Research, 5* (1962): 263–271.

Dodd, B., "Recognition and reproduction of words by Down's syndrome and non–Down's syndrome retarded children." *American Journal of Mental Deficiency, 80* (1975): 306–311.

Dubois, E., and J. Bernthal, "A comparison of three methods for obtaining articulatory responses." *Journal of Speech and Hearing Disorders, 43* (1978): 295–305.

Dunn, C., and L. Newton, "A comprehensive model for speech development in hearing-impaired children." *Topics in Language Disorders: Hearing Impairment: Implications from Normal Child Language, 6* (1986): 25–46.

Dworkin, J., "Protrusive lingual force and lingual diadochokinetic rates: A comparative analysis between normal and lisping speakers." *Language, Speech, and Hearing Services in Schools, 9* (1978): 8–16.

Dworkin, J., and R. Culatta, "Tongue strength: Its relationship to tongue thrusting, open-bite, and articulatory proficiency." *Journal of Speech and Hearing Disorders, 45* (1980): 227–282.

Eilers, R.E., and K.K. Oller, "The role of speech discrimination in developmental sound substitutions." *Journal of Child Language, 3* (1976): 319–329.

Eimas, P., E. Siqueland, P. Jusczyk, and J. Vigorito, "Speech perception in infants." *Science, 171* (1971): 303–306.

Everhart, R., "The relationship between articulation and other developmental factors in children." *Journal of Speech and Hearing Disorders, 18* (1953): 332–338.

Everhart, R., "Paternal occupational classification and the maturation of articulation." *Speech Monographs, 23* (1956): 75–77.

Everhart, R., "Literature survey of growth and developmental factors in articulation maturation." *Journal of Speech and Hearing Disorders, 25* (1960): 59–69.

Fairbanks, G., and B. Bebout, "A study of minor organic deviations in 'functional' disorders of articulation; 3. The tongue." *Journal of Speech and Hearing Disorders, 15* (1950): 348–352.

Fairbanks, G., and E. Green, "A study of minor organic deviations in 'functional' disorders of articulation; 2. Dimension and relationships of the lips." *Journal of Speech and Hearing Disorders, 15* (1950): 165–168.

Fairbanks, G., and M. Lintner, "A study of minor organic deviations in 'functional' disorders of articulation; 4. The teeth and hard palate." *Journal of Speech and Hearing Disorders, 16* (1951): 273–279.

Fey, M., Personal Communication, 1991.

Fitzsimons, R., "Developmental, psychosocial and educational factors in children with nonorganic articulation problems." *Child Development, 29* (1958): 481–489.

Fletcher, S., "Time-by-count measurement of diadochokinetic syllable rate." *Journal of Speech and Hearing Research, 15* (1972): 763–780.

Fletcher, S., R. Casteel, and D. Bradley, "Tongue-thrust swallow, speech articulation." *Journal of Speech and Hearing Disorders, 26* (1961): 201–208.

Fletcher, S., and J. Meldrum, "Lingual function and relative length of the lingual frenulum." *Journal of Speech and Hearing Research, 11* (1968): 382–399.

Flynn, P., and M. Byrne, "Relationship between reading and selected auditory abilities of third-grade children." *Journal of Speech and Hearing Research, 13* (1970): 731–740.

Factors Related to Phonological Disorders

Fucci, D., "Oral vibrotactile sensation: An evaluation of normal and defective speakers." *Journal of Speech and Hearing Research, 15* (1972): 179–184.

Gammon, S., P. Smith, R. Daniloff, and C. Kim, "Articulation and stress juncture production under oral anesthetization and masking." *Journal of Speech and Hearing Research, 14* (1971): 271–282.

Garrett, R., "A study of children's discrimination of phonetic variations of the /s/ phoneme." Ph.D. dissertation, Ohio University, 1969.

Gross, G., K. St. Louis, D. Ruscello, and F. Hull, "Language abilities of articulatory-disordered school children with multiple or residual errors." *Language, Speech, and Hearing Services in Schools, 16* (1985): 174–186.

Guyette, R., and W. Diedrich, "A critical review of developmental apraxia of speech." In N. Lass (Ed.), *Speech and Language: Advances in Basic Research and Practice*, Vol. 5. New York: Academic Press, 1981.

Hadden, W.B., "On certain defects of articulation in children with cases illustrating the results of education of the oral system." *Journal of Mental Science, 37* (1891): 96–100.

Hall, M., "Auditory factors in functional articulatory speech defects." *Journal of Experimental Education, 7* (1938): 110–132.

Hansen, B., "The application of sound discrimination tests to functional articulatory defectives with normal hearing." *Journal of Speech Disorders, 9* (1944): 347–355.

Hanson, M.L., "Orofacial myofunctional disorders: Guidelines for assessment and treatment." *International Journal of Orofacial Myology, 14* (1988a): 27–32.

Hanson, M.L., "Orofacial myofunctional therapy: Historical and philosophical considerations." *International Journal of Orofacial Myology, 14* (1988b): 3–10.

Haynes, S., "Developmental apraxia of speech: Symptoms and treatment." In D.F. Johns (Ed.), *Clinical Management of Neurogenic Communicative Disorders*. Boston: Little, Brown, 1985.

Haynes, S., D. Johns, and E. May, "Assessment and therapeutic management of an adult patient with developmental apraxia of speech and orosensory perceptual deficits." *Tejas, 3* (1978): 6–9.

Hilton, L., "Treatment of deviant phonologic systems: Tongue thrust." In W. Perkins (Ed.), *Phonological-Articulatory Disorders*. New York: Thieme-Stratton, 1984.

Hoffman, P., "Spelling, phonology, and the speech pathologist: A whole language perspective." *Language, Speech, and Hearing Services in Schools, 21* (1990): 238–243.

Hoffman, P., and J. Norris, "On the nature of phonological development: Evidence from normal children's spelling errors." *Journal of Speech and Hearing Research, 32* (1989): 787–794.

Hoffman, P., J. Norris, and J. Monjure, "Comparison of process targeting and whole language treatments of phonologically delayed children." *Language, Speech, and Hearing Services in Schools, 21* (1990): 102–109.

Hoffman, P., S. Stager, and R. Daniloff, "Perception and production of misarticulated /r/." *Journal of Speech and Hearing Disorders, 48* (1983): 210–214.

Holland, A., "Training speech sound discrimination in children who misarticulate. A demonstration of teaching machine technique in speech correction." Project No. 5007. Washington, D.C.: U.S. Department of Health, Education and Welfare, 1967.

Horii, Y., A. House, K. Li, and R. Ringel, "Acoustic characteristics of speech produced without oral sensation." *Journal of Speech and Hearing Research, 16* (1973): 67–77.

Hull, F., P. Mielke, R. Timmons, and J. Willeford, "The national speech and hearing survey: Preliminary results." *Asha, 13* (1971): 501–509.

Itoh, M., and S. Sasanuma, "Articulatory movements in apraxia of speech." In J. Rosenbek, M. McNeil, and A. Aronson (Eds.), *Apraxia of Speech: Physiology, Acoustics, Linguistics, Management*. San Diego: College-Hill Press, 1984.

Jaffe, M., "Neurological impairment of speech production: Assessment and treatment." In A. Holland and J. Costello (Eds.), *Handbook of Speech and Language Disorders*. San Diego: College-Hill Press, 1986.

Jann, G., M. Ward, and H. Jann, "A longitudinal study of articulation, deglutition and malocclusion." *Journal of Speech and Hearing Disorders, 29* (1964): 424–435.

Jenkins, E., and F. Lohr, "Severe articulation disorders and motor ability." *Journal of Speech and Hearing Disorders, 29* (1964): 286–292.

Johns, D., and F. Darley, "Phonemic variability in apraxia of speech." *Journal of Speech and Hearing Research, 13* (1970): 556–583.

Johns, D., and K. Salyer, "Surgical and prosthetic management of neurogenic speech disorders." In D. Johns (Ed.), *Clinical Management of Neurogenic Communicative Disorders*. Boston: Little, Brown, 1978.

Jordan, L., J. Hardy, and H. Morris, "Performance of children with good and poor articulation on tasks of tongue placement." *Journal of Speech and Hearing Research, 21* (1978): 429–439.

Kenney, K., and E. Prather, "Articulation in preschool children: Consistency of productions." *Journal of Speech and Hearing Research, 29* (1986): 29–36.

Koch, H., "Sibling influence on children's speech." *Journal of Speech and Hearing Disorders, 21* (1956): 322–329.

Koegel, L.K., R.L. Koegel, and J.C. Ingham, "Programming rapid generalization of correct articulation through self-monitoring procedures." *Journal of Speech and Hearing Disorders, 51* (1986): 24–32.

Koegel, R., L. Koegel, K. Van Voy, and J. Ingham, "Within-clinic versus outside-of-clinic self-monitoring of artic- ulation to promote generalization." *Journal of Speech and Hearing Disorders, 53* (1988): 392–399.

Kronvall, E., and C. Diehl, "The relationship of auditory discrimination to articulatory defects of children with no known organic impairment." *Journal of Speech and Hearing Disorders, 19* (1954): 335–338.

Lapko, L., and N. Bankson, "Relationship between auditory discrimination, articulation stimulability and consistency of misarticulation." *Perceptual and Motor Skills, 40* (1975): 171–177.

Lapointe, L., and R. Wertz, "Oral-movement abilities and articulatory characteristics of brain-injured adults." *Per- ceptual Motor Skills, 39* (1974): 39–46.

Lerea, L., and B. Ward, "The social schema of normal and speech-defective children." *Journal of Social Psychology, 69* (1966): 87–94.

Levitt, H., and H. Stromberg, "Segmental characteristics of speech of hearing-impaired children: Factors affecting intelligibility." In I. Hochberg, H. Levitt, and M. Osberger (Eds.), *Speech of the Hearing Impaired: Re- search, Training and Personnel Preparation.* Baltimore: University Park Press, 1983.

Lewis, B., B. Ekelman, and D. Aram, "A familial study of severe phonological disorders." *Journal of Speech and Hearing Research, 32* (1989): 713–724.

Lewis, B., and L. Freebairn-Farr, "Preschool phonology disorders at school age, adolescence, and adulthood." Paper presented at the annual convention of the American Speech-Language-Hearing Association, Atlanta, 1991.

Liberman, I., and D. Shankweiler, "Phonology and problems of learning to read and write." *Remedial and Special Education, 6* (1985): 8–17.

Ling, D., *Foundations of Spoken Language for Hearing-Impaired Children.* Washington, DC: Alexander Graham Bell Association for the Deaf, 1969.

Locke, J., "Oral perception and articulation learning." *Perceptual and Motor Skills, 26* (1968): 1259–1264.

Locke, J.L., "The inference of speech perception in the phonologically disordered child, part I: A rationale, some criteria, the conventional tests." *Journal of Speech and Hearing Disorders, 4* (1980): 431–444.

Locke, J., and K. Kutz, "Memory for speech and speech for memory." *Journal of Speech and Hearing Research, 18* (1975): 179–191.

Locke, J., and P. Mather, "Genetic factors in phonology. Evidence from monozygotic and dizygotic twins." Paper presented at the annual convention of the American Speech-Language-Hearing Association, New Orleans, 1987.

Love, R., *Childhood Motor Speech Disability.* New York: Macmillan, 1992.

Love, R., and M. Fitzgerald, "Is the diagnosis of developmental apraxia of speech valid?" *Australian Journal of Human Communication Disorders, 12* (1984): 71–82.

McDonald, E. T., *Articulation Testing and Treatment: A Sensory Motor Approach.* Pittsburgh, Pa.: Stanwix House, 1964.

McDonald, E.T., and L. Aungst, "Apparent impedence of oral sensory functions and articulatory proficiency." In J. Bosma (Ed.), *Second Symposium on Oral Sensation and Perception.* Springfield, Ill.: Charles C Thomas, 1970.

McEnery, E., and F. Gaines, "Tongue-tie in infants and children." *Journal of Pediatrics, 18* (1941): 252–255.

McNutt, J., "Oral sensory and motor behaviors of children with /s/ or /r/ misarticulations." *Journal of Speech and Hearing Research, 20* (1977): 694–703.

Majid, A., B. Weinberg, and V. Chalin, "Speech intelligibility following prosthetic obturation of surgically acquired maxillary defects." *Journal of Prosthetic Dentition, 32* (1974): 87–96.

Marquardt, T., and J. Saxman, "Language comprehension and auditory discrimination in articulation deficient kin- dergarten children." *Journal of Speech and Hearing Research, 15* (1972): 382–389.

Mase, D., "Etiology of articulatory speech defects." *Teacher's College Contribution to Education,* No. 921. New York: Columbia University, 1946.

Mason, R., "The examination and treatment concerns in cleft palate and maxillo-facial disorders." Tufts-New England Medical Center Lecture Series, Boston, October 1979.

Mason, R.M., "Orthodontic perspectives on orofacial myofunctional therapy." *International Journal of Orofacial Myology, 14* (1988): 49–55.

Mason, R., and W. Proffit, "The tongue-thrust controversy: Background and recommendations." *Journal of Speech and Hearing Disorders, 39* (1974): 115–132.

Mason, R., and N. Wickwire, "Examining for orofacial variations." *Communique, 8* (1978): 2–26.

Massengill, R., S. Maxwell, and K. Picknell, "An analysis of articulation following partial and total glossectomy." *Journal of Speech and Hearing Disorders, 35* (1970): 170–173.

Matheny, A., and C. Bruggeman, "Children's speech: Heredity components and sex differences." *Folia Phoniatrica, 25* (1973): 442–449.

Matheny, N., and J. Panagos, "Comparing the effects of articulation and syntax programs on syntax and articulation improvement." *Language, Speech, and Hearing Services in Schools, 9* (1978): 57–61.

Mills, A., and H. Streit, "Report of a speech survey, Holyoke, Massachusetts." *Journal of Speech Disorders, 7* (1942): 161–167.

Factors Related to Phonological Disorders

Moll, K., and F. Darley, "Attitudes of mothers of articulatory-impaired and speech-retarded children." *Journal of Speech and Hearing Disorders, 25* (1960): 377–384.

Monson, R., "The oral speech intelligibility of hearing-impaired talkers." *Journal of Speech and Hearing Disorders, 48* (1983): 286–296.

Morley, D., "A ten-year survey of speech disorders among university students." *Journal of Speech and Hearing Disorders, 17* (1952): 25–31.

Morley, M.E., *The Development and Disorders of Speech in Childhood.* London: Livingston, 1957.

Mowrer, D., R. Baker, and R. Schutz, "Operant procedures in the control of speech articulation." In H. Sloane and B. MacAulay (Eds.), *Operant Procedures in Remedial Speech and Language Training.* Boston: Houghton Mifflin, 1968.

Neils, J., and D. Aram, "Family history of children with developmental language disorders," *Perceptual and Motor Skills, 63* (1986): 655–658.

Netsell, R.A., *A Neurobiologic View of Speech Production and the Dysarthrias.* Boston: College-Hill Press, 1986.

Overstake, C., "Investigation of the efficacy of a treatment program for deviant swallowing and allied problems, part II." *International Journal of Oral Myology, 2* (1976): 1–6.

Paden, E.P., M.L. Matthies, and M.A. Novak, "Recovery from OME-related phonologic delay following tube placement." *Journal of Speech and Hearing Disorders, 54* (1989): 94–100.

Paden, E.P., M.A. Novak, and A.L. Beiter, "Predictors of phonologic inadequacy in young children prone to otitis media." *Journal of Speech and Hearing Disorders, 52* (1987): 232–242.

Palmer, J., "Tongue-thrusting: A clinical hypothesis." *Journal of Speech and Hearing Disorders, 27* (1962): 323–333.

Panagos, J., and P. Prelock, "Phonological constraints on the sentence productions of language disordered children." *Journal of Speech and Hearing Research, 25* (1982): 171–176.

Panagos, J., M. Quine, and R. Klich, "Syntactic and phonological influences on children's articulation." *Journal of Speech and Hearing Research, 22* (1979): 841–848.

Parlour, S., and P. Broen, "Environmental factors in familial phonological disorders: Preliminary home scale results." Paper presented at the annual convention of the American Speech-Language-Hearing Association, Atlanta, 1991.

Paul, R., and L. Shriberg, "Associations between phonology and syntax in speech delayed children." *Journal of Speech and Hearing Research, 25* (1982): 536–546.

Paul, R., and L.D. Shriberg, "Reply to Panagos and Prelock (Letter)." *Journal of Speech and Hearing Research, 27* (1984): 319–320.

Perkins, W., *Speech Pathology: An Applied Behavioral Science.* St. Louis: C.V. Mosby, 1977.

Powers, M., "Functional disorders of articulation-symptomatology and etiology." In L. Travis (Ed.), *Handbook of Speech Pathology and Audiology.* Englewood Cliffs, N.J.: Prentice Hall, 1957, 1971.

Prins, D., "Analysis of correlations among various articulatory deviations." *Journal of Speech and Hearing Research, 5* (1962a): 151–160.

Prins, D., "Motor and auditory abilities in different groups of children with articulatory deviations." *Journal of Speech and Hearing Research, 5* (1962b): 161–168.

Proffit, W.R., *Contemporary Orthodontics.* St. Louis: C.V. Mosby, 1986.

Prosek, R., and A. House, "Intraoral air pressure as a feedback cue in consonant production." *Journal of Speech and Hearing Research, 18* (1975): 133–147.

Reid, G., "The etiology and nature of functional articulatory defects in elementary school children." *Journal of Speech and Hearing Disorders, 12* (1947a): 143–150.

Reid, G., "The efficiency of speech re-education of functional articulatory defectives in elementary school." *Journal of Speech and Hearing Disorders, 12* (1947b): 301–313.

Ringel, R., K. Burk, and C. Scott, "Tactile perception: Form discrimination in the mouth." In J. Bosma (Ed.), *Second Symposium on Oral Sensation and Perception.* Springfield, Ill.: Charles C Thomas, 1970.

Ringel, R., and S. Ewanowski, "Oral perception: I. Two-point discrimination." *Journal of Speech and Hearing Research, 8* (1965): 389–400.

Ringel, R., A. House, K. Burk, J. Dolinsky, and C. Scott, "Some relations between orosensory discrimination and articulatory aspects of speech production." *Journal of Speech and Hearing Disorders, 35* (1970): 3–11.

Roberts, J.E., M.R. Burchinal, M.A. Koch, M.M. Footo, and F.W. Henderson, "Otitis media in early childhood and its relationship to later phonological development." *Journal of Speech and Hearing Disorders, 53* (1988): 424–432.

Roe, V., and R. Milisen, "The effect of maturation upon defective articulation in elementary grades." *Journal of Speech Disorders, 7* (1942): 37–50.

Rosenbek, J., and R. Wertz, "A review of fifty cases of developmental apraxia of speech." *Language, Speech, and Hearing Services in Schools, 1* (1972): 23–33.

Rosin, M., E. Swift, D. Bless, and D.K. Vetter, "Communication profiles of adolescents with Down's syndrome." *Journal of Childhood Communication Disorders, 12* (1988): 49–62.

Ruscello, D.M., "Articulation improvement and oral tactile changes in children." Thesis, University of West Virginia, 1972.

Sayler, H., "The effect of maturation upon defective articulation in grades seven through twelve." *Journal of Speech and Hearing Disorders, 14* (1949): 202–207.

Schlanger, B., "Speech examination of a group of institutionalized mentally handicapped children." *Journal of Speech and Hearing Disorders, 18* (1953): 339–349.

Schlanger, B., and R. Gottsleben, "Analysis of speech defects among the institutionalized mentally retarded." *Journal of Speech and Hearing Disorders, 22* (1957): 98–103.

Schmauch, V., J. Panagos, and R. Klich, "Syntax influences the accuracy of consonant production in language-disordered children." *Journal of Communication Disorders, 11* (1978): 315–323.

Schwartz, A., and R. Goldman, "Variables influencing performance on speech sound discrimination tests." *Journal of Speech and Hearing Research, 17* (1974): 25–32.

Schwartz, R., L. Leonard, M.K. Folger, and M.J. Wilcox, "Evidence for a synergistic view of linguistic disorders: Early phonological behavior in normal and language disordered children." *Journal of Speech and Hearing Disorders, 45* (1980): 357–377.

Scott, C., and R. Ringel, "Articulation without oral sensory control." *Journal of Speech and Hearing Research, 14* (1971): 804–818.

Shelton, R., "Science, clinical art, and speech pathology." Paper presented at Kansas University, Spring 1989.

Shelton, R., A. Johnson, and W. Arndt, "Delayed judgment speech sound discrimination and /r/ or /s/ articulation status and improvement." *Journal of Speech and Hearing Research, 20* (1977): 704–717.

Shelton, R.L., V. Willis, A.F. Johnson, and W.B. Arndt, "Oral form recognition training and articulation change." *Perceptual Motor Skills, 36* (1973): 523–531.

Sherman, D., and A. Geith, "Speech sound discrimination and articulation skill." *Journal of Speech and Hearing Disorders, 10* (1967): 277–280.

Shriberg, L.D., and J. Kwiatkowski, "Phonological disorders I: A diagnostic classification system." *Journal of Speech and Hearing Disorders, 47* (1982): 226–241.

Shriberg, L.D., and A.J. Smith, "Phonological correlates of middle-ear involvement in speech-delayed children: A methodological note." *Journal of Speech and Hearing Research, 26* (1983): 293–297.

Shriberg, L.D., and C. Widder, "Speech and prosody characteristics of adults with mental retardation." *Journal of Speech and Hearing Research, 33* (1990): 627–653.

Shriner, T., M. Holloway, and R. Daniloff, "The relationship between articulatory deficits and syntax in speech defective children." *Journal of Speech and Hearing Research, 12* (1969): 319–325.

Skelly, M., D. Spector, R. Donaldson, A. Brodeur, and R. Paletta, "Compensatory physiologic phonetics for the glossectomee." *Journal of Speech and Hearing Disorders, 36* (1971): 101–114.

Smit, A., L. Hand, J. Freilinger, J. Bernthal, and A. Bird, "The Iowa articulation norms project and its Nebraska replication." *Journal of Speech and Hearing Disorders, 55* (1990): 779–798.

Smith, B., and C. Stoel-Gammon, "A longitudinal study of the development of stop consonant production in normal and Down's syndrome children." *Journal of Speech and Hearing Disorders, 48* (1983): 114–118.

Smith, C., "Residual hearing and speech production in deaf children." Ph.D. dissertation, City University of New York, 1972.

Snow, K., "Articulation proficiency in relation to certain dental abnormalities." *Journal of Speech and Hearing Disorders, 26* (1961): 209–212.

Solomon, A., "Personality and behavior patterns of children with functional defects of articulation." *Child Development, 32* (1961): 731–737.

Sommers, R., C. Cockerille, R. Bowser, G. Fichter, A. Fenton, and F. Copetas, "Effects of speech therapy and speech improvement upon articulation and reading." *Journal of Speech and Hearing Disorders, 26* (1961): 27–38.

Sommers, R., J. Patterson, and P. Wildgen, "Phonology of Down's syndrome speakers." *Journal of Childhood Communication Disorders, 12* (1988): 65–88.

Sommers, R., R. Reinhart, and D. Sistrunk, "Traditional articulation measures of Down's syndrome speakers, ages 13–22." *Journal of Childhood Communication Disorders, 12* (1988): 93–108.

Sonderman, J., "An experimental study of clinical relationships between auditory discrimination and articulation skills." Paper presented at the annual convention of the American Speech and Hearing Association, San Francisco, 1971.

Spriestersbach, D., "Research in articulation disorders and personality." *Journal of Speech and Hearing Disorders, 21* (1956): 329–335.

Spriestersbach, D., and J. Curtis, "Misarticulation and discrimination of speech sounds." *Quarterly Journal of Speech, 37* (1951): 483–491.

Starr, C., "Dental and occlusal hazards to normal speech production." In K. Bzoch (Ed.), *Communicative Disorders Related to Cleft Lip and Palate*. Boston: Little, Brown, 1972.

Stelcik, J., "An investigation of internal versus external discrimination and general versus phoneme-specific discrimination." Unpublished thesis, University of Maryland, 1972.

Stoel-Gammon, C., "Phonological analysis of four Down's syndrome children." *Journal of Applied Psycholinguistics, 1* (1980): 31–48.

Stoel-Gammon, C., "Speech development of infants and children with Down's syndrome." In J. Darby (Ed.), *Speech Evaluation in Medicine*. New York: Grune and Stratton, 1981.

Strange, W., and P. Broen, "Perception and production of approximant consonants by 3-year-olds: A first study." In G. Yeni-Komshian, J. Kavanaugh, and C.A. Ferguson (Eds.), *Child Phonology*, Vol. 2. *Perception*. New York: Academic Press, 1980.

Subtelny, J., J. Mestre, and J. Subtelny, "Comparative study of normal and defective articulation of /s/ as related to malocclusion and deglutition." *Journal of Speech and Hearing Disorders, 29* (1964): 269–285.

Tabor, T., "Speech disorders associated with developmental facial anomalies." Lecture presented at Boston University, March 1979.

Templin, M., *Certain Language Skills in Children*. Institute of Child Welfare Monograph Series 26. Minneapolis: University of Minnesota, 1957.

Templin, M., "Development of speech." *Journal of Pediatrics, 62* (1963): 11–14.

Templin, M., *Longitudinal Study through the 4th Grade of Language Skills of Children with Varying Speech Sound Articulation in Kindergarten* (Final Report, Project 2220). Washington, D.C.: U.S. Department of Health, Education, and Welfare, Office of Education, 1968.

Tiffany, W., "Effects of syllable structure on diadochokinetic and reading rates." *Journal of Speech and Hearing Research, 23* (1980): 894–908.

Travis, L., and B. Rasmus, "The speech sound discrimination ability of cases with functional disorders of articulation." *Quarterly Journal of Speech, 17* (1931): 217–226.

Tyler, A., and K. Watterson, "Effects of phonological versus language intervention in preschoolers with both phonological and language impairment." *Child Language Teaching and Therapy, 7* (1991): 141–160.

VanDemark, A., and M. Mann, "Oral language skills of children with defective articulation." *Journal of Speech and Hearing Research, 8* (1965): 409–414.

Veatch, J., "An experimental investigation of a motor theory of auditory discrimination." Ph.D. dissertation, University of Idaho, 1970.

Velleman, S.L., "Children's production and perception of English voiceless fricatives." Unpublished Ph.D. dissertation, University of Texas at Austin, 1983.

Weaver, C., C. Furbee, and R. Everhart, "Paternal occupational class and articulatory defects in children." *Journal of Speech and Hearing Disorders, 25* (1960): 171–175.

Weinberg, B., R. Christensen, W. Logan, J. Bosma, and A. Wornall, "Severe hypoplasia on the tongue." *Journal of Speech and Hearing Disorders, 34* (1969): 157–168.

Weinberg, B., G.M. Liss, and J.A. Hillis, "Comparative study of visual, manual and oral form identification skills in speech impaired and normal speaking children." In J.F. Bosma (Ed.), *Second Symposium on Oral Sensation and Perception*. Springfield, Ill.: Charles C Thomas, 1970.

Weiner, P., "Auditory discrimination and articulation." *Journal of Speech and Hearing Disorders, 32* (1967): 19–28.

Wellman, B., I. Case, I. Mengert, and D. Bradbury, "Speech sounds of young children." *University of Iowa Studies in Child Welfare, 5* (1931).

Whitaker, J., H. Luper, and H. Pollio, "General language deficits in children with articulation problems." *Language and Speech, 3* (1970): 231–239.

Wilhelm, C.L., "The effects of oral form recognition training on articulation in children." Dissertation, University of Kansas, 1971.

Williams, G., and L. McReynolds, "The relationship between discrimination and articulation training in children with misarticulations." *Journal of Speech and Hearing Research, 18* (1975): 401–412.

Williams, R., R. Ingham, and J. Rosenthal, "A further analysis for developmental apraxia of speech in children with defective articulation." *Journal of Speech and Hearing Research, 24* (1981): 496–505.

Wilson, F., "Efficacy of speech therapy with educable mentally retarded children." *Journal of Speech and Hearing Research, 9* (1966): 423–433.

Winitz, H., "Language skills of male and female kindergarten children." *Journal of Speech and Hearing Research, 2* (1959a): 377–386.

Winitz, H., "Relationship between language and nonlanguage measures of kindergarten children." *Journal of Speech and Hearing Research, 2* (1959b): 387–391.

Winitz, H., *Articulatory Acquisition and Behavior*. Englewood Cliffs, N.J.: Prentice Hall, 1969.

Winitz, H., "Auditory considerations in articulation training." In H. Winitz (Ed.), *Treating Articulation Disorders: For Clinicians by Clinicians*. Baltimore: University Park Press, 1984.

Wolfe, V., and R. Irwin, "Sound discrimination ability of children with misarticulation of the /r/ sound." *Perceptual and Motor Skills, 37* (1973): 415–420.

Wood, K., "Parental maladjustment and functional articulatory defects in children." *Journal of Speech and Hearing Disorders, 11* (1946): 255–275.

Woolf, G., and M. Pilberg, "A comparison of three tests of auditory discrimination and their relationship to performance on a deep test of articulation." *Journal of Communication Disorders, 3* (1971): 239–249.

Yoss, K., and F. Darley, "Developmental apraxia of speech in children with defective articulation." *Journal of Speech and Hearing Research, 17* (1974): 399–416.

chapter
6

Phonological
Assessment Procedures

INTRODUCTION

Speech-language pathologists have made a unique contribution to the assessment of verbal behavior through the development of phonological assessment instruments. For several decades, phonological/articulation assessment procedures have remained almost the exclusive domain of speech-language clinicians, although linguists, child development specialists, psychologists, pediatricians, and special educators also use such tools.

Evaluation of an individual's phonological status involves description of his or her speech sound production system and relating this system to the adult standard of the speaker's linguistic community. This analysis is often done in the context of an overall communication evaluation that includes assessment of voice quality, fluency of speech, and aspects of language including syntax, semantics, pragmatics, and discourse. In addition, such related measures as hearing testing, oral cavity examination, and "perceptual testing" are usually included in a comprehensive assessment. As part of the evaluation, the clinician seeks to identify etiological factors that may be related to the presence and maintenance of the phonological disorder.

Phonological assessment is used to:

1. Describe the phonological status of an individual and determine if his or her speech sound system is sufficiently different from normal development to warrant intervention

2. Determine treatment direction and strategies to be used in the management of the client

3. Make predictive and prognostic statements relative to phonological change with or without intervention
4. Monitor change in phonological performance across time
5. Identify factors that may be related to the presence or maintenance of a phonologic disability.

The primary purposes of a comprehensive phonological assessment are to determine whether an individual needs remedial instruction, and if so, the direction of treatment. To make these determinations, the clinician engages in a multistep process that involves sampling the client's speech through a variety of procedures, analyzing the data gathered, interpreting the data that has been analyzed, and then making clinical recommendations and decisions. No hard and fast rules dictate when intervention is warranted or the type of treatment to be recommended. State guidelines often dictate when a child qualifies for services in the public schools. In this chapter, we will discuss various sampling and testing procedures and discuss factors and issues that should be taken into consideration when analyzing and interpreting phonological samples.

SCREENING FOR PHONOLOGICAL DISORDERS

Comprehensive phonological testing, including analysis and interpretation of results, often requires a considerable expenditure of time. Frequently, a clinician will do a *screening* to determine if a more comprehensive assessment of this nature is warranted. Screening procedures are not designed to determine the need or direction of therapy, but rather to differentiate individuals who merit further evaluation from those for whom further evaluation is not indicated. Typical screening situations might include (1) screening children at a preschool or "kindergarten roundup" to determine whether they have age appropriate phonological skills, (2) screening children in grade 3 (by which time maturation should have resolved most developmental errors), (3) screening college students preparing for occupations, such as teaching or broadcast journalism, which require certain speech performance standards, and (4) screening the phonological status of referred children and adults for a suspected communication impairment.

In screening, individuals are not identified as candidates for therapy, but rather are simply identified as needing further assessment. Additional testing is often required before statements about the presence or absence of a phonological disorder can be made, and certainly is required for determining the direction for treatment. Instruments used for screening consist of a limited sampling of speech sound productions, which can usually be administered in five minutes or less. Screening measures can be categorized as informal or formal.

INFORMAL SCREENING MEASURES

Informal screening measures are usually devised by the examiner and are tailored to the population being screened. For example, with a group of kindergarten children, the examiner might ask each child to

1. State his or her name and address
2. Count to ten; name the days of the week
3. Tell about a television show

If the subjects are adults, the examiner might ask them to do one or both of the following:

1. Read sentences designed to elicit several productions of frequently misarticulated sounds, such as /s/, /r/, /l/, and /θ/. For example, "I saw Sally at her seaside house; Rob ran around the orange car."
2. Read a passage with a representative sample of English speech sounds such as the "Grandfather Passage" or the "Rainbow Passage."

Grandfather Passage

You wish to know all about my grandfather. Well, he is nearly 93 years old, yet he still thinks as swiftly as ever. He dresses himself in an old black frock coat, usually several buttons missing. A long beard clings to his chin, giving those who observe him a pronounced feeling of the utmost respect. When he speaks, his voice is just a bit cracked and quivers a bit. Twice each day he plays skillfully and with zest upon a small organ. Except in winter when the snow or ice prevents, he slowly takes a short walk in the open air each day. We have often urged him to walk more and smoke less, but he always answers, "Banana oil." Grandfather likes to be modern in his language.

Rainbow Passage

When the sunlight strikes raindrops in the air, they act like a prism and form a rainbow. The rainbow is a division of white light into many beautiful colors. These take the shape of a long round arch, with its path high above, and its two ends apparently beyond the horizon. There is, according to legend, a boiling pot of gold at one end. People look, but no one ever finds it. When a man looks for something beyond his reach, his friends say he is looking for the pot of gold at the end of the rainbow.

Throughout the centuries men have explained the rainbow in various ways. Some have accepted it as a miracle without physical explanation. To the Hebrews it was a token that there would be no more universal floods. The Greeks used to imagine that it was a sign from the gods to foretell war or heavy rain. The Norsemen considered the rainbow as a bridge over which the gods passed from the earth to their home in the sky. Other men have tried to explain the phenomenon physically. Aristotle thought that the rainbow was caused by reflection of the sun's rays by the rain. Since then physicists have found that it is not reflection, but refraction by the raindrops which causes the rainbow. Many complicated ideas about the rainbow have been formed. The difference in the rainbow depends considerably upon the size of the water drops, and the width of the colored band increases as the size of the drop increases. The actual primary rainbow observed is said to be the effect of superposition of a number of bows. If the red of the second bow falls upon the green of the first, the result is to give a bow with an abnormally wide yellow band, since red and green lights when mixed form yellow. This is a very common type of bow, one showing mainly red and yellow, with little or no green or blue.

Criterion for failure of informal screening is usually determined by the examiner. An often used rule of thumb is "if in doubt, refer." In other words, if one suspects that the client's speech sound system is not appropriate for his or her age and/or language community, one should refer for a more complete assessment. Those individuals with the greatest need for additional testing and probable intervention will usually be obvious to the examiner from even a small sample of the individuals' speech and language.

Formal screening measures include published elicitation procedures for which normative data and/or cut-off scores are often available. These formal measures are of three types: (1) tests that are part of a more comprehensive single-word articulation test, (2) tests designed solely for screening phonology, and (3) tests which screen phonology as well as other aspects of language. Tests designed explicitly for screening phonology are most frequently used when screening phonology is the primary goal. Those instruments that combine phonological screening with other aspects of language screening are most commonly used for more general communication screening often conducted by child development specialists, pediatricians, and special educators.

The following are formal phonology screening tests:

Templin-Darley Screening Test (Templin and Darley, 1969). This test consists of 50 items, from the *Templin-Darley Tests of Articulation*, intended to elicit 22 single consonants, 26 consonant clusters, one vowel, and one consonant-vowel combination. Norms and suggested cut-off scores for children aged 3 through 8 years are provided.

Quick Screen of Phonology (QSP) (Bankson and Bernthal, 1990). This test consists of 28 picture-naming items, with each word assessing sounds in more than one context (usually initial and final). Twenty-three phonemes are screened plus three consonant clusters. These items were selected because of their correlation with the overall norms of the *Bankson-Bernthal Test of Phonology*. Percentile ranks and standard scores are provided for children ages 3;0 through 7;11 years on the QSP.

Denver Articulation Screening Test (Drumwright, 1971). This instrument was designed specifically for screening phonological status in Anglo, black, and Mexican-American children. Responses are elicited imitatively. The examiner is asked to judge intelligibility on a 4-point scale, with 1 being "easy to understand" and 4 being "can't evaluate." Children are ranked "normal to abnormal," depending on composite articulation and intelligibility scores.

Screening Deep Test Articulation (McDonald, 1968). This test consists of 90 items and is similar in form to the more complete *Deep Test of Articulation* (McDonald, 1964a). It uses pairs of pictures to elicit ten productions of each of nine commonly misarticulated consonants. This allows for production of specific consonants in a variety of contexts. The normative data provided for children from kindergarten through grade 3 are designed to identify those children unlikely to develop mature articulation without intervention.

Predictive Screening Test of Articulation (Van Riper and Erickson, 1969). This test, as its title implies, was designed not only for screening but also for predicting whether or not first-grade children are likely to correct their speech sound errors without intervention. In other words, it was designed both to indicate the need for additional testing for those who fail to obtain a cut-off score and to allow the examiner to make prognostic statements about the likelihood of self-correction of speech sound errors. Stockman and McDonald (1980) reported that this test may have greater predictive value for those first-graders who misarticulate specific consonant sounds (e.g., those with defective sibilant sounds, or defective liquids) since those sounds occur frequently in the test.

The following tests include screening of phonology as part of an overall speech and language screening:

Fluharty Speech and Language Screening Test for Preschool Children (Fluharty, 1978). This test was designed for children, ages 2 through 6 years. The phonology portion of the test uses 15 objects to elicit 19 target sounds. Some stimulus items are designed to assess a single segment; other items assess two sounds. Cut-off scores to indicate the need for further testing are included.

Preschool Language Scale (Zimmerman, Steiner, and Pond, 1979). This test was designed for children, ages 1 through 7. The phonology portion of the test consists of 20 imitated words that test 18 speech sounds in initial, medial, and final word-positions. Performance levels expected for children are provided.

As with informal screening measures, the criteria for failure on formal screening tests are often left up to the examiner. When available, standard scores and percentile ranks aid the examiner in establishing such criteria. It is not uncommon for a score one standard deviation below the mean to be used as a cut-off score. For some instruments, cut-off scores or age expectation scores are provided.

SAMPLING PROCEDURES INVOLVED IN A COMPREHENSIVE PHONOLOGICAL EVALUATION

Introduction

As indicated earlier, the two major purposes of a comprehensive phonological evaluation are to determine the need for and direction of treatment. It is to these purposes that most of the writings, research, and testing materials concerning phonological disorders have been addressed. In the following pages, we will discuss components of a phonological battery, with an emphasis on procedures for obtaining phonological samples. In Chapter 7 we will emphasize the analysis and interpretation of data collected through our sampling procedures. Throughout these discussions we will attempt to present a synthesis of the available literature, and in the absence of a data base, often make suggestions based upon our own clinical experience.

Sampling procedures involved in phonological assessment are more detailed and time-consuming than those described for screening. When doing testing of this nature, the clinician usually employs not just one, but rather a battery of assessment instruments and sampling procedures. A complete phonological evaluation typically involves phonological productions in samples of varying lengths, phonetic contexts, and in response to various elicitation procedures. This collection of samples is often referred to as an *Assessment Battery,* a framework for assessment based on the recognition that no one procedure provides all one needs to know in determining the direction that an intervention program should take.

As a student of speech-language pathology, you will likely learn a variety of assessment, analysis, and interpretation procedures. It is important to recognize that while certain procedures are used and have been found helpful, it does not follow that all procedures are as efficient or as scientific (data based) as we might like them to be. In the interest of scientific and professional advancement, the efficacy of our clinical practices must be carefully examined. Clinical assessment is an extremely complex area to investigate, with many important related variables. Much study is needed before definitive statements can be made on many assessment issues.

In the pages that follow, various types of samples that comprise a phonological assessment battery are described. Characteristics and elicitation procedures for each sample type will be presented.

TYPES OF ASSESSMENTS INCLUDED IN A BATTERY

CONNECTED SPEECH SAMPLES

All phonological evaluations should include a sample of connected speech. The ultimate objective of phonological treatment is correct production of sounds in spontaneous conversation; therefore, it is important that the examiner observe sound productions in as "natural" a speaking context as possible. Such samples allow one to observe phoneme productions in a variety of phonetic contexts, to observe error patterns, and to judge the intelligibility of the speaker in continuous discourse. Sounds produced in connected speech may also be studied in relation to other factors such as speech rate, intonation, stress, and syllable structure. This is typically not the case when sounds are sampled in isolated syllable or word productions. In addition, connected speech samples allow for multiple productions of sounds across lexical items.

Because spontaneous connected speech samples are the most valid or representative sample of phonological performance, some clinicians suggest that phonological analyses should almost exclusively be based on this type of sample (Shriberg and Kwiatkowski, 1980; Stoel-Gammon and Dunn, 1985). Connected speech samples have the advantage of allowing the examiner to observe sound productions within the context of the child's vocabulary and with natural prosodic patterns. In addition, these samples can be used for other types of language analysis. There are, however, sometimes practical problems associated with relying on such samples. Many individuals with severe phonological problems may be almost unintelligible, and it may be impossible or very difficult to reliably determine what they are attempting to say in a conversational speech sample. On the other hand, because clinicians may be quite familiar with a given child's speech patterns, they may be less capable of making independent and realistic assessments of intelligibility. Some children may be reluctant to engage in conversational dialogue with an adult they do not know. Simply eliciting single-word responses from some children may represent a challenge, even for a skilled clinician. It may also be an almost impossible task to obtain a spontaneous speech corpus that contains a truly representative sample of English phonemes.

Ingram (1989) has suggested that difficulty in obtaining a "cross-section of the sounds in English" (representative sample) may not be a critical issue. He argued that if a spontaneous sample is of "sufficient size," the child's preference for sounds is revealed. Sounds missing from the sample may reflect a "selective avoidance" by the child; that is, the child chooses not to produce them. He speculated that the "important sounds" will be produced a number of times in a spontaneous conversational speech sample and will provide a general picture of the child's phonological system. Words of caution regarding Ingram's speculations were offered by Bankson and Bernthal (1981). They argued that, first, the absence of specific sounds in a child's spontaneous speech may reflect an infrequent occurrence of those sounds in English rather than selective avoidance; and second, even if the assumption of selective avoidance is valid, clinicians may want the benefit of information about other articulatory productions.

Elicitation Procedures. The customary and preferred method for obtaining a sample of connected speech is to engage a client in spontaneous conversation. The clinician may talk with the client about such things as hobbies, television shows, or places the client has visited. The samples should be tape-recorded so that the clinician can play them back as often as required to accurately transcribe the client's utterances. Clinicians should make notes about topics covered and errors noted to facilitate later transcription.

Allen (1984) presented the following suggestions with respect to recording speech-language samples:

1. Avoid noise sources as much as possible. By using soft toys, soft books, and cloth-covered table tops, noises can be muted considerably. By not talking while the client is talking, the voice of interest will not be obscured, and, by recording in a closed room, other environmental noises can be kept off the tape.
2. Record in stereo. This procedure results in a wider dynamic range of voice signals being recorded and permits the use of binaural auditory acuity in later analyses.
3. Moderately priced equipment may be entirely satisfactory for the job. A stereo cassette recorder, two lavaliere microphones, low-priced tape, and light open-back headsets will deliver fully adequate recording and play-back performance. In addition, look for output level controls, a "review" button, and direct, sturdy, and convenient connectors. Take spares of anything you can afford to buy and manage to carry.

Some clinicians have the client read a passage orally as an alternative method for obtaining a connected sample of speech. Although this procedure provides a sample of connected speech, it has been demonstrated that, usually, fewer errors occur in a sample obtained in this manner than in a corpus of conversational speech (Wright, Shelton, and Arndt, 1969). Moreover, clinicians frequently test children who have not yet learned to read, in which case this procedure is obviously not a viable option.

Some speech sound inventories specify procedures for obtaining a sample of connected speech. For example, in the "Sounds-in-Sentences" subtest of the Goldman-Fristoe Test of Articulation (1969, 1986), the client listens to a story while viewing the accompanying pictures and is then asked to repeat the story. Such a delayed imitation task is designed to elicit particular sounds in certain phonetic contexts. A variation of the delayed imitation method is the sentence repetition technique in which the clinician verbalizes a sentence containing a target sound and instructs the client to repeat it.

Phonological Assessment Procedures

A more spontaneous method than either the immediate or delayed imitation technique is for the client to tell a story about a series of pictures selected to elicit target words and sounds. Dubois and Bernthal (1978) compared productions in the same word stimuli elicited through a picture-naming task, a delayed imitation task, and a storytelling task. They reported that the greatest number of errors were found on the storytelling task and the smallest number on the picture-naming task. These findings were not surprising since the task of naming single words requires different skills than the sequencing of words in phrases and sentences. Although the differences between the methods were statistically significant, the authors interpreted the differences as clinically nonsignificant. They did, however, report that some individuals varied from group trends in their production of certain sounds, depending on the task; for example, some children made significantly more errors on the delayed imitation task than on the picture-naming task.

It has been argued that when individuals know their speech is being recorded or observed, they may be more cautious in their speech patterns and, therefore, do not produce a true picture or valid sample of conversational speech. Bankson and Byrne (1972), in a study of five school-age children, reported differences between the spontaneous samples gathered when the clients were aware and those gathered when they were unaware that they were being tape-recorded. Their findings indicated that one could not, however, predict whether the number of correct productions would increase or decrease when the child was aware that his or her spontaneous speech was being recorded. Shriberg and Kwiatkowski (1985) reported that preschool children seem oblivious to the presence of micro-phones.

Summary. A connected speech sample is a crucial part of any phonological assessment battery because it allows (1) assessment of overall intelligibility, (2) determination of speech sound usage in its natural form, and (3) a data base from which to judge the accuracy of individual sounds, patterns of errors, and consistency of misarticulations. The preferred method for obtaining connected speech samples is to engage the client in spontaneous conversation. If, for some reason, this cannot be accomplished, alternate procedures that can be used include: (1) conversational responses elicited via picture stimuli or objects, (2) utilization of a reading passage, and (3) telling a story following the clinician's model (delayed imitation).

SINGLE-WORD PRODUCTIONS

From the standpoint of widespread usage, analyzing phoneme productions in a corpus of single-word productions (usually elicited by having an examinee name pictures) has been a common method for determining whether or not particular sounds are produced correctly by an individual. Single words provide a discrete, identifiable unit of production that examiners can usually readily transcribe. Since transcribers often are interested in observing the production of only one or perhaps two segments per word production, they are thus able to transcribe and analyze single-word samples much more quickly than multiple or connected word samples, where all phonemes are attended to. The efficiency of analyzing sound productions from single-word samples has resulted in widespread usage of such samples.

While examiners in some instances may be interested in transcribing all the phonemes in a single word, as stated above, it is more often the case that for a given word, only a sound in a particular word-position is transcribed or scored. The most widely used descriptors of sound-positions in a word are initial (sound at the beginning of a word, e.g., /b/ in /bot/), final (sound at the end of a word, e.g., /t/ in /ræbɪt/), and medial (all sounds between the initial and final sounds, e.g., /ɔ/, /k/, and /ɪ/ in /wɔkɪŋ/).

In some instances, the prefixes *pre-, inter-,* and *post-* are each combined with the term *vocalic* to describe the location of a target sound within syllables. Prevocalic position refers to consonants that precede a vowel (CV) and, therefore, initiate the syllable (e.g., *s*oap, *c*at). Postvocalic position refers to consonants that follow the vowel (VC) and, therefore, terminate the syllable (e.g., soa*p*, ca*t*). Intervocalic position involves a consonant that is embedded (VCV) between two vowels (e.g., ca*m*el, ea*g*er). Generally, a singleton consonant in the initial position of a word is prevocalic. Likewise a singleton sound in word-final position is generally postvocalic. Fisher and Logemann (1971) indicated that a consonant in the intervocalic position serves the dual function of ending the preceding syllable and initiating the following syllable. Ingram (1981) suggested that when one consonant occurs between two vowel nuclei, such "ambisyllabic" consonants may be viewed as being shared by both syllables. Grunwell (1982) indicated that if such consonants are allotted to one or the other of the syllables, the most often heard dictum is that the consonant should be viewed as beginning the second syllable (e.g., *ra-bbit; su-gar*). Only in a one-syllable word would the prevocalic position inevitably be word-initial position and the postvocalic, word-final position. The intervocalic consonant would be in the word-medial position since medial refers to somewhere between the first and the last sounds of the word. A medial consonant may stand next to another consonant and serve to initiate or terminate a syllable and, therefore, is not necessarily intervocalic. McDonald (1964b) used the term **releasor** to describe consonants in the prevocalic position (e.g., *b*at) and **arrestor** to describe consonants in the postvocalic position (e.g., ba*t*). Thus, references to initial, medial, and final positions refer to location of consonants in a word, whereas the terms *prevocalic, intervocalic, postvocalic, releasor,* and *arrestor* refer to consonant position relative to syllables.

It has been suggested that speech sound productions may be influenced by the complexity of the syllables and words in which they are produced. We know that the number and juxtaposition of segments make some syllables more difficult to produce than others. The first syllable shapes to develop are generally CV, VC, and CVCV, which constitute the simplest syllable shapes. It has also been reported that CV and CVC are the forms most frequently used by children with phonological disorders (Grunwell, 1981; Schwartz, Leonard, Folger, and Wilcox, 1980). It is to be expected that segmental productions fluctuate with syllable complexity when children name words.

One of the key issues in assessment concerns the correlation between phonological productions that occur in citation form (single words) and those that occur in connected speech. Most investigators have reported that, in general, the information obtained from naming pictures correlates fairly high with speech sound productions in spontaneous speaking situations although differences are frequently obtained in the two types of measures. Clinicians need to be aware that, sometimes, there may be relatively large differences between the two sampling procedures. Sound productions in single words may not accurately reflect

Phonological Assessment Procedures

the same sounds produced in a spontaneous speech context, especially in clients who have had experience with testing or been enrolled in therapy, since these clients often have learned to produce certain sounds correctly in single-word responses to picture stimuli.

Jordan (1960) reported a relatively high correlation between the listener's perception of articulation adequacy in a spontaneous sample and the number of speech sound errors identified by a single-word articulation test. Although the Jordan study is frequently cited as justification for the use of a single-word test to predict performance in spontaneous speech, it should be remembered that these correlations (1) did not compare the number of errors in single-word productions with the number in spontaneous speech, and (2) were based on group trends, which may not reflect the performance of a given individual.

A second issue concerning the use of single-word test stimuli arises from the fact, discussed in Chapter 1, that speech does not occur in single words but in syllable strings. Using single words to make inferences about performance during connected speech may be questionable since the speaking tasks are different. Faircloth and Faircloth (1970) and Dubois and Bernthal (1978) reported differences with respect to speech sound errors identified with single-word tests and those identified with conversational speech samples. In a study of natural processes, Shriberg and Kwiatkowski (1980) reported a nonsignificant correlation between responses obtained through single-word and connected speech samples.

Single-word testing does not provide the tester an opportunity to evaluate the effect of context on speech sound productions (coarticulation). As discussed in Chapter 1, coarticulatory effects transcend phonetic, syllabic, and lexical (word) boundaries. Gallagher and Shriner (1975) reported that children's /s/ productions were affected by position in CCV consonant clusters. Curtis and Hardy (1959) reported that /r/ was more likely to be produced correctly in consonant clusters than in single phoneme productions. Hoffman, Schuckers, and Ratusnik (1977) reported that /r/ was influenced by factors such as lexical constraints (within vs. across word boundaries) and phonetic contexts. For example, when /r/ was embedded in nonlexically constrained contexts (e.g., "the sick rat died"), production was facilitated in the environment of /s/ as compared to /n/, /p/, and /t/. Variations in consonant production when sounds are elicited in consonant plus vowel contexts rather than in consonant clusters are widely recognized.

Despite reservations concerning some of the inferences that can be made about conversational speech on the basis of single word samples, most clinicians value and include single-word productions in the assessment battery. Single-word tests can provide the clinician with information concerning phonetic skills, can be constructed to include all phonemes in a language, and can provide phonological data in a relatively short time. In addition, for unintelligible clients, the tester has the advantage of knowing the productions the client has attempted to say.

Elicitation Procedures. The customary way to elicit single-word productions is through the administration of a single-word articulation test (sometimes called a speech sound inventory), where a client names single words in response to picture stimuli. Single words may also be obtained by having a child name toys or objects. For young children the clinician may simply wish to transcribe single-word productions the child produces spontaneously. Since picture-naming tests are the typical method for sampling single words, the following discussion will focus on this type of sampling procedure.

Single-Word Articulation Tests. A commonly used speech sound test is based on single-word productions, and sometimes referred to as a phonetic or speech sound inventory. Such instruments typically sample consonants, consonant clusters, and occasionally vowels and diphthongs. Consonants are usually assessed in the initial, medial, and final positions of words, for example, /s/ in *saw*, pen*c*il, hou*s*e; /ʃ/ in *sh*oe, sta*t*ion, fi*sh* (see Figure 6-1). Some instruments elicit sounds only in the initial and final positions. The specific sounds included vary from test to test but almost always include those sounds that have a high frequency of error in children's speech. Winitz (1969) combined data on frequently defective sounds from Roe and Milisen (1942), with findings of Templin (1957) regarding later developing sounds and indicated there is agreement between the two regarding the following sounds: /s, z, θ, ð, ʃ, ʒ, tʃ, dʒ, v, r, hw/. With the exception of /hw/ (a phoneme that is occurring less frequently in our language), these sounds are among those items usually included in single-word tests.

Speech sound tests have enjoyed widespread popularity because they constitute an efficient way to sample sound productions. By focusing on particular word productions, the examiner knows what the child is attempting to say and that the client will produce (or attempt to produce) a particular set of sound productions. In contrast, with spontaneous speech samples, the examiner may not obtain a representative sample of sounds the child may be able to produce, and if intelligibility is a problem, will not know what the client has attempted to say.

A number of tests are commercially available. Despite the similarities between such tests, certain stimulus and response features differentiate one test from another. For example, one test may present items in a developmental sequence, another may organize the analysis according to place and manner of articulation. Still a third test may emphasize colored line drawings that are especially attractive to young children or include actual photographs.

It is sometimes recommended that clinicians construct their own articulation tests. Certainly for the student, the process of selecting and trying out test items provides important insights about phonological sampling. Emerick and Hatten (1974) pointed out that so-called "homemade" tests often have an intangible appeal not found in other instruments. Perhaps a more important reason for developing one's own test is that the data obtained will more readily lend itself to the kind of analysis one wishes to make. An example of this is the 306 Item Analysis Probe developed at Indiana University (Gierut, Elbert, and Dinnsen, 1987). Commercially available tests, however, can allow an examiner certain advantages: (1) They reduce the need to spend time selecting items, developing test stimuli, and preparing recording forms; (2) they lend themselves more readily to comparisons of data collected; (3) they may allow comparison of scores with normative data, which is frequently necessary to qualify children for services; and (4) they contain features that are difficult to replicate in self-constructed tests, such as pictures coordinated in style, size, and color.

Although phonological tests usually use pictures to elicit spontaneous responses, in some instances, imitation tasks are used. Studies comparing responses elicited via imitation with those elicited through spontaneous picture-naming have

Phonological Assessment Procedures

PAT RECORDING SHEET *

		Year	Month	Day
Name_____	Date	____	____	____
School_____	Birth	____	____	____
Grade_____	Age	____	____	____

Key: Omission (−); substitution (write phonetic symbol of sound substituted); severity of distortion (D1), (D2), (D3); ability to imitate (circle symbol or error).

Sound	Photograph	1	2	3	Vowels, Diph.		Comments
	I				**III**		
s	saw, pencil, house				aʊ	house	
s bl	spoon, skates, stars						
z	zipper, scissors, keys						
ʃ	shoe, station, fish				u	shoe	
tʃ	chair, matches, sandwich						
dʒ	jars, angels, orange						
t	table, potatoes, hat				æ	hat	
d	dog, ladder, bed				ɔ	dog	
n	nails, bananas, can				ə	bananas	
l	lamp, balloons, bell				ɛ	bell	
l bl	blocks, clock, flag				ɑ	blocks	
θ	thumb, toothbrush, teeth				i	teeth	
r	radio, carrots, car						
r bl	brush, crayons, train				e	train	
k	cat, crackers, cake				ɚ-ə	crackers	
g	gun, wagon, egg				ʌ	gun	
	II						
f	fork, elephant, knife						
v	vacuum, TV, stove				ju	vacuum	
p	pipe, apples, cup				aɪ	pipe	
b	book, baby, bathtub				ʊ	book	
m	monkey, hammer, comb				o	comb	
w-hw	witch, flowers, whistle				ɪ	witch	
	I						
ð	this, that, feathers, bathe						
h-ŋ	hanger, hanger, swing						
j	yes, thank you						
ʒ	measure, beige				ɔɪ	boy	
	(story)				ɝ-ɝ	bird	

SCORE

Sounds

I Tongue_____

II Lip _____

III Vowels_____

Total _____

FIGURE 6–1. **Three-position Speech Sound Test.**

produced inconsistent results. Investigators studying children between the ages of 5 and 8 years have reported that responses elicited via imitation tasks yield a greater number of correct responses than those elicited via spontaneous picture-naming (Siegel, Winitz, and Conkey, 1963; Smith and Ainsworth, 1967; Carter and Buck, 1958; Snow and Milisen, 1954). Other investigators who studied children ranging in age from 2 to 6 years reported no significant differences in results from elicitation via picture-naming and imitation (Templin, 1947; Paynter and Bumpas, 1977).

Harrington, Lux, and Higgins (1984) studied responses to different types of picture-naming tasks and reported that children produced fewer errors when items were elicited via photographs as compared to line drawings. These data again suggest that different response elicitation procedures frequently produce different findings.

In spite of their widespread use, single-word tests have a number of limitations. Some experimenters have questioned the use of such tests because such measures do not allow children to use their "own" words but rather a set of predetermined and sometimes complex syllable and word shapes. Speech sound tests typically include both monosyllabic and multisyllabic words. The use of multisyllabic words may make more demands on a child's productions and elicit more errors than would monosyllabic words or the words used in a child's own spontaneous speech. Ingram (1976) compared young children's productions of initial fricatives and affricates in word-pairs in which the two words differed in syllable structure and/or stress. He reported that when stimulus pairs were similar in stress pattern and syllable structure, phone productions tended to be similar, but when syllable structure and/or stress of the pairs differed, monosyllabic words were more likely to be produced correctly than were multisyllabic words. Clinicians should recognize that syllable shape and stress patterns of stimulus words may affect speech sound productions.

Another difficulty with tests which elicit a sample via picture-naming is that they typically elicit only a single production in each of the three word-positions. During phonological development, inconsistency in production is common, even in the same stimulus word. Since the production of a sound may fluctuate widely, the client's customary articulatory patterns should not be based on the production of a single stimulus item. The clinician can increase the number of sound samples obtained through a single-word picture-naming test by transcribing all the sounds in each stimulus (lexical) item, instead of focusing only on a single sound in each stimulus item.

Summary. Single-word samples, including speech sound tests, provide an efficient and relatively easy method for obtaining a sample of speech sound productions. Although they frequently are a valuable part of the phonological assessment battery, they should not constitute the only sampling procedure. Among their limitations are the small number of phonetic contexts sampled, the failure to fully reflect the effects of coarticulation, the questionable representatives of single-word naming responses, and the lack of consistency in factors such as syllable shape, prosody, word familiarity, and parts of speech (nouns, verbs, and so on). To increase the number of phonetic contexts sampled through such tests, the clinician is encouraged to transcribe entire stimulus words.

A third sample of speech sound productions frequently included in a test battery is obtained through stimulability testing; that is, sampling the client's ability to repeat the correct form (adult standard) of error sounds when provided with "stimulation." In essence, this testing examines how well an individual imitates correct models of speech sounds that he or she produced incorrectly in single-word productions or in a connected speech sample. Although definitions of what constitutes stimulability testing have varied in the literature, a commonly used procedure has the examiner asking the respondent to imitate an auditory and/or visual model of a sound, syllable, or word containing the adult form of the segment. The examiner may tell the client to "watch and listen to what I am going to say, and then you say it." It should be recognized, however, that there are no standardized procedures for conducting this type of testing. Some investigators have focused on a single type of response form (e.g., nonsense syllables), but in practice, examiners typically seek to stimulate production at three levels: sound in isolation, sound embedded in syllables, and sound embedded in words. The number of models provided by the examiner has typically varied from one examiner to another. Most simply provide one or two models in order to elicit a response, but recommendations in the literature vary from one to five models (Diedrich, 1983).

Stimulability testing has been used to predict (1) whether or not a sound is likely to be acquired without intervention, and (2) the level of phonetic production at which instruction might begin (e.g., isolation, syllables, or words). In other words, these data are often used when making decisions regarding case selection and speech sounds targeted for treatment.

Several investigators have reported that the ability of a child (ages 5 through 7 years) to imitate syllables or words containing a specific sound is related to the probability of that child spontaneously correcting his or her misarticulation of that sound (Carter and Buck, 1958; Farquhar, 1961; Sommers, Leiss, Delp, Gerber, Fundrella, Smith, Revucky, Ellis, and Haley, 1967). Carter and Buck (1958) reported, in a study of first-grade children, that stimulability testing can be used for such prognostic purposes. They inferred that first-grade children who correctly imitated error sounds in nonsense syllables 75 percent of the time were likely to correct those sounds without instruction. An example of the nonsense syllables used by Carter and Buck for the /f/ are the following: /fi/, /fae/, /fa/, /ifi/, /aefae/, /afa/, /if/, /aef/, /af/. Kisatsky (1967) compared the pre- to post-test gains in articulation accuracy over a six-month period of two groups of kindergarten children, one identified as a high stimulability group and the other as a low stimulability group. Although neither group received articulation instruction, results indicated that significantly higher correct scores were obtained by the high stimulability group in the six-month post-test.

Sommers et al. (1967) reported that children who had the poorest scores on stimulability or imitation measures were most likely to benefit from intervention. Using control and experimental groups, these investigators compared the results of articulation remediation for groups of children differentiated on the basis of grade (kindergarten, first, second), articulatory defectiveness (mild, moderate, severe), and stimulability scores. When untreated groups were compared, the greatest gains in articulation accuracy were made by first and second graders who had the highest stimulability scores; no differences in articulation gains were seen between untreated kindergartners with good and poor stimulability scores.

In a comprehensive review of literature concerning stimulability, Diedrich (1983) drew the following conclusions regarding stimulability testing as a prognostic measure:

1. For kindergarten, first-, and second-graders who received therapy, children with low stimulability scores (less than 25 percent correction) made significantly more improvement than those with high stimulability scores (greater than 60 percent correction) (Carter and Buck, 1958; Sommers et al., 1967).
2. For first- and second-graders who did not receive therapy, children with high stimulability scores (60 percent correction) demonstrated significant improvement in articulation (Snow and Milisen, 1954; Carter and Buck, 1958; Irwin, West and Trombetta, 1966; Sommers et al., 1967).
3. For kindergartners not in therapy, children with high stimulability obtained significant improvement in two studies (Farquhar, 1961; Kisatsky, 1967), but improvement was not significant in a third study (Sommers et al., 1967).

The use of stimulability for predicting spontaneous improvement or the rate of improvement in remediation has not been documented to the extent that definitive prognostic statements can be made, particularly with reference to an individual client. Diedrich (1983) suggested that a trial period of "diagnostic therapy" provides a stronger basis than do results of stimulability testing for predicting instructional needs.

Stimulability testing is, at best, only a general guide for the identification of clients who may correct their phonological errors without intervention. False positives (i.e., clients identified as needing instruction but who ultimately will outgrow their problems) and false negatives (i.e., clients identified as not needing instruction but who ultimately will require intervention) have been identified in all investigations focusing on stimulability as a prognostic indicator. These findings must be considered when results from stimulability testing are used to make predictive statements in clinical practice. Investigations of imitation as a prognostic indicator have looked at imitation in isolated sounds, syllables, and word productions as predictors of improvement on single-word tests.

Clinicians have also postulated that error sounds that can be produced through imitation are more rapidly corrected through intervention than sounds that cannot be imitated (Winitz, 1975). Diedrich (1983) indicated that even "if it failed to tell us whether the error would correct, the 'stimulation test' at least served to suggest a hierarchy of error sounds selected for treatment and/or to indicate whether the clinician should begin at the isolation, syllable, word, or phrase level of therapy" (297). Irwin, West, and Trombetta (1966) reported that stimulability, in addition to mental age and initial speech sound articulation scores, was predictive of successful remediation.

McReynolds and Elbert (1978) reported that once a child could imitate a sound, generalization occurred to other contexts. Thus, imitation served as a predictor of generalization. When a client is stimulable, the clinician does not have to teach the production of a sound, since the client can already produce the target sound. These two factors probably account in part for the finding that stimulability scores were predictive of successful treatment.

Pollack and Rees (1972) and Turton (1973) have suggested that since stim-

Phonological Assessment Procedures

ulability testing reflects the child's ability to produce speech sounds at an imitative level, such testing only reflects the child's phonetic skills. In other words, correct production of speech sounds on a stimulability task assesses only phonetic ability; it provides no information concerning appropriate linguistic usage. Pollack and Rees (1972) speculated that while poor stimulability may suggest a poor short-term prognosis, good stimulability does not necessarily suggest a good short-term prognosis since stimulability measurements do not reflect the child's appropriate phonological usage.

It has been postulated (Dinnsen and Elbert, 1984) that imitation of words by the child may also reflect correct underlying representations (storage of the adult form). One might speculate then, that if a child is able to imitate a word, this performance may indicate that the child has acquired at a cognitive level the linguistic contrasts of the language necessary to produce a sound in at least some appropriate contrastive contexts. From this perspective, correct imitation is a reflection not only of phonetic or motor skill but also of the child's possession of the adult's (correct) underlying form of the error word. Further investigation is necessary, however, before a more definitive statement can be made as to whether or not imitative utterances are reflective of underlying phonological representations, including knowledge of phonological contrasts.

Madison (1979), after a review of the literature concerning stimulability, made the following recommendations concerning the clinical applicability of stimulability testing: (1) sounds on which the client is stimulable in isolated productions (CV syllables in the case of stops and certain other sounds) should be given priority for instruction; (2) children who are stimulable on syllables (regardless of stimulability status in isolation or words) may self-correct without intervention and are likely to do well in instruction; and (3) children stimulable at the word level may self-correct although data are equivocal. In his summary of stimulability, Diedrich (1983) concluded that on the basis of the research reported, there appears to be no advantage of imitated nonsense syllables over imitated words in predicting future articulatory performance.

Elicitation Procedures. Stimulability assessment is perhaps the least structured assessment included in phonological evaluation. As stated in the paragraphs above, the examiner typically asks the client to look at the examiner's mouth or watch it in a mirror, listen to what is said, and then imitate the production. The examiner does not point out where teeth, tongue, or lips may be during production; the examinee is simply encouraged to listen and observe a production.

Stimulability testing usually includes imitative testing of those sounds produced in error in word and/or conversational samples. Such sounds are assessed in isolation, nonsense syllables (usually initial, medial, and final positions), and in monosyllabic words (again in the three word-positions). The number of productions at each level vary from one examiner to the next. Cooperation of the child, number of sounds produced in error, and success with the imitative task are factors the clinician should consider when deciding how extensive the stimulability assessment will be.

It is not uncommon for speech sound tests to include a place on the scoring form to record stimulability results, particularly for sounds in isolation. As suggested above, the clinician will usually want to probe imitative skills in syllables and words. The Carter-Buck (1958) procedure discussed earlier included the following format for testing sounds in nonsense syllables:

__i	i__i	i__
__ae	ae__ae	ae__
__a	a__a	a__

For each of the blanks, a consonant produced in error is inserted. For example, if a client misarticulated /k/, stimuli for the Carter-Buck protocol would be as follows:

*k*i	i*k*i	i*k*
*k*æ	æ*k*æ	æ*k*
*k*a	a*k*a	a*k*

Summary. Stimulability testing is useful in identifying those individuals most likely to need phonological intervention (those with poor stimulability scores), and for determining the level of linguistic production for initiation of instruction. Although stimulability scores have been found to have some prognostic value for identifying those children who will self-correct errors, research data do not indicate that such testing can be relied upon to identify clients that will self-correct their errors.

CONTEXTUAL ASSESSMENT

As indicated earlier, speech sound errors, especially in children, are often variable and inconsistent. It has been suggested that sounds are often easier to produce in some contexts as opposed to others, thus resulting in inconsistency in production during the phonological acquisition period. Knowledge of the consistency of phonological errors is a factor taken into consideration when deciding on the need for therapy and for making treatment decisions such as choosing a sound to work on in therapy or deciding on a particular phonetic context which may facilitate accurate sound production.

Assessing contextual influences is based on the concept that sound productions influence each other in the ongoing stream of speech. McDonald (1964a) suggested that valuable clinical information could be gained by systematically reviewing a sound as it is produced in varying contexts, and coined the term *deep test* to refer to the practice of testing a sound in a variety of phonetic contexts. McDonald was interested in the influence that adjacent sounds have on each other during speech production. For example, /s/ may be produced differently when preceded by /p/ in "capsun" than when it is preceded by /t/ as in "hatsun." Coarticulatory effects consist of mechanical constraints associated with adjacent sounds and simultaneous preprogramming adjustments for segments later in the speech stream. This overlapping of movements (preprogramming) may extend as far as six phonetic segments away from a given sound (Kent and Minifie, 1977). The result is that segments may be perceived by a listener as being produced correctly in one context but not in another. Such information is of value to the clinician who seeks to establish a particular segment in a client's repertoire.

McDonald (1964b) criticized assessment procedures where sounds are analyzed in three word-positions (initial, medial, final), and indicated that such word-positions are representative of sounds in written words rather than connected speech. He pointed out that individual phones are a series of overlapping syllable strings rather than individual sound productions. He further stated that consonants should be viewed as functioning as releasors (e.g., cup-*s*un) or arrestors (e.g., hou*s*e-pipe) of syllables, not as occurring in the initial, medial, or final position of words.

A second criticism McDonald makes with regard to traditional single-word articulation tests is that sounds are usually observed only in three phonetic contexts. He argued that in-depth contextual testing of a speech sound allows the examiner to obtain a sampling of sounds in a variety of phonetic contexts.

Elicitation Procedures. A procedure that has often been used to sample contextual influences is the *Deep Test of Articulation* (McDonald, 1964a). The Deep Test of Articulation is a series of phoneme-specific tasks designed to assess individual speech sounds in approximately 50 phonetic contexts. Deep testing is predicated on the hypothesis that when the consonants preceding or following the sound of interest are systematically altered, the client will usually produce the target sound correctly in at least one phonetic context. In the Deep Test of Articulation, each of the stimulus items contains two words, one of which has the target sound in either the arresting or releasing position. The two words are said together as a single bisyllable unit in order to assess the contextual influence. Phonetic context is varied by systematically changing the segment that immediately precedes or follows the target sound.

A second set of tools sometimes used for consistency–contextual testing are the *Sound Production Tasks* (SPT) developed by Elbert, Shelton, and Arndt (1967). Each imitative task assesses individual consonants in 30 contexts including a sound in isolation, syllables, words, and phrases. For example, items related to the /s/ include the following: /s/, /us/, hou*s*ehold, I like *s*oup.

Probably the most comprehensive set of materials that has been developed to assess consistency–contextual influences is the *Clinical Probes of Articulation Consistency* (C-PAC) by Secord (1981). Individual probes elicit responses containing a particular sound in the prevocalic and postvocalic positions, plus clusters, sentences, and storytelling contexts. Probes are developed for all consonant sounds and vocalic /ɝ/. Approximately 100 responses are elicited for each sound.

A fourth way of doing a contextual analysis is by reviewing a connected speech sample for contexts in which a target sound is produced correctly. Occasionally facilitating contexts can be found in conversation that are not observed in single words or word-pairs.

A type of contextual assessment that clinicians have borrowed from the field of linguistics is the examination of a phoneme in various morphophonemic alterations (the effect of morpheme structure on phonological production). Such alterations may be examined by having the client produce a sound in differing morphophonemic structures. For example, if word-final obstruent /g/ has been deleted in /dɔg/ (i.e., [dɔ]), the examiner might assess whether or not /g/ is produced in the diminutive /dɔgi/. Likewise, if the child misarticulates /z/ in the word /roz/, the examiner might observe /z/ production in the morphophonemic context of /rozəz/.

Summary. Contextual testing is done primarily to determine phonetic contexts in which a speech sound error may be produced correctly. These contexts may then be used as a starting point for remediation. Contextual testing is also used as a measure of consistency of misarticulation.

ASSESSMENT OF VOWELS

An area of phonological assessment that has received little attention in the literature is that of the assessment of vowels. Undoubtedly this is a reflection of the fact that most children with phonological disorders have problems primarily with consonants. In addition, vowels are typically mastered at a relatively early age and are seldom misarticulated by children.

Phonological assessment instruments have placed little emphasis on vowel assessment, although some speech sound tests do sample vowels (e.g., *Fisher-Logemann Test of Articulation Competence,* Fisher and Logemann, 1971; *Templin-Darley Tests of Articulation,* Templin and Darley, 1969). The Fisher-Logemann Test of Articulation Competence is one of the few measures that includes the assessment of commonalities among vowel errors (i.e., vowel height, place of articulation, degree of tension, lip rounding).

Pollock (1991) delineated the following suggestions regarding vowel sampling:

1. Clients should be provided with multiple opportunities to produce each vowel.
2. Vowels should be assessed in a variety of different contexts, including (a) monosyllabic and multisyllabic words, (b) stressed and unstressed syllables, and (c) a variety of adjacent preceding and especially following consonants.
3. Limits for the range of responses considered correct or acceptable should be established since cultural influences may affect what is considered "correct."
4. Recommended vowels and diphthongs to be assessed include the following:

Non-rhotic

/i/	/ou/
/ɪ/	/ɔ/
/ei/	/ɑ/
/ɛ/	/ʌ/ə/
/ae/	/aɪ/
/u/	/aʊ/
/ʊ/	/ɔi/

Rhotic

/ɝ,ɚ/	/ɔɚ/
/ɪɚ/	/ɑɚ/
/ɛɚ/	

To compensate for the lack of formal vowel assessment procedures, Pollock (1991) suggested that clinicians transcribe whole-word responses to the stimuli from commonly used articulation or phonological process tests. In order to get a comprehensive review of vowels and diphthongs, it may be necessary, however, to supplement existing stimuli with additional vowels–diphthongs and contexts not included in standard tests.

Several investigators have used acoustic analysis of phonologically disordered children's speech to supplement descriptive phonological analysis (Smit

Phonological Assessment Procedures

and Bernthal, 1983; Tyler, Edwards, and Saxman, 1990; Weismer, Dinnsen, and Elbert 1981). In several of these reports, children were found to show an acoustically measurable but auditorially imperceptible marking of certain sound productions. Phonetic distinctions identified by acoustic analysis provide data that are not available from phonetic transcription. While acoustical analysis is primarily a research tool to supplement perceptual analysis, the time is fast approaching when clinicians will have inexpensive technology available for doing selected acoustic measurements. Such information will hopefully lead to a better understanding of a child's speech sound system and more efficacious clinical decisions.

PHONOLOGICAL ASSESSMENT BATTERY

The four types of assessment instruments and procedures identified so far in this chapter—connected speech, single words, stimulability, and contextual—are all part of a phonological assessment battery. As stated in the introduction to the chapter, no one measure is likely to provide all the information needed by the clinician, and thus a battery of tools must be used. It is suggested that samples of each type be included in a comprehensive phonological assessment. Acoustic analysis, which is a tool that can enhance clinical judgments, is primarily used as a research tool at this time. It may eventually become a critical part of a phonological assessment battery.

TRANSCRIPTION AND SCORING PROCEDURES

TRADITIONAL METHODS FOR RECORDING RESPONSES

The recording systems used by clinicians vary according to the purposes of testing, the transcription skills of the examiner, and personal preferences. The type of response-recording employed by the examiner will, however, determine the type of analysis the clinician is able to do with the sample obtained. In turn, the treatment approach may be significantly influenced by the type of analysis conducted.

In the least sophisticated scoring level, phonological productions are simply scored as correct or incorrect, based on the examiner's perception of whether the sound produced is within the acceptable adult phoneme boundary for the sound. This type of judgment is often the first assessment skill that clinicians learn and may be adequate for screening purposes. This type of scoring, however, is not recommended for the clinician doing a phonological assessment to determine the direction of treatment where more detail is necessary.

A second scoring level is to identify error productions as **substitutions, distortions,** or **omissions** (deletions). Sound substitutions are the replacement (substitution) of incorrect sounds for target segments (correct sounds), as when a child substitutes *w*abbit for *r*abbit. Sound distortions are similar to substitutions, but the replacement phone is an unacceptable allophonic variation within the perceptual boundary of a target phoneme, and the transcriber does not have a symbol that adequately reflects the "distorted" production.

The most common and useful transcription system is the *International Phonetic Alphabet* (IPA), which includes a different symbol for each phoneme. As indicated in Chapter 1, for English, over 40 such symbols are utilized to identify the phonemes of the language. This broad transcription system supplemented with a set of **diacritics** (narrow markers) usually provides sufficient detail for speech-language clinicians to adequately describe speech sound productions. For example, in a broad transcription of the word *key*, one would transcribe the initial segment with the symbol /k/. A more precise transcription of the initial /k/ would include the diacritic for aspiration [ʰ] following word-initial [kʰ] since aspiration occurs in production of /k/ in word-initial contexts. The aspiration modifier [ʰ] in this transcription represents one example of a diacritic. Use of diacritics, sometimes called a **close transcription system,** allows for recording specific topographical dimensions of individual segments. We strongly recommend the use of such a transcription system during most assessment procedures. An example of diacritics that reflects an error seen in disordered phonology is the following: If /t/ in the word /tɪp/ is dentalized, the diacritic for dentalization [ɳ] is placed under the /t/, thus [t̪ɪp]. Edwards (1986) recommended the symbols and diacritics presented in Table 6–1 for clinical use. Shriberg, Kwiatkowski, and Hoffman (1984) categorized some diacritic symbols as typically either "non-error" symbols or "error" symbols. In other words, as reflected in the examples above, some diacritics are most commonly used to transcribe variations in correct or standard productions, while others are more frequently used when transcribing speech sound errors. Some clinicians prefer to utilize their own set of diacritics instead of published diacritics such as those presented in Table 6–1.

As stated above, close transcription is particularly useful for describing the speech of individuals whose speech sound productions cannot be adequately described by broad phonetic symbols. For example, when assessing the phonological status of an individual with a cleft condition who is unable to achieve velopharyngeal closure for certain speech sounds, diacritics indicating nasal emission (šnail), or nasalization (bãet), may be useful in the description of the client's production of certain segments. Similarly, when assessing the articulation of an individual with impaired hearing, symbols to indicate excessive breathiness on vowels (e.g., [ɪ̤]), inappropriate vowel duration (e.g., [si:] for lengthened, [we'] for shortened), devoicing (e.g., [b̥]), and denasalization (e.g., ræt) are recommended if these characteristics are present in productions. Likewise, with developmental articulation errors characterized by laterization (e.g., [s̺]), dentalization (e.g., [s̪]), and devoicing (e.g., [n̥]), diacritics should be utilized.

Accuracy of Transcriptions

One of the major concerns regarding transcription of responses relates to the accuracy of transcriptions. As clinicians, we must be concerned with whether or not our transcriptions are a valid representation of a client's productions. When making transcriptions, clinicians rely primarily upon auditory perceptual judgments. These judgments are sometimes supplemented with physiological measures (such as air pressure and flow information) and acoustical measures (such as that obtained from spectrographic analysis). These three types of data may not always be consistent with each other. For example, a glottal substitution for a stop in word-final position may be identified via a spectrographic analysis; and yet, the glottal production may not be heard by a listener and, thus, will be transcribed as a deletion (omission). It must be recognized, however, that even the

TABLE 6–1. **Symbols and Diacritics.**

[x]	voiceless velar fricative, as in *Bach*
[Φ]	voiceless bilabial fricative
[ß]	voiced bilabial fricative
[ɬ]	voiceless lateral fricative
[pf]	voiceless labial affricate
[ts]	voiceless alveolar affricate
[dz]	voiced alveolar affricate
[ʔ]	glottal stop, as in [mʌʔi]

Stop Release Diacritics

[ʰ]	aspirated, as in [tʰap]
[⁼]	unaspirated, as in [p⁼un]
[¬]	unreleased, as in [kʰæt¬]
[ʻ]	slightly aspirated

Diacritics for Lip Shape

[w]	labialized, as in [swit]
[ʮ]	protruded labialized
[ɯ] or [₀]	unrounded
[×]	produced with lip inversion
[ɔ]	a vowel produced with lip rounding
[c]	a vowel produced with less lip rounding than usual

Diacritics for Nasality

[~]	nasalized, as in [fæ̃n]
[⁓]	denasalized
[͌]	produced with nasal emission

Diacritics for Length

[:]	lengthened
[ʼ] or [˘]	shortened
[⌃] or [˯]	synchronous

Diacritics for Voicing

[ᵥ]	partially voiced, as in [k̬æt]
[̥]	partially devoiced, as in [spu̥ŋ]
[..]	produced with breathy voice (murmured)

Diacritics for Syllabicity

[ˌ]	a syllabic consonant, as in [bʌtŋ̩]
[˯]	a nonsyllabic vowel, as in [ðeə̯]

Diacritics for Stress

[ʹ], [ˈ], or [¹]	primary stress
[ˋ], [ˌ], or [²]	secondary stress
[.] or [³]	tertiary (weak) stress

Diacritics for Tongue Position or Shape

[ᴣ] or [ʲ]	palatalized, as in [sʲu]
[ ]	dentalized, as in [teŋ̪ə]
[-]	velarized, as in [tʰebɫ] (or pharyngealized)
[ₒ] or [ʳ]	/r/-colored, rhotacized, or retroflexed, as in [kʰa̠]
[c] or [ˌ]	lateralized, as in [sop]
[ʊ]	markedly grooved
[⊢⊣]	produced with a flattened tongue
[˟] or [¨]	centralized
[⊢] or [→]	retracted tongue, as in [s→op] or [sop]
[⊣] or [←]	advanced tongue, as in [ʃ←u] or [ʃu̯]
[⊥] or [ˆ]	raised tongue
[⊤] or [ˇ]	lowered tongue
[‹]	a fronted sound
[›]	a backed sound
[˳]	derhotacized or deretroflexed

TABLE 6-1. Continued

Other Diacritics

['], [?], or [.]	glottalized
[ₓ]	produced with frication
[„]	whistled
[√]	trilled

Juncture Markers

+	open juncture
|	internal open juncture
↓	falling terminal juncture
↑	rising terminal juncture
→	checked or held juncture

The additional symbols listed here are part of the International Phonetic Alphabet (1978). Some diacritics are also from the IPA. Others are adapted from Bush and colleagues (1973) and Shriberg and Kent (1982). This is not an exhaustive list of additional symbols and diacritics.
Source: From M. L. Edwards. *Introduction to Applied Phonetics: Laboratory Workbook*. San Diego, Calif.: College-Hill Press, 1986, 185–187 © 1986. Used with permission.

more objective measures of speech segments (i.e., acoustical and physiological recordings) are not devoid of human interpretation since no one-to-one correspondence exists between a phoneme production, perception, and/or acoustical and physiological measurements. For most aspects of clinical phonology, auditory perceptual judgments by the examiner form the basis for intervention decisions. Because of this, it is important for clinicians to establish the reliability of their perceptual judgments.

Interjudge Reliability. Traditionally, clinicians have used agreement between two independent transcribers as a means of establishing reliability of judgments. Interjudge agreement or reliability is determined by the comparison of one examiner's transcriptions with those of another, and is essential for reporting the results of phonological research. In addition, for students beginning to make judgments about accuracy of phonological productions, establishing interjudge reliability with a more experienced person establishes the accuracy of judgments. A commonly used method to determine interjudge reliability, called point-to-point agreement, compares the clinicians' judgments on each test item. The number of items judged the same is divided by the total number of items to determine a percentage of agreement between judges. As an example, consider the data contained in Table 6–2, which reflects independent judgments of articulatory productions made by two clinicians.

The two judges agreed on 17 of the 20 items and disagreed on 3. Hence, 17 divided by 20 is 0.85, which is then multiplied by 100 to obtain an interjudge reliability index of 85 percent. Such point-to-point, or item-by-item, reliability is a stringent method for establishing agreement between judges.

A second, less stringent method for determining interjudge reliability makes an overall comparison between examiners' judgments. Instead of comparing judgments on an item-by-item basis, the total number of items scored as correct or incorrect by each judge is compared. For example, in Table 6–2 Judge A scored 14 items correct and 6 items incorrect, and Judge B scored 13 items correct and 7 items incorrect. Thus, of the 20 items, both judges agreed that 13 items were correct and 6 items were incorrect, agreeing 19 times. Following the method described above, 20 is divided into 19, and then multiplied by 100, resulting in a percentage of agreement of 95 percent. It can readily be seen that the latter method

TABLE 6–2. Independent Judgments by Judges
A and B.

ITEM	JUDGE A	JUDGE B
1	correct	correct
2	correct	correct
3	correct	incorrect
4	correct	incorrect
5	incorrect	incorrect
6	incorrect	incorrect
7	correct	correct
8	correct	correct
9	correct	correct
10	incorrect	correct
11	correct	correct
12	correct	correct
13	correct	correct
14	incorrect	incorrect
15	incorrect	incorrect
16	correct	correct
17	correct	correct
18	correct	correct
19	correct	correct
20	incorrect	incorrect

is less stringent than the point-to-point method since a direct comparison of judgments on each item is not made. However, agreement between judges regarding overall performance (as opposed to performance on a specific item) was high.

Sometimes transcriptions are made by two or more examiners independently but simultaneously, with the final transcript arrived at by consensus (Shriberg, Kwiatkowski, and Hoffman, 1984). Discussion between examiners regarding what is heard occurs prior to a "final" judgment. This procedure, which typically involves a panel of examiners listening to tape-recorded responses, is used in difficult to judge situations. Obviously, independence of judgments is lost in such a procedure.

In Table 6–2 the reliability index was based on correct–incorrect judgments of sound productions. It is easier to reach agreement on binary right–wrong judgments than on judgments recorded phonetically. It is even more difficult to obtain high reliability when sounds are transcribed with close phonetic transcription. An interjudge reliability figure of at least 90 percent or above on an item-by-item right–wrong comparison is usually considered sufficient to ensure that one person's judgments of articulatory productions are similar to another's. For more difficult transcription tasks, such as those where diacritics are used, interjudge agreement percentages will likely be considerably lower than this figure.

Since phonetic transcription has excellent clinical utility, difficulty in obtaining high reliability should not discourage its use. As inexpensive instrumentation is developed to assist clinicians in recording and analyzing productions, some of the perceptual problems currently faced in transcription may be reduced (e.g., judging voicing errors). Acoustic instrumentation allows one to support perceptual judgments with acoustic data.

Intrajudge Reliability. Along with knowing that his or her judgments are in agreement with those of another examiner, the clinician will also want to know that his or her standards for judgments are consistent over time. Comparison of judgments made when scoring the same data on two separate occasions is referred to as intrajudge reliability. High reliability on such a measure is an indication that the examiner is consistent in his or her judgments. In rating intrajudge reliability, it is recommended that a point-to-point reliability index of 90 percent or above be achieved on a correct–incorrect judgment basis. When determining this type of reliability, tape recordings of responses are used since judgments are made twice of the same responses.

ADDITIONAL ASSESSMENT PROCEDURES

The assessment of a child with a phonological problem includes testing procedures supplemental to those focusing directly on phonological behavior. Information gathered from this supplemental testing is intended to provide a more comprehensive picture of an individual client and thereby contribute to a better understanding of his or her problem. It may also influence management recommendations that are made regarding a given client.

These additional assessment procedures typically include a case history; an oral cavity examination; and hearing, language, fluency, and voice screenings. These procedures can aid the clinician in the identification of factors that may contribute to or be related to the delay or impairment of phonology. Data gathered from these additional measures may lead to referral to other specialists and/or influence remediation decisions. If, for example, a child has a problem with closure of the velopharyngeal port, referral to a cleft palate team may result in pharyngeal flap surgery prior to speech intervention. Problems in communication additional to phonology will impact any therapy decisions that ultimately are made. Although they are routinely screened in phonological evaluations, language, fluency, and voice screening will not be covered in this text.

Case History

In order to facilitate an efficient and effective assessment, a case history is obtained from the client or a parent. This will allow the clinician to identify (1) possible etiological factors; (2) the family's or client's perception of the problem; (3) the academic, work, home, and social environment of the client; and (4) medical, developmental, and social information about the client. Case history information is usually obtained through a written form completed by the client or parents. It may also be obtained, or at least supplemented, by an interview. Specific questions regarding the phonological status of a young child might include the following: (1) Did your child babble? Can you describe it? (2) When did your child say his or her first words? What were they? When did he or she start putting words together? (3) Describe your child's communication problem, and your concerns about it. (4) How easy is your child to understand? By the family? By strangers? (5) What sounds does your child say? (6) What do you think caused your child's speech difficulty? While case histories obtained from the client or the client's family are products of memory and perception, and thus may not reflect total accuracy, parents and clients, in general, are reliable informants. In spite of its shortcomings, the case history provides the clinician with important background information that frequently influences assessment decisions and subsequent management recommendations.

ORAL CAVITY EXAMINATION

Oral cavity (oral peripheral) examinations are administered to describe the structure and function of the oral mechanism for normal speech purposes. In particular, dentition is observed for bite and missing teeth; hard and soft palates are examined for clefts, submucous clefts, fistulas, and fissures. Size, symmetry, and movement of the lips; the tongue; and symmetry, movement, and functional length of the soft palate are examined.

To examine the intraoral structures, it is recommended that the client be seated immediately in front of the clinician with his or her head in a natural upright position and at a level that allows easy viewing. The examiner should wear surgical gloves. If the client is a child, the examiner may have the child sit on a table or the examiner can kneel on the floor. Although it might seem that the oral cavity would be viewed best when the client extends his or her head backward, such a position can distort normal relationships of the head and neck. The client's mouth usually should be at the examiner's eye level. A flashlight, or other light source, together with a tongue blade will aid in the examination. Observations should start at the front of the oral cavity and progress to the back. Since the oral cavity examination is important in identifying possible etiological factors, a description of how an examination is conducted is presented below.

Dentition. In order for the examiner to evaluate the occlusal relationship (i.e., alignment of upper and lower jaws), the client should have the first molars in contact with each other since the occlusal relationships of the upper and lower dental arch are made with reference to these molar contacts. The upper dental arch is normally longer and wider than the lower dental arch; therefore, the upper teeth normally extend horizontally around the lower dental arch; and the maxillary (upper) incisors protrude about one-quarter inch in front of the lower teeth and cover about one third of the crown of the mandibular incisors. Such dental overjet or overbite is the normal relationship of the dental arches in occlusion.

The teeth are said to be in open bite when the upper teeth do not cover part of the lower teeth at any given point along the dental arch. Mason and Wickwire (1978) recommended that, when evaluating occlusal relationships, the clinician should instruct the client to bite on the back teeth and to separate the lips. They further started that

> . . . while in occlusion, the client should be asked to produce several speech sounds in isolation, especially /s/, /z/, /f/, and /v/. Although these sounds may not normally be produced by the client with teeth in occlusion, the standardization of airspace dimensions and increases in pressure in the oral cavity can unmask a variety of functional relationships. For example, the child who usually exhibits an interdental lisp may be able to articulate /s/ surprisingly well with teeth together. This occluded position can also unmask and/or counteract habit patterns related to the protrusion of tongue and mandible on selected sounds. (15)

Mason and Wickwire also suggested that when an individual with excessive overjet has difficulty with /s/, he or she should be instructed to rotate the mandible forward as a means of adaption to the excessive overjet. As pointed out in Chapter

5, however, dental abnormality and speech problems are frequently unrelated, and thus cause-and-effect between occlusion deviation and articulation problems should not be assumed.

Hard Palate. The hard palate (i.e., the bony portion of the oral cavity roof) is best viewed when the client extends his or her head backward. Normal midline coloration is pink and white. When a blue tint on the midline is observed, further investigation of the integrity of the bony framework is called for. Such discoloration may be caused by a blood supply close to the surface of the palate and is sometimes associated with a submucous cleft (an opening in the bony palatal shelf). But when a blue tint is seen lateral to the midline of the hard palate, it usually suggests only an extra bony growth, which occurs in approximately 20 percent of the population.

Where a submucous cleft of the hard palate is suspected, palpation (rubbing) of the mucous membrane at the midline of the most posterior portion of the hard palate (nasal spine) is recommended. Although many speech-language pathologists note the height of the hard palatal vault, it probably has little relationship to articulation deviations. The contour or height of the palatal vault may influence certain articulatory contacts, but most individuals with high palatal vaults use compensatory movements that allow for adequate speech sound production.

Soft Palate or Velum. The soft palate should be evaluated with the head in a natural upright position. When the head is not in that position, changes in the structural relationships in the oral cavity area may prevent the viewing of velar function as it occurs during speech.

Mason and Wickwire cautioned that the assessment of velar function, especially velar elevation, should not be done with the tongue protruded or with the mandible positioned for maximum mouth opening. They recommended a mouth opening of about three quarters of the maximum opening since velar elevation may be less than maximum when the mouth is open maximally.

The coloration of the soft palate like that of the hard palate should be pink and white. A midline bluish tint should alert the clinician to the possibility of a submucous cleft of the velum, in which case the surface of the velum is covered with mucous membrane, but the underlining layer of periosteum is absent.

The critical factor in velar function is the effective or functional length of the velum and not the velar length per se. Effective velar length is the portion of tissue that fills the space between the posterior border of the hard palate and the pharyngeal walls; it is measured in a line with the vertical plane of the hard palate. Unfortunately, effective length cannot be determined by an intraoral inspection because the velar contact is above the plane of the hard palate during velopharyngeal closure. Effective velar length is only one factor in adequate velopharyngeal sphincter function and provides little or no information concerning the function of the sphincter's pharyngeal component, another critical factor for adequate velopharyngeal valving.

The final velar observation typically made is velar symmetry and elevation. The elevation and posterior movement of the velum is also partially obstructed from view in an intraoral exam. But when the velum does not elevate to the plane of the hard palate during sustained vowel phonation, an inadequately functioning velopharyngeal sphincter should be suspected. It should also be remembered that

Phonological Assessment Procedures

if the observation is made with the tongue protruded, velar elevation can be restricted.

The posterior-most appendage or extension of the velum is the uvula, which has little or no role in speech production. However, a **bifid** uvula should alert the clinician to possible anatomical deviations. A bifid uvula appears as two appendages rather than one and is occasionally seen in the presence of submucous clefts and other abnormal anatomical findings.

Fauces. The next area to observe in the oral cavity is the faucial pillars and the tonsillar masses. Only in rare instances are these structures a factor in speech production. The presence or absence of tonsillar masses is noted and, if present, their size and coloration are observed. Redness or inflammation may be evidence of tonsillitis, and large tonsillar masses may displace the faucial pillars and reduce the isthmus.

Pharynx. The oropharyngeal area is difficult to view in an intraoral examination. The pharyngeal contribution to velopharyngeal closure cannot be assessed through intraoral viewing because pharyngeal valving occurs at the level of the nasopharynx, a level superior to that which can be observed through the oral cavity. In some individuals, movement of tissue to form a prominence or ridge (Passavant's Pad) can be seen on the posterior wall of the pharynx; Passavant's Pad is not visible at rest but can usually be seen during sustained phonation. Passavant's Pad is present in approximately one third of the individuals with cleft palates but is otherwise rare. Since its presence reflects a compensatory mechanism, the examiner should be alert to possible velopharyngeal valving problems. The presence of Passavant's Pad may suggest that adenoidal tissue is needed for velopharyngeal closure, and this factor should be considered in surgical decisions regarding adenoidectomies.

The pharyngeal gag response has been identified as a useful procedure to obtain an idea of the functional potential of the velum. We recommend that the gag response be used only in very rare instances since many clients have a strong aversion to the procedure, and velar function during gagging generally has little relationship to velopharyngeal valving during speech. Elicitation of a gag may provide some useful information in cases where lack of innervation and a paresis of the pharyngeal or palatal function is suspected. Gagging can be induced by pressing firmly on the base of the tongue or by touching the velum with a tongue blade. Gagging usually results in maximum velar excursion and maximum movement of the pharyngeal walls.

Tongue. As pointed out in Chapter 5, the tongue is a primary articulator, and individuals are able to modify tongue movements to compensate for many structural variations in the oral cavity. In terms of tongue size, two problematic conditions occasionally are found. The first, termed *macroglossia,* is an abnormally large tongue. Although this characteristic occurs frequently in certain populations (for example, those with Down's syndrome), the overall incidence is relatively low and research data do not point to the tongue as the cause of speech problems in Down's children. The condition where the tongue is abnormally small in relation to the oral cavity is termed *microglossia,* but this condition rarely, if ever, causes a speech problem.

It has been pointed out that tongue movements for speech activities show little relationship to tongue movements for non-speech activities. Unless motor problems are suspected, little is gained by having the client perform a series of tongue movements used for non-speech activities. But protrusion of the tongue or moving the tongue laterally from one corner of the mouth to the other may provide information about possible motor limitations or problems in control of the tongue.

The rapid speech movements observed in diadochokinetic tasks provide limited information with respect to speech function. Winitz (1969) pointed out that the child with a speech problem is at a distinct disadvantage on such tasks because he or she has had less experience producing phonemes correctly than normal developing children. The absolute number of syllables, such as /ta/ or /ka/, that an individual can produce in a given unit of time usually bears little relationship to articulatory proficiency except when gross motor problems are present. For a discussion of the relationship between diadochokinetic testing and articulation, see Chapter 5. Mason and Wickwire (1978) suggested that the clinician focus on the pattern of tongue movement and the consistency of contacts during diadochokinetic tasks.

A short lingual frenum can restrict movement of the tongue tip. Most individuals, however, acquire normal speech in spite of a short lingual frenum. If the client can touch the alveolar ridge with the tongue tip, the length of the frenum is probably adequate for speech purposes. In the rare instance where this is not possible, surgical intervention may be necessary.

Making Use of the Findings. In an oral cavity examination, in which the clinician notes an inadequacy of structure or function which might contribute to the articulation disorders, he or she has several options: (1) refer the client to other professionals (e.g., ENT physician, orthodontist) for assessment and possible intervention, (2) engage in further observation and testing to verify the earlier observation and note its impact upon speaking skills, and (3) provide instruction related to compensatory or remedial behaviors.

AUDIOLOGICAL SCREENING

The primary purpose of audiological screening is to determine whether a client exhibits a loss of auditory function, which could be an etiological factor associated with a phonological disorder. Audiological screening is usually conducted with pure tones and/or impedance audiometry.

Pure tone screening typically involves presentation of pure tone stimuli at 500, 1000, 2000, and 4000 Hz at a predetermined intensity level. Usually, a 20 dB level is used for screening, but this level may be altered to compensate for ambient noise in the room. The pure tone frequencies used in screening are those considered most important for receiving speech stimuli. The loudness of the pure tone stimuli reflects threshold levels needed to function adequately in the classroom.

Impedance screening measures eardrum compliance (movement of the eardrum) and middle-ear pressure as air pressure is altered in the external auditory canal. The acoustic reflex is a contraction of the stapedial muscle when the ear is stimulated by a loud sound; it serves as a protective device for the inner ear. The acoustic reflex can be measured by presenting a relatively loud signal to the ear and observing the presence or absence of a change in the compliance of the eardrum. Screening of the acoustic reflex usually involves the presentation of a

1000 Hz signal at 70 dB above a person's threshold. This screening test yields basic information about the functioning of the tympanic membrane and the middle ear. The client who fails a pure tone or impedance screening test should be referred to an audiologist for a complete audiological assessment.

SPEECH SOUND DISCRIMINATION TESTING

A review of the literature concerning the relationship between speech sound discrimination and articulation is presented in Chapter 5. The information presented in Chapter 5 provides background for the assessment of speech sound discrimination.

For many years, clinicians assumed that most children with articulation errors were unable to perceive the difference between the standard adult production and their own error production, and then inferred that many phonological problems were the result of this faulty perception. As a result of this assumption, speech sound discrimination testing became a standard procedure in the assessment battery. Research reported in the last two decades has cast doubt on the cause-and-effect relationship between faulty perception and phonological disorders. Thus, the routine use of speech sound discrimination tests has declined. At the present time, speech sound discrimination testing is typically done routinely only with those clients suspected of having a perceptual problem (e.g., collapsing of two or more adult contrasts into a single sound).

For many years, the most widely used speech sound discrimination tests were general tests of sound discrimination which did not reflect a child's specific speech sound errors. These tests typically involved a paired comparison task of minimal pairs (e.g., *coat–boat*) produced by the examiner or presented via audio tape. Most of the comparisons did not examine contrasts relevant to a particular child's error productions. Examples of general tests of discrimination include the *Auditory Discrimination Test* (Wepman, 1958) and the *Goldman-Fristoe-Woodcock Diagnostic Auditory Discrimination Test* (Goldman, Fristoe, and Woodcock, 1970).

Perceptual testing usually involves the client's differentiating the adult standard production from his or her error production, and/or assessment of the child's perception of phonological contrasts. In-depth perceptual testing of an error sound requirement assesses numerous phonemic contrasts, all focusing on a particular target sound.

Locke's Speech Production Perception Task. One perceptual measure of various phonemic contrasts is the *Speech Production Perception Task* (Locke, 1980), which was designed to assess a child's perception of his or her articulatory errors and involves no preselected stimuli. The stimuli presented are based on the child's error productions. The format for this task, along with an example of the scoring sheet, appear in Table 6–3.

Preliminary to the presentation of Locke's protocol, the child's speech sound errors must be identified. The child's error productions and the corresponding adult (correct) forms are then used to construct the perception task. In this procedure, the adult form is identified as the *production task stimulus,* and the child's substitution or deletion as the *production task response.* A perceptually similar control phoneme is entered as the *production task control phoneme.* For example, if the client substitutes [wek] for /rek/, the stimulus production (SP) would be

TABLE 6–3. **Speech Production Perception Task.**

CHILD'S NAME _____ SEX: M F BIRTHDATE: _____ AGE: ____ YRS. ____ MOS. _____

Date _____		Date _____		Date _____	
Production Task		Production Task		Production Task	
Stimulus	Response*	Stimulus	Response	Stimulus	Response
/θ ʌ m/ → /f ʌ m/		/r e i k/ → /w e i k/		/ʃ u/ → /s u/	
SP /θ/ RP /f/ CP /s/		SP /r/ RP /w/ CP /l/		SP /ʃ/ RP /s/ CP /t/	
Stimulus-Class	*Response*	*Stimulus-Class*	*Response*	*Stimulus-Class*	*Response*
1 /s/ – CP	yes NO	1 /r/ – SP	YES no	1 /s/ – RP	yes NO
2 /f/ – RP	yes NO	2 /l/ – CP	yes NO	2 /t/ – CP	yes NO
3 /θ/ – SP	YES no	3 /r/ – SP	YES no	3 /t/ – CP	yes NO
4 /θ/ – SP	YES no	4 /l/ – CP	yes NO	4 /ʃ/ – SP	YES no
5 /f/ – RP	yes NO	5 /w/ – RP	yes NO	5 /ʃ/ – SP	YES no
6 /s/ – CP	yes NO	6 /w/ – RP	yes NO	6 /s/ – RP	yes NO
7 /s/ – CP	yes NO	7 /r/ – SP	YES no	7 /s/ – RP	yes NO
8 /θ/ – SP	YES no	8 /w/ – RP	yes NO	8 /ʃ/ – SP	YES no
9 /f/ – RP	yes NO	9 /r/ – SP	YES no	9 /t/ – CP	yes NO
10 /θ/ – SP	YES no	10 /l/ – CP	yes NO	10 /ʃ/ – SP	YES no
11 /f/ – RP	yes NO	11 /l/ – CP	yes NO	11 /t/ – CP	yes NO
12 /s/ – CP	yes NO	12 /w/ – RP	yes NO	12 /s/ – RP	yes NO
13 /f/ – RP	yes NO	13 /t/ – SP	YES no	13 /ʃ/ – SP	YES no
14 /θ/ – SP	YES no	14 /l/ – CP	yes NO	14 /s/ – RP	yes NO
15 /s/ – CP	yes NO	15 /w/ – SP	YES no	15 /ʃ/ – SP	YES no
16 /f/ – RP	yes NO	16 /r/ – SP	YES no	16 /t/ – CP	yes NO
17 /θ/ – SP	YES no	17 /w/ – RP	yes NO	17 /t/ – CP	yes NO
18 /s/ – CP	yes NO	18 /l/ – CP	yes NO	18 /s/ – RP	yes NO
RP ____ CP ____ SP ____		RP ____ CP ____ SP ____		RP ____ CP ____ SP ____	

* The correct response is in upper case letters.

Source: Adapted by permission from J. Locke, "The Inference of Speech Perception in the Phonologically Disordered Child Part II: Some Clinically Novel Procedures, Their Use, Some Findings." *Journal of Speech and Hearing Disorders,* 45 (1980): 447.

rake /r/, the response production (RP) would be *wake* /w/, and an appropriate control production (CP) could be *lake* /l/.

To administer the task, the examiner presents a picture or an object to the child and names it, using either the correct (SP), incorrect (RP), or control sound (CP) in accord with the test protocol. After the examiner asks "Is this _____?", the child responds yes or no, indicating that he or she accepts or rejects the correct, incorrect, and control phonemes presented. Following administration of the 18 items included in the test, the number of correct responses to the three types of items (SP, RP, CP) are tabulated. A similar procedure would have to be constructed for each sound substitution in which perception is to be examined.

Winitz's Phonological Performance Test. Winitz (1984) suggested that speech sound perception may be adequate on word discrimination tasks but may break down in a conversational context. He described the following procedure for assessing discrimination at what he calls the "phonological level." He devised a mental perceptual measure that is phoneme-specific and designed to assess the contrast between a target sound and a perceptually similar sound in a sentence context. The clinician tells the child to listen to three sentences, each of which contains one example of a given target sound. When they are completed, two pictures will be presented and the child is instructed to select the picture which best represents the meaning of the three sentences. In each sentence the same

Phonological Assessment Procedures

FIGURE 6–2. **Phonological Performance Analysis Test.**
I was to wake it up.
I didn't want to wake it up.
Finally I was told to wake it up.

I was to rake it up.
I didn't want to rake it up.
Finally I was told to rake it up.

Source: Winitz, H., *Treating Articulation Disorders: For Clinicians by Clinicians.* Austin, Tex.: PRO-ED (1984), p. 35. Used with permission.

word (e.g., *rake*) of a minimal pair (e.g., *rake–wake*) is used. At a later point in testing, the contrastive word (e.g., *wake*) is examined within the same three sentences.

In Figure 6–2, items used to assess the /r/–/w/ contrast are presented.

Phonological Contrast Testing. An additional type of perceptual testing is the assessment of a child's perception of phonological contrasts. Grunwell (1982) indicated that the child with disordered phonology characteristically lacks perception of the phonological contrasts of the language. It has been hypothesized that one reason for this is the child's small phonetic inventory.

Assessment of a child's awareness of phonological contrasts provides the clinician with data relative to the child's phonemic system at a perceptual level. Although no formal perceptual measures of phonological contrasts have been published, most clinicians improvise assessment tasks requiring the child to indicate awareness that certain contrasts are in his or her perceptual repertoire. For example, a child may be shown pictures of the following pairs of words which contrast s/t, s/ʃ, and s/θ, and be asked to pick up one picture from each pair as it is named.

sea	sea	some
tea	she	thumb

In addition to testing contrasts perceptually, contrasts also can be assessed at a productive level. Maxwell and Rockman (1984) developed a delayed-imitation task, which included 89 words, and sampled contrasting sounds of adult English in near minimal pairs and some alternations (e.g., *miss* vs. *missing, try* vs. *tie, sigh* vs. *sly*). The task made it possible to examine how sounds change according to phonological context. For example, *dog* and *doggie* might be elicited to see what happens to a word-final consonant, or *try* and *tie* to examine the effect of word-initial consonant clusters. In contrast testing, the examiner usually is interested in assessing only those contrasts involving sounds on which the child produces errors.

Summary. Once it is determined that perceptual testing is appropriate, the primary concerns are the child's ability to differentiate between the adult standard and his or her error productions. At present, we have only a superficial understanding of the relationship between phonological production and perception. As a result, caution is required when interpreting perceptual test findings relative to performance on speech sound production tasks. Further research is necessary if we are to better understand the critical perceptual skills for the clinical management of the child with a phonological disorder.

CRITERIA FOR SELECTING PHONOLOGICAL ASSESSMENT INSTRUMENTS

Speech-language pathologists have at their disposal a variety of published phonological assessment instruments. Although clinicians often tend to use particular assessment tools, most recognize that no one test is appropriate for all purposes. The test instruments selected should be appropriate to the individual being tested and provide the information desired by the clinician. When selecting instruments for phonological assessment, the clinician will want to consider the sample the instrument is designed to obtain, the nature of the stimulus materials, and the scoring and analysis system. A practical consideration in test selection is the amount of time required to administer the instrument and analyze the sample obtained.

SAMPLE OBTAINED

A factor to consider in selecting a test instrument is the adequacy or representativeness of the speech sample obtained: the specific consonants, consonant clusters, vowels, and diphthongs tested as well as the units in which they are produced (i.e., syllables, words, sentences). The model of stimulus presentation–sample elicitation (e.g., picture-naming, imitation, delayed imitation, conversation) should also be considered when selecting instruments.

MATERIAL PRESENTATION

Another practical factor in test selection is the attractiveness, compactness, and manipulability of the test materials. Size, familiarity, and color of stimulus pictures and appropriateness for the child's age sometimes influence the ease with which one obtains responses to test stimuli. In addition, the organization and format of the scoring sheet are important for information retrieval. Tests with familiar and attractive stimulus items and score sheets that facilitate error analysis are desirable.

SCORING AND ANALYSIS

Because the scoring and analysis procedures that accompany a test instrument determine the type of information obtained from the instrument, they are important considerations in test selection. For example, a clinician would be likely to select different test instruments to obtain each of the following types of information: (1) survey of English consonant and vowel sounds; (2) evaluation of a particular sound in a variety of contexts; (3) place, manner, and voicing analysis; (4) phonological process analysis; and (5) comparison of scores with normative data. Various instruments have been designed to facilitate different types of analyses.

REFERENCES

Allen, G., "Some tips on tape recording speech-language samples." *Journal of the National Student Speech-Language-Hearing Association, 12* (1984): 10–17.

Bankson, N., and J. Bernthal, "Assessment of articulation." In L. Lass, J. Northern, D. Yoder, and L. McReynolds (Eds.), *Speech, Language, Hearing.* Philadelphia: W. B. Saunders, 1981.

Bankson, N., and J. Bernthal, *Quick Screen of Phonology.* Chicago: Riverside Press, 1990.

Bankson, N., and M. Byrne, "The effect of a timed correct sound production task on carryover." *Journal of Speech and Hearing Research, 15* (1972): 160–168.

Carter, E., and M. Buck, "Prognostic testing for functional articulation disorders among children in the first grade." *Journal of Speech and Hearing Disorders, 23* (1958): 124–133.

Curtis, J., and J. Hardy, "A phonetic study of misarticulations of /r/." *Journal of Speech and Hearing Research, 2* (1959): 224–257.

Diedrich, W., "Stimulability and articulation disorders." In J. Locke (Ed.), *Assessing and Treating Phonological Disorders: Current Approaches. Seminars in Speech and Language,* 4. New York: Thieme-Stratton, 1983.

Dinnsen, D., and M. Elbert, "On the relationship between phonology and learning." In M. Elbert, D. Dinnsen, and G. Weismer (Eds.), *Phonological Theory and the Misarticulating Child, ASHA Monographs,* 22, Rockville, Md.: ASHA, 1984.

Drumwright, A., *The Denver Articulation Examination.* Denver: Ladoca Project and Publishing Foundation, 1971.

Dubois, E., and J. Bernthal, "A comparison of three methods for obtaining articulatory responses." *Journal of Speech and Hearing Disorders, 43* (1978): 295–305.

Edwards, M.L., *Introduction to Applied Phonetics.* San Diego: College-Hill Press, 1986.

Elbert, M., R. Shelton, and W. Arndt, "A task for evaluation of articulation change: 1. Development of methodology." *Journal of Speech and Hearing Research, 10* (1967): 281–288.

Emerick, L., and J. Hatten, *Diagnosis and Evaluation in Speech Pathology.* Englewood Cliffs, N.J.: Prentice Hall, 1974.

Faircloth, M., and S. Faircloth, "An analysis of the articulatory behavior of a speech-defective child in connected speech and in isolated-word responses." *Journal of Speech and Hearing Disorders, 35* (1970): 51–61.

Farquhar, M.S., "Prognostic value of imitative and auditory discrimination tests." *Journal of Speech and Hearing Disorders, 26* (1961): 342–347.

Fisher, H., and J. Logemann, *The Fisher-Logemann Test of Articulation Competence.* Boston: Houghton Mifflin, 1971.

Fluharty, N., *Fluharty Preschool Speech and Language Screening Test.* Bingingham, Mass.: Teaching Resources Corporation, 1978.

Gallagher, R., and T. Shriner, "Contextual variables related to inconsistent /s/ and /z/ production in the spontaneous speech of children." *Journal of Speech and Hearing Research, 18* (1975): 623–633.

Gierut, J., M. Elbert, and D. Dinnsen, "Functional analysis of phonological knowledge and generalization learning in misarticulating children." *Journal of Speech and Hearing Research, 30* (1987): 462–479.

Goldman, R., and R. Fristoe, *Goldman-Fristoe Test of Articulation.* Circle Pines, Minn.: American Guidance Service, 1969, 1986.

Goldman, R., M. Fristoe, and R. Woodcock, *The Goldman-Fristoe-Woodcock Test of Auditory Discrimination.* Circle Pines, Minn: American Guidance Service, 1970.

Grunwell, P., "The development of phonology: A descriptive profile." *First Language, 3* (1981): 161–191.

Grunwell, P., *Clinical Phonology.* Rockville, Md.: Aspen, 1982.

Harrington, J., I. Lux, and R. Higgins, "Identification of error types as related to stimuli in articulation tests." Paper presented at the annual convention of the American Speech-Language-Hearing Association, San Francisco, 1984.

Hoffman, P.R., and G. Schuckers, and D. Ratusnik, "Contextual-coarticulatory inconsistency of /r/ misarticulations." *Journal of Speech and Hearing Research, 20* (1977): 631–643.

Ingram, D., *Procedures for the Phonological Analysis of Children's Language*. Baltimore: University Park Press, 1981.

Ingram, D., *Phonological Disability in Children*. New York: American Elsevier, 1976, 1989.

Irwin, R., J. West, and M. Trombetta, "Effectiveness of speech therapy for second grade children with misarticulations: Predictive factors." *Exceptional Children, 32* (1966): 471–479.

Jordan, E.P., "Articulation test measures and listener ratings of articulation defectiveness." *Journal of Speech and Hearing Research, 3* (1960): 303–319.

Kent, R., and F. Minifie, "Coarticulation in recent speech production models." *Journal of Phonetics, 5* (1977): 115–133.

Kisatsky, T., "The prognostic value of Carter-Buck tests in measuring articulation skills in selected kindergarten children." *Exceptional Children, 34* (1967): 81–85.

Locke, J., "The inference of speech perception in the phonologically disordered child. Part II: Some clinically novel procedures, their use, some findings." *Journal of Speech and Hearing Disorders, 45* (1980): 445–468.

McDonald, E., *A Deep Test of Articulation*. Pittsburgh: Stanwix House, 1964a.

McDonald, E., *Articulation Testing and Treatment: A Sensory Motor Approach*. Pittsburgh: Stanwix House, 1964b.

McDonald, E., *Screening Deep Test of Articulation*. Pittsburgh: Stanwix House, 1968.

McReynolds, L.V., and M. Elbert, "An experimental analysis of misarticulating children's generalization." *Journal of Speech and Hearing Research, 21* (1978): 136–150.

Madison, C., "Articulation stimulability review." *Language, Speech, and Hearing Services in Schools, 10* (1979): 185–190.

Mason, R., and N. Wickwire, "Examining for orofacial variations." *Comminique, 8* (1978): 2–26.

Maxwell, E.M., and B.K. Rockman, "Procedures for linguistic analysis of misarticulated speech." In M. Elbert, D. Dinnsen, and G. Weismer (Eds.), *Phonological Theory and the Misarticulating Child. ASHA Monographs, 22*. Rockville, Md: ASHA, 1984.

Paynter, W., and T. Bumpas, "Imitative and spontaneous articulatory assessment of three-year-old children." *Journal of Speech and Hearing Disorders, 42* (1977): 119–125.

Pendergast, K., S. Dickey, T. Selmar, and A. Soder, *The Photo Articulation Test*, 2nd ed. Danville, Ill.: Interstate Press, 1969.

Pollack, K., "The identification of vowel errors using traditional articulation or phonological process test stimuli." *Language, Speech, and Hearing Services in Schools, 22* (1991): 39–50.

Pollack, E., and N. Rees, "Disorders of articulation: Some clinical applications of distinctive feature theory." *Journal of Speech and Hearing Disorders, 37* (1972): 451–470.

Roe, V., and R. Milisen, "The effect of maturation upon defective articulation in elementary grades." *Journal of Speech Disorders, 7* (1942): 37–50.

Schwartz, R., L. Leonard, M. Folger, and M. Wilcox, "Early phonological behavior in normal-speaking and language disordered children; Evidence for a synergistic view of linguistic disorders." *Journal of Speech and Hearing Disorders, 45* (1980): 357–377.

Secord, W., *C-PAC: Clinical Probes of Articulation Consistency*. San Antonio, Tex.: Psychological Corporation, 1981.

Shriberg, L.D., and R.D. Kent, *Clinical Phonetics*. New York: John Wiley and Sons, 1982.

Shriberg, L.D., and J. Kwiatkowski, *Natural Process Analysis*. New York: John Wiley, 1980.

Shriberg, L.D., and J. Kwiatkowski, "Continuous speech sampling for phonologic analysis of speech-delayed children." *Journal of Speech and Hearing Research, 50* (1985): 323–334.

Shriberg, L.D., J. Kwiatkowski, and K. Hoffman, "A procedure for phonetic transcription by consensus." *Journal of Speech and Hearing Research, 27* (1984): 456–465.

Siegel, R., H. Winitz, and H. Conkey, "The influence of testing instruments in articulatory responses of children." *Journal of Speech and Hearing Disorders, 28* (1963): 67–76.

Smit, A., and J. Bernthal, "Performance of articulation disordered children on language and perception measures." *Journal of Speech and Hearing Research, 26* (1983): 124–136.

Smith, M.W., and S. Ainsworth, "The effect of three types of stimulation on articulatory responses of speech defective children." *Journal of Speech and Hearing Research, 10* (1967): 333–338.

Snow, J., and R. Milisen, "The influences of oral versus pictorial representation upon articulation testing results." *Journal of Speech and Hearing Disorders. Monograph Supplement, 4* (1954): 29–36.

Sommers, R.K., R. Leiss, M. Delp, A. Gerber, D. Fundrella, R. Smith, M. Revucky, D. Ellis, and V. Haley, "Factors related to the effectiveness of articulation therapy for kindergarten, first- and second-grade children." *Journal of Speech and Hearing Research, 10* (1967): 428–437.

Stockman, I., and E. McDonald, "Heterogeneity as a confounding factor when predicting spontaneous improvement of misarticulated consonants." *Language, Speech, and Hearing Services in Schools, 11* (1980): 15–29.

Stoel-Gammon, C., and C. Dunn, *Normal and Disordered Phonology*. Baltimore: University Park Press, 1985.

Templin, M., "Spontaneous vs. imitated verbalization in testing pre-school children." *Journal of Speech and Hearing Disorders, 12* (1947): 293–300.

Templin, M., *Certain Language Skills in Children*. Institute of Child Welfare Monograph Series, 26. Minneapolis: University of Minnesota, 1957.

Templin, M., and F. Darley, *The Templin-Darley Tests of Articulation*. Iowa City, Iowa: Bureau of Educational Research and Service, University of Iowa, 1969.

Turton, L.J., "Diagnostic implications of articulation testing." In W.D. Wolfe and D.J. Goulding (Eds.), *Articulation and Learning*. Springfield, Ill.: Charles C Thomas, 1973.

Tyler, A., M.L. Edwards, and J. Saxman, "Acoustic validation of phonological knowledge and its relationship to treatment." *Journal of Speech and Hearing Disorders, 55* (1990): 251–261.

Van Riper, C., and R. Erickson, "A predictive screening test of articulation." *Journal of Speech and Hearing Disorders, 34* (1969): 214–219.

Weismer, G., D. Dinnsen, and M. Elbert, "A study of the voicing distinction associated with omitted, word-final stops." *Journal of Speech and Hearing Disorders, 46* (1981): 320–327.

Wepman, J., *Wepman Auditory Discrimination Test*. Chicago: Language Research Association, 1958.

Winitz, H., *Articulatory Acquisition and Behavior*. Englewood Cliffs, N.J.: Prentice Hall, 1969.

Winitz, H., *From Syllable to Conversation*. Baltimore: University Park Press, 1975.

Winitz, H., "Auditory considerations in articulation training." In H. Winitz (Ed.), *Treating Articulation Disorders: For Clinicians by Clinicians*. Austin, Tex: PRO-ED, 1984.

Wright, V., R. Shelton, and W. Arndt, "A task for evaluation of articulation change: III. Imitative task scores compared with scores for more spontaneous tasks." *Journal of Speech and Hearing Research, 12* (1969): 875–884.

Zimmerman, I., V. Steiner, and R. Pond, *Preschool Language Scale*. Columbus, Ohio: Charles E. Merrill, 1969, 1979.

chapter

7

Analysis and Interpretation of Assessment Data

INTRODUCTION

After the clinician has collected the phonological sample, the data gathered during the assessment is analyzed and interpreted to determine (1) whether or not there is a phonological problem; (2) the nature of the problem, if there is one; (3) whether or not the client should be seen for treatment; and (4) if treatment is indicated, an initial remediation plan. The primary goal of the *analysis* is to describe phonological performance. The purpose of *interpretation* is to examine the results of the phonological analysis and determine what course of action should be taken. Based on the interpretation of the phonological analysis, the clinician must determine whether or not the client needs instruction, and, if so, select target behaviors for treatment and appropriate intervention strategies. In summary, the clinician reviews responses to the phonological assessment tasks and interprets the analysis of these data in order to make appropriate and efficacious decisions.

Phonological data may be subjected to an **independent analysis** and/or a **relational analysis** (Stoel-Gammon and Dunn, 1985). An independent analysis consists of a delineation of the speech sound found in a child's repertoire without regard to the mature phonological system seen in adult speech. In this type of analysis, the speech sounds used by the child are viewed as a self-contained system. This type of analysis is usually done with very young children or those clients with a very limited phonological repertoire. An independent analysis usually would include some description of the frequency with which a sound is observed in the sample, the effect of word-position on the sound, the syllable shapes (CVC, CV, VC, CCV) in which the sound is used, and the constraints imposed by particular sound sequences. In short, an independent analysis reveals the sounds and sound sequences produced by the child without reference to the adult standard.

In a relational analysis the client's productions are compared to the target forms seen in the adult standard. Relational analysis is the most commonly employed type of analysis, probably because it is focused on identification of sounds produced in error and/or error patterns based on a comparison of the client's productions to the adult target forms. By comparing a client's way of saying a word with the adult standard form, one may find evidence of patterns such as substitution of stops for fricatives or deletion of word-final consonants. It should be pointed out that a relational analysis does not assign a cause for a mismatch but only identifies the mismatches and relates them to other error patterns. Frequently it is unclear if an error production is the result of a perceptual problem, a motor production problem, or lack of a particular phonological rule. Most of the analysis procedures and the subsequent interpretations discussed in this chapter focus on relational analyses.

ANALYSIS AND INTERPRETATION OF INTELLIGIBILITY AND SEVERITY JUDGMENTS

INTELLIGIBILITY

A most important consideration for determining the phonological status of an individual and the need for intervention is the intelligibility of the client's spontaneous speech. The intelligibility of spontaneous speech is a reflection of the client's verbal communication in a natural speaking situation and is very important when determining the need for intervention. Intelligibility of the speaker is the factor most frequently cited by both speech-language pathologists and naive listeners when judging the severity of a phonological problem (Shriberg and Kwiatkowski, 1982).

The degree of speech intelligibility is a subjective judgment made by a listener and is based, to a large extent, on the percentage of words in a speech sample which were understood by the listener. Intelligibility of speech reflects a continuum of judgment ranging from unintelligible (where the message is not understood) to totally intelligible (where the message is completely understood by the listener). Intermediate points along such a continuum might include the following: Speech is usually unintelligible, speech is partially intelligible, speech is intelligible although noticeably in error, or speech sound errors are occasionally noticed in continuous speech.

A major factor influencing speech sound intelligibility is the number and nature of speech sound errors a speaker makes. The larger the number of a speaker's productions which differ from the adult standard, the more intelligibility is reduced. However, a simple tally of the number of sounds in error is not an adequate index of intelligibility. As Shriberg and Kwiatkowski (1982) reported, there is a low correlation (r = .42) between the percentage of consonants correct and the intelligibility of a speech sample. The nature of the clients' errors relative to the target form will also affect intelligibility. For example, deleting a sound will affect intelligibility more than will a mild distortion of the same sound.

Intelligibility is also affected by the consistency of misarticulated sounds and the frequency with which an error sound occurs in the language. The more consistently a target sound is produced in error and the more frequently the target sound occurs in the language, the more likely the listener will perceive the speaker's speech as defective.

There are many extraneous factors that may influence intelligibility judgments. These factors include the listener's familiarity with the speaker's speech pattern; the speaker's rate, inflection, and stress patterns; the linguistic experience of the listener; the social environment of the communication act; the message content; the communication cues available to the listener; and the characteristics of the transmission media. The complexity of these factors probably accounts for the finding that intelligibility ratings are not highly correlated with the percentage of consonants correct.

A seven-point scale described by Fudala (1970) suggested that a child's speech rating on an intelligibility continuum could be based on the number of speech sound errors a client made in single-word productions, with the target sounds weighted according to their probable frequency of occurrence in American speech. Although such rating scales may have some value, especially in interpreting the effect of speech errors on intelligibility to the layman, they should be used with caution because of the many factors which influence intelligibility judgments.

In summary, a variety of factors have been identified that may influence clinicians' subjective judgments of intelligibility. In case selection, a general principle of operation is that the poorer the ratings of intelligibility, the more likely the need for intervention. It is generally recognized that a client 3 years of age or older who is unintelligible is a candidate for treatment and that intelligibility expectations increase with age. For clients exhibiting some intelligible problems, additional factors discussed below will need to be considered in deciding on the need for intervention.

SEVERITY OF INVOLVEMENT

The severity of a phonological disorder frequently needs to be addressed by speech-language clinicians. Shriberg and Kwiatkowski (1982) proposed a metric for quantifying the severity of involvement of children with a developmental phonological disorder. The term *severity of involvement* was used to reflect disability (degree to which a performance characteristic is subnormal), intelligibility (usually the percentage of intelligible words in continuous speech), and handicap (degree to which a disability impedes effective functioning). Shriberg and Kwiatkowski recommended the calculation of **percentage of consonants correct** (PCC) as an index to quantify severity of involvement. The percentage of consonants correct requires the examiner to make correct–incorrect judgments of individual sounds produced in a continuous speech sample. Such judgments were found to be a fairly reliable measure for the classification of most children's speech as mild, mild-moderate, moderate-severe, or severe.

Procedures outlined by Shriberg and Kwiatkowski (1982; 267) for determining PCC are as follows:

> Tape record a continuous speech sample of a child following sampling procedures. Any means that yield continuous speech from the child are acceptable, provided that the clinician can gloss each child-utterance. The clinician can tell the child that

his exact words will be repeated onto the "tape machine" so that the clinician is sure to "get things right."

I. Sampling Rules
   A. Consider only intended (target) consonants in words. Intended vowels are not considered.
      1. Addition of a consonant before a vowel, for example, *on* [hon], is not scored because the target sound /ɔ/ is a vowel.
      2. Postvocalic /r/ in *fair* [feir] is a consonant, but stressed and unstressed vocalics [ɝ] and [ɚ], as in *furrier* [fɝiɚ], are vowels.
   B. Do not score target consonants in the second or successive repetitions of a syllable, for example, *ba-balloon*—score only the first /b/.
   C. Do not score target consonants in words that are completely or partially unintelligible or whose gloss is highly questionable.
   D. Do not score target consonants in the third or successive repetitions of adjacent words unless articulation changes. For example, the consonants in only the first two words of the series [kæt], [kæt], [kæt] are counted. However, the consonants in all three words are counted if the series were [kæt], [kæk], [kæt].

II. Scoring Rules
   A. The following six types of consonant sound changes are scored as incorrect:
      1. Deletions of a target consonant
      2. Substitutions of another sound for a target consonant, including replacement by a glottal stop or a cognate
      3. Partial voicing of initial target consonants
      4. Distortions of a target sound, no matter how subtle
      5. Addition of a sound to a correct or incorrect target consonant, for example, *cars* said as [karks]
      6. Initial /h/ deletion (*he* [i]) and final n/ŋ substitutions (*ring* [rin]) are counted as errors only when they occur in stressed syllables; in unstressed syllables they are counted as correct, for example, *feed her* [fidɚ]; *running* [rʌnin].
   B. Observe the following:
      1. The response definition for children who obviously have speech errors is "score as incorrect unless heard as correct." This response definition assigns questionable speech behaviors to an "incorrect" category.
      2. Dialectal variants should be glossed as intended in the child's dialect, for example, *picture* "piture," *ask* "aks," and so on.
      3. Fast or casual speech sound changes should be glossed as the child intended, for example, *don't know* "dono," and "n," and the like.
      4. Allophones should be scored as correct, for example, *water* [warɚ], *tail* [teɪɫ].

III. Calculation of Percentage of Consonants Correct (PCC)

   Calculated by the formula:

   $$\text{PCC} = \frac{\text{Number of Correct Consonants}}{\text{Number of Correct Plus Incorrect Consonants}} \times 100$$

ANALYSIS AND INTERPRETATION OF NORMATIVE PHONOLOGICAL DATA

A second factor to consider in deciding if a client is a candidate for intervention is the age appropriateness of his or her productions. The need for intervention in children is frequently determined on the basis of phoneme acquisition data. If a child misarticulates sounds that are ordinarily produced by children at that age, or if a child's total number of correct speech sounds produced is below the age norm, the child is identified as having a developmental delay. How much delay is necessary before a child is considered a candidate for intervention is a judgment the clinician must make.

Two methods traditionally have been employed to compare articulation performance and chronological age: (1) the number of correct responses on a speech sound articulation test are tabulated and then compared with normative data for a given age level on the same test (e.g., *The Templin-Darley Tests of Articulation*, Templin and Darley, 1969; *Bankson-Bernthal Test of Phonology*, Bankson and Bernthal, 1990); and (2) a comparison is made of the child's individual segmental productions with developmental norms for individual sounds. In addition, there are instruments (e.g., *Khan-Lewis Phonological Analysis*, Khan and Lewis, 1986; *Bankson-Bernthal Test of Phonology*, Bankson and Bernthal, 1990) which include normative data on phonological processes so that a client's repertoire can be compared with the ages at which processes typically are no longer used by normal developing children. This topic will be discussed later in this chapter under the heading Pattern Analysis.

The number of correct speech sound productions in relation to age is a metric frequently used to qualify children for speech services in the public schools. For example, if a 4-year-old child produces 32 target items correctly, and the mean number of correct responses for children of the same age is 49, with a standard deviation of 12, the child's speech would usually be identified as phonologically delayed. Likewise, if a 5-year-old child uses final consonant deletions, stopping, and backing, he or she would be identified as phonologically delayed since these phonological patterns are no longer operating in normally developing children of that age.

NORMATIVE DATA FOR INDIVIDUAL SOUNDS

The comparison of a child's articulatory productions with acquisition norms for individual sounds is a second way developmental norms are used. Although this appears to be a simple task, one must be cautious when assigning an age norm to a particular sound. Normative data are only statistical averages and reflect general patterns of acquisition. One must also remember that children learn sounds at different rates and in different sequences. Thus caution is required in the application of these normative data for individual sounds produced by a child.

As discussed earlier, investigators have attached an age expectation to specific speech sounds by listing the age levels at which 75 percent and 90 percent of the children in a normative group mastered each sound tested. Sander (1972) pointed out that such normative data are group standards which reflect upper age limits rather than average performance and suggested instead that the concept of customary production be used. He defined customary production as the point at which 51 percent of the children correctly produced a sound in two of the three word-positions. Sander (1972) also argued that "variability among children in the ages at which they successfully produce specific sounds is so great as to discourage pinpoint statistics" (58).

Prather, Hedrick, and Kern (1975) reported speech sound acquisition norms for children from age 2 through 4 years on a test designed to elicit consonants in

Analysis and Interpretation of Assessment Data

the prevocalic and postvocalic positions. With respect to the age levels at which 75 percent of the children had mastered specific sounds, these investigators reported earlier age levels than Templin although the sequence of acquisition was similar in both studies. They pointed out that the differences in findings could be due to their use of two-position versus Templin's three-position testing. A useful set of normative data for individual sound acquisition, which reflects an age range for sound development, is shown in Figure 7–1.

Smit (1986) reanalyzed the data from Prather et al. (1975) and Templin (1957) and found that methodological differences could account for the apparent downward shift in ages of acquisition reported by Prather et al. She reported that when two-position data sets from Prather et al. were compared with two-position results from Templin, the findings were similar; and in fact, in a few instances the ages of acquisition for specific sounds reported by Prather et al. were later than those reported by Templin.

Smit, Hand, Freilinger, Bernthal, and Bird (1990) gathered three-position data from children in two midwestern states. Using a 75 percent criterion level, they reported that children acquire sounds at ages equal to or younger than ages reported by Templin. They found that /ŋ/ and /r/ reached the 75 percent criterion later than reported by Templin. They also found that clusters tended to reach the 75 percent criterion at the same age or later than singletons contained in the cluster. It is interesting to note the overall similarity between Smit et al.'s data and those of Templin gathered 33 years earlier.

The clinician should keep in mind that in using the data from any large group study, individual subject data are obscured. Although the precise sequence and nature of phonological development varies from one person to another, in general, certain segments are mastered earlier than others, and this information is used in determining presence of phonological delay and the direction of treatment. For example, if 6-year-old Kirsten says all sounds usually produced by 75 percent of 3-year-old children, but is not yet using sounds commonly associated with 4-, 5-, and 6-year-olds, her phonological productions would be considered delayed. This developmental aspect of phonological acquisition makes age a useful factor in determining whether a child has a phonological delay.

A second way to compare articulation and chronological age is to compare a child's phonological performance with test norms (as opposed to individual segmental norms). In this procedure, the number of speech sound productions produced correctly on a specific test are compared with normative data for that instrument. In other words, the number of sounds that the child produces correctly are compared with normative data to determine whether a child's articulatory performance is typical for the child's age. This analysis is appropriate for children 8 years old and younger since correct production of speech sound segments is usually expected by age 8 in normal children. This procedure is the basis by which many states and school districts determine if children with phonological delay and disorders qualify for services.

Comparison of age and phonological development is widely practiced and certainly such data must be taken into consideration in recommending intervention. Justifiable criticism has been made of using such data as the single criterion for case selection (Turton, 1980; Sander, 1972; Winitz, 1969). Criticism is based on the following factors: (1) Speech sound developmental norms typically reflect

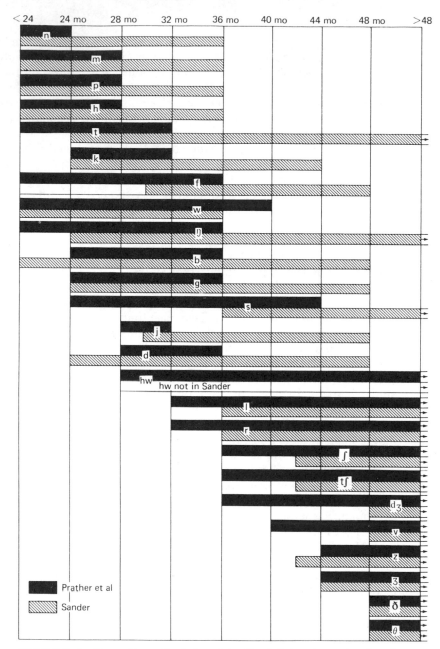

FIGURE 7–1. **Normative articulation data. The left-hand margin of each bar represents the age at which 50 percent of the children in a normative study used the specified sound correctly. The right-hand margin shows the age at which 90 percent of the children used the sound correctly.** Data reported in the lower bars are from Sander (1972). Data in the black bars are from the work of Hedrick, Prather, and Tobin (1975). Adapted by permission from E. M. Prather, D. L. Hedrick, and C. A. Kern, "Articulation Development in Children Aged Two to Four Years," *Journal of Speech and Hearing Disorders, 40* (1975): 179–191 (p. 186).

Analysis and Interpretation of Assessment Data

upper age limits of customary consonant production (between 75 and 100 percent of children produce the sounds correctly) rather than average age estimates; (2) the norms are based on production in the initial, medial, and final positions of single words rather than spontaneous speech; (3) there is a great deal of variability across children; (4) norms frequently are based on a single production of a particular sound in one context; (5) norms represent a statement of average performance by age, but the resulting sequence of acquisition may not be applicable to a given individual; (6) although sounds generally appear to be acquired in a sequence, prior acquisition of certain sounds is not necessarily required for the learning of other sounds; and (7) the nature of the error may be a critical factor. For example, Stephens, Hoffman, and Daniloff (1986) reported that unlike most errors, lateralization of /s/ did not spontaneously improve with age. As a result of this finding, together with our clinical experience, we do not consider such errors developmental. We would concur with the suggestion of Smit et al. (1990) that lateralized /s/ errors be treated earlier than other /s/ errors because unlike most speech sound errors they do not generally spontaneously correct with age.

As a general guideline for initiating intervention, the child should be at least one standard deviation (some guidelines call for 1.5 to 2 standard deviations) below his or her age norm in the number of sounds produced correctly. The clinician should recognize, however, that this is only a general guideline and other considerations, e.g., intelligibility, speaker's perception of his or her problem, nature of the error, consistency, and other speech patterns may also be important. In the case of an unintelligible child, the use of normative data may have minimal value because the concern is not to determine whether the child has a problem, but rather to understand the nature of the problem and to delineate the error patterns. It is for this type of child that knowledge of phonological patterns may be of greatest benefit.

ANALYSIS AND INTERPRETATION OF ERROR PATTERNS

PATTERN ANALYSIS

After the examiner has reviewed a speaker's phonological profile in terms of intelligibility and/or severity and age appropriateness, the next step is to further review the nature and patterns of the error productions to determine the nature of a client's phonological system. Procedures designed to provide a composite of individual productions are sometimes referred to as pattern analysis, and are particularly appropriate for those clients with multiple errors. In such procedures the clinician reviews the sampling data in an effort to categorize errors according to commonalities or patterns. This type of analysis is based on the assumption that children's speech sound errors are not random, but represent systematic variations from the adult standard. Phonological patterns that describe several individual speech sound errors can often be identified with careful examination. These error patterns frequently affect entire sound classes, particular sound sequences, or the syllable structure of words. Clinicians compare the child's productions with the adult standard (ambient or correct sound productions), and then categorize individual errors (mismatches with the adult standard) into phonological patterns.

The notion of an analysis of error patterns is not a new one. Van Riper

(1939), in his book *Speech Correction: Principles and Methods,* talked about substitution analysis and the need to organize speech sound errors into patterns. But it was not until the 1970s and 1980s that clinicians began to emphasize the identification of phonological patterns, processes, and rules.

One of the reasons pattern analysis procedures have appeal is that they often provide a better description of the child's phonological system than does a traditional categorization of errors as substitutions, distortions, and omissions. Khan (1982) furnished the following illustration of this point. A child who substitutes /wawa/ for *water* might be described in a traditional substitution analysis as substituting [w] for /t/ and substituting [a] for final /ɚ/. On the basis of what we know about phonological acquisition, the [wawa] for *water* substitution is more accurately described as syllable reduplication. The child in this instance is probably repeating the first syllable of the word *water* rather than using sound substitutions for target sounds in the second syllable. A second reason for doing a pattern analysis is the potential for treatment efficacy. When a pattern reflecting several sound errors is targeted for treatment, there is the potential for rapid generalization across sounds related to that pattern.

Determination of a child's phonological system usually is based on both a connected speech sample and productions obtained from a single-word articulation test. Included in an analysis of a phonological system is a delineation of a client's phonetic inventory, a determination of phonemes used contrastively, and an identification of phonological patterns. Phonological process analysis is a common method for identifying error patterns, including the influence of sound position within word and syllable shapes. In other words, since speech sound productions are affected by such factors as phonetic context, position in words, and syllable structure of words, these factors are reviewed for any systematic influence they may have.

Stoel-Gammon and Dunn (1985) developed a protocol based on the work of Shriberg and Kwiatkowski (1980) designed to facilitate organization and analysis of a child's phonological productions. This coding system organizes the words produced by a child and includes a separate coding sheet for different sound classes (i.e., stops, fricatives, affricates, and so on). The variables coded include (1) sound class, (2) word-position (initial, medial, final), and (3) different word structures (consonant singletons; consonant clusters; abutting consonants, i.e., two adjacent consonants that cross a syllable boundary; multisyllabic words). Figure 7–2 provides an example of a coding sheet for stops. This protocol may be particularly useful when analyzing a connected speech sample in young children and demonstrates how clinicians can organize sampling data to facilitate the identification of patterns present in the child's phonological system.

When to Use a Pattern Analysis. Systems of pattern analysis, whether based on a place-manner-voicing analysis, distinctive feature analysis, or more recent phonological process analysis procedures, are most appropriate for the client who has multiple errors. The intent of the analysis is to determine if there are patterns or relationships among speech sound error productions which differ from the adult standard; usually for individuals who have moderate to severe intelligibility problems. If only a few speech sounds are in error, one may not need to do a pattern analysis of a child's speech. For example, if a client is misarticulating only two consonants, for example, /s/ and /ʃ/, the clinician would not do a pattern analysis.

Name: DE
Age: 4;6

Sampling condition: *The Assessment of Phonological Processes*
Date of sampling: 11/24/82

Stops	Initial			Medial		Final		
	1. CV(c)	2. CⁿV(C)	3. Multisyllabic	4. -C-	5. -Cⁿ-	6. (C)VC	7. (C)VCⁿ	8. Multisyllabic
p	page [seɪʤ]	spoon [sũn] spring [swĩn]	paper ['fæfɚ]	open ['oʊʔɛn] paper [fæfɚ] zipper ['zɪpɚ]	airplane ['ɛɚsɛ̃n]	cup [sʌp] rope [rop] soap [sop]	jump [ʒʌp]	makeup ['meɪəp]
b	bed [bid] Bo [bo] book [but]	brown [bɑ̃n]	baseball ['bæbʌ] basket ['bæsɪt]	cowboy ['sobɔɪ]	baseball ['bæbʌ] football ['fʌtba] toothbrush ['tʰusrəʃ]	tub [sʌb]		
t	ten [zɛ̃n] tub [sʌb] two [tsu]	star [sɑʌ] stick [tʰɪ] string [swĩn] truck [tʰʌt]	TV [sivi] television ['tsɛzĩn] toothbrush ['tʰusrəʃ]	glitter ['zɪdə] scooter ['zʌdə] water ['wɑə]	football ['fʌtba] quarter ['tʃwʌdə]	hat [æt]	shirt [ʃɝt]	basket ['bæsɪt] minutes ['mĩnəz]
d	doll [dɑʌ]				screwdriver ['ʤudaɪbɚ] candle ['sɛ̃ndl]	bed [bid] sled [sɛd]	and [ʌ] closed [sozd] hand [æ̃n]	
k	couch [tʂɑʊtʂ] cup [sʌp]	Claus [sɔz] clothes [soz] closed [sozd] squirrel [swɛl]	candle ['sændl] coffee ['sɔsi] cowboy ['sobɔɪ] colors ['sʌzɚz] scooter ['zʌdə] screwdriver ['ʤudaɪbɚ]	makeup ['meɪəp] wrecker ['wɛdə]	basket ['bæsɪt]	book [but] like [lɛt] Luke [zʌt] snake [set] stick [tʰɪ] truck [tʰʌt]	fork [sɔɪt]	music ['musɪt]
g	gun [zʌ̃n]	glove [sʌz] green [wĩn, sĩn]	Christmas ['sɪtmʌs] quarter ['tʃwʌdə] glasses ['sæzɪz] glitter ['zɪdə]		Fall Guy [sʌ daɪ] finger ['fĩdə]	rug [wʌd]		

FIGURE 7–2. **Data organization for selecting words for analysis.** *Source:* Stoel-Gammon, C., and C. Dunn, *Normal and Disordered Phonology in Children,* 1985 (Austin, Tex.: PRO-ED.), p. 137. Used with permission.

In this instance, the clinician would develop a remediation plan where both consonants are targeted for instruction.

Phonological patterns identified during analysis become the focus for determining target behaviors for remediation. For example, if a child has eight speech sound substitutions reflecting three error patterns (e.g., stopping of fricatives, gliding of liquids, and fronting), remediation would likely focus on the reduction of one or more of these phonological patterns (processes). The modification of one or more speech sounds (exemplars) reflecting a particular error pattern frequently results in generalization to other speech sounds reflecting the same error pattern. For example, establishment of final /p/ may generalize to all other stops deleted in word-final position. Another example of a remediation strategy would be to target for instruction all speech sounds that reflect a given pattern; that is, all the speech sound errors that appear to be simplified in a similar manner (same phonological process). If fricatives were being substituted for stops, the clinician might focus on the contrast between stops and fricatives. By focusing on sounds that reflect a similar error pattern, treatment should be more efficient than if it focuses on individual sounds without regard to phonological patterns.

Types of Pattern Analysis.

Place-Manner-Voicing. Perhaps the most basic type of pattern analysis involves classifying substitution errors according to place, manner, and voicing characteristics. A place-manner-voicing analysis facilitates the identification of patterns such as voiced for voiceless sound substitutions (e.g., voicing errors—/v/→[f]/d/→[t]), replacement of fricatives by stops (e.g., manner errors—/ð/→[d] /s/→/t/), or substitution of lingua-alveolar sounds for linguavelar sounds (e.g., place errors—/t/→[k] /d/→[g]). The scoring form for the *Fisher-Logemann Test of Articulation Competence* (1971) is an example of how data can be organized to do a place-manner-voicing type analysis (see Figure 7–3).

Consider a child with several speech sound errors whose speech patterns reflect correct manner and voicing but errors in place of articulation, such as backing of consonants. This child substitutes /t/→[k] /d/→[g] /b/→[g] /p/→[k] /θ/ →[s] /ð/→[z]; and substitutes back sounds for front sounds (velars for alveolars and bilabials, alveolars for linguadentals). In this instance, the clinician's strategy might be to teach the client to focus on the place of production. Some clinicians might choose to teach a single sound, for example, /t/, as an exemplar of the correct place of production and then probe for generalization to other sounds, whereas others might choose to teach simultaneously all of the misarticulated stop sounds (same sound class) that reflect the error pattern. When selected exemplars are taught with the assumption that generalization will occur to other untrained sounds, the clinician should not assume that generalization will always occur, especially if the errors occur across sound classes. Generalization from trained to untrained sounds is difficult to predict. In addition, there is a great deal of individual variability in such generalization (Elbert, Powell, and Swartzlander, 1991).

The distinctive feature and phonological process analysis procedures are extensions of analyses based on manner of production, place of production, and voicing. These procedures are discussed below.

Distinctive Feature Analysis. In this second type of pattern analysis, speech

FIGURE 7–3. **The Fisher-Logemann Test of Articulation Competence.** *Source:* Reproduced with permission of The Riverside Publishing Company.

CARD #	IPA PHONEME	COMMON SPELLING	DEV. AGE	PLACE OF ARTICULATION	VOICING	Stop Pre	Stop Inter	Stop Post	Fricative Pre	Fricative Inter	Fricative Post	Affricate Pre	Affricate Inter	Affricate Post	Glide Pre	Glide Inter	Glide Post	Lateral Pre	Lateral Inter	Lateral Post	Nasal Pre	Nasal Inter	Nasal Post
1	p	p	3	Bilabial	∀	/p	/p	/p															
2	b	b	5	Bilabial	v	/b	/b	/b															
3	ʍ	wh	3	Bilabial	∀				/ʍ¹														
4	w	w		Bilabial	v										/w	/w							
5	m	m	3	Bilabial	v																/m	/m	/m
6	f	f	4	Labio-dental	∀				/f	/f	/f												
7	v	v	7	Labio-dental	v				/v	/v	/v												
8	θ	th	7	Tip-dental	∀				/θ	/θ	/θ												
9	ð	th	8	Tip-dental	v				/ð	/ð	/ð												
10	t	t	6	Tip-alveolar	∀	/t	/t²	/t															
11	d	d	5	Tip-alveolar	v	/d	/d	/d															
12	l	l	6	Tip-alveolar	v													/l	/l	/l			
13	n	n	3	Tip-alveolar	v																/n	/n	/n
14	s	s	7	Blade-alveolar	∀				/s	/s	/s												
15	z	z	7	Blade-alveolar	v				/z	/z	/z												
16	ʃ	sh	6	Blade-prepalatal	∀				/ʃ	/ʃ	/ʃ												
17	ʒ	zh	7	Blade-prepalatal	v					/ʒ	/ʒ³												
18	tʃ	ch	6	Blade-prepalatal	∀							/tʃ	/tʃ	/tʃ									
19	dʒ	j	7	Blade-prepalatal	v							/dʒ	/dʒ	/dʒ									
20	j	y	5	Front-palatal	v										/j	/j							
21	r	r	6	Central-palatal	v										/r	/r	/r⁴						
22	k	k	4	Back-velar	∀	/k	/k	k															
23	g	g	4	Back-velar	v	/g	/g	/g															
24	ŋ	ng	5	Back-velar	v																	/ŋ	/ŋ
25	h	h	3	Glottal	∀		/h	/h	/h														

sound substitutions are reviewed for presence or absence of particular distinctive features. The idea underlying distinctive features is that a combination of elements or features characterize a given sound segment and that such features can distinguish one sound from other sounds within and across languages. Distinctive features are based on acoustic, perceptual, or articulatory characteristics. From a clinical perspective, distinctive features most easily adapted to assessment and treatment of phonological problems are those based primarily on articulatory characteristics. As discussed in Chapter 1, distinctive features typically include between 13 and 16 bipolar characteristics which are used to distinguish speech sound segments.

While there are a variety of ways to do a distinctive feature analysis, one feature analysis procedure designed for children's speech sound errors was published by McReynolds and Engmann (1975). They published a manual which described, step by step, how to conduct a substitution analysis based on distinctive features. When a deletion occurs, all the features in the target sounds are scored as absent or in error. A treatment program based on distinctive features is described in Chapter 10.

Some of the applications that speech-language pathologists have made of distinctive feature analysis have been the subject of criticism. It has been suggested that distinctive features, although helpful in classifying sounds of languages, may not be suited to the analysis of speech sound errors. Since distinctive feature systems were developed to classify the speech sounds of languages, they do not accurately describe many nonstandard (error) productions (e.g., certain sound distortions). The binary (plus or minus feature value) nature of the distinctive features may not reflect the varied productions seen in the speech of children with phonological disorders. A further problem is that the features of a deleted target sound are scored as errors although the sound and, as a result, the features were never attempted. For a critical discussion of the issues regarding the application of distinctive features to clinical analysis and intervention, the reader is referred to the papers by Walsh (1974), Parker (1976), and Foster, Riley, and Parker (1985).

Phonological Process Analysis. Since the late 1970s, several analysis procedures have been published that are based on the notion of phonological processes. Phonological analysis procedures have been published by Compton and Hutton (1978), Weiner (1979), Hodson (1986), Shriberg and Kwiatkowski (1980), Ingram (1981), Khan and Lewis (1986), and Bankson and Bernthal (1990). In all of these procedures, phonological patterns are described as phonological processes.

A phonological process or pattern is typically defined as a systematic sound change or simplification that affects a class of sounds, or a particular sequence of sounds. This general definition reflects the way the concept has been used by most clinical phonologists. As stated earlier, some authors limit their definition of processes to "natural" phonological processes (Shriberg and Kwiatkowski, 1980; Stampe, 1969, 1973). According to these authors, for a phonological pattern to be considered a "natural" phonological process, it cannot be merely a pattern reflecting simplification of a more complex articulatory gesture; it must also occur in sound changes documented in at least some other phonological phenomenon, such as historical language changes, slips of the tongue, dialectical variation, as well as in normal phonological acquisition.

As stated earlier, the child's underlying representation or knowledge about a sound is assumed to be similar to the adult form in most phonological process analysis procedures. The examiner's task then, is to note the speech sound mismatches with the adult standard, and identify the phonological patterns that may be present among these mismatches.

Some investigators have called for quantitative criteria to be used in the determination of phonological processes. McReynolds and Elbert (1981) suggested that some percentage of occurrence of a process be applied in determining if a given error pattern constitutes a phonological process. As a guideline for identifying error patterns as phonological processes, they recommended that an error pattern occur in at least four instances and in at least 20 percent of the items that could be affected by the process. McReynolds and Elbert (1981) also urged that certain qualitative conditions be met before a pattern is considered a process. For example, they recommended that the error sound be produced correctly and used contrastively in some context but not necessarily in the context in which the process appeared to be operating. For example, if /k/ is deleted in the word-final position but is used appropriately in word-initial position, this observation would indicate that the client can make the /k/ and a process is operating in the word-final position.

Phonological Process Delineation. Chapter 3 listed common phonological processes seen in the normal development of children's phonology. They are presented here in greater detail so that you can become more familiar with them. Although the process listings of different authors may vary, most resemble this listing.

Word and syllable structure processes. Syllable structure processes are changes that affect the syllabic structures of the target word.

1. *Final consonant deletion*. Deletion of the final consonant in a word.
   e.g. *book* [bu]
   cap [ka]
   fish [fɪ]

2. *Unstressed syllable deletion* (weak syllable deletion). An unstressed syllable is deleted, often at the beginning of a word, sometimes in the middle.
   e.g. *telephone* [tɛfon]
   potato [teto]
   elephant [ɛfʌnt]

3. *Cluster simplification*. A consonant cluster is simplified in some manner. The cluster can be reduced to one member of the consonant cluster, the entire cluster can be deleted, another sound can be substituted for the entire cluster, one member of the cluster is retained and a sound substitution is made for the other member of the cluster. Characteristics of features from two adjacent sounds combined so that one sound replaces two other sounds (*coalescence*).
   e.g. *stop* [tap]   *brown* [bwon]   *swim* [fɪm]
   milk [mɪ]   *park* [pak]   *snow* [n̥ou]
   tree [fi]   *skate* [at]

4. *Reduplication*. A syllable or a portion of a syllable is repeated or duplicated or

a portion of a target word (monosyllabic word) is repeated or duplicated; for example, a CV or CVC is produced as syllable utterances (CVCV).

  e.g. *dad* [dada]
     water [wawa]
     cat [kaka]

5. *Epenthesis*. A segment, usually the unstressed vowel [ɚ], is inserted.

  e.g. *black* [bɚlak]
     sweet [sɚwit]
     sun [sθʌn]

6. *Metathesis*. There is a transposition or reversal of two segments (sounds) in a word.

  e.g. *basket* [bæksɪt]
     spaghetti [pʌsgɛti]
     elephant [ɛfɚlʌnt]

Harmony processes. One sound is influenced by another sound where a sound assumes features or becomes similar to a second sound. Thus, the two segments become more alike (hence the term *harmony*) or, frequently, become identical. These sound changes are sometimes termed **progressive assimilation** if the sound that causes the sound change precedes the affected sound (*gate* [geɪk]) and **regressive assimilation** if the sound that causes the sound change follows the affected sound (*soup* [pup]).

1. Assimilation
 a. *Velar assimilation*. A nonvelar sound is assimilated (changed) to a velar sound because of the influence, or dominance, of the velar.

   e.g. *duck* [gʌk] (regressive assimilation)
      take [kek] (regressive assimilation)
      coat [kok] (progressive assimilation)

 b. *Nasal assimilation*. A nonnasal sound is assimilated because of the influence, or dominance, of a nasal consonant.

   e.g. *candy* [næni] (regressive assimilation)
      lamb [næm] (regressive assimilation)
      fun [nʌn] (regressive assimilation)

 c. *Labial assimilation*. A nonlabial sound is assimilated to a labial consonant because of the influence of a labial consonant.

   e.g. *bed* [bɛb] (progressive assimilation)
      table [bebu] (regressive assimilation)
      pit [pip] (progressive assimilation)

2. Voicing Changes
 a. *Prevocalic voicing*. Voicing of voiceless consonants (obstruents) in prevocalic position.

   e.g. *paper* [bepɚ]
      Tom [dam]
      table [debi]

 b. *Devoicing of final consonants*. Voiced obstruents are devoiced in final position.

   e.g. *dog* [dɔk]
      nose [nos]
      bed [bɛt]

Segment change (substitution) processes. One sound is substituted for another, with the replacement sound reflecting changes in place of articulation, manner of articulation, or some other change in the way a sound is produced in a standard production.

1. Place Changes
   a. *Fronting.* Substitutions are produced anterior, or forward of, the standard production.
      e.g. *shoe*   [su]   (palatal replaced by alveolar)
           key   [ti]   (velar replaced by alveolar)
           pitch [pɪts] (palatal replaced by alveolar)
   b. *Backing.* Sounds are substituted or replaced by segments produced posterior to, or further back in, the oral cavity than the standard production.
      e.g. *tan* [kæn]
           do   [gu]
           sip [ʃɪp]
2. Manner Changes
   a. *Stopping.* Fricatives or affricates are replaced by stops.
      e.g. *sun*   [tʌn]
           peach [pit]
           that   [dæt]
   b. *Affrication.* Fricatives are replaced by affricates.
      e.g. *saw*   [tʃau]
           shoe [tʃu]
           sun   [tʃʌn]
   c. *Gliding of liquids.* Prevocalic liquids are replaced by glides.
      e.g. *run*   [wʌn]
           yellow [jɛwo]
           leaf   [wif]
   d. *Vocalization.* Liquids or nasals are replaced by vowels.
      e.g. *bird*   [bɛd]
           table   [tebo]
           mother [mʌðɚ]
   e. *Denasalization.* Nasals are replaced by homorganic stops (place of articulation is similar to target sound).
      e.g. *moon* [bud]
           nice [deis]
           man   [bæn]
   f. *Deaffrication.* Affricates are replaced by fricatives.
      e.g. *chop* [sap]
           chip [ʃɪp]
           page [pez]
   g. *Glottal replacement.* Glottal stops replace sounds usually in either intervocalic or final position.
      e.g. *cat*   [kæʔ]
           tooth   [tuʔ]
           bottle [baʔl]

Multiple Pattern Occurrence. The examples of phonological patterns given above typically included lexical items in which only a single pattern was used. In reality, the child may produce forms that reflect more than one process, including some that are not reflected in the definitions and descriptions above. A single lexical item may have two or even more processes interacting. When such productions occur, they are more complex and difficult to unravel than words which reflect a single process. For example, in the production of [du] for *shoe*,

Edwards (1983) pointed out that the [d] for /ʃ/ replacement reflects the phonological processes of (1) depalatalization, which changes the place of articulation; (2) stopping, which changes the manner of articulation; and (3) prevocalic voicing, which changes a voiceless consonant target to a voiced consonant. In the substitution of [dar] for *car*, the [d] for /k/ substitution is accounted for by the processes of velar fronting and prevocalic voicing. The identification of the sequence of steps describing how interacting processes account for substitutions is called a **derivation** or **process ordering**. Determining process derivations within a speaker can be difficult and is beyond the scope of this textbook.

Unusual Pattern Occurrence. As indicated throughout this book, a great deal of individual variation exists in the phonological development of children. Although there are common developmental phonological patterns used by many children, the patterns observed across individuals vary. Unusual phonological patterns (e.g., use of a nasal sound for /s/ and /z/), called idiosyncratic processes or patterns, differ from the more common phonological processes and are seen in both children with normal and delayed phonological development. The greatest variation in phonological pattern usage occurs during the early stages of development and is probably influenced, in part, by the lexical items the child uses when acquiring his or her first words. When idiosyncratic patterns persist after age 3.0 to 3.5 years, they likely reflect a phonological disorder.

Conditions of Occurrence. In order to more accurately describe the child's phonological system, one should specify the conditions of occurrence in which a child's error or process is used. In the case of final consonant deletions, for example, the sound classes reflecting the process should be listed (e.g., stops, fricatives, and nasals). Likewise, in the case of assimilation, the clinician should determine which sounds or sound classes are being assimilated or influenced. Similarly, if velar fronting is observed, the clinician will need to indicate the word-positions in which the fronting occurs. Treatment planning is enhanced when the condition of occurrence of a process or the positional constraints of a phonetic production are identified.

Sound Preferences. Another type of sound pattern that some clinicians have reported is called sound preference. In these situations, children seem to have a segment or two that they use for a large number of sounds or sound classes. Sometimes a particular sound is substituted for several or even all phonemes in a particular sound class (e.g., fricatives). Other children will substitute a single consonant for a variety of segments, such as [h] for /b, d, s, ʒ, z, dʒ, tʃ, ʃ, l, k, g, r/ (Weiner, 1981). It has been postulated that some children avoid the use of certain sounds in their productions and, instead, use those sounds they find easiest to produce. The phenomenon of sound preference is not viewed as a phonological process by most clinicians.

The list of phonological processes presented above is not exhaustive but represents most of the common patterns seen in normally developing children. These phonological processes have also been used in analyzing the sound errors of phonologically delayed children. Several procedures designed to assist the clinician in the identification of phonological processes in children's speech have been published in monograph or kit form. Included in these procedures are various groupings, as well as additions and deletions to the processes listed above. At first glance, these procedures seem quite similar, but a closer examination reveals

Analysis and Interpretation of Assessment Data

significant differences among them. Table 7–1 reflects a modified version of Edwards' (1983) listing of the characteristics of published phonological assessment procedures.

Normative Data Regarding Process Usage. Preisser, Hodson, and Paden (1988), in a cross-sectional study, examined phonological process usage in young children. Between 24 and 29 months, the most commonly observed processes were cluster reduction, liquid deviation (which included deletions of a liquid in a consonant cluster, e.g., *black* → [bæk]), vowelization (e.g., *zipper* → [zɪpɚ]), and gliding of liquids (e.g., *red* → [wɛd]). Next most common were patterns involving the strident feature.

Roberts, Burchinal, and Footo (1990) observed a group of children between 2.5 and 8 years in a quasi-longitudinal study, that is, children were tested a varying number of times over the course of the study. They reported a marked decrease in process use between the ages of 2.5 and 4 years. They also reported percentage of occurrence (i.e., dividing the total number of occurrences for each process by the total number of opportunities for the occurrence of that process) of 20 percent or more for cluster reductions, deletion of final consonants, syllable reductions, liquid gliding, fronting, stopping, deletion of medial consonants and deaffrication. By age 4, only cluster reduction, liquid gliding, and deaffrication had a percentage of occurrence of 20 percent or more. They also reported that at 2.5 years the percentage of occurrence was less than 20 percent for the following processes: reduplication, assimilation, deletion of initial consonants, addition of a consonant, labialization shifts, metathesis, and backing.

Stoel-Gammon and Dunn (1985) reviewed studies of process occurrence and identified those processes which typically are deleted by age 3 and those that persist after 3 years. Their summary is presented below:

Processes Disappearing by 3 Years	Processes Persisting after 3 Years
Unstressed syllable deletion	Cluster reduction
Final consonant deletion	Epenthesis
Consonant assimilation	Gliding
Reduplication	Vocalization
Velar fronting	Stopping
Diminutization	Depalatalization
Prevocalic voicing	Final devoicing

Table 7–2 from Grunwell (1981) reflects "simplifying processes" used by young children in normal phonological development. The table is derived largely from data reported by Ingram (1976) and Anthony, Bogle, Ingram, and McIsaac (1971) and is based on a relatively small number of subjects. The solid lines reflect typical ages at which particular processes are evidenced, and the broken lines reflect the approximate ages at which the processes are modified or begin to disappear.

Bankson and Bernthal (1990) reported data on the processes most frequently observed in a sample of over 1,000 children, 3 to 9 years of age, tested during the standardization of the *Bankson-Bernthal Test of Phonology (BBTOP)*. The BBTOP ultimately included the 10 processes that appeared most frequently in children's productions during standardization testing. The processes which per-

TABLE 7–1. Characteristics of the Published Phonological Assessment Procedures.

BASIS OF COMPARISON	WEINER (1973)	SHRIBERG AND KWIATKOWSKI (1980)	HODSON (1986)	KHAN-LEWIS (1986)	BANKSON AND BERNTHAL (1990)
Stimuli	"Action" pictures	No specific stimuli	3-dimensional objects	Pictures from the *Goldman-Fristoe Test of Articulation*	Pictures from the *Bankson-Bernthal Test of Phonology*
Elicitation procedures	Delayed imitation and sentence recall	Continuous speech samples	Object-naming; no set order	Picture-naming in citation form	Picture-naming in citation form
Sample size	136 target words, said twice and control items	80–100 different words from 200–250 word sample	50 single words	44 single words	80 single words
Transcription	Live and from recordings	Narrow "on-line" and from tapes	Broad transcriptions are modified; audio taped for reference	Narrow "on-line" and from recordings	Live and from recordings
Number of processes	16	8 "natural" processes	30 processes	12 developmental processes 3 nondevelopmental processes	10 most frequently occurring processes in standardized samples
Target population	Unintelligible children, ages 2–5	Children with severely delayed speech	Children with multiple articulation errors	Normally developing and phonologically disordered children	Normally developing children and phonologically disordered children
Time (total)	±45 minutes with a cooperative child	About 1½ hours	±50 minutes	±35 minutes	±30 minutes
Number of processes per word	One test process; others noted	Two processes coded for some words	More than one process per word	All that apply are coded	All that apply are coded
Process descriptions	Conditions of occurrence noted	Organized by sound and position on summary sheet	Number of occurrences tabulated across sounds and positions	Organized by sounds and word-position	Organized by sounds and word-position
Frequency of occurrence	Percent calculated for each test process	Approximate frequency indicated on summary sheet	Calculation for 10 basic processes	Frequency of each of the 15 processes calculated	Frequency of each of the 10 processes calculated
Interacting processes	Not discussed	Only two combinations are coded	Errors coded under all appropriate processes	Errors coded under all appropriate processes	Errors coded under all appropriate processes

Analysis and Interpretation of Assessment Data

TABLE 7−2. **Chronology of Phonological Processes.**

	2;0–2;6	2;6–3;0	3;0–3;6	3;6–4;0	4;0–4;6	4;6–5;0	5;0→
Unstressed Syllable Deletion	▬▬▬	▬▬▬	▬▬▬	▬▬			
Final Consonant Deletion	▬▬▬	▬▬▬	▬				
Reduplication	▬▬						
Consonant Harmony	▬▬▬	▬▬					
Cluster Reduction (Initial)							
Obstruent— Approximant	▬▬▬	▬▬▬	▬▬▬	▬			
/s/ + Consonant	▬▬▬	▬▬▬	▬▬▬	▬			
Stopping /f/	▬▬▬	▬▬					
/v/		▬▬▬	▬▬				
/θ/ θ → [f]	▬▬▬	▬▬▬	▬▬▬	▬▬▬	▬▬▬	▬▬▬	▬▬▬
/ð/ /ð/ → [d] or [v]	▬▬▬	▬▬▬	▬▬▬	▬▬▬	▬▬▬	▬▬▬	▬▬▬
/s/	▬▬▬	▬▬▬	▬				
/z/			▬▬▬	▬			
/ʃ/ Fronting '[s] type'	▬▬▬	▬▬▬	▬▬▬	▬▬▬	▬		
/tʃ, dʒ/ Fronting [ts, dz]	▬▬▬	▬▬▬	▬▬▬	▬▬▬	▬▬▬	▬	
Fronting/k, g, ŋ/	▬▬▬	▬▬▬	▬				
Gliding r → [w]	▬▬▬	▬▬▬	▬▬▬	▬▬▬	▬▬▬	▬▬▬	▬▬▬
Context-Sensitive Voicing	▬▬▬	▬▬▬	▬				

Source: Adapted by permission from P. Grunwell, "The Development of Phonology: A Descriptive Profile." *First Language, 3* (1981): 161–191. Used with permission.

sisted the longest in children's speech were gliding of liquids, stopping, cluster simplification, vocalization, and final consonant deletion. These data are identical to those reported by Khan and Lewis (1986) in the standardization of the *Khan-Lewis Test of Phonological Processes,* except their results also included velar fronting as a process persisting in young children's speech.

The comparison of a client's use of phonological processes with normative data can be used in target selection. The processes used by a phonologically delayed child can be compared with those that might be expected in the speech of normally developing children. Those processes which usually are not present in normal children are targeted for intervention. One caution regarding this procedure should be pointed out. There are few, if any, data which would suggest that reduction in the use of phonological processes occurs in a prescribed order, although some processes tend to persist in older children and others tend to occur only in younger children. Moreover, there are no data suggesting that the elimination of one process in a child's speech should occur before another process is targeted for treatment. There are some general trends that may be helpful in targeting processes for treatment, but a universally prescribed development order for the deletion of processes has not been established.

Theoretical Considerations Regarding Phonological Processes

Description versus explanation

Some speech-language clinicians have suggested that the presence of phonological processes is evidence of a cognitive-linguistic deficit, thereby providing an *explanation* of the phonological errors. This is an inappropriate interpretation since phonological process analysis procedures are only *descriptive* devices and do not reveal causes or provide explanations of the error patterns. Smith (1981) warned that when studying phonological development with a linguistic-based pattern analysis, ". . . one must avoid falling into the trap of believing that a child's behavior has been *explained* by having written a series of formal rules or a list of processes relating to particular phonological observations" (11).

An example demonstrating the inherent difficulty in arriving at an explanatory statement for a given phonological process was provided by Hoffman and Schuckers (1984). One explanation for the occurrence of that process might be that the child misperceives the adult word, for example, perceives [dɔg] as [dɔ]. A second explanation might be that the child's underlying lexical representation for *dog* is [dɔ], so the closest match in his store of lexical items is [dɔ]; thus [dɔg] becomes [dɔ]. A third possible explanation is that the child's perceptual system functions appropriately and the lexical match between what the child perceives and what he or she has stored is consistent with the adult standard, but he or she has a phonological production rule that calls for the deletion of word-final stops. A fourth possibility is that the child has a motor production problem; in this case the child may have the appropriate perception but does not possess the necessary motor skill to make the articulation gesture to produce the sound.

This discussion is not intended to minimize the value of the information provided from a phonological process analysis, but rather to emphasize that when such procedures are used to analyze a child's speech, they serve to describe, not explain, behavior. In other words, when doing an analysis, one cannot assume that because a phonological process (e.g., final consonant deletion) has been identified, that such patterns can be attributed to specific cognitive-linguistic, perceptual, or motor explanations.

Underlying representation in phonological processes

Shelton (1986) has identified three different theoretical interpretations of phonological processes in the speech-language pathology literature. One view is that phonological processes constitute a taxonomy or listing of speech sound error patterns, a catalog of descriptors that can be used to identify the simplifications or modifications used by children. This view makes no speculations or assumptions regarding the child's underlying representations (mental images or internal knowledge of the lexical items) in relation to the adult standard; it simply describes behavior at the observable or surface level. This atheoretical perspective posits nothing about the operation of processes, the nature of phonological structure, the relationship of surface forms and underlying representations, or even the relationship of production and perception.

A second view of phonological processes assumes that the child has underlying representations of lexical forms that are similar to those of the adult surface forms. This view, which comes from work in normal phonological development, assumes that the child is attempting to produce the adult form of the word and has an adult-like mental image of the lexical item. The surface forms produced by the child, however, reflect an immature development. The child changes the target production in some manner during the production of the word.

Analysis and Interpretation of Assessment Data

It is these simplifications that are identified as errors in the individual's speech. The mismatches between the child's productions and his or her underlying representations (which are the same as the adult standard) are expressed as phonological processes.

The third theoretical position acknowledges the existence of underlying representations but makes no assumptions concerning their form. The clinician examines the child's surface forms (the child's articulatory productions) to determine the status or nature of the child's underlying representations. If a child uses a phoneme contrastively, it is assumed that he or she has the adult underlying form. If the child misarticulates a sound, and there is no evidence from phonological testing or acoustical analysis that the sound is in the child's repertoire, it is not assumed the child has the adult-like underlying representation of the sound. For example, if a child says [dɔ] for [dɔg] but uses [g] in the diminutive *doggy* [dɔgi], one can assume that the child has the underlying form for [g] since /g/ is produced in the form [dɔgi]. On the other hand, if /g/ is not observed in any of the child's utterances, no assumption is made regarding the underlying form for /g/. Thus, this view of underlying structures differs from the second view, described above, in that it makes no assumptions concerning the underlying representations; the second assumes the child has the adult form.

Elbert and Gierut (1986) have sought to provide data to support their concept of underlying forms. On the basis of observed phonological productions, they described what they call children's "phonological knowledge," and made inferences from these data about underlying forms. From their perspective, the more knowledge a child has about sounds, the more inferences can be made with respect to the child's underlying forms. Phonological knowledge was determined in a variety of ways, including (1) correct use of the error phoneme in other word-positions; (2) correct use of the error phoneme in different contexts; (3) stimulability testing; (4) morphophonemic alternation tasks, for example, [dɔ] for *dog* but [dɔgi] for *doggy*, [pɪ] for *pig* but [pɪgi] for *piggy*; and (5) acoustic analysis, for example, evidence of a glottal gesture in the word-final position on a spectrogram when the examiner transcribed the final consonant as a deletion. When a child demonstrated phonological knowledge on one of the tasks, the investigators inferred that the child's underlying representation was similar to the adult.

CONTEXTUAL ANALYSIS

As stated in Chapter 6, contextual testing is concerned with the influence of surrounding sounds on a particular sound that is not produced correctly. Contextual testing may identify facilitating phonetic contexts in which surrounding sounds have a positive influence on the production of error sounds. Contextual testing provides data on phonetic contexts in which an error sound may be produced correctly and be helpful in determining a treatment program. Thus, contextual testing is to determine the *focus* of treatment rather than the *need* for treatment. Through the identification of such contexts, the clinician may find that a specific sound doesn't have to be taught because it is already in the client's repertoire. Both the client and clinician may save time and frustration that often accompany initial attempts to produce a speech sound by focusing first on a certain context in which a sound is produced correctly and then gradually shifting to other contexts. In general, when contexts can be found where target sounds are produced correctly, such sounds take less time to correct in remediation. The number of contexts in which a child can produce a sound correctly on a deep test may provide some indication of the stability of the error. It seems logical that the less stable the error, the easier it may be to correct. However, some clinicians find that a stable error pattern is easier to focus on than is a more "elusive" error. The clinician can utilize those contexts in which a segment is produced correctly to reinforce correct production and facilitate generalization to other contexts. If a client's error tends to be inconsistent across different phonetic contexts, one might assume that the chances for improvement are better than if the error tends to persist across different phonetic contexts or situations. This assumption, however, has yet to be demonstrated. For a more complete discussion of contextual testing, see the discussion in Chapter 6.

OTHER PHONOLOGICAL CONSIDERATIONS IN TARGET BEHAVIOR SELECTION

STIMULABILITY DATA

Stimulability testing consists of assessing client performance when the client is asked to imitate the adult form of speech sound errors in isolation, syllables, or words. Stimulability testing has been used as a prognostic indicator for (1) self-correction of individual segments (sounds), (2) contextual generalization, (3) evidence of the child's phonological knowledge (through imitation at the word level), and (4) response to instruction. Thus, results from this type of testing are considered in case selection decisions. The main purpose of stimulability testing, however, is to aid in selecting target behaviors for instruction and determining the direction of treatment. A more complete discussion of the clinical utilization of stimulability testing was presented in Chapter 6, and the reader is encouraged to review the section on stimulability assessment in that chapter.

Intervention should be initiated at the level of the most complex linguistic unit the client can imitate (i.e., isolation, syllable, word, phrase). In choosing target behaviors for instruction, it may be useful to select exemplars on which the child is stimulable in order to facilitate generalization. Sounds from different sound classes are usually chosen as examplars, with stimulability data aiding in their selection. For example, if word-final stops, fricatives, and nasals are all deleted, the clinician might target one stimulable stop, fricative, and nasal as exemplars.

FREQUENCY OF OCCURRENCE

A factor used in target behavior selection is the frequency with which the sounds produced in error occur in the language. Obviously, the greater the frequency of a sound in a language, the greater its potential effect on intelligibility. Thus, treatment will have the greatest impact on a client's overall intelligibility if frequently occurring segments produced in error are selected for treatment.

Table 7–3 lists the rank order and frequency of occurrence of the 24 most frequently used consonants in conversational American English (Shriberg and Kwiatkowski, 1983). These statistics are based on a collection of natural speech data from a variety of sources. Mines, Hanson, and Shoup (1978) noted a relatively

TABLE 7–3. Percentage of Occurrence of (Intended) English Consonants in Continuous Speech.

SOUND	MEAN Rank	MEAN %	HOFFMANN (1982)	IRWIN AND WONG (1983)*	CARTERETTE AND JONES (1974)	MADER (1954)	SHRIBERG AND KWIATKOWSKI (1982)	SHRIBERG AND KWIATKOWSKI (1983)	MINES ET AL. (1978)
n	1	12.01	11.22	9.84	13.63	13.14	11.7	13.04	11.49
t	2	11.83	12.43	14.05	7.91	11.74	13.7	13.08	9.88
s	3	6.90	6.78	6.66	6.94	6.50	7.1	6.43	7.88
r	4	6.68	7.06	5.99	8.20	7.83	5.2	5.84	6.61
d	5	6.41	4.26	6.89	6.31	10.25	5.8	5.33	5.70
m	6	5.93	5.20	5.52	7.49	4.63	5.6	7.97	5.11
z	7	5.36	8.69	4.88	4.58	3.70	3.0	3.97	4.70
ð	8	5.32	6.90	6.04	4.42	6.40	4.1	4.04	5.37
l	9	5.25	3.42	5.41	4.96	5.55	5.6	5.59	6.21
k	10	5.13	4.60	5.20	4.96	4.25	6.0	5.57	5.30
w	11	4.88	4.19	4.70	5.57	5.33	4.8	4.79	4.81
h	12	4.38	7.47	5.17	3.37	3.33	4.2	4.97	2.23
b	13	3.28	2.84	3.40	3.18	2.97	3.5	3.92	3.24
p	14	3.12	2.98	3.12	2.12	2.73	3.9	3.90	3.07
g	15	3.08	3.93	3.29	2.90	2.38	4.1	2.93	2.02
f	16	2.07	2.38	1.64	2.21	1.83	2.4	1.37	2.65
ŋ	17	1.58	.94	1.86	1.05	1.61	2.5	1.24	1.85
j	18	1.56	1.22	1.49	1.41	0.77	2.2	1.94	1.87
v	19	1.52	1.03	1.46	1.64	1.91	1.2	0.42	2.97
ʃ	20	0.93	0.87	1.14	0.84	0.84	1.5	0.38	0.95
θ	21	0.89	0.59	0.84	1.03	0.93	0.9	0.76	1.19
dʒ	22	0.58	0.62	0.50	0.53	0.69	0.6	0.19	0.95
tʃ	23	0.55	0.34	0.31	0.51	0.55	0.7	0.56	0.85
ʒ	24	0.03	0.01	0.01	0	0.01	0	0	0.15

* Data calculated from page 156, Table 8.4 to reflect only children aged 3, 4, and 6 years.
Source: L. Shriberg and F. Kwiatkowski, "Computer-Assisted Natural Process Analysis (NPA): Recent Issues and Data." In Assessing and Treating Phonological Disorders: Current Approaches. J. Locke (Ed.), Seminars in Speech and Language, 4 (1983): 397. Used by permission.

high correlation among all frequency counts, based on both spoken and written expression. Seven consonants /n, t, s, r, d, m, z/ account for over half of all consonant occurrences in our language. However, consonants /n, t, s, r, l, d, ð, k, m, w, z/ occur very frequently in connected speech and errors on these sounds will adversely affect intelligibility. Other data reported in the table showed that almost two thirds of the consonants used are voiced, 29 percent are stops, 19 percent are sonorants, and 18 percent are nasals. Moreover, three of the six stops /t, d, k/, three of four sonorants /r, l, w/, and two of three nasals /n, m/ are among the 11 most frequently occurring consonants. Dental and alveolar consonants accounted for 61 percent of the productions and labial and labiodental sounds, 21 percent. In other words, over four fifths of consonant occurrences are produced at the anterior area of the mouth.

EASE OF PRODUCTION

Sounds produced in error may also be analyzed in terms of ease of production. Adult speakers' subjective ratings regarding the amount of effort required to produce certain sounds have been recorded (Malecot, 1970; Locke, 1972; Parnell and Amerman, 1977). In general, speakers have judged early appearing sounds and frequently occurring sounds as easiest to produce.

Locke (1983) explained continuity between babbling and the child's success with particular phonemes in early lexical productions in terms of similarity between phonetic forms used in prelexical babbling and those appearing in early lexical productions. Babbling repetitions of "mamamama," for example, are similar in form to the lexical "mama." In other words, the early lexical productions of "mama" seem to differ very little, if any, from prelexical productions. The child finds certain forms communicatively useful and then produces them. One might hypothesize that the phonetic productions (e.g., [mama] or [dada]) that are almost universally seen in babbling and early lexical productions may be easier for the client to learn than a phonetic form such as [dʒ], which occurs infrequently in communication, is used in a minority of languages of the world, and is not heard in deaf babbling at 6 months. Natural productions like [d], seen in babbling and early lexical productions, may be less difficult phonetic productions. A clinical implication of this concept is that easier-to-produce sounds require less instructional time to modify than more-difficult-to-produce sounds.

CONTRAST TRAINING TARGETS

A phonological treatment approach designed to establish phonemic contrasts, is frequently employed with phonologically delayed children. There are two common strategies in selection of targets to be used in therapy designed to establish contrasts. One strategy is that the phonemic contrast targeted for treatment should reflect minimal feature differences (e.g., *p*ig–*b*ig), while another is that sounds targeted for contrast training should reflect maximal contrasts (e.g., *s*ad–*m*ad). Both minimal contrast treatment and maximal contrast treatment have been reported to be effective in the modification of the phonological systems of children displaying speech sound errors (Weiner, 1981; Gierut, 1989).

Although these contrast training strategies share certain similarities, Gierut (1989) has indicated that they differ in two basic ways: (1) the number of distinctive oppositions (features) that are contrasted in a given word-pair as delineated in

Analysis and Interpretation of Assessment Data

the preceding paragraph and (2) the relationship of the sounds contrasted to the child's existing grammar (phonology). Thus, minimal and maximal opposition strategies differ in the number of feature differences between sound pairs (one vs. several), and the nature of these relative to the child's phonology, i.e., minimal pairs (error vs. target production); maximal pairs (target production vs. another sound already in the child's repertoire).

Minimal pair contrast training typically involves having a child distinguish (first through perception, then imitation and then spontaneous production) between pairs of syllables or words that differ along a single feature contrast, such as manner, place, or voicing. For example, the word pairs *coat–goat* and *gate–date* each differ by a single feature.

Maximal feature contrast training uses word-pairs that encompass several feature differences (e.g., *tell–shell, can–van*). In other words, the contrastive sounds for maximal feature contrast training differ in several features.

Clinicians more commonly employ minimal as opposed to maximal contrasts in target selection, although both procedures are designed to reduce homonymy by increasing contrast usage. Based on the limited data available (Gierut, 1990), maximal contrasts may be a more efficacious strategy for enhancing some children's phonological systems.

ASSESSMENT OF PHONOLOGICAL KNOWLEDGE

Elbert and Gierut (1986) suggested that phonological assessment should include a determination of a client's "productive phonological knowledge" (child's cognitive awareness of a particular sound at a linguistic level). These authors have postulated that the consistency with which a phoneme is used across morphemes and word-positions is a reflection of the child's phonological knowledge of that phoneme. In Table 7–4 Gierut (1986) identified a continuum of knowledge types, with 1 representing "most knowledge" about a sound and 6 representing "least knowledge" of a sound. As can be seen in Table 7–4, a child displaying Type 2 knowledge of [s] would produce the sound correctly for all morphemes and word-positions, with the occasional substitution of /t/ for /s/ in word-final position. By contrast, a child displaying Type 5 knowledge of [s] would inconsistently produce this sound correctly in the initial position, while [s] morphemes in word-final positions would always be produced incorrectly.

Gierut, Elbert, and Dinnsen (1987) reported that when phonological intervention was directed toward those error sounds that evidenced "least knowledge" (as opposed to "most knowledge"), the greatest changes in a child's phonology occurred. In the continuum of knowledge, as reflected in Table 7–4, it is assumed that the extent of misarticulation is a reflection of the degree of an individual's phonological knowledge. In terms of making the most efficacious decisions relative to target behavior selection, Elbert and Gierut (1986) suggested selecting those sounds for treatment that reflect the least phonological knowledge. They observed greater generalization to untrained sounds when they targeted sounds reflecting least phonological knowledge than when they targeted those with most phonological knowledge. They hypothesized that focusing on least knowledge resulted in greater overall reorganization of a child's phonological system, and thus greater generalization.

Gierut (1986) outlined several steps involved in determining a person's pho-

TABLE 7–4. **Phonological Knowledge Continuum.**

KNOWLEDGE TYPE	DESCRIPTION	EXAMPLE		
1	A child displaying Type 1 knowledge of target [s] would produce this sound correctly in all word-positions and for all morphemes; [s] would never be produced incorrectly.	[sʌn] [sup] [mɛsi] [mɪsɪŋ] [mɪs]	sun soup messy missing miss	
2	A child displaying Type 2 knowledge of target [s] would produce this sound correctly for all morphemes and positions. However, a phonological rule would apply to account for observed alternations between, for example, [s] and [t] in morpheme-final position.	[sʌn] [sup] [mɛsi] [aɪs; BUT: 	sun soup messy ice [mɪs]–[mɪt] [kɪs]–[kɪt]	 miss kiss
3	A child displaying Type 3 knowledge of target [s] would produce this sound correctly in all positions. However, certain morphemes that were presumably acquired early and acquired incorrecly (i.e., "fossilized") would always be produced in error.	[sʌn] [mɛsi] [mɪs] BUT: 	sun messy miss [nænə] [wu]	 Santa juice
4	A child displaying Type 4 knowledge of target [s] would produce this sound correctly for all morphemes in, for example, initial position. However, production of [s] would be incorrect for all morphemes in medial and final positions.	[sʌn] [sup] BUT: 	sun soup [mɛti] [mɪtɪŋ] [mɪt] [kɪt]	 messy missing miss kiss
5	A child displaying Type 5 knowledge of]target [s] would produce this sound correctly in, for example, initial position. However, only some morphemes in this position would be produced correctly. All [s] morphemes in postvocalic positions would be produced incorrectly.	[sʌn] [sup] BUT: 	sun soup [top] [tak] [mɛti] [kɪt]	 soap sock messy kiss
6	A child displaying Type 6 knowledge of target [s] would produce this sound incorrectly in all word-positions and for all morphemes; [s] would never be produced correctly.	[tʌn] [tup] [mɪtɪŋ] [mɪt] [kɪt]	sun soup missing miss kiss	

Source: Description and examples of six types of productive knowledge. From J. Gierut, "On the Assessment of Productive Phonological Knowledge." *NSSLHA Journal,* 14 (1986), p. 88.

nological knowledge at a productive level. Included among these steps are the following:

1. Obtain a representative sample of speech. Ideally this would include both connected speech and spontaneous single-word utterances in order that a sample of all English sounds in at least three word-positions can be obtained. Sounds should be sampled more than once in each position.

2. Determine the type of knowledge that a child displays for each target sound according to the continuum of knowledge (Table 7–4).

3. Establish what the child has yet to learn. This is done by ranking a child's phonological knowledge on a continuum ranging from "most" to "least" phonological knowledge for each target phoneme.

4. Select treatment sounds and goals based on the treatment continuum.

OTHER FACTORS TO CONSIDER IN CASE SELECTION— CLINICAL MANAGEMENT DECISIONS

DIALECTAL CONSIDERATIONS

The linguistic culture of the speaker is a factor which must be considered when deciding on the need for speech-language intervention, particularly for those clients from ethnic or minority populations, where standard English may not be the norm. Dialect refers to a consistent variation of a language, reflected in pronunciation, grammar, or vocabulary, that is used by a particular subgroup of the general population. Although many dialects are identified with a geographical area, those of greatest concern to clinicians are dialects related to sociocultural or ethnic identification.

The phonological patterns of a particular dialect will differ to some degree from the general cultural norm, but these variations reflect only *differences* and not delays or deficiencies in comparison to the so-called standard version of the language. To view the phonological or syntactic patterns used by members of such subcultures as delayed, deviant, or substandard is totally inappropriate. As Williams (1972) put it, "The relatively simple yet important point here is that language variation is a logical and expected phenomenon, hence, we should not look upon nonstandard dialects as *deficient* versions of a language" (111). This perspective has obvious clinical implications since persons whose speech and language patterns reflect a cultural dialect should not be considered for remediation unless their phonological patterns are outside the cultural norm for the region or ethnic group, or the individual wishes to learn a standard dialect.

Phonological differences may also occur in the speech of individuals within subcultures. The language patterns of inner-city African-Americans in New York City, for example, may be quite different from those in New Orleans. The point, then, is that (1) one cannot use normative data based on general American English to judge the phonological status of individuals of some subcultures, and (2) one should not assume that members of certain subcultures have homogeneous linguistic patterns, especially when geographic or ethnic factors are considered. The phonological characteristics of selected dialects with implications for treatment are discussed in Chapter 4. The reader should refer to this chapter for further information on this topic.

SOCIAL–VOCATIONAL EXPECTATIONS

Another factor to consider in the analysis and interpretation of a phonological sample is the attitude of the client or the client's parents toward the individual's phonological status. In borderline cases (those for whom a treatment recommendation is debatable), attitude may be a factor in decisions for or against intervention. Extreme concern over a relatively minor articulatory difference by the client or the client's parents may convince the clinician to enroll an individual for instruction. For example, the child who has a frontal lisp and also has a name that begins with /s/ may feel very strongly that the error is a source of embarrassment. Kleffner (1952) found that fourth-grade children react unfavorably to children who have only one or two frequently occurring speech sound errors. There are many reports in the literature wherein elementary children have recounted negative experiences in speaking or reading situations when they produced only a few speech sounds in error. Even "minor distortions" can influence how one is perceived. Silverman (1976) reported that when a female speaker simulated a lateral lisp, listeners judged her more negatively on a personality characteristics inventory than when she spoke without a lisp.

The standard for acceptance of communication depends, to a large extent, on the speaking situation. People in public speaking situations may find that even minor distortions detract from their message. Some vocations, for example, radio and television broadcasters, may call for very precise pronunciations, and thus, some individuals may feel the need for intervention for what may be relatively minor phonetic distortions. We suggest that if an individual, regardless of age, feels handicapped by speech errors, treatment should usually be provided.

OTHER CONSIDERATIONS

In addition to the factors delineated above, the results of related tests (e.g., hearing and the oral cavity examination) are reviewed in making case selection decisions. Presence of suspected sensory, structural, or neurological deficiencies must be corroborated by appropriate related personnel (e.g., audiological, medical) and recommendations from those sources are taken into consideration. Any of these factors may be important in decisions regarding the need for therapy, the point at which therapy should begin, and the treatment to be prescribed. Related testing was discussed in greater detail in Chapter 6.

GUIDELINES FOR INTERVENTION

1. Clients, age 3 years or older, who evidence pronounced intelligibility and/or severity problems are priority candidates for intervention; children younger than 2.5 years and candidates for intervention are usually recommended for parent stimulation programs.
2. Children, age 8 and below, whose phonological performance is at least one standard deviation below the mean for their age are candidates for intervention.
3. Most children 9 years or older are candidates for intervention if they have consistently produced speech sound errors.
4. Adults who perceive that their phonological errors constitute a handicap should be considered for instruction. Likewise, children should be considered for intervention when they or their parents are very concerned about their speech sound productions.
5. Individuals whose phonological patterns reflect cultural or regional dialects are not considered to have communication disorders. If phonological differences occur that are outside their linguistic cultural norm, the individual may be a candidate for therapy. Individuals who reflect dialectical variation and wish to learn standard American dialect may also be candidates for intervention.
6. When selecting target behaviors, consideration is given to sounds that are in the client's repertoire, sounds with a high frequency of occurrence in the language, age of acquisition, phonological patterns, and some would suggest productive phonological knowledge.
7. Phonological patterns given priority for intervention are (a) those that may interfere the most with intelligibility, (b) those that cut across sound classes, and (c) those that tend to disappear at the earliest age from a normal child's speech.
8. Perceptual training is recommended when it has been ascertained that a client has a perceptual problem.

Analysis and Interpretation of Assessment Data

REFERENCES

Anthony, A., D. Bogle, T. Ingram, and M. McIsaac, *Edinburgh Articulation Test*. Edinburgh: Churchill Livingstone, 1971.

Bankson, N.W., and J.E. Bernthal, *Bankson-Bernthal Test of Phonology*. Chicago: Riverside Press, 1990.

Compton, A., and S. Hutton, *Compton-Hutton Phonological Assessment*. San Francisco: Carousel House, 1978.

Edwards, M., "Issues in phonological assessment." In J. Locke (Ed.), *Assessing and Treating Phonological Disorders: Current Approaches. Seminars in Speech and Language, 4*. New York: Thieme-Stratton, 1983.

Elbert, M., and J. Gierut, *Handbook of Clinical Phonology Approaches to Assessment and Treatment*. San Diego: College-Hill Press, 1986.

Elbert, M., T.W. Powell, and P. Swartzlander, "Toward a technology of generalization: How many exemplars are sufficient?" *Journal of Speech and Hearing Research, 34* (1991): 81–87.

Fisher, H.B., and J.A. Logemann, *The Fisher-Logemann Test of Articulation Competence*. Boston: Houghton Mifflin, 1971.

Foster, D., K. Riley, and F. Parker, "Some problems in the clinical applications of phonological theory." *Journal of Speech and Hearing Disorders, 50* (1985): 294–297.

Fudala, J., *Arizona Articulation Proficiency Scale: Revised*. Los Angeles: Western Psychological Services, 1970.

Gierut, J.A., "On the assessment of productive phonological knowledge." NSSLHA Journal, *14* (1986): 83–100.

Gierut, J.A., "Maximal opposition approach to phonological treatment." *Journal of Speech and Hearing Disorders, 54* (1989): 9–19.

Gierut, J.A., "Differential learning of phonological oppositions." *Journal of Speech and Hearing Research, 33* (1990): 540–549.

Gierut, J.A., M. Elbert, and D.A. Dinnsen, "A functional analysis of phonological knowledge and generalization learning in misarticulating children," *Journal of Speech and Hearing Research, 30* (1987): 462–479.

Grunwell, P., "The development of phonology: A descriptive profile." *First Language, 3* (1981): 161–191.

Hodson, B., *The Assessment of Phonological Processes*. Danville, Ill.: Interstate Press, 1986.

Hoffman, P.R., and G.H. Schuckers, "Articulation remediation treatment models." In R.G. Daniloff (Ed.), *Articulation Assessment and Treatment Issues*. San Diego: College-Hill Press, 1984.

Ingram, D., *Phonological Disability in Children*. New York: American Elsevier, 1976.

Ingram, D., *Procedures for the Phonological Analysis of Children's Language*. Baltimore: University Park Press, 1981.

Khan, L.M., and N.P. Lewis, *Khan-Lewis Phonological Analysis*. Circle Pines, Minn.: American Guidance Service, 1986.

Kleffner, F., "A comparison of the reactions of a group of fourth grade children to recorded examples of defective and nondefective articulation." Ph.D. thesis, University of Wisconsin, 1952.

Locke, J.L., "Ease of articulation." *Journal of Speech and Hearing Research, 15* (1972): 194–200.

Locke, J.L., *Phonological Acquisition and Change*. New York: Academic Press, 1983.

McReynolds, L.V., and M. Elbert, "Criteria for phonological process analysis." *Journal of Speech and Hearing Disorders, 46* (1981): 197–204.

McReynolds, L., and D. Engmann, *Distinctive Feature Analysis of Misarticulations*. Baltimore: University Park Press, 1975.

Malecot, A., "The Lenis-Fortis opposition: Its physiological parameters." *Journal of the Acoustical Society of America, 47* (1970): 1588–1592.

Mines, M., B. Hanson, and J. Shoup, "Frequency of occurrence of phonemes in conversational English." *Language and Speech, 21* (1978): 221–241.

Parker, F., "Distinctive features in speech pathology: Phonology of phonemics?" *Journal of Speech and Hearing Disorders, 41* (1976): 23–39.

Parnell, M., and J. Amerman, "Subjective evaluation of articulatory effort." *Journal of Speech and Hearing Research, 20* (1977): 644–652.

Prather, E., D. Hedrick, and C. Kern, "Articulation development in children aged two to four years." *Journal of Speech and Hearing Disorders, 40* (1975): 179–191.

Preisser, D.A., B.W. Hodson, and E.P. Paden, "Developmental phonology: 18–29 months." *Journal of Speech and Hearing Disorders, 53* (1988): 125–130.

Roberts, J.E., M. Burchinal, and M.M. Footo, "Phonological process decline from 2½ to 8 years." *Journal of Communication Disorders, 23* (1990): 205–217.

Sander, E., "When are speech sounds learned?" *Journal of Speech and Hearing Disorders, 37* (1972): 55–63.

Shelton, R., Personal Communication, 1986.

Shriberg, L., and J. Kwiatkowski, *Natural Process Analysis*. New York: John Wiley, 1980.

Shriberg, L.D., and J. Kwiatkowski, "Phonological disorders III: A procedure for assessing severity of involvement." *Journal of Speech and Hearing Disorders, 47* (1982): 256–270.

Shriberg, L., and J. Kwiatkowski, "Computer-assisted natural process analysis (NPA): Recent issues and data." In J. Locke (Ed.), *Assessing and Treating Phonological Disorders: Current Approaches. Seminars in Speech and Language, 4.* New York: Thieme-Stratton, 1983.

Silverman, E., "Listeners' impressions of speakers with lateral lisps." *Journal of Speech and Hearing Disorders, 41* (1976): 547–552.

Smit, A.B., "Ages of speech sound acquisition: Comparisons and critiques of several normative studies." *Language, Speech, and Hearing Services in Schools, 17* (1986): 175–186.

Smit, A.B., L. Hand, J.J. Freilinger, J.E. Bernthal, and A. Bird, "The Iowa articulation norms project and its Nebraska replication." *Journal of Speech and Hearing Disorders, 55* (1990): 779–798.

Smith, B.L., "Explaining the development of speech production skills in young children." *Journal of the National Student Speech-Language-Hearing Association, 9* (1981): 9–19.

Stampe, D., "The acquisition of phonetic representation." Papers from the Fifth Regional Meeting of the Chicago Linguistic Society, 1969.

Stampe, D., "A dissertation on natural phonology." Ph.D. thesis, University of Chicago, 1973.

Stephens, M.I., P. Hoffman, and R. Daniloff, "Phonetic characteristics of delayed /s/ development." *Journal of Phonetics, 14* (1986): 247–256.

Stoel-Gammon, C., and C. Dunn, *Normal and Disordered Phonology in Children.* Baltimore: University Park Press, 1985.

Templin, M., *Certain Language Skills in Children.* Institute of Child Welfare Monograph Series, 26. Minneapolis: University of Minnesota, 1957.

Templin, M., and F. Darley, *The Templin-Darley Tests of Articulation.* Iowa City, Iowa: Bureau of Educational Research and Service, University of Iowa, 1969.

Turton, L.J., "Developmental bases of articulation assessment." 129–155. In W.D. Wolfe and D.J. Goulding (Eds.), *Articulation and Learning.* 2nd Ed. Springfield, Ill.: Charles C Thomas, 1980.

Van Riper, C., *Speech Correction: Principles and Methods.* Englewood Cliffs, N.J.: Prentice Hall, 1939.

Walsh, H., "On certain practical inadequacies of distinctive feature systems." *Journal of Speech and Hearing Disorders, 39* (1974): 32–43.

Weiner, F., *Phonological Process Analysis.* Baltimore: University Park Press, 1979.

Weiner, F.F., "Systematic sound preference as a characteristic of phonological disability." *Journal of Speech and Hearing Disorders, 46* (1981): 281–286.

Williams, F., *Language and Speech: Introductory Perspectives.* Englewood Cliffs, N.J.: Prentice Hall, 1972.

Winitz, H., *Articulatory Acquisition and Behavior.* Englewood Cliffs, N.J.: Prentice Hall, 1969.

chapter

8

Computerized
Phonological Analysis

Julie J. Masterson, Department of Speech and Hearing Science, Arizona State University

Steven H. Long, Department of Speech Pathology and Audiology, Ithaca College

INTRODUCTION

Talking with speech-language pathologists over the years, we have heard various descriptions of a dream for clinical technology. In this dream a clinician records a child's speech sample, drops the tape into a sleek hi-tech box, presses a few buttons, and then collects a printed phonetic transcript and analysis of phonological patterns. Regrettably, this IS only a dream and we have little idea when, if ever, it will be realized. In the meantime, clinicians should become aware of computerized methods for phonological analysis (CPA) that DO exist and the different ways in which they work. This knowledge will help practitioners to make wise consumer decisions in acquiring computer hardware and software and to make appropriate clinical use of the available technology.

A number of advantages have been claimed for CPA, but, for clinicians, two stand out ahead of the others: (1) it saves time and (2) it provides greater detail of analysis. Clinicians usually have large caseloads and it is impossible to spend several hours analyzing samples from each client. Some CPA packages can derive a phonetic inventory and perform a substitution and phonological rules analysis on a 400-word sample in less than a minute! Although some time is required for data entry, this leaves most of the clinician's time available for interpretation of results and planning of appropriate therapy, two things that a computer alone cannot do.

To organize our discussion of CPA we have identified five parameters by which various programs can be evaluated and judged. These parameters are (1) the method of data entry, (2) the method of data processing, (3) the options for output of analyses, (4) hardware requirements, and (5) documentation and support. From the consumer's perspective, these five features largely determine whether a program is affordable, whether it is practical to use, and whether it yields analyses that are clinically valuable. In the second half of this chapter, we review seven currently available CPA packages in relation to each of these five issues. The CPA programs we examine are Computer Analysis of Phonological Processes Version 1.0 (CAPP) (Hodson, 1985), Computerized Profiling (CP) (Long and Fey 1988; in press, a and b), Logical International Phonetic Programs Version 1.03 (LIPP) (Oller and Delgado, 1990), The Macintosh Interactive System for Phonological Analysis (Mac-ISPA) (Masterson and Pagan, in press), Process Analysis Version 2.0 (PAC) (Weiner, 1986), Pye Analysis of Language Version 2.0 (PAL) (Pye, 1987), and Programs to Examine Phonetic and Phonologic Evaluation Records Version 4.0 (PEPPER) (Shriberg, 1986).

DATA ENTRY

From the user's perspective, a critical feature of any CPA program is its scheme of data entry. This scheme determines, in large part, how easy the software is to learn and to use. Below we discuss some of the variables in organization of data entry used by different CPA programs.

LIMITATIONS OF THE KEYBOARD

CPA software must provide a means for inputting phonetic transcriptions from a computer keyboard, displaying these data on the screen, and printing the transcriptions on paper. Microcomputers can be programmed to work with either text (letters and numbers) or graphics ("pictures" composed of dots). Text programs are simpler and require less hardware to operate than graphics programs. Text characters are entered by pressing keys on the keyboard and are represented on the screen and on paper by using a set of codes stored in the machine. The limitations of text programming for CPA software are that (1) not all IPA characters and diacritics are available as text characters, and (2) characters must be displayed in a left-to-right sequence. This left-to-right display does not permit diacritics to be positioned above, below, or to the upper right of sound segments.

A programmer has two solutions for these keyboard limitations. In the first solution, letters and symbols that are present on the keyboard are substituted for those international phonetic alphabet (IPA) symbols that are not available (e.g., the schwa vowel may be represented with the symbol "@"). Diacritics are always placed to the right of the consonant or vowel segments they modify. To operate a program written in this way, the user must apply the symbol substitution scheme in order to input data and to read and interpret the output. Essentially, the user must learn an alternate system of phonetic representation and be able to switch back and forth between this system and the IPA. When programs of this kind are first used, there is likely to be some confusion and mental effort, which decreases as the user becomes more familiar with the other transcriptional system.

The second solution for keyboard limitations is to use graphics to represent all IPA symbols. This method requires special hardware that allows the computer to create "pictures" on both the screen and the printer. It also requires a system for inputting each IPA symbol. The usual technique for inputting phonetic symbols is to retain all the key-to-symbol correspondences that exist on the computer keyboard (e.g., typing a lower case "p" inputs the symbol for a /p/) and to use unique key combinations for entering all other symbols (e.g., holding down the "control" key while typing "s" may produce the symbol for a /ʃ/). The user must learn the keyboard mapping scheme of the software, and touch typing may be somewhat difficult because of the need to press more than one key simultaneously.

CORRESPONDENCE BETWEEN TARGET AND PRODUCTION FORMS

Substitution and omission analyses are accomplished by comparing target sounds with transcriptions of a client's productions. CPA software must be able to determine "what corresponds to what." For example, if [ti] was produced for the target /klin/, the program must recognize that the target cluster /kl/ was realized as [t], the target vowel /i/ as [i], and the /n/ was omitted.

Software must either automatically establish correspondences between target sounds and production forms or rely on the user to specify the correspondences. If the user is to specify the correspondences, the data must be entered in a format that somehow indicates the boundaries of phonological units in both the target and production forms. One way to accomplish this is to require that the two forms be vertically aligned. For example, in the case of /smok/ → [mot] the forms are entered as:

Target: smok
Production: mot

In this format, target and production units can be compared column by column in order to determine which sounds have changed and which have been produced correctly (/sm/ → [m], /o/ produced correctly, /k/ → [t]).

If a CPA program is to determine correspondences automatically, it might do so by identifying the vowels in a string of sounds and then considering everything else to be a consonant. For example, in the case of /wægən/ → [wædə], the program can scan both the target and production forms for vowels:

Target: wægən
                 V √
Production: wædə
                 V √

All other segments are then identified as consonants and the two forms are aligned in accordance with their vowels:

Target: wægən
                 CVCVC
Production: wædə
                 CVCV

If the program finds that the number of vowels in the target and production forms differ, it will know that a change in syllable structure has occurred (e.g., unstressed syllable deletion) or that a mistake was made in data entry.

This need for one-to-one correspondence between target forms and client productions poses several difficulties for computer-aided phonological analysis. One difficulty occurs when consonants are deleted or added. For example, when clusters are reduced, it must be decided which segment(s) are deleted. If /ski/ were produced as [ti], both user-determined and automatic methods of correspondence establishment would identify cluster reduction. However, the classification of the error as stopping or fronting would depend upon whether correspondence was established between [t] and /s/ or [t] and /k/. This, in turn, might lead to slightly different judgments about the nature of a client's phonological difficulties.

Another problem inherent in segmental comparisons is the occurrence of errors that are not based upon segment-to-segment relationships. For example, in coalescence, features of each consonant in the cluster are included in a third consonant that is substituted for the entire cluster, for example, /slip/ → [zip]. Segmental comparison would count one segment as being deleted and may not even recognize the relationship between the remaining cluster member and the substituted sound.

Every CPA program contains a set of definitions (which may or may not be modifiable) for determining phonological rules. These definitions are often stated in terms of specific segmental change patterns. For example, a program may count any occurrence of a /k/ → [t] change as fronting of velars. Occasionally, this approach can be misleading. A child might produce /kot/ as [tot] because of alveolar assimilations rather than velar fronting. Velars produced in words that did not contain alveolar targets would be produced correctly if the pattern was alveolar assimilation. Many programs will count such an error as assimilation but also will count it as an occurrence of velar fronting. If results are offered only in terms of percentages, the user may misinterpret the child's phonological pattern. Some programs, such as PAC, set priorities for process assignment; this approach would result in the above example being classified as assimilation only and not as fronting. The problem with the priority approach, however, is that some errors do indeed represent the operation of multiple processes and these would be missed. Consequently, programs such as PEPPER and Mac-ISPA count the above substitution as an example of both fronting and assimilation. These programs output all words that have been classified as being affected by a particular process. The user can then determine whether the classifications are appropriate.

SINGLE-WORD OR CONNECTED SPEECH

CPA software can be designed from the perspective of single-word or connected speech production. Both methods can analyze data consisting of single words or connected speech; however, each method approaches the task in a different manner. For instance, data from a standardized single-word articulation test are entered word by word in a single-word program:

Entry #1	horse
Phonetic Target:	hors
Transcription:	hot

Entry #2	pig
Phonetic Target:	pɪg
Transcription:	pɪd

In a connected speech program, these two words (and other items) are entered as a single item:

Entry #1	horse	pig	clock	host	yellow	block
Phonetic Target:	hors	pɪg	klak	gost	jɛlo	blak
Transcription:	ho t	pɪd	k ak	gʊs	jɛwo	b at

Similarly, data from a spontaneous speech sample are entered as follows for a connected speech program:

Entry #1	he	raises	horses
Phonetic Target:	hi	rezɪz	horsɪz
Transcription:	hi	redɪ	hortɪ

The sentence must be broken up and treated as a series of individual items when using a program designed to analyze single words.

Entry #1	he
Phonetic Target:	hi
Transcription:	hi

Entry #2	raises
Phonetic Target:	rezɪz
Transcription:	redI

Entry #3	horses
Phonetic Target:	horsɪz
Transcription:	hortɪ

To our knowledge, none of the programs on the market analyze rules that operate across word boundaries (though LIPP has the potential to do so). Thus, even a program designed to allow connected speech input ultimately segments each sentence into individual words and performs the analysis based on word-to-word comparisons. A connected speech program is advantageous only in that it maintains the integrity of the utterances as they were transcribed.

CLOSED VERSUS OPEN SET OF TARGETS

CPA software is designed either to handle a specific set of targets (closed set) or to allow users to enter their own targets (open set). If the software employs a closed set, it may not allow missing data (null responses); that is, the clinician must obtain a response for every item in the data set or else the program will not yield accurate analyses.

It is considerably easier to create a CPA program that works only with a closed set of targets. Because the targets do not change from one analysis to the next, the program operates with a smaller set of variables, which leads to faster data output. For example, the segmentation of each target into individual sounds can be stored in the program so that the information is already available for data analysis. In addition, analyses based on phonetic or feature classes are greatly simplified because the program will "know" which word items are relevant to a particular analysis. If the program contains a closed set of 75 words, and only items 9, 16, 33, 37, 48, and 64 contain velar consonants, then only these items need to be examined for velar substitution and velar fronting.

A closed set of targets also allows the CPA software to perform normative analysis. Standardization data can be incorporated into the program so that, given identification data about the client (age, sex, language background, and the like), percentiles and standard scores can be identified.

In sum, closed-set programs have three main advantages for the user: (1) They are generally easy to operate, as one interacts only with the production data; (2) they perform their analyses rapidly; and (3) they often yield a normative analysis. The disadvantages of using closed-set programs are that (1) the stimulus set available in the program may not be appropriate for a particular patient; (2) the limited number of stimuli may not allow for an adequate sample; (3) they usually require a complete set of production forms, which may be difficult to obtain; and (4) they cannot be used to analyze connected speech. A sample collected from spontaneous conversation can be analyzed only with an open-set program.

TIME-SAVING FEATURES

As shown in the examples above, CPA data entry involves at least two and sometimes three types of entries: the gloss (orthographic) form, the target (phonetic) form, and the production (phonetic) form. Program features that automatically supply one or more of these items can result in considerable time savings.

If a program works with a closed set of targets, the target forms are embedded in the program and are not modifiable. If, however, the program allows an open set of target forms, it stores these forms on disk. This feature allows the user to create files consisting of gloss and/or target forms for use with different clients.

Some CPA programs include a phonetic dictionary that contains pairs of gloss and target forms. The user enters the orthographic forms of the words produced in a sample and the program looks up the corresponding target forms in the dictionary. If a word is not in the dictionary, the user has to enter the phonetic target.

DATA PROCESSING

All CPA programs perform a relational (substitution and omission) analysis and many perform an independent (phonetic) analysis as well. The manner in which these analyses are done varies because of differences in program assumptions or models. In the paragraphs that follow, four such assumptions are discussed.

THE STRUCTURAL UNIT

The structural unit of phonological analysis is either the syllable or the word. CPA software will analyze sound-positions in words and consonant clusters differently depending upon which structural unit is employed. For example, as shown below, the words *grandmother, spoonful,* and *airplane* all contain adjacent consonants that would be analyzed as medial consonant clusters if the program considers the structural unit to be the word:

graendmʌðɚ   spunfʊl   ærpleˡn
—CCC—   —CC—   —CC—

If the syllable is assumed to be the structural unit, however, the consonants are classified as initial, medial, and final singletons, or clusters, based on their position in the syllable:

grænd mʌðɚ   spun fʊl   ær pleˈn
—CC C—   —C—   —CC—

A word-based structure allows a programmer to use a straightforward logic: Consonants at the beginning of a word are identified as initial, those at the end of a word as final, and all others as medial. In contrast, a syllable-based structure requires phonotactic information (sound sequences that are permitted in English). The program might, for instance, consult a list of "allowable" consonant clusters whenever a word-medial sequence of consonants is encountered. If a sequence is not on the list but consists of more than two consonants, then a search commences to find any juxtaposed sounds that are on the list. For example:

grændmʌðɚ   sequence of consonants [ndm] found;
                   [ndm] not on list; [nd] on list
grænd mʌðɚ   word sequenced as shown

Another syllable-based program could leave the decision up to the user. A juncture symbol could be entered that would cause the program to separate units appropriately. For instance, if the word *grasshopper* were entered as

Target: græs + hapɚ
Production: gwæs + hapɚ

the program would analyze the sound change in /græs/ → [gwæs].

It is crucial that the user learn, by reading the documentation and experimenting with data files, whether the CPA software is syllable or word based. If the program makes segmentation decisions automatically, the user should take special note of multisyllabic word targets. If the program treats all word-medial consonants as medial position, one can work around this limitation by entering portions of the target as separate items. For example:

Entry #1   butter-   Entry #2   -fly
Target: bʌɾɚ   Target: flaɪ

This tactic will work as long as the user is careful to segment the production form correctly and to remember that any statistics based upon word counts will be inflated.

OPERATION OF MULTIPLE RULES

Some sound changes reflect the operation of more than one phonological rule. For example, one might find a child who produces /slip/ as [tip]. The initial sound change, from a cluster to a stop, can be interpreted as resulting from two underlying processes: one that simplifies clusters to singletons (cluster simplification) and one that substitutes stops for fricatives. Ideally, CPA software should be able to identify such instances of multiple-step sound changes.

Phonological rule identification can be accomplished in more than one way. In the simplest method, which applies only to sound substitutions, a program will search for all the substitution patterns that serve as manifestations of a particular phonological pattern. For example, a program can identify instances of velar fronting by locating the following substitutions: /ŋ/ → [n], /k/ → [t] , /g/ → [d] (other substitutions also might be included /ŋ/ → [d], /k/ → [d], and so forth, depending on how the process is defined). This method is effective in detecting single-step patterns of substitution or omission. However, it may not identify sound changes that occur as a result of more than one rule. It is possible to assign definitions for two-step patterns. For instance, a program could search for /ʃ/ → [t] and always categorize it as an instance of palatal fronting and stopping. One might be dissatisfied with this interpretation, however, unless there was evidence that these two processes were operating independently in other substitution patterns. The program would need to cross-check other patterns in the data, which becomes a formidable programming task. In another method, the program would work from a featural description of each phone and a featural description of the phonological rule (e.g., velar → alveolar). Rule identification would then occur in two steps: First, the program would scan the target forms for phones that match the featural description (e.g., all velar sounds); then the program would scan the corresponding production forms for a match with the other term in the featural description (e.g., all alveolar sounds). In this manner a segment could serve as an opportunity for multiple rules and a substitution could be counted as representing more than one rule. For example, final /g/ in the word *log* would be classified as a velar, and thus an opportunity for fronting; a final consonant and thus an opportunity for final consonant deletion; and a voiced segment and an opportunity for devoicing of final consonants. This method does allow the determination of multiple-step rules but has the disadvantage of potentially inflating percentages of occurrence for individual rules.

It is evident that both methods have associated pros and cons. Clinicians should remember that the purpose of CPA software is to organize the data in a way that aids interpretation. It is not surprising that a given program may not perform the organization and interpretation in a manner that suits all users. The key to using CPA software effectively is to recognize the prescribed organization. Multiply determined sound simplifications are a good example. If these are not analyzed, then the user should find out what the program does with them. If such sound simplifications are listed in a general category such as "idiosyncratic" or "other" substitutions, it is possible for the user to complete the analytical work.

USER-DETERMINED PROCESSING

Clinicians have their own needs and preferences in phonological assessment and analysis. If these preferences are not met by a specific CPA program, then the user must either adapt to the program or modify the software.

Modifications of a program may range from customizing the output to altering the basic decisions made in the program. Users may wish to change terminology in the output so that it conforms to their preferences. For example, one might prefer *plosive* to *stop, cluster* to *blend,* or *liquid simplification* to *gliding.* Clinicians also may wish to redefine certain categories. For example, a user may want to exclude the omission of postvocalic liquids in the analysis of final consonant deletion. Finally, a user may want to change the keyboard correspondence scheme used by the program or even to change the appearance of the phonetic symbols themselves. LIPP allows the user to actually construct and then define the phonetic symbols to be used in the program.

The simplest way to create an open design for CPA software is to organize the program so that selected variables are stored on disk and loaded each time the program is run. It is then possible for the user either to modify variables directly (e.g., by editing them with a word processor) or by means of a utility module. Programs that allow for this kind of user input are more difficult to create because they must ensure that the user cannot inadvertently crash the program as modifications are made. Modifications of any program should always be done on a working copy of the master program disk(s). Hence, no user-modifiable program should be copy protected.

SPEED

One of the principal reasons for using CPA software is the potential for time savings. Compared to analysis by hand, all CPA software will provide greater efficiency. Various CPA programs have large differences in processing time. Programs developed some years ago took as long as 25 minutes to process a sample, whereas more recent programs can process a sizable sample in less than a minute.

The speed of a program is the product of factors related to both hardware and software. The language in which a program is written will have some effect on how quickly it will run. All recent programs are compiled, however, which tends to minimize such speed differences.

The speed of a computer's microprocessor will determine the rate at which a program's instructions are executed. As improved microprocessors have been developed, they have been incorporated into newer model microcomputers. In some instances it is possible to enhance performance of an older microcomputer by adding accelerator boards that contain the newer microprocessor.

The speed of input/output operations may be of little or great consequence, depending on the design of a particular CPA program. If the program performs a large number of disk operations such as reading in data and variables, storing data in temporary files, and writing the program output to a disk file, then more efficient input/output will have a significant effect. The greatest variable in input/output is the speed with which the disk drives operate. A hard disk drive will perform much faster than a floppy drive. RAM disks or RAM caches—bits of electronic memory that simulate a mechanical disk drive—will also improve speed, though they carry the risk of information loss in the event of a power outage or machine malfunction.

The user can be given some control over the speed of an analysis by organizing a program so that its various analyses (phonetic inventory, correspondence, rule structure, and so on) are performed in a series of independent operations. The user can then select which of the analyses are to be done and eliminate time spent on unwanted analyses.

Users should consider the issue of speed in relation to their own time requirements and work habits. CPA software might be used with the intention of rapidly analyzing test data so that results can be interpreted and presented to clients. In this case speed is a very important requirement and may even outweigh other considerations in the selection of a program. On the other hand, when the primary purpose of CPA software is to gain greater detail of analysis, speed of execution is less significant.

If speed is important, the user might consider enhancement through hardware upgrades. The cost of a hard disk drive or accelerator board may be small compared to the improved efficiency it can bring to a frequently used program.

OUTPUT

The types of output available and the format in which they may be viewed are important considerations for CPA software. Optimally, output should be under the control of the user and permit querying of results. It should be possible to have the results shown only on the screen, printed, or stored in a disk file.

USER CONTROL

Some programs offer phonetic, substitution, and rules analyses. The user may not need all of these analyses and the option to select only the ones desired is therefore valuable.

QUERYING OF RESULTS

Many times clinicians will examine preliminary results from the phonetic or rules analysis and desire additional information. For example, they may want to query the data for selected subsets of the findings, such as substitutions or phonological rules that occurred in specific phonetic contexts or under phonotactic constraints. Users may want to look at all words in which a certain substitution was used, or in which a certain target phoneme or feature occurred. They may also be interested in examining groups of words in which a particular rule was potentially operative. Upon selection of one of the subsets, the availability of further analysis options (e.g., effects of phonetic environment) may assist the user in determining the contexts in which the rules or substitutions occur.

OUTPUT FORMATS

CPA software should allow users to output results to a monitor, printer, or disk file. If data output are in graphics mode, screen and printer compatibility are important. Analysis results stored on a disk are particularly beneficial because they can be imported by most word processing programs and included in reports, IEPs, manuscripts, and the like.

HARDWARE REQUIREMENTS AND COST

CPA packages are designed to run on Apple II-series (II, IIe, IIc, IIGS), IBM-compatible, or Macintosh microcomputers. There is a range of prices for phonological analysis programs and, as with many other products, a high cost does not ensure a quality program nor one that is well suited to an individual clinician's needs. Cost and features, therefore, must be evaluated by each potential user. The expense involved with a software package includes more than just the cost of the package. Some programs may involve special hardware components and the cost of these should be considered.

Computerized Phonological Analysis

DOCUMENTATION AND SUPPORT

Documentation and support are often referred to as hidden considerations in software evaluation because they are so easily overlooked. The clarity and thoroughness of the manual, the provision of a tutorial program, and the availability of technical support are all important program features.

THE MANUAL

Adequate documentation for a computer program is essential. The level of knowledge expected on the part of the user should be clearly stated and the manual written accordingly. Most manuals assume at least a basic familiarity with phonological analysis and include few suggestions regarding collection and preliminary transcription of the sample. These manuals typically provide basic information on how to use the software to facilitate analyses with which users are already familiar. Thus, these manuals will not contain information about the theoretical background or applicability of phonological analysis. However, because the definitions of specific rules may vary from one researcher to another, all manuals should state the program's criteria for assigning phonological rules.

The manual also should contain straightforward instructions for operating the software. This should include definitions and functions associated with each menu choice. Examples of option sequences used to perform various analyses should be provided. The user should not have to wade through a lot of information before understanding the basic operation of the program.

TUTORIAL PROGRAM

The provision of a tutorial program is another desirable component of a software package. The tutorial is designed to walk the user through the operation of the program. The hands-on experience often makes subsequent use more easily understood.

TECHNICAL SUPPORT

The price of software makes it a substantial investment. All packages should include an address and telephone number to contact in case additional support is needed. The provision of adequate technical support to registered purchasers is one way that software developers have hoped to discourage illegal software copying.

REVIEWS OF CURRENT CPA PACKAGES

We have included information on seven currently available CPA packages and have reviewed the packages according to the principles described previously. The software industry is constantly changing, and as a result, we anticipate the appearance of new programs on the market. The reader is encouraged to examine and evaluate any new programs or updates of current packages using the principles previously discussed.

COMPUTER ANALYSIS OF PHONOLOGICAL PROCESSES VERSION 1.0 (Hodson, 1985)

Computer Analysis of Phonological Processes (*CAPP*) yields data on percentage of occurrence for 10 phonological processes described by Hodson (1985). In Hodson's analysis approach, target classes are listed and any error (substitution or deletion) is considered a single category for deviations. For example, the omission of an /s/ and a substitution of a [t] for an /s/ would both be considered occurrences of stridency deletion. Hodson states that CAPP was designed to provide a rapid phonological process analysis.

Data Entry and Processing. CAPP includes a closed set of 50 words for which the user enters the transcription form produced by the client in a modified IPA format. IPA characters that are included on a standard keyboard are used. Those that are not are entered with alternate symbols. For example, a "?" is used to denote a glottal stop /ʔ/ and a "T" is used for both the /θ/ and the /ð/. Vowels are entered with a semicolon symbol or one of the vowels included on the keyboard. Vowel characters are not analyzed, so the symbols used do not really matter. The orthographic gloss of each word and the phonetic target form are provided. A space corresponding to each target character is provided and the user enters the client's transcription form. The space bar is used to denote deletions. The program does not accept a transcription form entry until characters corresponding to each of the target characters have been entered. A transcription form must be entered for all target words. An editing function is available to users before the analysis is performed. However, once the analysis is completed, users cannot access the data that were entered.

Data cannot be saved to a disk file. Consequently, users cannot enter transcriptions for part of the words at one time and finish at a later time, nor can data be saved for future comparisons. The program contains no utility for printing or viewing the entire data file at once.

Output. The program yields the following:

1. Percentage of occurrence for 10 target patterns: syllables, prevocalic singletons, postvocalic singletons, consonant sequences, stridents, velars, liquid (l), liquid (r), nasals, and glides
2. Overall average percentage of occurrence of phonological processes
3. Phonological deviance score
4. Severity interval
5. List of target patterns that should be initially targeted as goals in therapy

No information regarding conventions used in process assignment is included. The program does not allow the user to view words containing errors classified as an occurrence of a phonological process. The formulas for determining deviance scores and severity intervals are described.

Hardware and Software Requirements. CAPP runs on any of the Apple II series computers. The program disk is self-booting, so no additional software is necessary. Hodson (personal communications) is currently developing an IBM-compatible version of CAPP.

Documentation. CAPP includes a small manual describing steps involved in operation of the software. Additionally, a chapter and an appendix describing phonological remediation fundamentals are included.

Discussion. CAPP is easy to use and data can be entered quickly. Clinicians with little or no experience with microcomputers should be readily able to use this software. A client's responses to the 50 word items can usually be entered in less than 10 minutes, and the computer takes about a minute to complete the analysis. However, CAPP's simplicity has some disadvantages: Because the words are a closed set, spontaneous speech data cannot be analyzed. No phonetic information, such as consonant inventory, is provided. Words classified as containing an error are not displayed so users cannot judge for themselves whether the classification is appropriate. Finally, deviations of all types are grouped by the structure or manner of classifications of the targets. No differentiation between simplifications of various types is provided. For example, stopping of fricatives, deletion of the /s/ in a consonant cluster, and deletion of a plural marker are all counted as occurrences of stridency deletion.

COMPUTERIZED PROFILING (Long and Fey, 1988; in press, a and b)

Computerized Profiling (*CP*) is a diverse set of programs that can be used to perform various analyses of speech sample data. Included in the software is a set of modules for doing a *Profile of Phonology* (PROPH). PROPH was developed by Crystal and Fletcher (in Crystal, 1982) and the computer program is derived from their manual procedure. The major difference in the computerized version is the omission of a syllable stress analysis and the replacement of the distinctive feature analysis by a phonological process analysis based on the descriptions by Grunwell (1987).

Data Entry and Processing. CP runs on different types of microcomputers, and data entry varies according to the version of the program. In the MS-DOS (IBM-compatible) and ProDOS (Apple II series) versions, a transliterated version of the IPA is used. Phonetic symbols that are identical with English letters (e.g., *t, k, m, s*) or standard keyboard symbols (e.g., +, =) are entered by pressing the appropriate key. All other symbols are entered with one- or two-character sequences that either closely resemble the phonetic symbol (e.g., ''?'' for glottal stop /ʔ/, ''d3'' for /ʤ/) or the most common corresponding grapheme (e.g., ''sh'' for /ʃ/, ''th'' for /θ/). In the Macintosh version, nonalphabetic phonetic symbols are entered by means of special keystroke combinations (e.g., option ''s'' for /ʃ/) and are represented on the screen and on all printouts with a special phonetic font. It is possible to customize the keystroke combinations by using special macros which accompany the Macintosh program.

For each item to be analyzed, the program requires three forms to be entered: the gloss, the target form, and the transcription form produced by the client. To simplify the task of data entry for articulation tests, gloss and target forms may be stored in disk files and then retrieved for each client. Thus the user needs to enter only the transcription form. To simplify entry of connected speech data, the program includes a modifiable phonetic dictionary. The user enters the gloss forms as a transcript and then invokes the program to find the corresponding target forms in the dictionary. Prompts appear for any words not contained in the dictionary. Both articulation test and connected speech transcription data are entered phonetically. The program has a maximum sample size of 300 words for the Macintosh version, 200 words for the MS-DOS version, and 125 words for the ProDOS version. It is not necessary to align individual segments in the target and transcription forms, so omitted phones need not be marked with special symbols. The program automatically determines consonant-vowel boundaries and then analyzes the correspondence between segments in the two forms. If the syllable structure of the target and transcription forms is found to be different, the program automatically excludes that word from the correspondence analysis.

Output. CP offers nine options for its analysis of the data:

1. Listing of gloss, target, and transcription forms
2. Word shape analysis
3. Classification of correct vowel productions and vowel changes
4. Classification of consonant productions as correct, substituted, or omitted, and organized by sound-position and manner
5. Percentage consonants correct (Shriberg and Kwiatkowski, 1982)
6. Phonetic inventory, organized by sound-position and manner class
7. Phonological process analysis, organized by sound-position and developmental order
8. Alphabetized word listing
9. Printing of a diacritics key

The user may select any or all of these options to be included in a profile report.

The phonological process analysis only classifies sound changes that result from a single rule. Hence, sound changes that might be analyzed in terms of two or more ordered processes are not attributed to any of those processes. Instead they are classified in a residual "other substitutions" category and left to the user's judgment. Phonological processes are identified from a set of substitution and omission definitions contained in a disk file. Within certain limits, this file may be modified so that the process definitions applied in the analysis will conform to the views of the user.

In addition to its standard analyses, CP also permits three types of data base searches. The user may specify any set of correctly produced phones, substituted or omitted phones, or word shapes. The program will then list all such instances that occurred in the data set.

A supplementary PROPH module allows the user to combine the data from more than one sample, up to the limit on sample size. Another module displays the transcriptions of all words found in common in up to five data files. Such a comparison is useful for tracking longitudinal changes in a single subject.

All output from the program is automatically saved in text files, which may be viewed on the screen, printed, or loaded into other applications such as a word processor.

Hardware and Software Requirements. The MS-DOS version of the program operates on all IBM-compatible computers with at least 256K of RAM and DOS version 2.0 or higher. The ProDOS version runs on Apple IIe, IIc, and IIGS computers and includes the necessary ProDOS software. The Macintosh version requires a minimum 512K of RAM and must be run under Finder rather than Multifinder. Any printer or monitor type may be used.

Documentation. The user's manual explains the operation of the program by means of a guided tutorial. Additional details are contained in an appendix. The program defers most issues of phonological analysis and interpretation to the original sources on which the program is based (Crystal, 1982; Grunwell, 1987).

Discussion. The simplified procedures for data entry make the program very accessible to beginning clinicians and save time for all users. The analyses generated by the program are adequate for the majority of clinical cases but are not equivalent to some of the extensive analyses that appear in the clinical phonology literature. CP also includes modules for semantic, syntactic, pragmatic, and prosodic analyses. Thus, users need only enter a sample once to obtain results regarding not only phonology but also other linguistic skills. This may be attractive for individuals in both research and clinical settings. The transliteration of phonetic symbols used in the MS-DOS and ProDOS versions may be disconcerting to some users. The multiple-key input scheme used in the Macintosh version may be confusing at first to inexperienced computer users.

LOGICAL INTERNATIONAL PHONETIC PROGRAMS VERSION 1.03 (Oller and Delgado, 1990)

Logical International Phonetic Programs (*LIPP*) is a highly innovative and flexible approach to computerized phonological analysis. Unlike other software developed for this purpose, nearly every feature of LIPP—the phonetic alphabet it uses, the arrangement of symbols on the keyboard, the number and type of analyses it performs—can be modified by the user. This design virtually assures that LIPP will meet or can be made to meet any individual's analysis needs.

Data Entry and Processing. Data are entered on three lines representing the gloss, target, and transcription forms, respectively. Each data item is entered in a 40-column screen display, with words separated by special boundary markers. This arrangement allows users to enter words as individual items or to enter strings of words (as would occur in the transcription of connected speech) up to the width of the display. Gloss forms are enclosed within quotation marks but are otherwise typed in normally. Target and transcription forms are entered in phonetic symbols by using the shift, control, and alternate keys in conjunction with the letter and number keys. The user must ensure that all three data forms are vertically aligned in order to generate an accurate analysis of segmental correspondences.

LIPP provides two phonetic alphabets. Both are closely based on the 1989 revision of the IPA and include symbols for consonant and vowel segments, diacritics, and "global" symbols that may be used for superbroad transcription. Differences between the two alphabets are slight and are explained in the manual. Either alphabet may be modified to suit the views and clinical needs of the user and entirely new alphabets also may be created.

LIPP is well-designed for the analysis of both articulation test and connected speech data. A template file containing the gloss and target forms from any test can be created and stored. To enter a client's data, this file is retrieved, the transcription forms are entered, and the file is saved under a different name. To simplify the analysis of connected speech, LIPP contains a modifiable phonetic dictionary. The user enters the first few letters of a word on the gloss line and then invokes the dictionary. The dictionary shows entries beginning with those letters. If the desired word is present, it is selected and the appropriate target form is entered into the data automatically.

Phonetic and phonological analyses are produced by comparing the information entered on the target and transcription lines. LIPP has a very sophisticated scheme for representing phonetic values. Every symbol in a phonetic alphabet is assigned a value for 16 different phonetic parameters. This allows a user to define individual sounds, diacritics, and sound classes in terms of unique parameter configurations. Once these basic phonetic variables have been defined, LIPP allows the user to write a series of rule statements that detail certain kinds of sound equivalences or sound changes. It is these rule statements that the program evaluates and that determine its analyses.

Output. LIPP produces two types of analyses: (1) an inventory analysis, which compares the corresponding segments on the target and transcription lines; and (2) rule-driven analyses, which are flexible and may be used to count sounds, calculate percentage of correctness, evaluate structural characteristics of the sample, perform phonological process analyses, and many other tasks. The inventory analysis can be used to generate a list of correspondences between target and transcription segments; for example, [p] was produced correctly twice, was omitted three times, and was substituted by a glottal stop once. The analysis also can be done in the opposite direction; for example, LIPP will display how many times [t] occurred as a substitution for [p], for [k], for [s], and so forth. For research purposes, inventory analysis may be used to determine the reliability between two transcriptions of the same phonetic sample.

All other analyses generated by LIPP are rule-driven. The program comes with certain rule statements already written, but these may be modified and new ones may be written if the user invests the time to learn the necessary procedures. Among the analyses included with LIPP are a phonetic inventory by position, a correctness analysis by segment and sound class, and an extensive phonological process analysis. LIPP also includes rule statements for evaluating a sample's "phonological adequacy." This ratio is designed to reflect the combined effect of a child's simplification processes on his speech intelligibility.

Hardware and Software Requirements. LIPP is sold in three packages: The low-end version (Thin LIPP) includes only the modules for creating transcription data files; the middle version (Lower LIPP) adds a set of rule-statement files along with the modules needed to execute the analyses; and the complete version (Upper LIPP) adds the modules that allow users to modify symbols and alphabets and to write their own rule statement files. All versions of LIPP require an IBM-compatible computer with 640K of RAM, a hard disk drive, and an EGA or VGA graphics monitor. The Upper LIPP modules for modifying phonetic alphabets require a mouse. Most dot matrix and non-Postscript laser printers are supported by the program.

Documentation. The LIPP manual contains sections that explain the overall design of the program and how to install the program on a hard disk. A tutorial section guides the user through the steps of program operation. This section is well organized and easy to follow for a user with some computer experience. Sample printouts of all program data files, analyses, and rule statements are included in appendices. The manual deals exclusively with the LIPP program and does not discuss general issues of phonological analysis or interpretation.

Discussion. LIPP is a unique program because of the amount of flexibility it offers to the user. This flexibility, however, comes at a price. Upper LIPP, the complete version of the program that allows the user to make modifications, is an expensive product. There is also a price in terms of time. Though LIPP is extremely well-designed to take advantage of menus and word processing editing features, it remains an elaborate program and takes time to master. Moreover, LIPP assumes that the user is well versed in phonetic symbology and phonological theory and terminology. Clinicians with limited backgrounds in these areas may find LIPP overwhelming. Although the program can be used at a simple level (that is, using broad transcription and generating basic accuracy counts), the "stock" LIPP dictionaries and rule-statement files are written in a more complex way. Since the manual does not serve as a primer on clinical phonology, some users may need some additional guidance in order to take full advantage of LIPP.

Given the complexity of what the program does, LIPP generally operates in an extremely elegant and intuitive way. Nevertheless, some of the design features involve trade-offs in user-friendliness. For example, all of the analysis reports are output as ASCII files. This is an advantage in that they can be loaded, edited, and printed out from a word processor program. It is a disadvantage in that the reports cannot contain phonetic symbols and therefore must resort to creative ways of spelling each segment name (e.g., [t] = "tee," [θ] = "theta," [tʃ] = "Tsh").

THE MACINTOSH INTERACTIVE SYSTEM FOR PHONOLOGICAL ANALYSIS (Masterson and Pagan, in press)

The *Macintosh Interactive System for Phonological Analysis* (*Mac-ISPA*) was designed to provide the user with maximum flexibility in performing various phonological analyses. The program performs three basic analyses, which are based on the procedures described by Ingram (1981), and then allows the user a series of interactive options to explore the data further.

Data Entry and Processing. Data are entered as IPA characters via a standard Macintosh keyboard. Mac-ISPA includes a phonetic font, and a keyboard chart corresponding to IPA symbols for phones and diacritics is contained in the manual. Most symbols correspond to the standard keyboard characters and some attempt is made to make the mapping of non-keyboard characters intuitive (e.g., /ʃ/ is entered by depressing the shift key and typing "s"). Phonetic symbols and diacritics appear on the screen and are printed.

Each entry consists of two parts: the target form and the corresponding transcription form produced by the client. The entries consist of single words rather than sentences. Both the target and the transcription forms are entered in phonetic symbols. The phonetic segments in the target and transcription forms must correspond in both number and type (vowel versus consonant). Thus, if a phoneme is omitted, the user must enter a null symbol (0) in its place in the transcription form.

Mac-ISPA can accommodate an open set of targets, so that words elicited during connected speech or articulation test data may be analyzed. The user can construct and store files containing target items from standard articulation tests or other protocols of interest. Transcription forms that are correct do not have to be entered because the program uses the entered target form as the default for the transcription form. The user need only enter productions that contain an error.

Output. Mac-ISPA performs three basic analyses:

1. Phonetic, which includes three inventories: word-initial phones, word-medial phones, and word-final phones. The inventories include the following for each phone: frequency counts; stability classification as marginal, used, or frequent based on Ingram's (1981) criteria; and lists of each unique word-form containing the phone in the indicated position. Frequencies for various syllabic structures (e.g., CV, CVC, CVCVC) are also provided.

2. Substitution, which provides inventories of all initial, medial, and final phonemes

attempted; each target's corresponding substitutions; and the words manifesting correct use or substitution. Quantitative data include a "percentage consonants correct" (Shriberg and Kwiatkowski, 1982) and a "proportion of matches" (Ingram, 1981).

3. Phonological process, which yields percentage-of-occurrence data for 27 different phonological rules. The user also may view word-pairs in which a rule was operative and those in which a rule could have been operative but was not.

In addition to the above analyses, Mac-ISPA offers the user several options for more detailed inspection of the sample. Sets of data can be defined and accessed according to the following parameters:

1. Sounds in the target or production forms (e.g., place, manner, voice classification); for example, all target words containing velars in the initial position
2. Sounds in the target and their corresponding substitutions; for example, velar targets might be found to have bilabial and alveolar substitutions and the user could access words containing either type of substitution
3. Words in which a specified substitution occurred, for example, all words in which a glottal stop or a nasal was used as a substitution
4. Words in which a phonological rule was operative or nonoperative

Once a set of data have been selected, the user is offered several options for further analysis including percentage sample affected, vowel or consonant environment, phonemic length, and syllabic structure.

The phonetic analysis is based upon identification of consonant singletons and clusters in the initial, medial, and final word-positions. Successive consonants are treated as "clusters" in the phonetic and substitution analyses. However, the process analysis only analyzes true clusters as opportunities for cluster simplification. Phonological processes are identified by rule statements that allow for a substitution to be classified as the operation of more than one rule. For example, /ki/ → [di] would be classified as an occurrence of both velar fronting and prevocalic voicing. This allows for the identification of simultaneous operation of multiple rules; however, it also requires caution in interpretation by the user. For example, /dom/ → [mom] would be classified as both nasal assimilation and labialization. Perhaps labialization is not really an appropriate description of the error, but instead is an artifact of nasal assimilation. Some of the Mac-ISPA querying options facilitate the user's determination of appropriate rule assignment.

Output from Mac-ISPA can be viewed on the screen, sent to the printer, or saved as a text file for use with other applications such as word processing.

Hardware and Software Requirements. Mac-ISPA operates on any Macintosh system and compatible printer.

Documentation. Mac-ISPA comes with a manual that covers procedures for operation. A tutorial that outlines procedures for use and provides examples is included. A limited amount of information regarding background and suggested interpretation for each analysis is provided. However, users are referred to other sources (e.g., Ingram, 1981; Shriberg and Kwiatkowski, 1982) for detailed information regarding analysis procedures and implications of output. Prerequisite knowledge (e.g., of Macintosh utilities, and so on) required of the user is specified.

Discussion. Mac-ISPA is a fast and comprehensive phonological analysis program. On a low-end Macintosh system (e.g., an enhanced 512 Mac), the program will perform a phonetic, substitution, and process analysis on a 250-word sample in about one minute. The extensive automatic analyses allow beginning clinicians to use Mac-ISPA readily. However, those with limited background in phonological analysis may find the program's terminology initially difficult. The highly flexible search features make Mac-ISPA especially appealing for use with complex clinical cases or for research applications that require analytical detail.

PROCESS ANALYSIS VERSION 2.0 (Weiner, 1986)

Process Analysis (PAC) analyzes phonetic responses to a closed set of 59 monosyllabic words. The program yields a phonetic inventory of initial and final sounds and a frequency count of several phonological processes.

Data Entry and Processing. Words elicited via formal tests or during conversational speech cannot be analyzed by PAC. The program user is shown the gloss form of each word and then must enter a transcription of the client's production. Consonants entered appear as IPA symbols on the screen. The user must become familiar with how phonetic symbols are entered via the keyboard. The letter "x" is used for all vowels, and vowels are not considered in the analyses. The number of consonants in the transcription form must equal the number included in the target; deletions are designated with a "★" symbol. If the user attempts to enter more or fewer consonants than are included in the target word, the computer will beep and display a reminder message to enter the response correctly. As a result, PAC cannot process transcription forms that involve errors of addition. Decisions regarding correspondence between target and production characters are left to the user. For example, if "skip" is produced as [tɪp], the user can enter the form as "★tɪP" in which the [t] would count as a replacement for the [k], or as "t★ɪp", in which [t] would count as a replacement for the /s/.

The user must enter a response for each of the 59 words; however, this need not be done at one sitting. PAC offers the user the option to save data files to a disk so that they can be updated or viewed at a later time. PAC also includes an editing feature that can be employed with files that are currently being constructed or those that have been saved at an earlier time.

Output. Output includes phonetic inventories with frequency counts for each initial and final sound that appears in a transcription form. The number of possible occurrences and corresponding percentages are provided for approximately 15 phonological processes, including deletion of initial or final consonants, stopping, fronting, assimilation, cluster simplification, and gliding of liquids. The program does not list the words in which specific phones or phonological processes were found.

Phonological process assignment is done in a specified hierarchical fashion, and an error can be attributed to only one process. For example, if a child produced /kip/ as [dib], the /k/ → [d] substitution would be counted as prevocalic voicing only; the instance of velar fronting would be ignored. The manual provides the priority of process assignment.

Analysis results can be viewed on the screen and/or printed. PAC does not allow the results of an analysis to be saved to a disk. However, the analyses performed are completed rapidly, so little time is lost in repeating the analysis of a previously saved file.

Hardware and Software Requirements. PAC requires an Apple II family microcomputer and one disk drive. A printer is optional. The program is self-booting, so no additional software is required.

Documentation. PAC includes a brief manual that includes clear instructions for using the software. Between the information provided in the manual and the on-screen instructions, a user should be able to enter and analyze data quite readily. The manual also lists the definitions the program employs for assigning an error to a process category.

Discussion. PAC is simple to use. It provides information regarding both independent and relational analyses. Additionally, the manual includes information about the decisions made in the analyses, such as process definition and priority of assignment.

PAC's primary weakness is its inability to handle words elicited spontaneously or via formal tests. The stimulus set included consists of monosyllabic words only, so word-medial consonant production is not considered. Further, the use of only simple phonological structures prohibits the exploration of the influence of increased phonological complexity on the occurrence of errors or the contents of phonetic inventories. The assignment of an error to only one process precludes identification of any processes that may be operating simultaneously.

PYE ANALYSIS OF LANGUAGE VERSION 2.0 (Pye, 1987)

The *Pye Analysis of Language* (*PAL*) is a set of programs for carrying out linguistic analyses of transcript data. The PHONIX program, in particular, is intended to facilitate a number of phonological analysis procedures recommended by Ingram (1981).

Data Entry and Processing. PAL is designed to analyze the information contained in transcript files that have been created with a word processor. The transcript conventions that must be observed are illustrated in the program manual and are easily learned. Phonetic transcription forms are entered on one line and the corresponding orthographic gloss forms are entered on the line below. Either single-word or connected speech data may be analyzed. A transliterated form of the IPA is used to enter phonetic segmental information (e.g., *wagon* is transcribed as [wAg6n]). A small number of diacritics are allowed and unassigned symbols may be used to represent unusual vowel or consonant phones.

Analysis of a sample occurs in five steps. First, a transcript is created and saved in text (ASCII) format. This file is then input to the FORMIX module of PAL and checked for format errors. If errors are found, they must be edited with a word processor. Otherwise, the third step is to input the file to the PHONIX module of PAL and create a phonological lexicon file. This lexicon lists all the word types that occurred in the sample along with their phonetic token(s). The file, in the form of a report, must then be edited with a word processor so that it contains only the data the user wishes to analyze. The fourth step is to run this edited file through a phonetic dictionary, which automatically finds the target form for each of the words in the sample. For words not contained in the dictionary, the user must add the target form to the file with a word processor. Finally, the file containing the lexical, target, and production forms is submitted for phonological analysis by the program.

Output. PAL's phonological analysis consists of a phonetic inventory and a substitution analysis. Both analyses display initial consonants, vowels, and final consonants separately. Word-medial consonants are not analyzed. The phonetic inventory does not yield a count for each sound but rather lists all of the production forms in which the sound occurred. The program does calculate the number of phonetic types occurring for each sound class (vowel, consonant) and position (initial, final). Clusters are analyzed in terms of the individual segments they contain; for example, the production form [stov] would be listed under both initial [s] and initial [t].

The substitution analysis is a cross-listing of each target-production pair according to the sounds contained in the target form. Thus all target forms containing an initial [p] (this would include clusters such as [sp], [pr], and the like) are listed along with their corresponding production forms. The user must scan these listings by hand and mark—for example, by circling—those words in which errors occurred and those that were produced correctly.

Hardware and Software Requirements. PAL will run on any IBM-compatible with 256K of RAM and the MS-DOS operating system. Both hard and floppy disk operation are possible. The user must possess a word processing program capable of producing ASCII file output in order to create and edit the necessary PAL data files. PAL outputs its analyses in the form of ASCII files, which may be printed out on any model of printer.

Documentation. The PAL manual contains basic instructions for running the program and includes appendices with printouts of a sample data file and all of its associated analyses. These sample files are also contained on the program disk itself. The manual is written in a straightforward style and provides a very useful commentary on the many practical issues involved in creating a computer program to do phonological analysis. Unfortunately, from the user's standpoint, the manual is written so concisely that it is easy to miss or misunderstand some of the steps for running the program.

Discussion. PAL may be viewed as a program that can provide assistance to a clinician doing a phonological analysis by hand. Unlike other programs, PAL is not designed to yield a finished phonological analysis. Instead, it helps the user with several of the most time-consuming and tedious tasks of organizing a data set: alphabetizing the word list, finding and listing all productions of the same word, organizing and listing all the sounds contained in the transcription forms, and so on. The program does not identify or count specific sound changes that occur in a sample, search for certain common patterns of sound substitution or omission, nor calculate statistics that reflect the patient's overall accuracy of production. PAL does have the following strengths: (a) It is able to analyze any set of words, including connected speech data; (b) it analyzes vowels; (c) it is extremely fast; and (d) it handles very large data sets.

The transliterated IPA used by PAL must be learned by the user. PAL also assumes that the user has enough computer experience to cope with tasks such as using a word processor, viewing or printing files from the operating system, and naming files according to MS-DOS conventions. The computer novice should master these skills before attempting to use PAL.

Programs to Examine Phonetic and Phonologic Evaluation Records Version 4.0 (Shriberg, 1986)

Programs to Examine Phonetic and Phonologic Evaluation Records (*PEPPER*) is a comprehensive approach to the analysis and interpretation of phonological data. The manual includes a thorough review of the conceptual and procedural issues surrounding phonological analysis. The software provides information about an individual's phonetic abilities and the phonological simplifications used.

Data Entry and Processing. Three lines of data are entered: (1) the orthographic gloss form, (2) the phonetic target form, and (3) the phonetic transcription form produced by the subject. Entry lines can accommodate either single words or connected speech. PEPPER employs a graphics mode which allows data for the target and transcription lines to be entered in IPA symbols. Diacritics also are allowed, as are several other useful symbols to represent segments as on- or offglides, unintelligible, and so on, or to indicate suprasegmentals. Users also have the option of entering comments on the gloss line, which allows the marking of additional linguistic or nonlinguistic variables of interest. "Protocol" files consisting of the orthographic and phonetic representations of target forms can be constructed and saved on disk. Once a protocol is completed, the user need only enter a client's productions of each target item. This makes possible the efficient entry of articulation test data. Data from individuals may be grouped in order to determine characteristics of an entire sample.

Although data may be entered as connected speech, analyses are performed by comparing corresponding single words in the target and transcription lines. The number of segments in the transcription form must match the number of segments in the target form. Thus, the user enters an underbar to represent a deleted phoneme and additions are entered as on- or offglides. PEPPER includes several worksheets or forms to facilitate data entry into the computer. However, users may wish to skip the use of the forms and enter data directly into the computer when transcribing.

Output. The software yields the following:

1. Structural statistics, which include the syllabic structures intended and obtained, average words per utterance, and type-token percentages
2. Artic tests, which provide percentages of occurrence for correct use, deletion, substitution, and distortion for each individual consonant and vowel and for each class, place, manner, and voicing classification of consonants and vowels; and an item analysis that lists each target word along with the correct, omitted, substituted, or distorted phonemes it contains
3. Percentage consonants correct figures for various data sets (i.e., singletons, clusters, word-positions)
4. Phonetic inventories for word-initial and -final phones
5. Phonological process analysis, which includes percentage of occurrence of each of the eight natural phonological processes described in Shriberg and Kwiatkowski (1980), a listing of words by vowels and canonical form, and phonological processes occurring in each word

In addition to the output provided by the software, the PEPPER manual contains several tables that are beneficial in interpretation of results. The documentation contains explicit definitions that are used by the software to classify errors as phonological processes. PEPPER does not perform any specific searches of results; however, a table containing guidelines for viewing the output from PEPPER to determine factors such as phonetic influences and the like is included. For example, users are instructed to consult the printouts regarding structural statistics and percentage consonant correct figures to identify avoidance in a client. The contrastive status of phonemes within a child's system may be determined by viewing the word lists provided in the natural process analysis section.

Documentation. The PEPPER manual is very comprehensive, including chapters on conceptual and procedural issues surrounding phonological analysis, recording and transcribing speech samples, use of the software package, and interpretation of results. Several appendices are included, which contain examples of the forms used with PEPPER, sample outputs, reference data, installation procedures, technical limitations, and interpretation of results. One appendix is designed as a tutorial; however, the instructions may be somewhat difficult to follow for inexperienced users.

Hardware and Software Requirements. PEPPER requires an IBM-compatible computer with at least 640K on-board memory and DOS 2.1 or higher. The program will operate from two floppy disk drives, but the use of a hard drive allows for greater ease of use and speed. The software requires specific display devices (monitors), printers, and a math co-processor. Potential users should consult the publisher to determine if their hardware is compatible before purchasing this package.

Discussion. PEPPER has been reviewed twice (Pollock, 1988; Wynne, 1987) and received excellent ratings. Additionally, PEPPER has been employed as an analysis tool in published studies regarding phonology (e.g., Campbell and Dollaghan, 1990). The documentation for PEPPER is comprehensive, and a thorough reading will acquaint users with considerations for phonological analysis performed both by the computer and by hand. In general, a user can find most prerequisite knowledge regarding phonological analysis contained in the manual, so it is not necessary to consult other sources for this information. The manual really consists of two types of information: (1) issues surrounding phonological analysis and (2) procedures for running PEPPER. Because the material is not clearly divided, the reader must sort through information concerning the former to determine the latter. This can be difficult even for users with a fair degree of experience with microcomputers. However, once the user has mastered the logistics of running PEPPER, the program's output is very useful. The interpretative material included in the manual is particularly valuable.

As with any alternate symbol set, keyboard entry and the conventions used in editing data are initially awkward. However, these problems are quickly overcome as the user gains experience with the package. The screen graphics for data entry and display are quite good; however, analysis results displayed on the screen are displayed sideways and are difficult to read. Results are best viewed in printed form. Output of results does require considerable time on any printer other than a laser printer, but choices for several reports can be made at one time so that it is unnecessary for the user to be present while information is being printed.

TABLE 8–1. Descriptions of CPA packages.

FEATURE	SOFTWARE PACKAGES							
	PAC	CAPP	PEPPER	PAL 2.0	CP-Mac	CP-DOS	Mac-ISPA	LIPP
Symbols	IPA*	Translit.	IPA	Translit.	IPA	Translit.	IPA	IPA/User-Determined
Level of Representation	Broad	Broad	Broad/Narrow	Broad/Narrow	Broad/Narrow	Broad/Narrow	Broad/Narrow	Broad/Narrow Superbroad
Data Set	Fixed	Fixed	Open	Open	Open	Open	Open	Open
Multiple Rules	No	No	No	No	No	No	Yes	Yes
Analysis Unit	Word	Word	Word	Word	Word/Syllable	Word/Syllable	Word/Syllable	User-Determined
Phonetic Dictionary	No	No	No	Yes	Yes	Yes	No	Yes
User-Modifiable Features	None	None	Num. of Analyses	None	Keyboard† Num. of Analyses	Num. of Analyses; Rule Defs.	Num/Type of Analyses; Keyboard†	Number/Type of Analyses$; Keyboard
Output Device	Monitor Printer*	Monitor Printer	Monitor& Printer Disk file	Monitor Printer Disk file	Monitor Printer Disk file	Monitor Printer Disk file	Monitor Printer Disk file	Monitor Printer Disk file
Hardware Requirements	Apple II 1 floppy	Apple II 1 floppy	IBM/com; 640K RAM; 2 fl. drives or hard dr.; Math proc. Specific monitors/printers	IBM/com. 256K RAM; Floppy or hard dr.	Mac Plus or higher; Hard dr.	IBM/com. 256K RAM; 2 fl. drives or hard dr.	Mac Plus or higher; Floppy or hard dr.	IBM/com. 640K RAM; EGA/VGA; Mouse

* Printed output uses transliteration; not IPA symbols.
† Keyboard remapped with MacroMaker files.
& Reports appear sideways on the monitor.
$ Available only with Upper LIPP.

Computerized Phonological Analysis

SUMMARY

Table 8–1 summarizes the symbol set used, level of phonetic transcription allowed, data set, method for handling multiple rules, analysis unit, incorporation of a phonetic dictionary, user-modifiable features, output devices, and hardware requirements for each of the CPA packages reviewed.

CPA software offers numerous benefits to the clinician. The savings in time are accompanied by a depth of analysis that may otherwise be difficult to achieve. Although there are problems inherent to CPA, most can be overcome by awareness and good judgment on the part of the user. We have tried to illustrate the power and desirability of CPA software while at the same time emphasizing the clinician's responsibility for accurate data entry and interpretation of results. The microcomputer can be a very rapid counter and efficient organizer, but it offers little flexibility. Thus, CPA software can function only as an aide to the professional who must make the decisions regarding the status of a client's phonological system.

REFERENCES

Campbell, T., and C. Dollaghan, "Expressive language recovery in severely brain-injured children and adults." *Journal of Speech and Hearing Research, 55* (1990): 567–581.

Crystal, D., *Profiling Linguistic Disability*. London: Edward Arnold, 1982.

Grunwell, P., *Clinical Phonology*, 2nd ed. Baltimore: Williams & Wilkins, 1987.

Hodson, B., *Computerized Assessment of Phonological Processes: Version 1.0* (Apple II series computer program). Danville, Ill.: Interstate, 1985.

Ingram, D., *Procedures for Phonological Analysis of Children's Language*. Baltimore: University Park Press, 1981.

Long, S., and M. Fey, *Computerized Profiling* (Apple II series computer program). Ithaca, N.Y.: Department of Speech Pathology and Audiology, Ithaca College, 1988.

Long, S., and M. Fey, *Computerized Profiling* (Macintosh computer program). San Antonio, Tex.: Psychological Corporation (in press, a).

Long, S., and M. Fey, *Computerized Profiling* (MS-DOS computer program). San Antonio, Tex.: Psychological Corporation (in press, b).

Masterson, J., and F. Pagan, *The Macintosh Interactive System for Phonological Analysis* (Macintosh computer program). San Antonio, Tex.: Psychological Corporation (in press).

Oller, K., and R. Delgado, *Logical International Phonetic Programs: Version 1.03* (MS-DOS computer program). Miami, Fla.: Intelligent Hearing Systems, 1990.

Pollock, K., "Review of Shriberg, L. (1986), *Programs to Examine Phonetic and Phonologic Evaluation Records*." *Asha, 30* (1988): 57–58.

Pye, C., *Pye Analysis of Language: Version 2.0* (MS-DOS computer program). Lawrence, Kan.: 200 Arrowhead Dr., 1987.

Shriberg, L., *Programs to Examine Phonetic and Phonologic Evaluation Records: Version 4.0* (MS-DOS computer program). Hillsdale, N.J.: Lawrence Erlbaum, 1986.

Shriberg, L., and J. Kwiatkowski, *Natural Process Analysis (NPA): A Procedure for Phonological Analysis of Continuous Speech Samples*. New York: Macmillan, 1980.

Shriberg, L., and J. Kwiatkowski, "Phonological disorders III: A procedure for assessing severity of involvement." *Journal of Speech and Hearing Disorders, 51* (1982): 140–161.

Weiner, F., *Process Analysis: Version 2.0* (Apple II series computer program). State College, Pa.: Parrot Software, 1986.

Wynne, M., "Review of Shriberg, L. (1986), *Programs to Examine Phonetic and Phonologic Evaluation Records*." *Review of Journal of Computer Users in Speech and Hearing, 2* (1987): 148–158.

chapter

9

Remediation Concepts
and Principles

INTRODUCTION

In most instances, the long-range objective of remediation for phonological disorders or delay is the client's spontaneous use of speech sounds that reflect the adult standard of his or her linguistic community. Once a speech-language clinician has determined that an individual's phonology is disordered or otherwise warrants intervention, assessment data are used in the planning of management strategies to accomplish this objective. As described in Chapter 6, phonological analyses are designed to assist the clinician in identifying appropriate target behaviors for instruction as well as in determining intervention strategies and approaches that will facilitate the accomplishment of treatment goals and objectives.

The treatment process can be viewed as a continuum comprising three stages—establishment, facilitation of generalization, and maintenance. Such a temporal continuum may also be viewed as an ordered sequence of short-range goals that ultimately lead to the terminal objective for remediation. This continuum, applicable to most types of speech and language disorders, constitutes a framework for a wide variety of specific teaching techniques and procedures.

The goal of the first phase of instruction, called **establishment,** is to elicit target behaviors from a client and then stabilize such behaviors at a voluntary level, and/or establish phonological contrasts lacking in a client's rule system. Establishment procedures are often based on production tasks, as in the example of a clinician teaching a child who does not produce /l/, where to place his tongue to say /l/. In addition, for a child who can say /l/ but deletes it in the final position (e.g., *bow* for *bowl*), the contrast between word-pairs, such as *bow* and *bowl*, may need to be taught during the establishment phase.

The second phase of instruction, called **generalization,** is designed to facilitate transfer or carry-over of behavior at several levels—positional generalization, contextual generalization, linguistic unit generalization, sound and feature generalization, and situational generalization. The treatment process includes instructional activities or strategies designed to facilitate generalization of correct sound productions to sound contrasts, words, and speaking situations that have not been specifically trained. An example of a context generalization activity would be practicing /s/ in a few key words with high vowels (e.g., *see, sit, seek*) and then determining whether /s/ is produced correctly in words where /s/ is followed by low vowels (e.g., *soft, sock, sat*). An example of a situational generalization activity would be practicing /l/ in sentences in the treatment setting and then observing whether the child uses /l/ in sentences produced in his or her classroom or home.

The third phase of remediation, **maintenance,** is designed to stabilize and facilitate retention of those behaviors acquired during the establishment and generalization phases. Instructional activities related to the generalization and maintenance phases of treatment generally overlap. Frequency and duration of instruction are often reduced during maintenance, and the client assumes increased responsibility for "maintaining" correct speech patterns. The client may also engage in specific activities designed to habituate or automatize particular speech patterns. A maintenance activity may consist of a client keeping track of his or her /s/ productions at mealtime or use of *r*-clusters during five-minute phone conversations every evening for a week.

A traditional approach to remediation has been to focus on correcting a single sound, move it through the treatment continuum to the maintenance phase, and then initiate the correction of another sound. Some clinicians prefer to focus on several error sounds or phonological patterns simultaneously, proceeding along the treatment continuum with several segments or processes. Once the client is able to produce the correct form of an error sound and is aware of how it is used contrastively, he or she is ready to move into the generalization phase of instruction.

Clients may enter the treatment continuum at different points, the exact point being determined by the individual's current articulatory skills and phonological rules. Consider these two examples: Mark is able to produce a sound correctly in certain words and is able to perceive the target contrastively. Mark therefore begins instruction at the generalization stage. Kristy is able to produce a sound imitatively in syllables, perceives the sound contrast in word-pairs, but fails to incorporate the target production of the sound into words. She also enters the treatment continuum at the generalization stage, but at an earlier point than Mark. The clinician must identify not only the appropriate phase of the treatment continuum but also the appropriate level within a phase at which to begin instruction. In the cases of Mark and Kristy, the clinician determined from assessment data that instruction for Kristy might start at the syllable level to reinforce correct target sound production at that level, while Mark would start on words that contained facilitating contexts.

STAGES OF THE TREATMENT CONTINUUM

ESTABLISHMENT OF TARGET BEHAVIORS

The first phase of remediation for clients who do not produce target behaviors upon request, or who have perceptual and/or production difficulty with particular adult phonological contrasts, is called *establishment*. During this phase of instruction, the clinician seeks to teach target behaviors and/or establish phonological contrasts. Thus, the focus in this treatment phase is usually the production of a sound in "isolation," syllables, words, and/or the perception of sound contrasts in words. Clients that enter the treatment continuum at the establishment phase are those who (1) do not have a specific sound in their repertoire and are not stimulable on it, (2) produce a sound in their repertoire (produced only in a limited number of phonetic contexts or occasionally in conversation) but are not able to produce the segment on demand, (3) are unable to perceive the sound in minimal pairs, (4) do not use the segment in a particular context or position (positional, sequential, or contextual constraints), and (5) produce a sound on demand but do not easily incorporate the sound into syllabic units.

Two basic teaching strategies are used to establish target behaviors. The first involves perceptual training prior to production training. The second strategy focuses almost exclusively on production tasks. Perceptual training may be described as including conceptualization or phonological contrast training (e.g., sorting word-pairs such as *two* and *tooth* into two categories that reflect the presence of the final consonant and the deletion of the consonant) as well as traditional discrimination tasks (e.g., discrimination of [s] from [θ]).

Discrimination Training. The type of perceptual training that historically was used most commonly is called ear training or speech sound discrimination training. Instructional tasks designed to teach discrimination stem from the traditional motor approach to articulation treatment and typically involve making same–different judgments about what is heard (e.g., "Tell me if these are the same or different—*rake–wake*"). In the next chapter you will find a more complete presentation of procedures for speech sound discrimination training.

Van Riper and Emerick (1984), Winitz (1975, 1984), and Powers (1971) recommended that discrimination training occur prior to production training during the establishment phase of the treatment continuum. Winitz (1975) stated, "A child who does not hear differences between sounds hardly can be expected to produce sounds precisely" (48). Van Riper (1978) made a similar statement: "We [speech clinicians] must help him [child] know how it [the sound] looks, and especially how it sounds" (183). Only sounds produced in error should be included in speech sound discrimination training since little, if any, relationship is reported between an individual's misarticulation of speech sounds and his or her performance on general speech sound discrimination tasks (Aungst and Frick, 1964; Monnin and Huntington, 1974; Locke, 1980).

Traditionally, speech sound (auditory) discrimination training has focused on judgments of external speech sound stimuli. Client productions tape-recorded and played back to the client, as well as ongoing self-judgments (internal speech sound perception or monitoring) by the client of his or her own speech, have also been suggested as training activities. Speech sound discrimination training procedures are often sequenced so that the client goes from external discrimination

Remediation Concepts and Principles

(judgments of another speaker's productions) to delayed external self-discrimination (judgments of one's own tape-recorded productions) to simultaneous productions and monitoring of sounds (judgments of one's own sounds as they are produced).

Winitz (1984) suggested that several weeks or more of auditory discrimination training precede articulation production training, and also be concurrent with production training at each stage of production. In such a procedure, the child does not work on production at a particular production level (e.g., isolation, syllable, word, sentence, conversation) until he or she can make the appropriate speech sound discrimination easily at that level. See the presentation of a traditional discrimination treatment approach in Chapter 10 for an outline of the protocol used in such treatment.

The idea that discrimination training should precede production training is based on the assumption that certain perceptual distinctions are prerequisites for establishing the production of a speech sound in the child's phonological system. This assumption is not universally accepted, either in terms of developmental theory or in intervention models. Regarding the latter, a critical question that remains to be answered is whether or not speech sound discrimination training has an impact on the establishment or production of a target sound.

The extent to which perceptual instruction is an inherent aspect of production training is not clear. For example, when a client is asked to say *house* and he or she says *hout*, the clinician may say "no, not *hout* but *house*." In this instance, instruction is production-oriented, but perceptual training becomes an inherent part of the task. Williams and McReynolds (1975) reported that production training generalized to speech sound discrimination tasks. They also found that sound discrimination training had little initial effect on production of sounds. Shelton, Johnson, and Arndt (1977) reported that production training did not significantly affect speech discrimination scores and discrimination training did not affect production scores. Although there is a lack of evidence regarding the precise nature of the relationship between sound discrimination and the establishment of correct productions, it frequently has been assumed that perceptual training is an inherent part of teaching articulatory productions.

The reported failure of discrimination training to influence phonological productions may be related to the nature of the training task. Savin (1972) questioned children's ability to analyze syllables into phone-size units (individual segments) before 5 or 6 years. Based on that assumption, Shelton (1978) has inferred that speech sound discrimination training focused on segmentation of phones from "larger units" may be of questionable value in children younger than 6 years. Likewise, Bernthal, Greenlee, Eblen, and Marking (1987) found that 4- to 6-year-old normal children with age appropriate phonology had difficulty identifying certain speech sound errors in sentences.

Conceptualization Training. A second type of perceptual training that has gained increased acceptance in recent years is conceptualization or contrast training. The idea of conceptualization training was proposed by La Riviere, Winitz, Reeds, and Herriman (1974) as a strategy for the treatment of certain phonological problems. For example, they recommended that when consonant clusters are reduced the child be taught to sort contrasting word-pairs (e.g., *led–sled*) into categories that reflect simplification of a consonant cluster and those that reflect appropriate production of the target consonant cluster.

Auditory conceptualization was also discussed by Winitz (1975), who emphasized the child's discrimination of auditory features. He pointed out that some children with phonological errors may not have a true speech sound discrimination problem, but rather are simply not able to conceptualize and use sound contrasts ranging from word-pair contrasts to running speech. For example, the client who may be lacking the phonological concept of word-final consonant usage (i.e., the client evidences final consonant deletion—*so* and *soul*; *tea* and *teeth*). In order to facilitate the reduction of the final consonant deletion process, Winitz (1975) suggested conceptualization training. In conceptualization training, the child is trained to contrast and compare speech sounds and syllable structures at the word level and in sentence contexts. Other clinicians (Weiner, 1981; Elbert, Rockman, and Saltzman, 1980) have labeled treatment of this nature as contrast training. In conceptualization training, the client is taught to work contrasting words or syllables into two classes or categories. As suggested above, such training might include a task in which the client raises his or her right hand when a final stop is present in a target word and his or her left hand when a final stop is deleted. The intent of this training is to develop a perceptual awareness of similarities and differences between minimal pairs. It is hypothesized that this awareness will help the client to establish and produce the appropriate phonological contrasts.

In summary, many speech clinicians teach their clients to perceive the distinction between target error sounds, or to identify phonemic contrasts as part of the establishment process. Such training activities may precede and/or accompany production training. Traditional discrimination training has been questioned because many individuals with phonological disorders do not reflect discrimination problems. In addition, production training not accompanied by direct discrimination training has been shown to modify phonological errors. The type of perceptual training that appears most useful during the establishment phase is that of conceptualization or contrast training (for those clients who have not established phonemic contrasts). While there is little data to support the direct influence of conceptualization training on the client's productions, the procedure is a logical requisite to production training, especially when the target sound is produced in other word-positions or contexts. Thus, the face validity of conceptualization training is strong and the instructional procedures have been found useful.

Production Training. Many clinicians begin phonological intervention by focusing on production and postpone or delete perceptual training as part of establishing a new behavior. Whether or not perceptual training precedes or is interwoven with production training, the goal during the establishment phase of production training is to elicit a target behavior from a client, stabilize it at a voluntary level, and make certain that the target segment (speech sound) is perceived in minimal pair contrasts.

When a sound is not in a person's repertoire, it is sometimes taught in isolation or syllables rather than words. It should be remembered that it is nearly impossible to teach speech sounds such as stops in isolation, since by their physical nature, stops are produced in combination with a vowel or vowel approximation. Glides likewise involve production of more than one sound when they are produced.

Whether sounds should be taught initially in isolation, syllables, or words is a matter of some controversy. McDonald (1964) urged that syllables be used in production training since he assumed that the syllable is the basic unit of motor speech production. Some clinicians (e.g., Van Riper and Emerick, 1984) argue that since isolated sounds or syllables are the least complex units of production, and afford the least interference between the client's habitual speech sound error and the learning of a correct production in a meaningful context, they should be taught first. Words sometimes elicit interference from old error patterns and in such cases are not a good place to initiate instruction. Others advocate words (lexical items) as the best place to begin instruction because the client can benefit from contextual influences in meaningful productions.

Four methods are commonly employed by speech-language clinicians to establish the motoric production of a target sound: imitation, contextual utilization, phonetic placement, and successive approximation. Each of these approaches is discussed below.

1. Imitation. We recommend that the clinician attempt to elicit responses through imitation as an initial instructional method for production training. Usually the clinician presents several auditory models of the desired behavior (typically a sound in isolation, syllables, or words), instructs the client to watch his or her mouth and listen to the sound that is being said, and then asks the client to repeat the target behavior. Sometimes, the clinician may wish to amplify the model through an auditory trainer or by simply rolling a sheet of paper into a funnel, placing it against the side of the client's head surrounding the ear, and speaking into the other end. Following this auditory stimulation, the client is asked to produce the sound, syllable, or word. Often, imitation is used in conjunction with phonetic placement (described below) to establish a sound. Correct productions are sometimes tape-recorded by the clinician so that the client may play back and evaluate his or her own productions. Clients may also be asked to focus on how a sound feels during correct production and to modify their productions to maintain this kinesthetic awareness.

When an individual can imitate a target sound, the goal during establishment is to stabilize target productions. Subsequent instruction should begin at the most complex linguistic level at which the client is able to imitate, whether it be isolation, syllables, words, phrases, or sentences. This should have been determined during stimulability testing. Even if the client was not stimulable on a sound during assessment, it is recommended that the clinician begin remediation by asking the client to imitate target productions using auditory, visual, and tactile cues. Milisen (1954) called such multisensory instruction "integral stimulation."

2. Contextual utilization. As a second approach to establishment, especially when the client does not imitate the target behavior, we recommend that the clinician look for contexts in which the target sound can be produced correctly. As indicated earlier, correct sound productions can frequently be elicited through contextual testing since segments are affected by phonetic and positional context. In Chapter 6, contextual or deep testing was recommended for many clients selected for remediation. The intent of such testing is to identify environments and instances where correct production of target behaviors occurs. It is also recommended that when the clinician listens to the client's spontaneous speech that he or she note any words in which misarticulated sounds are produced correctly. Production training would then begin on such a "key" word.

As previously pointed out, although consonants are less likely to be in error when they appear as singles, correct consonant productions are occasionally elicited in clusters even when absent in singles. Therefore, clusters should also be included in contextual testing. Curtis and Hardy (1959) reported that more correct responses of /r/ were elicited in consonant clusters than in consonant singles.

Usually, less than 30 minutes are needed to do a systematic search for correct productions through contextual testing of an individual sound. If a particular context can be found in which the target behavior is produced correctly, it can be used to facilitate correct production in other contexts. For example, if /s/ is produced correctly in the context of the word-pair *bright sun*, the /t/ preceding the /s/ may be viewed as a facilitating context. As a treatment methodology, the client can be instructed to say these two words and prolong the /s/. Later, surrounding sounds may be changed to represent other contexts (e.g., *watch–sun, weep–sun*). By modifying the context, correct productions may become stabilized in the client's repertoire.

The rationale for using phonetic context is similar to that presented for the use of imitation as an instructional method. Because contextual utilization allows the clinician to capitalize on a behavior already in the client's repertoire, it can be an efficient means of establishing the target behavior. McDonald (1964) developed an articulation remediation program based on the assumption that establishment can be accomplished in most clients via context utilization. We recommend that the clinician use imitation and context utilization as the first two procedures in production training.

3. Phonetic placement. When the client is unable to imitate a target sound and no contexts are identified where the target is produced appropriately, the clinician can instruct the client about how to produce a particular sound. This type of instruction is called phonetic placement. In teaching phonetic placement, the clinician

1. Instructs the client where to place the articulators to produce a specific speech sound
2. Provides verbal descriptions of how to make the sound
3. Provides visual and tactile cues to supplement verbal description
4. Analyzes and describes differences between the error production and the target production

The phonetic placement method has probably been used for as long as clinicians have attempted to modify speech patterns. Over a half century ago, Scripture and Jackson (1927) published *A Manual of Exercises for the Correction of Speech Disorders* that included phonetic placement techniques for speech instruction. These authors suggested

1. Mirror work
2. Drawings designed to show the position of the articulators for the production of specific sounds
3. "Mouth gymnastics"; that is, movements of the articulators (lips and tongue) in response to models and verbal cues and instructions
4. The use of tongue blades in order to teach placement of sounds

Remediation Concepts and Principles

The phonetic placement approach involves explanations and descriptions of idealized phoneme productions. The verbal explanations provided to the client include descriptions of motor gestures or movements and the appropriate points of articulatory contact (tongue, jaw, lip, and velum) involved in producing the target segments. This approach to teaching sounds frequently is used alone or in combination with imitation and context utilization. The Appendix describes techniques for teaching various consonants, some of which utilize phonetic placement cues. The following description is an example of a phonetic placement approach to teaching [s]:

> The entire tongue is raised so that its sides are firmly in contact with the inner surface of the upper back teeth. The front of the tongue is slightly grooved along the midline. A tongue depressor is inserted along the midline of the tongue to provide the client a tactile cue as to the place to form the groove. The tip of the tongue is placed immediately behind the upper or lower teeth. The clinician shows the client in a mirror where he or she places the tongue tip. The front teeth (central incisors) are brought in alignment (as much as possible) so that a narrow small space between the rows of teeth is formed. The air stream is directed along the groove of the tongue toward the cutting edges of the teeth.

4. Successive approximation. Complex behavioral responses such as speech sound productions often need to be broken down into a series of successive steps or approximations that lead to the production of the target behavior(s). A teaching method that utilizes successive approximation is termed **shaping.** The shaping process begins with the elicitation or imitation of a response that the client can emit and proceeds through a series of graded steps or approximations, each progressively closer to the target behavior. Shaping has been found to be an efficient method for teaching complex behavioral tasks but requires careful planning in the sequencing of events to be used for treatment.

The first step in shaping is to identify an initial response that the client can produce and one that is related to the terminal goal. One common way this method can be initiated is by the modification of other speech sounds already in the repertoire. Instructional steps move successfully from the initial response to the desired behavior. For example, a client who is unable to produce /s/ could be instructed to:

1. Make [t] (the place of constriction is similar for both sounds)
2. Make [t] with a strong aspiration on the release, prior to the onset of the vowel
3. Prolong the strongly aspirated release
4. Remove the tip of the tongue slowly during the release from the alveolar ridge to make a [ts] cluster
5. Prolong the [s] portion of the [ts] cluster in a word like *oats*
6. Practice prolonging the last portion of the [ts] production, and finally
7. Produce [s]

Likewise, for a child who produces [ɝ] in error, the clinician might shape the child's production according to the evocation program reported by Shriberg (1975):

1. Stick your tongue out (model provided),
2. Stick your tongue out and touch the tip of your finger (model provided),

3. Put your finger on the bumpy place right behind your top teeth (model provided),
4. Now put the tip of your tongue ''lightly'' on that bumpy place (model provided),
5. Now put your tongue tip there again, and say [l] (model provided),
6. Say [l] each time I hold up my finger (clinician holds up finger),
7. Now say [l] for as long as I hold my finger up, like this: (model provided for 5 seconds). Ready. Go.
8. Say a long [l] but this time as you're saying it, drag the tip of your tongue slowly back along the roof of your mouth—so far back that you have to drop it. (Accompany instructions with hand gestures of moving fingertips back slowly, palm up.) (104)

The two examples above reflect ways that clinicians typically capitalize on successive approximations: by shaping behaviors from a sound in the client's repertoire (e.g., /t/), and by shaping from a nonphonetic behavior in the client's repertoire (e.g., protruded tongue). Once the client produces a sound that is close to the target, the clinician can use other techniques, such as auditory stimulation, imitation, and phonetic placement cues to reach the target production. Descriptions of the other possible ways to elicit various sounds are provided in the Appendix.

Establishment Guidelines. Although we have attempted to formulate the following guidelines on the basis of available literature, more often than not, they reflect our own clinical biases. Recognizing that individual variations among clients preclude a detailed set of specific instructions applicable to all clients, these guidelines are general.

1. Perceptual training, particularly contrast training employing minimal pairs, is suggested as part of establishment when there is evidence that the client is unable to perceive appropriate phonological contrasts or that the error pattern is based on a phonological rule.
2. When teaching the production of a target sound,
   a. The recommended sequence for eliciting sounds is (1) imitation (verbal stimulation), (2) contextual utilization, (3) phonetic placement, and (4) successive approximation (shaping).
   b. Look for the target sound in the client's response repertoire through stimulability (imitation) testing, contextual testing (including consonant clusters and other word-positions), and connected speech samples. Stabilize these productions and use them as a starting point for production training.
   c. When several sounds are in error and such errors reflect underlying patterns, the clinician should look for correct production of at least one sound (exemplar) within each sound class during stimulability testing, contextual testing, or in a spontaneous speech corpus. The exemplar(s) should then be stabilized and used to facilitate generalization.
   d. When correct productions of the target patterns are not located via stimulability, contextual testing, or in the speech corpus, such productions may have to be taught.

In summary, imitation, phonetic placement, contextual utilization, and successive approximation are all methods that can be used to establish speech sound productions. Perceptual training should be utilized when appropriate phonological contrasts are not made. If the target behavior can be elicited via imitation, instruction should then proceed to the generalization and maintenance phases of the treatment continuum. For the client who is unable to imitate target sounds

Remediation Concepts and Principles

correctly, context utilization, phonetic placement, and successive approximation should be used.

Generalization

As stated earlier, an articulatory behavior may be considered established in a person's repertoire when that behavior can be produced on demand, and the client is able to make appropriate perceptual judgments of minimal pair contrasts involving the target sound. Once a sound or target behavior has been established, the next task is to facilitate generalization to other linguistic contexts and non-clinical settings. It should be pointed out that in contrast to establishment, generalization is a process that is facilitated rather than taught. Our discussion of generalization will include an introduction to the concept followed by a review of (1) across position generalization, (2) across context generalization, (3) across linguistic unit generalization, (4) across sound and feature generalization, and (5) across situation generalization.

Generalization has been defined by Stokes and Baer (1977) as follows:

> The occurrence of relevant behavior under different non-training conditions (i.e., across subjects, settings, people, behavior, and/or time) without the scheduling of the same events in those conditions as had been scheduled in the training conditions. Thus, generalization may be claimed when no extratraining manipulations are needed for extratraining changes (350).

In other words, generalization (sometimes called transfer) refers to the principle that learning of one behavior in a particular environment often carries over to other similar behaviors, environments, or untrained contexts. For example, if one learns to drive in a Ford automobile, there is a high probability that one can also drive a Plymouth. Generalization of training occurs from one stimulus—driving apparatuses in the Ford—to another—driving apparatuses in the Plymouth. In terms of articulation remediation, if a client learns to produce /f/ in the word *fish*, that [f] production will probably generalize to other words that contain /f/, such as *fun*. If generalization did not occur, it would be necessary to teach a sound in every word and context—an impossible task.

The clinician must rely on a client's ability to generalize in order to effect a change in phonological usage. Generalization, however, does not occur automatically, nor do all persons have the same aptitude for it. People vary in their ability to achieve generalization, but certain activities can increase the likelihood of generalization.

One type of generalization is **stimulus generalization,** which occurs when a learned response to a particular stimulus is evoked by similar stimuli. The importance of reinforcement in such generalization cannot be overemphasized. Behaviors that have been reinforced in the presence of a particular stimulus may be said to have generalized when they occur in the presence of novel but similar stimuli even though the response was not reinforced. Consider this example: A client who utilizes the process of "fronting" has been taught, through the use of an auditory model and appropriate reinforcement, to produce /k/ correctly at the word level in response to the auditory stimulus, "say kangaroo." The client is later shown a picture of a kangaroo and asked to name it, but no model is provided. If the client says "kangaroo" with [kʰ] produced correctly, in response to the picture, stimulus generalization may be said to have occurred.

Response generalization is another type of generalization that is especially relevant to speech remediation. It refers to the process in which responses that are taught carry over to other behaviors that are not taught. An example of response generalization is as follows: A client with /s/ and /z/ errors is taught to say [s] in response to an auditory model of [s]. He or she is then presented with an auditory model [z] and asked to imitate it. If the client emits a correct [z], response generalization may be said to have occurred. Such generalization is well documented in the literature, including an early study by Elbert, Shelton, and Arndt (1967) in which children with /s/, /z/, and /r/ errors were taught to say [s] correctly. Generalization was evident by correction of the untrained /z/, which has many features in common with /s/. However, no generalization to the untrained [r] was noted. Obviously, sounds in the same sound class and having similar features with the target sound are those where response generalization is most likely to occur.

Several different types of generalization may occur during phonological remediation, including generalization from one position to another, from one context to another, to increasingly complex linguistic levels, to nontrained words, to other sounds and features, and to various speaking environments and situations. Clinicians often attempt to facilitate generalization by sequencing instructional steps from simple to more complex behaviors. By proceeding in small progressive steps, the clinician seeks to gradually extend the behavior developed during the establishment period to other contexts and situations.

The amount of training required for generalization has not been established and seems to vary considerably across subjects. Elbert and McReynolds (1978) have reported data from five children indicating that from 5 to 26 sessions were required before generalization occurred. They speculated that the error patterns exhibited by children affected both the time required and the extent of transfer which occurs.

For those clients who begin remediation with an established target behavior in their repertoire, generalization may be the primary task of instruction. Following is a discussion of the various types of generalization that are expected in the articulation remediation process.

Across Word-Position Generalization. Generalization of correct sound productions across word-positions is well documented (Elbert and McReynolds, 1975, 1978; Powell and McReynolds, 1969). This term refers to generalization from a word-position that is taught (initial, medial, or final) to a word-position that is not taught. By teaching a sound in a particular position (e.g., initial position), generalization may occur to a second position (e.g., final position). Speech-language pathologists have traditionally taught target sounds first in the initial position of words, followed by either the final or medial position. One rationale for beginning with the initial position is that, for most children, many sounds are first acquired in the prevocalic position (the most notable exception is certain fricatives which appear first in word-final position).

In the process of investigating the paired-stimuli approach to articulation remediation, Weston and Irwin (1971) examined position generalization. They observed that when a sound was taught in the prevocalic position, generalization usually occurred to the postvocalic position. Similarly, they observed that sounds taught in the postvocalic position usually generalized to the prevocalic position.

In contrast, McLean (1970) found, in a study involving retarded children, that although instruction and practice in the initial (prevocalic) position resulted in generalization to initial position in other words, little transfer occurred to other word-positions. Likewise, Compton (1975) reported little generalization from initial to final word-position in a case study involving a child with normal intelligence.

Ruscello (1975) studied the influence of training on generalization across word-positions. Two groups, each containing three subjects, were presented training programs that differed with respect to the number of word-positions practiced in each session. Ruscello reported significantly more generalization across training sessions for those subjects who practiced a target sound in the initial, medial, and final word-positions than the group who practiced a target sound only in the word-initial position.

Olswang and Bain (1985) reported different amounts of position generalization for /s/ and /l/ in two subjects. For both subjects, improvement in initial /l/ had little influence on final /l/. In other words, improvement on initial /l/ did not seem to facilitate improvement of final /l/. By contrast, when /s/ was trained in one word-position in one subject, it seemed to facilitate production of the sound to other positions. They attributed the differences in position generalization between /l/ and /s/ to the greater allophonic variation between initial and final /l/ compared to that of initial and final /s/.

It can be inferred from the available data that for children with normal intelligence, generalization from initial to final position is just as likely to occur as generalization from final to initial. A preferred word-position that would maximally facilitate position generalization has not been established. Thus the word-position in which a target sound is trained does not seem to be a factor in position generalization. In terms of clinical management, unless the pattern of errors suggests a particular word-position for initial training (such as final consonant deletion), it is recommended that the clinician train the word-position that the client finds easiest to produce, check for generalization to other positions, and then proceed to train the other word-positions if generalization has not already occurred. Except for selected fricative sounds, the easiest position to teach often is the initial position. However, contextual testing may result in the identification of contexts that are more facilitating for an individual child than those which can be predicted from developmental phonological data.

Across Context Generalization. Technically, position generalization may be viewed as a type of contextual generalization. The term *contextual generalization*, however, more commonly refers to phonetic context transfer; for example, generalization from /s/ in *ask* to /s/ in *biscuit* or to /s/ in *fist*. This type of generalization where a production transfers to other words without direct treatment is an example of response generalization as described above.

When preliminary testing has indicated specific contexts in which an error sound may be produced correctly, clinicians will frequently attempt to stabilize such productions—that is, see that a target sound can be consistently produced correctly in that context—and then provide instruction designed to facilitate generalization of the correct sound to other contexts. As with all types of generalization, the client must exhibit transfer to untrained contexts at some point for the remediation process to be complete.

In a study of phoneme generalization, Elbert and McReynolds (1978) reported that although facilitative phonetic contexts have been posited as a factor in generalization, their data did not support the idea that certain contexts facilitate generalization across subjects. Instead, they found a great deal of variability in facilitative contexts across subjects. The authors also reported that once a child imitated the sound, generalization occurred to other contexts. They concluded that the client's possession of the sound in his or her productive repertoire had more to do with generalization than did contextual factors.

Elbert, Powell, and Swartzlander (1991) examined the number of minimal word-pair exemplars necessary for phonologically impaired children to meet a generalization criterion. They reported that for most children, generalization occurred using a small number of word-pair exemplars (five or less for 80 percent of the children) but there was substantial variability across subjects. The occurrence of response generalization subsequent to teaching a small number of exemplars is consistent with findings from previous treatment reports (Elbert and McReynolds, 1978; Weiner, 1981).

Across Linguistic-Unit Generalization. A third type of generalization involves shifting correct sound productions from one level of linguistic complexity to another (e.g., from syllables to words). For some clients, the first goal in this process is to transfer isolated sounds to syllables and words; others begin at the syllabic or word level and generalize target sound productions to phrases and sentences.

Van Riper and Emerick (1984) recommended that the transfer sequence be initiated with sounds in isolation, followed by syllables, words, and finally sentences. This hierarchy of production complexity has been widely adhered to as a treatment sequence.

Instruction at the transfer phase of the instructional continuum begins at the highest level of linguistic complexity at which a client can produce a target behavior on demand. Instruction progresses from that point to the next level of complexity. Winitz (1975) speculated that when sounds are taught in isolation, the effects of coarticulation are absent, and therefore, the potential for generalization to syllables and words is relatively poor. This notion received some support from a study reported by McReynolds (1972), in which the transfer of /s/ productions to words was probed after each of four sequential teaching steps: (1) /s/ in isolation, (2) /sa/, (3) /as/, and (4) /asa/. Although no transfer to words was observed following training on /s/ in isolation, over 50 percent transfer to words was observed following training on /sa/. It should be recognized, however, that the training of /s/ in isolation prior to syllables may have had a learning effect and influenced the generalization observed following syllable instruction.

Some clinicians prefer to initially teach sounds in isolation or in syllables rather than in words in order to decrease interference from previous learning. To avoid interference from previously learned behaviors, the use of nonsense syllables or nonsense (nonce) words to facilitate generalization has been recommended. A child may consistently say *dye* for *bye* and yet, be able to produce the nonsense syllable /baɪ/ because this consonant + diphthong response has not been habituated in a meaningful context and does not reflect interference from previous learning when produced in a series of nonsense syllables.

Van Riper and Emerick (1984) and Winitz (1975) recommended that sounds be taught in nonsense syllables before they are practiced in meaningful words, thereby reducing the interference of previous error productions on the target sound. This view contrasts with another notion that phonological contrasts are more readily established at the word or lexical level since meaningful contrasts are a key to normal phonological acquisition.

When nonsense syllable and/or nonsense word sequences have been taught, the next step is to facilitate generalization to meaningful words. In this phase of instruction, the clinician structures training tasks from less complex to more complex contexts.

Powell and McReynolds (1969) studied generalization in four subjects who misarticulated /s/. They reported that when two of the subjects were taught consonant productions in nonsense syllables, transfer of the target sound to words occurred without additional training. The other two subjects had to be provided instruction at each level of linguistic behavior as generalization from nonsense syllables to words did not occur.

Elbert, Dinnsen, Swartzlander, and Chin (1990) reported that when preschool children were taught target sounds within a minimal pair contrast training paradigm, generalization occurred to other single-word productions as well as to conversational speech. These findings would suggest that these children learned more than motor production skills during treatment as correct forms were stored and retrieved on demand. Based on a three-month post-treatment probe, they reported that subjects continued to improve and increase the number of correct productions.

Shriberg and Kwiatkowski (1987), in a retrospective study of efficacy of intervention strategies, identified self-monitoring procedures as a potentially effective component to facilitate generalization to continuous speech. A subsequent experimental study (Shriberg and Kwiatkowski, 1990) included self-monitoring instruction. They reported that seven of the eight preschool subjects generalized from such self-monitoring instruction to spontaneous speech. They concluded, however, that while self-monitoring facilitated generalization, it varied in terms of type, extent, and point of onset. Thus, while self-monitoring would appear to be a critical skill in generalization, these data did indicate that speech sound generalization could not be predicted from the onset of self-monitoring behaviors.

To facilitate generalization, Gerber (1973) outlined an instructional sequence that relied heavily on the use of nonsense syllables. Gerber arranged nonsense materials according to a hierarchy of complexity in the following sequence:

1. Simple CV, VCV, and VC syllables
2. More complex syllables, including consonant clusters in the pre-, post-, and intervocalic positions: CCV, VCC, and VCCV
3. Simple nonsense words: CVC
4. More complex nonsense words specifically tailored to contexts difficult for the client
   a. Multisyllabic configurations such as *sikesoo, lanasos*
   b. Variations in abutting consonants in releasing and arresting positions such as *kapset, kikso*
5. "Phrases" composed of nonsense words
6. "Conversations" in nonsense words
7. Embedding nonsense material in meaningful units

In summary, it appears that some clients will generalize from one linguistic unit to another without specific training; others will require specific instructional activities for transfer from one linguistic unit to another. The process of generalization seems to vary across individuals for most types of generalization and is true also for linguistic unit generalization.

Across Sound and Feature Generalization. A fourth type of generalization is observed when correct production of a target sound generalizes from one sound to another. Generalization most often occurs within sound classes and/or between sounds that are phonetically similar (e.g., /k/ to /g/; /s/ to /z/ and /ʃ/). Clinicians have long observed that training on one sound in a cognate pair frequently results in generalization to the second sound (e.g., Elbert, Shelton, and Arndt, 1967).

Powell and Elbert (1984) investigated the generalization patterns of two groups of three children each with misarticulations. Specifically, they wanted to see if the group receiving instruction on earlier developing consonant clusters (stop + liquid) would exhibit generalization patterns different from the group receiving instruction on later developing consonant clusters (fricative + liquid). The authors reported that no clear overall pattern was observed; instead, the six subjects exhibited individual generalization patterns. All subjects evidenced some generalization to both the trained and untrained consonant clusters. The most interesting finding was that generalization to both cluster categories occurred on the final probe measure in five of six subjects, regardless of the treatment received. Powell and Elbert (1984) attributed the across sound-class generalization seen in three subjects, in part, to their good pretreatment stimulability skills.

Weiner (1981) also reported across sound generalization in teaching final consonants to children who deleted them. He trained subjects to produce word-final stops and found generalization to word-final fricatives. He also showed that when stopping of fricatives was reduced, the process of fronting of stops was also reduced.

Elbert and Gierut (1986) suggested that generalization across sounds that have little apparent relationship might reflect the child's phonological knowledge of the untreated sounds. They also pointed out that generalization across sound classes has only been reported in cases where the errors were related in terms of phonological processes or rules.

Generalization of correct production from one sound to another is an inherent part of remediation approaches based on place, manner, and voicing analysis, distinctive feature analysis, or phonological process analysis. Often in these approaches, target behaviors, or exemplars, reflecting processes common to several error productions are selected for training. This is done on the assumption that generalization will occur from exemplars to other error sounds within the same sound class or, in some instances, across sound classes.

Sound generalization, as described above, is sometimes explained on the basis of feature similarity among sounds. An underlying assumption of distinctive feature analysis and remediation is that features will generalize from one sound production to another production containing the same features. An example of such generalization can be seen in the client who initially did not correctly produce any sounds containing [+ stridency], yet after learning to produce /s/, was able to correctly articulate /ʃ/ and /z/, which also contain the feature [+ stridency].

A client can learn a feature and transfer the feature without necessarily correcting a sound. For example, a client who substitutes stops for fricatives may learn to produce /f/ and begin using it in his or her speech for several fricative sounds. Although the client no longer substitutes stops for fricatives, he or she now substitutes /f/ for other fricatives (e.g., [sʌn] → [fʌn]; [ʃou] → [fou]); in other words, the client has incorporated a feature into his or her productions but still misarticulates several of the same sounds.

McReynolds and Bennett (1972) studied three subjects who received training to facilitate feature generalization. Instruction for each subject focused on a specified sound that was selected to reflect a particular feature. Specifically, one subject was taught an exemplar containing the [+ stridency] feature, another the [+ voicing] feature, and the third the [+ continuancy] feature. Feature generalization to other error sounds was assessed through deep testing of those phonemes not taught. Results for the three subjects indicated that the feature generalized to several sounds even though training was limited to a single sound (exemplar).

Feature generalization is a critical element in most treatment based on a phonological process approach since elimination of a process may be dependent upon acquisition of a feature in a client's repertoire. The examples presented previously in which stops were substituted for fricatives (stopping) reflect this phenomenon: By teaching the [+ frication] feature, the client acquired a feature that resulted in the reduction of the stopping in untrained fricatives.

Frequently, the establishment of feature contrasts is part of the effort to reduce and eliminate process usage; thus, feature teaching and process reduction approaches are inextricably intertwined. In our later discussion of distinctive feature and contrast therapy, this relationship should become more apparent. The notion of feature and sound generalization, like other types of generalization, is critical to the remediation process.

Across Situations Generalization. The fifth and final type of generalization to be discussed in this chapter is called situational generalization, which involves transfer of behaviors taught in the clinical setting to other situations and locations, such as school, work, or home. This type of generalization is critical to the remediation process because it represents the terminal objective of instruction (i.e., correct phonological productions in conversational speech in nonclinical settings). Such generalization has also been called *carry-over* or "extra therapy generalization" in the speech-language pathology literature.

Most clinicians focus on activities to facilitate situational transfer during the final stages of remediation. Some, including the authors, have argued that clinicians should incorporate these activities into early stages of instruction. For example, once a client can produce single words correctly, efforts should be made to incorporate these words into nonclinical settings. Although much emphasis is placed on facilitating situational generalization, little experimental data are available to provide specific guidance to the clinician.

Studies by Costello and Bosler (1976) and Bankson and Byrne (1972) have shown that situational generalization can be facilitated through training, but the extent of such transfer varies greatly from one individual to another. Costello and Bosler (1976) investigated whether certain situations were more likely to facilitate generalization than others. Using a program designed by Carrier (1970), they observed the extent of transfer that occurred from training in the home environment to probes obtained in the following four settings:

1. A mother administered the probe while sitting across from her child at a table in a treatment room of the speech clinic.
2. An experimenter (who was only vaguely familiar to the child) administered the probe while sitting across from the child at the same table in the same room as #1.
3. The same experimenter administered the probe while she and the child were seated at separate desks facing each other in a large classroom outside of the speech clinic.
4. A second experimenter (unknown to the child prior to the study) administered a probe while she and the child were alone and seated in comfortable chairs in the informal atmosphere of the clinic waiting room.

Although all three subjects generalized from the teaching setting to one or more experimental settings, there was no evidence that one setting was more facilitative than another. These findings point out the complexity of the transfer process. It may be that the variables differ so much from person to person that it is impossible to predict which environments are most likely to facilitate situational transfer.

Costello and Bosler (1976) also reported more situational generalization of training words than untrained words. One might infer from this finding that more situational generalization might be facilitated through the use of a large number of training words than fewer words.

Olswang and Bain (1985) monitored situational generalization for three 4-year-old children in two different settings during speech sound remediation. They examined connected speech samples recorded in conversational activities in a clinic treatment room and connected speech samples audio recorded by parents during conversational activities at home. They reported similar rates and amount of generalization of target sounds for both settings.

Bankson and Byrne (1972) reported that four out of five subjects generalized correct sound production in words from a motor-based remediation procedure to conversational samples gathered both in the training setting (school) and the home environment. While the amount of generalization seen in the home and school training probes varied from day to day for each subject, the daily fluctuations were consistent between settings for each subject. The overall extent to which generalization occurred varied greatly across individuals and fluctuated within subjects from day to day.

One strategy which has been suggested to facilitate situational generalization is the use of self-monitoring (self-evaluation). Self-monitoring techniques have included hand raising (Engel and Groth, 1976), charting (Diedrich, 1971; Koegel, Koegel, and Ingham, 1986), and counting of correct productions, both within and outside the clinic (Koegel, Koegel, Van Voy, and Ingham, 1988). Koegel et al. (1988) examined generalization of /s/ and /z/ in seven children. They reported that when children self-monitored their conversational productions in the clinic, no generalization of the correct target production outside the clinic occurred. However, when children were required to monitor their conversational speech outside the clinic, "rapid and widespread generalization" occurred across subjects although at slightly different rates. They reported high levels of generalization for all subjects.

Despite a paucity of data regarding situational generalization, available evidence indicates that, as with other forms of generalization, the extent to which it occurs in different settings varies greatly among individuals. There is also the suggestion that situational generalization may be influenced by age and how intact the child's phonological system is (Elbert et al., 1990).

Several investigators have suggested that productive phonological knowledge influences children's generalization learning (Dinnsen and Elbert, 1984; Elbert and Gierut, 1986; Gierut, Elbert, and Dinnsen, 1987; Gierut, 1989). They have inferred that phonological knowledge accounts for some of the individual differences that occur in generalization. Gierut, Elbert, and Dinnsen (1987) reported that greater generalization occurred on sounds where children exhibited the most knowledge as opposed to the least knowledge, but was restricted to those sounds for which training was provided. They also reported that when intervention was directed toward sounds where the child evidenced the least phonological knowledge, generalization learning occurred across the child's phonological system. These investigators recommended that clinicians choose sounds for treatment that reflect the least phonological knowledge. The children who demonstrated least phonological knowledge displayed inventory constraints on those sounds. Even though training on sounds in which children showed most knowledge (e.g., positional constraints) facilitated greater generalization within a sound class, training on sounds for which children exhibited least knowledge resulted in more broad-based generalization. Gierut et al. (1987) inferred from these findings that training on sounds in which children displayed least knowledge resulted in more system-wide changes and reorganization of the child's phonological system than did training on sounds in which children showed most knowledge.

Williams (1991) examined generalization of nine children who exhibited least phonological knowledge as reflected by inventory constraints (i.e., the children did not produce /s/ and /r/ on a conversational sample or on a 306-item probe test). The misarticulated [s] and [r] were trained in consonant clusters. Williams reported three different generalization and learning patterns across the subjects, and hypothesized that differences in generalization reflected different levels of phonological knowledge, even though all error targets were classified in the least phonological knowledge category. Williams questioned if Gierut, Elbert, and Dinnsen's (1987) category of least knowledge was too broad to capture subtle differences in children's knowledge and recommended acoustical measurements to supplement transcription to further differentiate the amount of phonological knowledge demonstrated for sounds in the least knowledge category of this system. This observation is consistent with recommendations from Weismer, Dinnsen, and Elbert (1981), Smit and Bernthal (1983), and Tyler, Edwards, and Saxman (1990).

Parental Assistance with Generalization. Clinicians have long recognized that the generalization process in articulation remediation might be facilitated if individuals from the client's environment could be drawn into the generalization phase of the treatment process. The assumption has been that persons significant to the client—parents, spouse, teachers, or peers—could engage in selected activities designed to extend what the clinician was doing in the clinical setting. Several programs include instructional activities designed for parents to use with their children at home (Mowrer, Baker, and Schutz, 1968; Gray, 1974). Sommers (1962) and Sommers, Furlong, Rhodes, Fichter, Bowser, Copetas, and Saunders (1964) studied several variables related to articulation instruction. Greater improvement between pre- and post-test scores was reported for children whose mothers were trained to assist with instruction than for a control group of children whose mothers had not received training. Carrier (1970) reported a study comparing a group of ten children 4 to 7 years old who participated in an articulation training program administered by their mothers and a similar control group who received minimal assistance from their mothers. The experimental group obtained significantly higher scores on four phonological measures than the control group.

Other investigations in which parents provided directed articulation instruction for their children were reported by Shelton, Johnson, and Arndt (1972) and Shelton, Johnson, Willis, and Arndt (1975). In the first investigation, eight school-age children received instruction and monitoring by their parents in the home. Repeated measures involving baseline and treatment probes on sound production tasks, reading samples, and conversational samples reflected varying results. Significant changes on the sound production tasks were not found although scores were higher on the post-test. On the other hand, significant differences were found between mean baseline scores and scores on final reading samples and conversational samples. Four-month post-treatment scores indicated that gains made during the program were maintained.

The second investigation was similar to the first, but younger children (4- to 6-year-olds) were studied. In contrast to the earlier study, these children improved significantly on the sound production tasks. It should be pointed out that the pretest scores for these younger children were lower than for the older group; in other words, the younger group had more room for improvement and, hence, a higher probability of significant differences. The younger children, however, showed less improvement on the conversational samples. Shelton and his colleagues (1975) speculated that the monitoring-reinforcement procedure had greater influence on the conversational scores of subjects who had higher scores on the sound production task at the time the procedure was initiated.

Hodson and Paden (1983) published an approach to remediation that includes parental assistance throughout the treatment process. Parents routinely read a 15-item word list to the child for auditory stimulation and have the child produce the 5 target words for the week. Additional details of this approach are included in the next chapter.

Generalization Guidelines.

1. To facilitate position and context generalization, the clinician usually begins instruction with target behaviors in positions or contexts in the client's repertoire.
2. Since word productions form the basis of position generalization, productions at this level should be incorporated into the instructional sequence as quickly as possible.
3. The more alike that two or more sounds are in terms of phonetic characteristics, the more likely that generalization will occur from one to another. For example, teaching [ɝ] usually results in generalization to the unstressed [ɚ] and the consonantal [r]; teaching one member of a cognate sound-pair, e.g., [s], will usually result in the client's use of the cognate [z].
4. Teaching a distinctive feature in the context of one sound, e.g., continuancy in [f], should result in some generalization of that feature in other untreated sounds, e.g., [ʒ], especially within the same sound class.
5. Data are lacking to support a particular order for teaching sounds in various

Remediation Concepts and Principles

word-positions. The traditional procedure of teaching sounds first in the initial position, and then in the final and medial positions is not supported by available research (even though the initial position develops earliest in most sounds, except for fricatives). Teaching a sound in all positions simultaneously may be an approach to more rapid sound position generalization.

6. To facilitate generalization, target behaviors selected for remediation should represent exemplars of error patterns in clients with multiple errors. When selecting sounds to target for reduction of phonological processes, select at least one sound for each sound class in which the process occurs because generalization is most likely to occur among sounds in the same sound class.

7. Nonsense syllables may facilitate production of sounds in syllable contexts during establishment of sound production because nonsense syllables pose less interference with previously learned behaviors than words. Meaningful words may generalize more rapidly than nonsense syllables because they reflect actual phonemic contrasts and are reinforced in the environment.

8. Activities to facilitate situational generalization are suggested as soon as the client can say a sound in words, rather than waiting until sounds are produced at the sentence level.

9. When sounds are taught in which the client demonstrates least knowledge, they are more likely to generalize to correct production of other sounds than when clients are taught sounds in which they demonstrate most knowledge. More rapid generalization to other words and contexts occurs when sounds which reflect most knowledge are treated.

10. Parents and others in the child's environment can be used effectively to facilitate phonological change in children. The clinician must be sensitive to the role parents or other nonprofessionals can assume in the treatment process. First, if parents are to judge the accuracy of sound productions, they must be able to discriminate the sounds correctly. Second, the clinician must demonstrate to the parents the procedures to be used in the program; then the parents must demonstrate to the clinician the procedures to be used to insure that parents can carry out the procedures. Third, recognize that parents have only a limited amount of time; consequently, programs should be designed for short periods. Fourth, written instructions of the specific tasks should be provided to the caregivers–parents. Finally, clinicians should keep in mind that parents probably function better as monitors of productions than as teachers. Often, parents lack the patience and objectivity necessary to teach their own child. However, if parents or other individuals in the child's environment have the desire, skill, time, and patience to work with their children, the clinician may have a helpful facilitator of the generalization process.

Maintenance and Dismissal

Maintenance. The third phase of phonological instruction, called *maintenance*, is the stage where the client habituates the target behavior and assumes increased responsibility for self-monitoring of target phonological productions. This phase of therapy is an extension of the generalization phase, with considerable overlap between the two. For some individuals, the two phases cannot be distinguished.

During the maintenance phase, clients decrease their contact with the clinician, and sometimes this phase is viewed as the final stage of instruction. Shelton (1978) labeled the terminal objective of articulation remediation as **automatization** and described it as automatic usage of standard articulation patterns in spontaneous speech. The term *automatization* implies that phonological productions can be viewed as motor behavior that develops into an automatic response. When phonological errors are linguistic in nature, maintenance may be viewed as the mastery of phonological rules and phonemic contrasts. In reality, both the motor production and phonological rules become part of a person's everyday productive behavioral responses by this point in treatment. The maintenance phase may be considered complete once the client can consistently use target behaviors in spontaneous speech.

During maintenance, the client usually receives intermittent reinforcement for the new speech patterns because this type of schedule results in behavior that is most resistant to extinction. Clients are also required to monitor their own articulation procedures during maintenance. Self-monitoring tasks can be checked by having the client keep track of target productions during specified periods of the day.

To determine the extent to which a client has maintained target behaviors, the clinician must assess a client's behavior during conversational speech. Diedrich (1971) described procedures for counting and charting speech behaviors but recognized that there are many times when speech patterns cannot be externally monitored. He suggested that three-minute "Talk" samples are a good way to begin monitoring speech during conversation and that counting correct and incorrect target sound productions during a three-minute time period is an effective way to monitor productions. He also suggested that, prior to dismissal from treatment, the monitoring period should be increased to include a majority of the speaking time.

In a study cited earlier, Bankson and Byrne (1972) reported a treatment procedure designed to facilitate generalization and maintenance of correct target sound productions. This procedure involved repetitive readings of a list of target words at increasingly rapid rates. Although generalization to conversational speech occurred from this motor task, none of the subjects developed correct target sound productions to the point of producing their error sounds correctly 95 percent of the time or more in conversation.

Manning and his colleagues (1976, 1977) have suggested that the extent to which a client automatizes a response is related to his or her ability to articulate correctly under conditions of noise. These authors measured the articulatory skills of children who misarticulated either /s/ or /r/. Subjects were divided into a low acquisition group (score below 80 percent correct on the *Deep Test of Articulation*) and a high acquisition group (score above 80 percent correct on the *Deep Test of Articulation*). The children were administered the *Deep Test of Articulation* while competing speech noise was presented binaurally through earphones. Subjects were also administered the same task in a quiet condition (absence of noise). A difference score, based on the articulation test scores under the two conditions, was obtained. Children in the high acquisition group demonstrated a significantly smaller difference score between the noise and quiet conditions than the children in the low acquisition group. The authors concluded that as children acquired correct production of /s/ and /r/, they simultaneously automatized the correct articulatory gestures for sounds, as evidenced by higher test scores and less influence of the noise. These data must be interpreted cautiously, however, because noise was not presented at a constant hearing level and the stimulus conditions were not counterbalanced.

Information from the learning literature offers insights into the maintenance or retention of newly acquired phonological patterns. **Retention,** in the context of phonological remediation, refers to the continued and persistent use of responses learned during instruction. Once an individual learns a new phonological pattern or response, he or she must continue to use (retain) the response. In clinical literature, retention is sometimes discussed in terms of intersession retention and sometimes in terms of habitual retention. *Intersession retention* refers to the ability to produce recently taught responses correctly. Speech clinicians frequently observe "between-session forgetting" in many clients. Mowrer (1977) pointed out that lack of intersession retention is a particular problem with mentally retarded children. *Habitual retention* is the persistent and continued use of the response after instruction has been terminated. The term *maintenance* is frequently used to refer to this phenomenon. Speech clinicians occasionally dismiss clients from instruction only to have them return for additional therapy some months later. Such individuals obviously did not habituate or retain their newly learned responses.

Sommers (1969) reported that articulation errors are particularly susceptible to regression. In a follow-up study of 177 elementary school children who had been dismissed from articulation instruction during a six-month period, he found that approximately one third had regressed. Based on conversational samples of target sound productions, 59 percent of those who had worked on /s/ and /z/ had regressed, but only 6 percent of those who had worked on /r/ had regressed. He does not report dismissal criteria or the level of performance prior to dismissal.

In contrast, Elbert et al. (1990) reported that in preschool children learning continued beyond treatment as subjects' speech continued to improve on both single-word and conversational speech samples obtained three months post-treatment. These data support the idea that young children are actively involved in the learning process and seem to make changes more easily in their phonological system. Such changes seemed to occur even after treatment was terminated.

Little is known about the reasons for regression in habitual retention or maintenance, but it is quite likely that variables affecting habitual retention affect intersession retention as well. On the basis of memory studies, Winitz (1969) proposed that interference, which results in competition between the error sound and the newly acquired sound, may explain why individuals forget articulatory responses. Winitz pointed out that the years of motor production practice using an incorrect articulatory gesture, such as /t/ for /tʃ/, will interfere with the individual's ability to produce a newly learned /tʃ/. Similarly, speech clinicians frequently observe individuals who, during the early stages of instruction, insert a /θ/ following a newly learned /s/ in a word context (e.g., [sθup]).

Mowrer (1982) pointed out several factors that have been shown to influence the degree to which information will be retained, whether in the child who is dismissed from therapy but returns for lack of long-term maintenance or the child who seems to have forgotten previous learning in the three days between sessions. First, the meaningfulness of the material used to teach the new responses may affect retention, although there is little empirical evidence in the articulation learning literature regarding this point. In general, as the meaningfulness of the material increases, the rate of forgetting tends to decrease, and thus, the use of meaningful material is recommended during remediation. Thus, names of friends, family members, pets, familiar objects, and animals are appropriate choices. Although meaningfulness of material may be an important aid to long-term retention, the clinician may find, as stated earlier, that nonmeaningful material (e.g., nonsense syllables) may be useful during earlier phases of instruction (i.e., establishment). Leonard (1973) reported that when /s/ had been established in meaningful words, fewer training trials were required to transfer to other words than when nonsense items were utilized. But this finding regarding generalization must be distinguished from the finding presented earlier in our discussion of interference, that acquisition or establishment of new responses can be accomplished in fewer trials with nonsense items than with meaningful items.

A second factor believed to affect retention is the degree or extent to which something has been learned. In general, the greater the number of trials during the learning process, the greater the retention. Retention improves when some overlearning of verbal material takes place. To avoid unnecessary practice, it is important to determine the minimum amount of learning needed to provide a satisfactory level of retention. The optimum point for stopping instruction occurs when additional training does not produce sufficient change in performance to merit additional practice; however, there is little data to provide guidance to the clinician as to where this point may be.

A third factor affecting retention is the frequency of instruction or the distribution of practice. Retention is superior when tasks are practiced during several short sessions (distributed practice) than during fewer, longer sessions (massed practice). On the basis of this fact, frequent, short practice sessions are recommended. In his review of this topic, Mowrer (1982) concluded that "On the basis of controlled learning experiments in psychology alone, it could be recommended that clinicians could increase retention by providing frequent instruction; but bear in mind that no data are available from speech research that confirms this recommendation . . . the important factor in terms of frequency of instruction is not how much instruction . . . but the total number of instruction periods" (259).

A fourth factor shown to affect retention is the individual's motivational state. The more motivated a person, the greater the retention of the material that has been learned. Little, if any, experimental work reported in the phonological literature has attempted to examine motivational state during speech instruction.

Dismissal Criteria. The maintenance phase provides a period for monitoring retention, and it is during this period that dismissal decisions are made. Limited data on dismissal criteria have been reported, and thus, evidence is lacking to support a single dismissal criterion. Elbert (1967) suggested dismissal might be based on two questions: (1) Has the maximum change in this individual's speech behavior been attained? (2) Can this individual maintain this level of speech behavior and continue to improve without additional speech instruction? Whatever criteria are used for dismissal, they should be based upon periodic samples of phonologic behavior over time. The maintenance phase provides the final opportunity for the clinician to monitor, reinforce, and encourage the client to assume responsibility for habituation of the new speech patterns.

Diedrich and Bangert (1976) reported data on articulatory retention and dismissal from treatment. Some of the children studied were dismissed after reaching a 75 percent criterion level for correct /s/ and /r/ productions, as measured on a 30-item probe word test plus a three-minute sample of conversational speech.

Four months later, 19 percent of the subjects had regressed below the 75 percent criterion level. No greater retention was found, however, among those children who remained in treatment until achieving higher than 75 percent criterion level on the probe measure. Diedrich and Bangert concluded that most speech clinicians tend to retain children with /s/ and /r/ errors in articulation instruction longer than necessary. It is unclear whether similar conclusions would have been reached if a higher criterion level (e.g., 95 to 100 percent) had been used.

Maintenance and Dismissal Guidelines.

1. Because the client is seen less frequently for clinical instruction during the maintenance phase, the client should assume responsibility for self-monitoring.
2. The reinforcement schedule for correct responses should be intermittent during maintenance, just as during the latter stages of generalization. Either a variable ratio or variable interval schedule of reinforcement is recommended.
3. Little information is available regarding dismissal criteria; therefore, the matter is left up to clinicians and clients. It has been suggested that clinicians may tend to keep clients enrolled for phonological remediation longer than is necessary. In other words, the cost–benefit ratio for intervention may significantly decline after a certain point is reached in treatment.

MEASURING CHANGES IN PHONOLOGICAL BEHAVIOR

Phonological assessments are used not only to determine the need for intervention and to plan treatment but also to measure changes brought about by intervention and maturation. Clinicians must have the knowledge and techniques to assess the results of their work so that they can monitor performance and demonstrate accountability for their services.

The traditional procedure for measuring the effectiveness of treatment was to compare a client's performance on a test administered before treatment with performance on the same test after a given span of time. Pre- and post-test comparisons were utilized almost exclusively in clinical practice prior to the 1970s as the basis for determining progress during an interval of clinical instruction.

Three-position speech sound tests have been used most commonly for pre- and post-test comparisons although spontaneous speech samples, contextual tests, and individually designed probes have also been used. Pre- and post-test comparisons with three-position tests provide the clinician with only general indices of client progress. Pre- and post-test comparisons using probes, contextual samples, or conversational samples may provide greater measurement sensitivity. However, they do not provide data regarding changes in production over short-term time intervals, such as a week or a month.

To obtain a more sensitive index of client change during instruction than is possible through pre- and post-testing, the clinician should make repeated measurements at daily, weekly, or biweekly intervals during intervention. Such repeated samplings of phonological behavior provide clinicians with better feedback about client progress.

Keeping track of client responses during an instructional session is an additional method whereby the clinician may assess client progress. Keeping track of responses provides the clinician with data for determining the percentage of correct and incorrect responses made during instruction. By noting each response, the clinician accumulates intrasession feedback on the appropriateness of the training tasks being used with the client. If the client is not experiencing an appropriate degree of success, the clinician may consider modifying instruction—perhaps increasing the number of stimulus cues, simplifying the task, changing the reinforcement schedule, or increasing the strength of reinforcement. Extraneous factors, such as time of day or week that sessions are scheduled or problems at school or home, can also affect success. Mowrer (1969) suggested that the error rate should not exceed 25 percent during the establishment phase of phonological remediation.

Counting correct and incorrect responses can also help the clinician determine whether a client has reached a particular level of achievement, that is, a criterion level. The clinician may, for example, require a client to produce a sound correctly in syllables on at least 18 out of 20 attempts (90 percent criterion level) before proceeding to production in words. In this hypothetical instance, the clinician may collect data on syllable productions in blocks of 20 trials. Since treatment programs are generally sequenced from easy to more complex tasks, movement from one level to the next is usually based upon the attainment of a particular criterion level.

A second sampling technique used to obtain repeated measures is the administration of a generalization probe that typically samples a target sound in a number of non-trained items. Some probes may assess several target sounds. An example of a generalization probe is the *Sound Production Task* (*SPT*) developed by Elbert, Shelton, and Arndt (1967) to assess phoneme productions on an in-depth basis. The Sound Production Task is a 30-item task requiring the client to imitate a particular sound in a variety of phonetic contexts, including isolation, syllables, words, and sentences (see Table 9–1). Elbert, Shelton, and Arndt reported that when variations of such tasks for /s/ and /z/ were repeatedly admin-

TABLE 9–1. **Sound Production Task Sheet.**

/S/ RANDOM ARRANGEMENT I	
1. /us/	16. classday
2. musty	17. Please breathe softly.
3. /sae/	18. He has on a clean suit.
4. household	19. passthat
5. glasszoo	20. iceroom
6. I'm on your side.	21. Will he be home soon?
7. placemat	22. husky
8. missing	23. /is/
9. The dog sits up.	24. Will you be up Sunday?
10. houseknife	25. asleep
11. /s/	26. Who took his seat?
12. I will get some.	27. I like soup.
13. Bob sent me.	28. The dress is all silk.
14. /sa/	29. icewater
15. busboy	30. I lost my red socks.

istered to children receiving instruction on these sounds, the probes were sensitive to changes in articulatory behavior. Subsequent investigators have also reported these tasks to be useful in assessing articulatory change (Diedrich, 1971; Turton, 1973). Similar measures for determining progress are the *Deep Test of Articulation* and the *C-Pak* described in Chapter 6. As with the SPT, these measures assess productions of a single phoneme in a variety of phonetic contexts.

Probably the most commonly used generalization tasks are specialized probe lists which reflect the behavior being taught in a variety of untrained stimulus contexts. For example, in a study to examine the potential effect of repeated probes, Winner and Elbert (1988) developed 36-item probe lists for each subject in the study. Each list consisted of stimulus items which contained the treatment sound in several different contexts: (1) consonant-vowel (CV) and vowel-consonant (VC) syllables, (2) vowel-consonant-vowel (VCV) nonsense syllables, (3) monosyllabic words, (4) bisyllabic words, and (5) short phrases. While training probes occasionally include both trained and non-trained items, generalization can only be determined through the non-trained items.

A third sampling procedure often used as a generalization probe technique is the collection of connected speech samples. Diedrich (1971) suggested that the clinician engage the client in a three-minute conversation, tabulate the number of correct and incorrect productions of target sounds, and then determine percentage of correct and incorrect productions. Winitz (1975) suggested weekly or biweekly conversational speech probes of five to ten minutes in length.

Generalization probes are a commonly used method for measuring behavioral changes during treatment. As discussed earlier, generalization may occur across phoneme positions and context (e.g., from initial to final position), across levels of articulation program steps (e.g., from words to phrases), across different evoking stimuli (e.g., from auditory model to picture), across different words (e.g., from a noun to a verb), from structured to spontaneous speech (e.g., from describing a picture to conversation), and from the clinical setting to the natural environment.

To effectively document changes in articulation, generalization measures should include enough items to provide a sensitive assessment of target sound production and should usually be administered on a weekly or biweekly basis. The following sections—on tabulating data and determining functional relationships—will provide further information on the measurement of articulatory performance.

Tabulating Data

Once phonological samples designed to measure clinical progress have been collected, the data must be analyzed and interpreted. Three common methods of reporting articulatory changes are (1) reporting the ratio of right–wrong responses, (2) reporting the percentage of correct responses, and (3) reporting the rate at which particular responses occur within a given time period.

When data are presented as the number of correct responses, all samples must contain the same number of target sound productions to allow meaningful comparisons. This is not a problem when a measure is employed which utilizes a standard number of items, but in spontaneous samples, the number of target sounds is likely to vary and a numerical count of the correct responses may be misleading. If the total number of target sounds varies from sample to sample, it is preferable to convert the ratio of right–wrong productions into a percentage score so that the data are comparable. Consider the following example: Susie produced 8 out of 30 sounds correctly on the first phonological sample, with the following correct/incorrect ratios: 8/36, 7/25, 9/23, 12/24, and 6/10. Presenting the right–wrong ratios in this form makes it difficult to determine if Susie is making progress. When these figures are translated into percentages—22 percent, 28 percent, 39 percent, 50 percent, and 60 percent—it becomes clear that this client's articulatory skill is improving. The expression of scores in a common scale or through conversion to percentages also makes it easier to chart progress. As a result, phonological behavior is commonly expressed as a percentage of correct items attempted even when articulatory samples or probes contain the same total number of responses.

A third method sometimes used to tabulate responses is the calculation of the rate of correct responses. In this system, the clinician records the number and rate of correct and incorrect responses during a given time period and then determines the rate of correct as well as incorrect responses per minute. For progress to be shown, the rate of correct responses must increase while the rate of incorrect responses decreases. Consider Figures 9–1 and 9–2. In Figure 9–1, although the rate of correct responses increased, the rate of incorrect responses also increased. In Figure 9–2, the rate of correct responses increased and the rate of incorrect responses decreased while the overall rate of responding remained stable across all four samples. Figure 9–2 thus reflects improvement in articulatory performance; Figure 9–1 reflects only an increase in the response rate. These examples illustrate the necessity of recording the rate of both correct and incorrect behaviors when using the rate of correct responses to measure change in articulation performance.

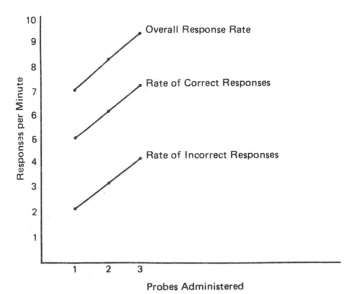

FIGURE 9–1. Correct responses only.

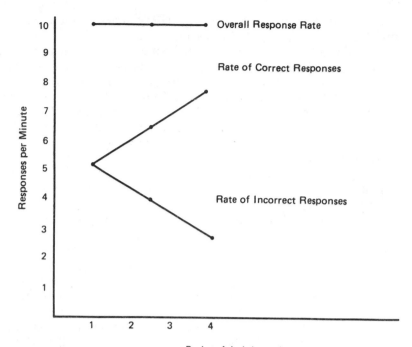

FIGURE 9–2. Correct and incorrect responses.

Client-Based Research: Determining Functional Relationships

To document client change, it is recommended that clinicians follow certain research principles. Adherence to these principles can enhance the certainty with which one can claim a relationship between instruction and changes in phonological performance.

A traditional research method for determining the effectiveness of treatment has been to compare progress made on pre- and post-test measures by a group of clients that receive treatment and a control group that does not. If the group receiving instruction made greater improvement than the control group, it was concluded that intervention was effective. This type of research design, however, is usually not practical for the practicing clinician because of the difficulties with matching groups, the heterogeneity of subjects, and obtaining appropriate control subjects. More viable designs are single-subject designs in which a client can serve as his or her own control.

To establish a functional relationship between treatment and changes in phonological behavior, using a single-subject research design, the clinician must first measure the level of performance before intervention. Performance can be measured with repeated probes such as conversational samples, number of consonants correct, or whole-word accuracy. Such repeated measures are used to establish a **baseline.** A stable performance baseline is desirable so that measures obtained during treatment can be compared with it. Three or four samples within ±10 percent of a mean are usually considered a stable baseline. Once a baseline is established, the treatment program is administered. During the treatment stage, the clinician periodically probes articulatory generalization, and data from these probes are compared with the baseline data.

Although intervention data may reflect changes in behavior, some might argue that improvement from baseline performance during treatment may result from factors other than treatment. Changes in phonological performance across time might result from maturation or from the fact that the child's classroom teacher has worked on sound productions during reading class. Such possibilities point out the necessity of using a control procedure to establish a functional relationship between treatment procedures and phonological change. Accordingly, if it can be demonstrated that when intervention is withdrawn or terminated, the performance regresses or maintains at the same level, then a functional relationship may be assumed to exist between intervention techniques and the behavior of interest.

The graph in Figure 9–3 reflects baseline, intervention, and the withdrawal or termination of treatment. By comparing performance level during the baseline condition and following withdrawal of treatment with that which occurred during intervention, the clinician may be able to determine if treatment affected the phonological behaviors being measured. This design is called an **A-B-A design.** A variation of this design is an **A-B-A-B design** where the treatment is later reinstated following the termination of the treatment to see if the percent of correct responses increases when treatment is reinstated. While this type of design is useful in certain types of behavioral research, it does not lend itself well to clinical phonology. Because phonological instruction is designed to facilitate continuance of behavior without contingencies, it is sometimes difficult and usually undesirable to get a behavior back to baseline status once progress has begun to occur. As a result of this phenomenon, other designs are more appropriate for demonstrating a functional relationship between instruction and changes in phonology.

Another research design which allows for control procedures more appropriate to phonological intervention is called a **multiple baseline design.** A multiple

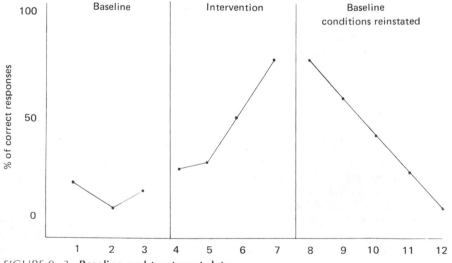

FIGURE 9–3. Baseline and treatment data.

baseline design allows one to determine if a particular treatment is effective in changing two or more behaviors (sounds) in a subject. The phonemes selected for treatment need to have enough featural dissimilarity so that treatment of one does not influence production of another (i.e., generalization is not predicted to occur from one segment to another). For example, treatment which focused on a distorted /s/ would not likely generalize to /r/ but such training would likely generalize to /z/.

Initially, baseline measurements are taken on two to four target phonemes.

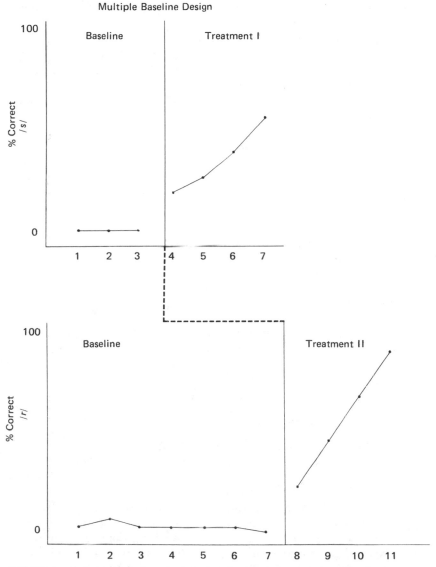

FIGURE 9–4. **A multiple baseline design for investigating the effects of a phonological intervention procedure.**

Treatment is then initiated for one target while performance on the other targets continues to be assessed through ongoing probe measures. Once treatment on the first behavior reaches a predetermined criterion, treatment is shifted to the second behavior. It is expected that the second, third, or fourth behavior will continue to show little, if any, change in the ongoing baseline measurements until treatment activities are focused on that particular behavior. A stable baseline for the second behavior (and subsequent additional behaviors) prior to direct intervention demonstrates that the treatment affected only the treated behavior (i.e., a functional relationship exists between the treatment and a change in behavior). It also demonstrates that time, maturation, and/or other variables did not change the behavior before treatment initiation.

The graph in Figure 9–4 reflects similar baseline levels for both /s/ and /r/. During Treatment Phase I, /s/ is taught and /r/ remains in baseline. Note that during this phase, /s/ improved and /r/ did not. During Treatment Phase II, however, the clinician trained /r/, and this time, production of /r/ improved. Such data support the assertion of a functional relationship between treatment and changes in articulatory behavior. A multiple baseline design provides stronger documentation of treatment effectiveness than a simple comparison of baseline and treatment measures for a single experimental phoneme. Procedures like these allow the clinician to approach each client as a mini-research endeavor and to personify what is often referred to as a clinician-researcher. Individuals who are interested in other single-subject designs are referred to references such as McReynolds and Kearns (1983).

ADMINISTRATIVE CONSIDERATIONS RELATED TO PROVISION OF INSTRUCTION

Several administrative or treatment related organizational matters should be presented in a discussion of clinical intervention for communication disorders. Establishing treatment objectives, developing individual educational plans (IEPs), temporal sequencing of instructional components, principles of behavioral management, strategies for attacking treatment goals, scheduling of treatment, determining whether individual or group treatment is appropriate, and intervention style are topics we want to briefly discuss in this section. These concerns are relevant for most treatment approaches being employed.

ESTABLISHING TREATMENT OBJECTIVES

Before initiating treatment, the clinician targets behaviors for instruction and then develops an overall plan of action. Typically, this involves formulating short-term and long-term goals for instruction plus precise goals for initial instruction. It is often helpful to state goals as *behavioral objectives* since the specificity required to present goals in this fashion makes evaluation and measurement of progress less subjective and provides a mechanism for modifying treatment as needed.

Short-term goals represent objectives for a single week or month of therapy, whereas long-term goals are the terminal objectives of remediation and usually result in dismissal from instruction. Successful performance on short-term goals leads to completion of long-term goals. This hierarchical relationship allows progress to be monitored in order to modify instruction as needed. The following statement provides an example of a short-term goal:

> The child will use final consonant sounds with 50 percent accuracy in target words while reading 10 sentences.

Diedrich and Gerber (1974) presented this example of a terminal objective:

> The child will produce words containing /r/ in a Sound Production Task and three-minute talk task administered by the clinician during two consecutive probes which are given one or two weeks apart. At least 75 percent of the child's /r/ sounds must be judged as correct.

Behavioral Objectives. Mowrer (1982) stated that behavioral objectives serve three main functions: (1) They provide direction in the formation of goals for instruction; (2) they provide a way to determine whether goals have been met; and (3) they facilitate the student's learning. They also provide a mechanism for deciding when to alter treatment. Behavioral objectives should be formulated so that they delineate what the client will be able to do as a result of the learning experience. In his presentation on how to write objectives, Mager (1962) recommended that the definition of instructional objectives include (1) what the learner is supposed to be doing, (2) the conditions under which he or she will be doing it, and (3) a criterion to indicate how well he or she will be doing it.

When identifying the first component—what the client is to do, the clinician should choose verbs that specify behaviors that can be counted or measured (such as *say, write, point*) rather than behaviors that are more difficult to document (such as *know, understand, feel*). As a guideline for developing objectives, the clinician should view behavior as having a beginning and an ending. Terms like *enjoy, understand*, and *appreciate* do not have such beginnings and endings; they are difficult to measure or count and should be avoided when writing behavioral objectives. Another point to keep in mind is that behavioral objectives should delineate what the client is to do, not what the clinician is to do.

The following statements are behavioral objectives that are difficult to count:

1. Have the client learn /s/.
2. Have the client discriminate /r/.
3. Have the client know the phonetic placement for /s/.

Note the change when verbs describing countable or measurable behaviors are substituted:

1. Have the client say /s/.
2. Have the client raise his or her hand when /r/ is heard.
3. Have the client place his or her tongue behind the alveolar ridge.

The second component of a behavioral objective states the conditions under which the behavior is to be performed. The underlined words in the following examples specify the conditions:

1. Have the client say /s/ <u>following the clinician's model</u>.
2. Have the client raise his or her hand <u>each time /r/ is produced in the clinician's reading of the "My Grandfather" passage</u> (Fairbanks, 1960).

3. Have the client place his or her tongue behind the alveolar ridge <u>each time the clinician requests it</u>.

The third component of a behavioral objective establishes the criterion for successful completion of the objective; that is, it indicates the performance level required of the client. The criterion is often a specific number or percentage of correct responses, a time limit, or a minimum number of actions. The underlined words in the following examples establish the criterion measures:

1. Have the client say /s/ following the clinician's model <u>with 19 out of 20 correct</u> (criterion is based on the number of correct responses).
2. Have the client raise his or her hand each time /r/ is produced in the clinician's reading of the "My Grandfather" passage <u>with 60 percent accuracy</u> (criterion is based on percentage of correct responses).
3. Have the client place his or her tongue behind the alveolar ridge each time the clinician requests it <u>during a two-minute interval</u> (criterion is based on performance in a unit of time).

As can be observed in the examples above, these three components allow the clinician to formulate a behavioral objective that clearly states *what* the client is to accomplish, the *conditions* under which he or she is to accomplish it, and the *criterion* for success. Once the behavioral objectives of remediation have been determined, specific instructional methodologies should be developed and implemented.

Developing Individual Education Programs

Individualized instruction has been an inherent part of specific education and rehabilitation services for many years. The philosophy of an educational plan based on individual needs of children is reflected in Public Law 94-142, Education for All Handicapped Children Act, initially enacted into law in 1975 and amended and reauthorized several times. The most recent reauthorization was the 1990 Individuals with Disabilities Education Act (IDEA). One of the provisions of this act was the requirement that an individual education program (IEP) be developed for each child between 3 and 21 years enrolled in a public school special education program, including speech or language remediation programs. The IEP is a written statement of an individually designed instructional program which incorporates behavioral objectives as discussed above. In essence, this is a statement of the plans to achieve certain instructional objectives for a given child. The law stipulates that the following team of individuals will be involved in the development of the IEP:

1. A representative of the local education agency who is qualified to provide or supervise the provision of special education (e.g., the speech-language pathologist)
2. Teacher(s) of the child
3. The parents or guardian of the child
4. Whenever appropriate, the child
5. Other individuals (i.e., physical therapist or social worker) at the discretion of the parent or agency.

The function of the multidisciplinary team is to (1) develop the IEP and

Remediation Concepts and Principles

determine the education program, (2) specify the necessary related services (e.g., speech-language services), and (3) establish monitoring procedures for the implementation and revision of the plan.

The basic IEP contents must include:

1. A statement of the child's present levels of educational performance
2. A statement of annual goals, including short-term instructional objectives
3. A statement of the specific special-education and related services to be provided the child
4. The projected dates for initiation of services and the anticipated duration of the services
5. Appropriate objective criteria and evaluation procedures and schedules for determining, on at least an annual basis, whether the short-term instructional objectives are being achieved

In summary, the IEP must include a statement of annual goals including short-term objectives. The behavioral objectives required by the IEP can be formulated on the basis of information discussed above under the heading *Behavioral Objectives*. It will be remembered that the statement of behavioral objectives should include the circumstances surrounding the performance, what the child is to do, and the degree of proficiency the child is expected to achieve in performing the tasks.

A brief IEP for a child in need of phonological remediation might include the following:

PRESENT LEVEL OF PERFORMANCE	ANNUAL GOAL	INSTRUCTIONAL OBJECTIVES	EVALUATION PROCEDURES
Speech is intelligible (understandable) only 60 percent of the time in conversational speech	Increase speech intelligibility to 85 percent of the time in conversational speech	Reduce final consonant deletion of stops from 90 percent to 10 percent, and fricatives from 90 percent to 30 percent in conversational speech; reduce gliding of liquids from 100 percent to 30 percent in conversational speech	Tape-record and analyze a three-minute conversational sample; identify the possible occurrence of final consonant deletion in stops and fricatives and gliding of liquids and the percent of time child uses the patterns

Temporal Sequencing of Instructional Components

Once the instructional objectives have been determined, the clinician formulates an instructional plan that spells out the temporal sequence of instructional components. The typical sequence of clinical speech instruction is as follows:

Antecedent events: stimulus events designed to elicit particular responses

Responses: the behavior elicited

Consequent events: the reinforcement, punishment, or neutral consequences that follow the response

TABLE 9–2. **Temporal Sequence of Instructional Component.**

ANTECEDENT EVENT	RESPONSE	CONSEQUENT EVENT	CRITERION
Picture of sun + Verbal Instruction—"Say 'sun' 5 times."	"sun"	"good" + chip	5 out of 5 correct
	"sun"	"good" + chip	
	"sun"	"good" + chip	
	"sun"	"good" + chip	
	"sun"	"good" + chip	criterion met
Picture of sun + Verbal Instruction—"Name this picture 5 times."	"sun"	"good" + chip	5 out of 5 correct
	"sun"	"good" + chip	
	"sun"	"good" + chip	
	"sun"	"good" + chip	
	"sun"	"good" + chip	criterion met
Say "hot sun."	"hot thun"	"no—you didn't keep your teeth together."	1 out of 1 criterion not met

Antecedent events are the stimulus events present during or just prior to a response. Such events typically consist of a verbal model, a picture, printed material, or verbal instructions designed to elicit particular verbal responses.

Responses are the behaviors the client produces. They may range from approximations of the desired behavior (e.g., movement of the tongue backward) to production of the correct behavior (e.g., production of /k/ in connected speech). The clinician is concerned with the functional relationship between an antecedent event and a response or, in other words, the likelihood that a given stimulus will elicit the desired response.

The third aspect of the sequence is the *consequent events*. Consequent events occur following a particular response and usually are labeled reinforcement or punishment. Whether or not a response is learned (and how quickly it is learned) is closely related to the nature and frequency of the consequent events.

An example of the three instructional components in a temporal sequence of responses is reflected in Table 9–2.

An expansion of the treatment model described above was reported by Shriberg and Kwiatkowski (1982). They identified ten basic elements that are part of treatment programs and organized them under four components of therapy. The following is a listing of these elements:

1. Target Response
   a. *intended target response(s)*: phonological element selected for intervention—phoneme, cluster, process
   b. *response definition(s)*: Observable behavioral features required to produce the target response
   c. *obtained target response(s)*: behavioral response(s) from a client
2. Training Stimuli
   a. *training stimuli (individual)*: individual linguistic units in which the target response is embedded
   b. *training stimuli (block)*: refers to a list of training stimuli (e.g., list or block of words)
   c. *termination criterion*: performance level that is necessary and sufficient for advancing to the next step
3. Instructional Events
   a. *antecedent instructional event(s)*: clinician, material, and instrumental events designed to elicit a target response

Remediation Concepts and Principles

b. *subsequent instructional event(s)*: all clinician, material, and instrumental stimuli that occur after the target response

4. Motivational Events
   a. *antecedent motivation event(s)*: events that occur before or concurrently with the target response and motivate a response and/or learning (e.g., spinning a spinner)
   b. *subsequent motivational event(s)*: a consequating event that is intended as a reinforcer

While this model reflects a behavioral orientation to therapy, portions of it may also be applied to other intervention approaches.

Principles of Behavioral Management

McReynolds (1970) suggested that the major emphasis in the modification of verbal behavior should not be on the preparation and presentation of stimulus materials, but rather on the effective and efficient utilization of consequent events. Consequences which follow target behaviors are critical for increasing the likelihood of a response reoccurring in the future.

The administration of positive reinforcement is the most frequently used consequent event in clinical speech instruction. When a consequence is presented contingent upon or immediately following a behavior, and the behavior increases in frequency, the contingent consequence is termed a positive reinforcer.

To insure the efficient use of positive reinforcement, clinicians should keep three points in mind. First, a consequent event must be something that is reinforcing for the child; that is, it must increase the probability that a behavior will reoccur. Reinforcement is a highly individual matter, and thus, the nature of appropriate reinforcers will vary across individuals. Verbal reinforcement may give excellent results with some children; toys or food may be more effective with others. For some clients, tangible reinforcers can be paired with verbal or token reinforcement to establish nontangible consequences as reinforcers. Often, backup reinforcers, such as food, toys, or privileges must be used with token and/ or social consequences to maintain the reinforcing properties of the nontangible reinforcers. In these situations, tokens are traded in for some type of backup reinforcement (e.g., food, toys).

A second important point is that the reinforcer must be presented immediately after the desired behavior occurs. If a delay is allowed between the response and the presentation of the reinforcer, any intervening behavior that takes place will likely be reinforced and strengthened. In addition, any delay between a behavior and its reinforcement results in a decrement in learning, thus, reducing the effectiveness of the reinforcer.

The third point is that the reinforcer must be clearly identified. A clinician's smile that inadvertently occurs after the client makes an error may reinforce the error production. Thus, reinforcers with well-identified visual or auditory characteristics are recommended (e.g., tokens, stars, point counters that make loud clicks, and the like).

A second type of consequent event is called *punishment*. Punishment is the opposite of positive reinforcement and occurs when a consequence following a behavior decreases the probability of that behavior reoccurring. Punishment has very limited use in speech remediation primarily because (1) the ethics of using punishment are frequently questioned; (2) the long-term effectiveness of punishment has been questioned; and (3) the elimination of one undesirable behavior sometimes will result in the acquisition of a second undesirable behavior (symptom substitution).

A consequent event that functions like punishment is termed *time-out* from positive reinforcement. This procedure is effective only if some consequent event has previously been established as a positive reinforcer. In time-out from positive reinforcement, the behavior to be modified is followed by a withdrawal of the opportunity to receive positive reinforcement. A clinical example of this occurs when, following an undesirable behavior like putting feet on the table, the clinician stops instruction and looks at the floor until the client again places his or her feet on the floor.

Still another type of consequent event that reduces the probability of a response recurring is termed *response cost*. It consists of withdrawing previously accumulated positive reinforcement following an undesirable behavior. This procedure can be used only when reinforcers that can be accumulated are given out during a session and can therefore be removed; these reinforcers cannot be social or consumable because they cannot be accumulated and taken away.

The consequent event of choice and the most frequently employed in clinical speech instruction is positive reinforcement. An important variable when using reinforcement is the schedule of its presentation—that is, how the reinforcement is programmed to occur relative to the number of responses, the interval between responses, or other temporal features of the responses. The basic schedules of reinforcement are *continuous*, *fixed ratio*, *fixed interval*, *variable ratio*, and *variable interval*. When positive reinforcement is administered each time the client emits the desired behavior, the client is said to be under a continuous reinforcement schedule. The other four major reinforcement schedules are intermittent schedules. Intermittent reinforcement schedules have been shown to produce behaviors with greater resistance to extinction than continuous schedules of reinforcement and to reduce the probability of satiation.

Intermittent schedules can be categorized as ratio or interval, and each can be administered on either a fixed or variable basis. Under a fixed ratio schedule, the individual is reinforced only after he or she emits a specific number of responses. For example, a child who is reinforced regularly after every three correct responses is under a fixed ratio schedule. Under a variable ratio schedule, reinforcement occurs after a number of responses, and the number varies semirandomly around a mean value. A variable ratio schedule is illustrated in this example: A salesperson is told that she will make one sale for every 10 times a particular sales pitch is presented. In practice, however, she may make a sale on the fifth and ninth presentations. In terms of phonological remediation, a subject who is reinforced on a variable ratio schedule of 1 to 5 may, on a 15-item task in which all responses are correct, be reinforced on items 8, 12, and 13.

Under a fixed interval schedule, reinforcement is repeated after a specified time interval has elapsed since the previous reinforcement. For example, a client in the final stages of remediation of /s/ might be reinforced after each five-minute period of conversational speech contingent upon a correct [s] production immediately following each interval. With a variable interval schedule, reinforcement of a response occurs at random intervals around a specified mean time interval. This schedule differs from the fixed interval schedule in that the reinforcement randomly varies around a mean of five-minute intervals rather than occurring precisely every five minutes.

In practice, a continuous reinforcement schedule tends to be used during the establishment phase of treatment. During subsequent treatment stages, reinforcement is then modified to a variable ratio schedule and then, finally, to a variable interval schedule.

Program planning, in which the kind of detail described above is delineated, may be somewhat time-consuming, but the clinician knows the target behaviors to be focused upon, how to measure the effectiveness of instruction, and when to proceed to subsequent steps in the treatment continuum. In the long run, this initial planning will save the clinician time, facilitate greater instructional effectiveness and efficiency, and allow the clinician to be more accountable.

Strategies for Attacking Treatment Goals

Fey (1986) has outlined "goal attack strategies" for working with children who are language delayed that have application to children with phonological disorders. The first strategy is called a *vertically structured program* where one or two goals (targets) are trained to some performance criterion prior to proceeding to another target. The traditional approach to treatment of phonological disorders (see Chapter 10) is an example of a vertically structured program. In this approach, one or two phonemes are targeted for treatment and worked on to the point where they are produced in sentences, prior to initiation of training on other target sounds. Likewise, if the client used five different phonological processes, the clinician would target one process and focus treatment on that process until some criterion level were reached prior to proceeding to the next target process. If the target were final consonant deletions, only one or two exemplars would be the focus of the training. Elbert and Gierut (1986) termed this vertical type of strategy *training deep*. The assumption behind the vertical strategy is that mass practice on a restricted number of target sounds with a limited number of training items will facilitate generalization to other non-trained items. For examples of this type of training, see Elbert and McReynolds (1975, 1978) and McReynolds and Bennett (1972).

A second instructional strategy is a *horizontal approach to treatment* (Fey, 1986), or what Elbert and Gierut (1986) have called *training broad*. Using this strategy, the clinician works on several targets at the same time. Obviously, the time needed to reach a specific performance level will vary across targets. An example of this approach in which the clinician selects several sounds for simultaneous treatment is the multiphonemic approach (see Chapter 10). By working on several sounds simultaneously, the assumption is that the client will learn commonalities or relationships among target sound productions and treatment will be more efficient. In other words, the client receives less training about more aspects of the target sound system than in the vertical approach. Several related target sounds are taught in many treatment items. The concept behind training broad is that limited practice with a wide range of exemplars is an efficient way to modify a child's phonological system. The goal is to expose the child to a wide range of target sound productions so that this broad-based training will facilitate simultaneous acquisition of several treatment targets.

A third strategy, which combines aspects of the vertical and horizontal approaches, is a *cyclical approach* (Hodson and Paden, 1991; see Chapter 10). In this approach, the clinician works with the child on a specific goal in a cyclical schedule (three to four days per week, two to four weeks per cycle). Hodson and Paden (1991) recommended structuring treatment so that each cycle focuses on a specific error pattern (process). Within each pattern, instruction is focused on two to five exemplars the child can produce in which a process is not operating. Regardless of the progress at the end of a particular cycle, the next cycle focuses on a second process. It may be necessary, however, to come back to certain targets in subsequent cycles. The important difference between this strategy and the previously discussed vertical and horizontal strategies is that regardless of the progress at the end of the cycle, treatment proceeds to another goal (target process).

The most common strategy that has been employed in remediation is that of a vertical approach but, as in language treatment, the horizontal approach is gaining favor as is the related cyclical approach. Our preference is the horizontal and cyclical approaches although all three approaches have been shown to result in improved phonological productions.

Scheduling of Treatment

Variables potentially related to the success of intervention are the duration and scheduling of treatment sessions. While treatment should ideally be scheduled to meet the needs of the individual client, this may not occur. One reason for this is that sufficient research has not been reported to determine which scheduling arrangements are most desirable, and second, it is often not practical to schedule treatment sessions on an "ideal" basis. Relatively little is known about the influence that scheduling of instruction has upon remediation efficacy. Any consideration of this topic is intimately connected to the treatment methodology employed, the type of client treated, and other such variables.

Investigators who have studied scheduling have generally been concerned with the efficacy of intermittent scheduling versus block scheduling of treatment sessions. *Intermittent scheduling* usually refers to twice weekly scheduling over an extended period of time (such as eight months); *block scheduling* refers to daily sessions for a shorter temporal span (such as two eight-week blocks).

Several investigators, during the 1960s, compared dismissal rates associated with traditional (intermittent) and block scheduling primarily for public school students with articulation disorders (Van Hattum, 1969). A typical study compared dismissal rates for two groups of clients, one of which received treatment twice weekly for eight months, and the other four times per week for eight consecutive weeks in two separate eight-week cycles during an eight-month period. Unfortunately, variables like articulation severity, phonological knowledge, stimulability, and treatment methodology employed were not well controlled. In commenting on these studies, Van Hattum (1969) stated: "Research reports relating to scheduling are usually confusing and seldom conclusive. Further, research methodology, due to the complexity of the problem and the number of variables involved, is open to question" (171). Within the limitations of such experimental procedures, however, the following observations on scheduling of articulation intervention can be made:

1. Scheduling of intervention four to five times per week for eight to ten weeks would appear to result in slightly higher dismissal rates than intermittent scheduling for a longer period of time, the greater gains being made early in the treatment process.
2. Intensive scheduling on a short-term basis does not appear to be as successful with articulation disorders associated with organic impairment as with those without obvious organic impairment.

In a study of articulation change associated with treatment, Shelton, Elbert, and Arndt (1967) investigated whether or not articulatory improvement occurred between treatment sessions. Specifically, they compared articulatory changes across several subjects between Tuesday and Thursday with changes between Thursday and the following Tuesday. According to performance on probe measures (sound production tasks), no significant differences were noted in the amount of articulatory change between the two session intervals.

Other aspects of scheduling have received even less attention in the literature than session frequency. Powers (1971) suggested that for children under age 8, treatment sessions should probably not exceed one half hour, and if they do, the type of activity should be varied considerably after the first half hour. Older children may be able to work effectively for 40 minutes or more; however, even most adults cannot be expected to maintain sustained attention or effort for longer than one hour at a time. In addition to Powers' suggestions, we would recommend that sessions generally last at least 20 minutes, except in some cases of individual instruction during the establishment phase. At least twice weekly treatment sessions are advisable, except during the maintenance phase.

Group and Individual Treatment

Phonological instruction is often conducted in small groups to increase efficiency of remediation. Although group instruction is sometimes conducted because of large caseloads, reports have indicated that group instruction may well be as effective as individual instruction in the remediation of articulation disorders (Sommers et al., 1964; Sommers et al., 1966).

Sommers et al. (1964) reported that 50-minute group instruction resulted in as much articulatory change as 30-minute individual instruction when both group and individual sessions were conducted 4 times per week for 4 weeks. In a subsequent study (Sommers et al., 1966), similar results were obtained from group sessions held 45 minutes each week and individual instruction sessions held 30 minutes each week over a period of 8½ months. The investigators concluded that group and individual sessions were equally effective and that the results were not influenced by the grade level (fourth to sixth grade versus second grade) or the severity of the phonological disorder.

Articulation remediation groups usually contain three or four clients of about the same age who work on similar target behaviors. Van Hattum (1969) pointed out that, unfortunately, such sessions may become so regimented that all individuals work on the same activity, the same target behavior, and the same level of behavior; they are even given the same homework assignments. Many clinicians have reported success working with small groups where the clients reflect different target behaviors and different training levels.

It should be pointed out that *group instruction* should be different from *individual instruction* in a group. Often, the beginning clinician has had experience primarily in treating individual clients. When assigned a group of clients, the clinician may simply work with each client individually while remaining group members observe. Group instruction can and should be structured so that individuals in the group can benefit from interaction with other members and from activities that involve the entire group. For example, individuals can monitor and reinforce each other's productions and can serve as correct models for each other.

The trend for speech-language pathologists working in the schools to function in a collaborative consultative role with the classroom teacher (in contrast to the traditional pull-out model) has added new emphasis and direction to the concept of group instruction. In terms of phonological intervention, this approach emphasizes the use of particular targets in the context of expressing concepts and vocabulary related to the curriculum in a group setting. By working with groups of students (including clients) on academic material that allows emphasis on communication skills, the clinician can address phonological carry-over in a way not possible in individual instruction.

Powers (1971) stated that a combination of group and individual sessions would be most advantageous for individuals with phonological problems. She also recommended that instructional groups be limited to three or four individuals whose ages do not exceed a three-year range.

Intervention Style

Earlier, we talked about specific stages of remediation as well as particular approaches to intervention. A factor closely related to intervention approaches used in therapy is *intervention style*. In addition to selecting target behaviors and training stimuli to be used in treatment, the clinician must also consider the management mode or style most appropriate for a given client. A key issue in this regard is the amount of structure that may be prescribed for or tolerated by a given client.

Shriberg and Kwiatkowski (1982) described the continuum of therapy structure as ranging from drill (highly structured therapy) to play (little structure to therapy), with combinations of these two representing in-between stages on the continuum. These authors described the following four modes of management:

1. *Drill.* This type of therapy relies heavily on presentation by the clinician or some form of instrumentation of antecedent instructional events, followed by client responses. The client has no control over the rate and presentation of training stimuli.
2. *Drill play.* This type of therapy is distinguished from drill by the inclusion of an antecedent motivational event (e.g., activity involving a spinner; card games).
3. *Structured play.* This type of activity is structurally similar to drill play. However, training stimuli are presented as play activities. In this mode, the clinician moves from formal instructional antecedent events to play-like activities when the child becomes unresponsive to more formal stimuli presentations.
4. *Play.* The child perceives what he or she is doing as play. However, the clinician arranges activities so that target responses will occur as a natural component of the activity. Clinicians may also use modeling, self-talk, and other techniques to elicit responses from a child.

Shriberg and Kwiatkowski (1982) conducted several studies with young children to compare the relative effects of these four treatment modes. Their data

Remediation Concepts and Principles

indicated that drill and drill play modes were more effective and efficient than structured play and play modes. In addition, drill play was as effective and efficient as drill.

Clinicians' evaluation of the four modes indicated that they felt drill play was most effective and efficient for their clients, and they personally preferred it. They also urged that three factors be considered when making a choice of management mode: (1) a general knowledge of the child's personality, (2) the intended target response, and (3) the stage of therapy (Shriberg and Kwiatkowski, 1982).

As may be gathered from the above discussion, clinical management of phonological disorders involves not only technical and professional knowledge but also sensitivity in choice of treatment styles as well as sensitivity to the clients' needs and one's own personality. Thus, both science and art are involved in planning and executing remediation programs.

CONCLUSION

Phonological instruction, although practiced for decades, still lacks a unifying theoretical base from which remediation can be formulated and systematically tested. A number of models and atheoretical clinical approaches have been proposed with only limited documentation to support them. In spite of this absence of research data, clinicians must make certain decisions on the basis of experience and their professional judgment. Unresolved issues which continue to pose dilemmas for speech-language pathologists include:

1. The relationship between auditory perceptual skills and correction of phonological errors
2. The patterns of generalization that may be expected for a given client
3. Determination of the appropriateness of motor and/or cognitive-linguistic approaches to remediation with particular types of errors and disorders
4. The relative merits of one intervention approach as opposed to another
5. The relationship between intervention strategies and phonological knowledge

REFERENCES

Aungst, L., and J. Frick, "Auditory discrimination ability and consistency of articulation of /r/." *Journal of Speech and Hearing Disorders, 29* (1964): 76–85.

Bankson, N.W., and M.C. Byrne, "The effect of a timed correct sound production task on carryover." *Journal of Speech and Hearing Research, 15* (1972): 160–168.

Bernthal, J.E., M. Greenlee, R. Eblen, and K. Marking, "Detection of mispronunciations: A comparison of adults, normal-speaking children, and children with articulation errors." *Journal of Applied Psycholinguistics, 8* (1987): 209–222.

Carrier, J.K., "A program of articulation therapy administered by mothers." *Journal of Speech and Hearing Disorders, 33* (1970): 344–353.

Compton, A.J., "Generative studies of children's phonological disorders: A strategy of therapy." In S. Singh (Ed.), *Measurements in Hearing, Speech, and Language.* Baltimore: University Park Press, 1975.

Costello, J., and C. Bosler, "Generalization and articulation instruction." *Journal of Speech and Hearing Disorders, 41* (1976): 359–373.

Curtis, J.R., and J.C. Hardy, "A phonetic study of misarticulation of /r/." *Journal of Speech and Hearing Research, 2* (1959): 244–257.

Diedrich, W.M., "Procedures for counting and charting a target phoneme." *Language, Speech, and Hearing Services in the Schools, 2* (1971): 18–32.

Diedrich, W.M., and J. Bangert, "Training speech clinicians in recording and analysis of articulatory behavior." Washington, D.C.: U.S. Office of Education Grant No. OEG-0-70-1689 and OEG-0-71-1689, 1976.

Diedrich, W.M., and A. Gerber, "Analyses and management of articulation learning." Short course presentation at the annual convention of the American Speech-Language-Hearing Association, Las Vegas, 1974.

Dinnsen, D., and M. Elbert, "On the relationship between phonology and learning." In M. Elbert, D. Dinnsen, and G. Weismer (Eds.), *Phonological Theory and the Misarticulating Child*, ASHA Monographs. Rockville, Md.: ASHA, 1984.

Elbert, M., "Dismissal criteria from therapy." Unpublished manuscript, 1967.

Elbert, M., D.A. Dinnsen, P. Swartzlander, and S.B. Chin, "Generalization to conversational speech." *Journal of Speech and Hearing Disorders, 55* (1990): 694–699.

Elbert, M., and J. Gierut, *Handbook of Clinical Phonology Approaches to Assessment and Treatment*. San Diego: College-Hill Press, 1986.

Elbert, M., and L.V. McReynolds, "Transfer of /r/ across contexts." *Journal of Speech and Hearing Disorders, 40* (1975): 380–387.

Elbert, M., and L.V. McReynolds, "An experimental analysis of misarticulating children's generalization." *Journal of Speech and Hearing Research, 21* (1978): 136–149.

Elbert, M., T.W. Powell, and P. Swartzlander, "Toward a technology of generalization: How many exemplars are sufficient?" *Journal of Speech and Hearing Research, 34* (1991): 81–87.

Elbert, M., B. Rockman, and D. Saltzman, *Contrasts: The Use of Minimal Pairs in Articulation Training*. Austin, Tex.: Exceptional Resources, 1980.

Elbert, M., R.L. Shelton, and W.B. Arndt, "A task for education of articulation change." *Journal of Speech and Hearing Research, 10* (1967): 281–288.

Engel, D.C., and L.R. Groth, "Case studies of the effect on carry-over of reinforcing postarticulation responses based on feedback." *Language, Speech, and Hearing Services in Schools, 7* (1976): 93–101.

Fairbanks, G., *Voice and Articulation Drill Book*. New York: Harper & Row, 1960.

Fey, M.E., *Language Intervention with Young Children*. San Diego: College-Hill Press/Little, Brown, 1986.

Gerber, A., *Goal: Carryover*. Philadelphia: Temple University Press, 1973.

Gierut, J., "Maximal opposition approach to phonological treatment." *Journal of Speech and Hearing Disorders, 54* (1989): 9–19.

Gierut, J., M. Elbert, and D. Dinnsen, "A functional analysis of phonological knowledge and generalization learning in misarticulating children." *Journal of Speech and Hearing Research, 30* (1987): 462–479.

Gray, B., "A field study on programmed articulation therapy." *Language, Speech, and Hearing Services in the Schools, 5* (1974): 119–131.

Hodson, B., and E. Paden, *Targeting Intelligible Speech: A Phonological Approach to Remediation*. San Diego: College-Hill Press, 1983.

Hodson, B., and E. Paden, *Targeting Intelligible Speech: A Phonological Approach to Remediation*, 2nd ed. Austin, Tex: PRO-Ed, 1991.

Koegel, L.K., R.L. Koegel, and J.C. Ingham, "Programming rapid generalization of correct articulation through self-monitoring procedures." *Journal of Speech and Hearing Disorders, 51* (1986): 24–32.

Koegel, R., L. Koegel, K. Van Voy, and J. Ingham, "Within-clinic versus outside-of-clinic self-monitoring of articulation to promote generalization." *Journal of Speech and Hearing Disorders, 53* (1988): 392–399.

La Riviere, C., H. Winitz, J. Reeds, and E. Herriman, "The conceptual reality of selected distinctive features." *Journal of Speech and Hearing Research, 17* (1974): 122–133.

Leonard, L.B., "The nature of deviant articulation." *Journal of Speech and Hearing Disorders, 38* (1973): 156–161.

Locke, J.L., "The inference of speech perception in the phonologically disordered child. Part I. A rationale, some criteria, the conventional tests." *Journal of Speech and Hearing Disorders, 40* (1980): 431–444.

McDonald, E.T., *Articulation Testing and Treatment: A Sensory Motor Approach*. Pittsburgh: Stanwix House, 1964.

McLean, J.E., "Extending stimulus control of phoneme articulation by operant techniques." In *ASHA Monographs, 14*. Washington, D.C.: American Speech-Language-Hearing Association, 1970.

McReynolds, L., "Contingencies and consequences in speech therapy." *Journal of Speech and Hearing Disorders, 35* (1970): 12–24.

McReynolds, L.V., "Articulation generalization during articulation training." *Language and Speech, 15* (1972): 149–155.

McReynolds, L.V., and S. Bennett, "Distinctive feature generalization in articulation training." *Journal of Speech and Hearing Disorders, 37* (1972): 462–470.

McReynolds, L.V., and K.P. Kearns, *Single-Subject Experimental Designs in Communicative Disorders*. Baltimore: University Park Press, 1983.

Mager, R.F., *Preparing Behavioral Objectives*. Palo Alto, Calif: Fearon, 1962.

Manning, W.H., N. Keappock, and S. Stick, "The use of auditory masking to estimate automatization of correct articulatory production." *Journal of Speech and Hearing Disorders, 41* (1976): 143–150.

Manning, W.H., M.L. Wittstruch, R.R. Loyd, and T.F. Campbell, "Automatization of correct production at two levels of articulatory acquisition." *Journal of Speech and Hearing Disorders, 42* (1977): 77–84.

Milisen, R., "A rationale for articulation disorders." *Journal of Speech and Hearing Disorders Monograph Supplement, 4* (1954): 5–18.

Monnin, L., and D.A. Huntington, "Relationship of articulatory defects to speech-sound identification." *Journal of Speech and Hearing Research, 17* (1974): 352–366.

Mowrer, D.E., "Evaluating speech therapy through precision recording." *Journal of Speech and Hearing Disorders, 34* (1969): 239–243.

Mowrer, D.E., *Methods of Modifying Speech Behaviors.* Columbus, Ohio: Charles E. Merrill, 1977.

Mowrer, D.E., *Methods of Modifying Speech Behaviors,* 2nd ed. Columbus, Ohio: Charles E. Merrill, 1982.

Mowrer, D.E., R. Baker, and R. Schutz, *S-Programmed Articulation Control Kit.* Tempe, Ariz.: Educational Psychological Research Associates, 1968.

Olswang, L.B., and B.A. Bain, "The natural occurrence of generalization articulation treatment." *Journal of Communication Disorders, 18* (1985): 109–129.

Powell, J., and M. Elbert, "Generalization following the remediation of early and later-developing consonant clusters." *Journal of Speech and Hearing Disorders, 49* (1984): 211–218.

Powell, J., and L. McReynolds, "A procedure for testing position generalization from articulation training." *Journal of Speech and Hearing Research, 12* (1969): 625–645.

Powers, M.J., "Clinical and educational procedures in functional disorders of articulation." In L. Travis (Ed.), *Handbook of Speech Pathology and Audiology.* Englewood Cliffs, N.J.: Prentice Hall, 1971.

Ruscello, D.M., "The importance of word position in articulation therapy." *Language, Speech, and Hearing Services in Schools, 6* (1975): 190–196.

Savin, H.B., "What the child knows about speech when he starts to learn to read." In J.F. Kavanaugh and I.G. Mattingly (Eds.), *The Relationships between Speech and Reading.* Cambridge, Mass.: M.I.T. Press, 1972.

Scripture, M.K., and E. Jackson, *A Manual of Exercises for the Correction of Speech Disorders.* Philadelphia: F.A. Davis, 1927.

Shelton, R., "Disorders of articulation." In P. Skinner and R. Shelton (Eds.), *Speech, Language, and Hearing.* Reading, Mass.: Addison-Wesley, 1978.

Shelton, R.L., M. Elbert, and W.B. Arndt, "A task for evaluation of articulation change: II. Comparison of task scores during baseline and lesson series testing." *Journal of Speech and Hearing Research, 10* (1967): 578–585.

Shelton, R.L., A.F. Johnson, and W.B. Arndt, "Monitoring and reinforcement by parents as a means of automating articulatory responses." *Perceptual and Motor Skills, 35* (1972): 759–767.

Shelton, R., A. Johnson, and W. Arndt, "Delayed judgment speech sound discrimination and /r/ or /s/ articulation status and improvement." *Journal of Speech and Hearing Research, 20* (1977): 704–717.

Shelton, R.L., A.F. Johnson, V. Willis, and W.B. Arndt, "Monitoring and reinforcement by parents as a means of automating articulatory responses: II. Study of pre-school children." *Perceptual and Motor Skills, 40* (1975): 599–610.

Shriberg, L., "A response evocation program for /ɝ/." *Journal of Speech and Hearing Disorders, 40* (1975): 92–105.

Shriberg, L.D., and J. Kwiatkowski, "Phonological disorders III: A procedure for assessing severity of involvement." *Journal of Speech and Hearing Disorders, 47* (1982): 256–270.

Shriberg, L.D., and J. Kwiatkowski, "A retrospective study of spontaneous generalization in speech-delayed children." *Language, Speech, and Hearing Services in Schools, 18* (1987): 144–157.

Shriberg, L.D., and J. Kwiatkowski, "Self-monitoring and generalization in preschool speech-delayed children." *Language, Speech, and Hearing Services in Schools, 21* (1990): 157–170.

Smit, A.B., and J. Bernthal, "Voicing contrasts and their phonological implications in the speech of articulation-disordered children." *Journal of Speech and Hearing Research, 26* (1983): 19–28.

Sommers, R.K., "Factors in the effectiveness of mothers trained to aid in speech correction." *Journal of Speech and Hearing Disorders, 27* (1962): 178–186.

Sommers, R.K., "The therapy program." In R. Van Hattum (Ed.), *Clinical Speech in the Schools.* Springfield, Ill.: Charles C. Thomas, 1969.

Sommers, R.K., A.K. Furlong, F.H. Rhodes, G.R. Fichter, D.C. Bowser, F.H. Copetas, and Z.G. Saunders, "Effects of maternal attitudes upon improvement in articulation when mothers are trained to assist in speech correction." *Journal of Speech and Hearing Disorders, 29* (1964): 126–132.

Sommers, R.K., M.H. Schaeffer, R.H. Leiss, A.J. Gerber, M.A. Bray, D. Fundrella, J.K. Olson, and E.R. Tomkins, "The effectiveness of group and individual therapy." *Journal of Speech and Hearing Research, 9* (1966): 219–225.

Stokes, T.F., and D.M. Baer, "An implicit technology of generalization." *Journal of Applied Behavior Analysis, 10* (1977): 349–367.

Turton, L., "Diagnostic implications of articulation testing." In W.D. Wolfe and D.J. Goulding (Eds.), *Articulation and Learning.* Springfield, Ill.: Charles C. Thomas, 1973.

Tyler, A., M. Edwards, and J. Saxman, "Acoustic validation of phonological knowledge and its relationship to treatment." *Journal of Speech and Hearing Disorders, 55* (1990): 251–261.

Van Hattum, R.J., "Program scheduling." In R. Van Hattum (Ed.), *Clinical Speech in the Schools*. Springfield, Ill.: Charles C Thomas, 1969.

Van Riper, C., Speech Correction: Principles and Methods, 6th ed. Englewood Cliffs, N.J.: Prentice Hall, 1978.

Van Riper, C., and L. Emerick, *Speech Correction: An Introduction to Speech Pathology and Audiology*. Englewood Cliffs, N.J.: Prentice Hall, Inc., 1984.

Weiner, F.F., "Treatment of phonological disability using the method of meaningful minimal contrast: Two case studies." *Journal of Speech and Hearing Disorders, 46* (1981): 97–103.

Weismer, G., D. Dinnsen, and M. Elbert, "A study of the voicing distinction associated with omitted, word-final stops." *Journal of Speech and Hearing Disorders, 46* (1981): 91–103.

Weston, A.J., and J.V. Irwin, "Use of paired-stimuli in modification of articulation." *Perceptual and Motor Skills, 32* (1971): 947–957.

Williams, A.L., "Generalization patterns associated with training least phonological knowledge." *Journal of Speech and Hearing Research, 34* (1991): 722–733.

Williams, G., and L.V. McReynolds, "The relationship between discrimination and articulation training in children with misarticulation." *Journal of Speech and Hearing Research, 18* (1975): 401–412.

Winitz, H., *Articulatory Acquisition and Behavior*. Englewood Cliffs, N.J.: Prentice Hall, 1969.

Winitz, H., *From Syllable to Conversation*. Baltimore: University Park Press, 1975.

Winitz, H., "Auditory considerations in articulation training." In H. Winitz (Ed.), *Treating Articulation Disorders for Clinicians by Clinicians*. Baltimore: University Park Press, 1984.

Winner, M., and M. Elbert, "Evaluating the treatment effect of repeated probes." *Journal of Speech and Hearing Disorders, 53* (1988): 211–218.

chapter
10

Remediation Systems and Approaches

In Chapter 9 general concepts and principles of remediation were discussed. This chapter will be more specific and focus on various systems and approaches to phonological remediation. These approaches are organized under two broad categories: **Motor Approaches to Phonological Treatment** and **Cognitive-Linguistic Approaches to Phonological Treatment.** Information about intervention is presented in this manner to assist the reader with integration of clinical phonology literature which, from our perspective, tends to reflect this dichotomy. It should be remembered, as stated earlier, that procedures described under either heading are not mutually exclusive.

Historically, speech-language pathologists approached the correction of phonological errors from the standpoint of teaching a motor behavior since sound production errors were thought to reflect an individual's inability to perform the complex motor skills required for the articulation of speech sounds. In recent years, clinicians have come to view many developmental phonological disorders from a cognitive-linguistic perspective rather than a motor perspective. The cognitive-linguistic approach is based on the notion that some individuals produce phonological errors because they have not learned to use certain phonological rules, such as sound contrasts, in accord with the adult norm. In other words, some clients have not acquired the rules for appropriate sound usage such as the phonemic contrasts of the language.

Although it is convenient to dichotomize the **motor** and **cognitive-linguistic** aspects of phonology for organization purposes, in reality, normal phonological use involves both the production of sounds at a motor level and their use in accordance with the rules of the language. Thus, the two skills are intertwined and may be described as two sides of the same coin. At a clinical level, it is often difficult or impossible to determine whether a client's errors reflect a lack of motor skills, a lack of linguistic knowledge, or deficiencies in both. It may be that, in a given client, some errors relate to one factor, some to another, and some to both.

Even though a disorder may be related primarily to either the motor or cognitive-linguistic aspects of phonology, instructional programs typically involve elements of both. It should be recognized that although often it is difficult to determine whether a given instructional procedure is primarily a motor-based or a linguistic-based technique, some activities undoubtedly assist the client in both the development of linguistic knowledge and the development of appropriate motor skills. We recommend that activities of both types (motor and linguistic) be a part of most therapy programs. One notable exception is the case of a phonetic distortion (e.g., lateral /s/), where a motor approach is the treatment of choice since the "higher level" cognitive-linguistic aspects of the sound can be assumed (i.e., the child uses lateral /s/ in all rules where /s/ is to be used). By careful observation of a client and the nature of his or her problem, the clinician may be able to determine when one approach should be emphasized to a greater degree.

Although we have categorized the treatment approaches presented in this chapter as motor or cognitive-linguistic, that does not mean that the approaches were necessarily developed from a particular theoretical perspective. In fact many phonological treatment approaches have emerged from pragmatic origins and continue to be used simply because "they work." On the pages that follow, several approaches to remediation are described. Some of these can be related to theory, some are atheoretical, and others seem to be somewhere in-between. In the summary of each approach, we have presented a "Background Statement," which reflects our perception of the theoretical perspective from which the approach has emerged. A challenge for future scholars is to develop, refine, and revise theories that provide rationale, support, explanations, and direction for intervention procedures. Ingram (1986) reflected this concern when he stated that ". . . language intervention can only be pursued rationally within a theory of language" (1).

MOTOR APPROACHES

The remediation approaches we are about to describe were designed to focus primarily on the motor skills involved in producing target sounds and frequently include perceptual tasks as part of the treatment procedures. Most of them represent variations of the "traditional approach" to remediation. Remediation based on a motor perspective views phonological errors as motor based, with treatment focused on the placement and movement of the articulators so that segmental productions no longer violate adult standard pronunciations. The usual remediation approach involves the selection of a to-be-corrected target speech sound or sounds, with instruction proceeding through a sequence of increasingly complex linguistic units (e.g., isolation, syllables, words, phrases) until target sounds are used appropriately in spontaneous conversation. Thus, speech production is viewed as a learned motor skill, with remediation requiring repetitive practice at increasingly complex motor levels until the targeted articulatory gesture becomes automatic.

Ruscello (1984) has indicated that phonological errors may be modified in two ways when viewed from a motor perspective: (1) movements may be taught to replace incorrect movements, or (2) movements may be taught where they were formerly absent. On the basis of the literature related to motor skill learning, Ruscello has outlined the following critical features in motor skill development:

1. Cognitive analysis. A mental or cognitive analysis is important in the early phase of movement formation. In this process, the learner evaluates his or her anticipated performance mentally and then incorporates those adjustments necessary for appropriate execution of the movement. Once stabilization of the movement occurs, such cognitive planning is minimized. It is the internalization of a skilled movement which is thought to contribute to the generalization of skilled movement across a variety of contexts. Based on experimental data, Ruscello and Shelton (1979) reported that mental planning was helpful in the acquisition of articulatory skills in a treatment paradigm.

2. Practice. Practice is the key variable thought necessary for mastery of any skilled motor behavior. As the learner practices a particular motor skill, modifications based on internal and/or external feedback are made so that accuracy of performance is increased. A motor skill is best practiced in limited contexts until correct execution of the movement is achieved. Early treatment sessions involve discrete productions, such as isolated sound or word practice, while later sessions introduce more advanced tasks in the context of continuous discourse.

3. Stages of motor skill development. Initially there is a sluggishness in the execution of motor skills because the learner is acquiring the movement. With practice, the motor skill is perfected and stabilized. Ultimately, the skill becomes a part of the learner's repertoire of skilled movements and becomes automatic for the speaker.

4. Feedback. Sensory feedback processes (internal and external) are described in the motor learning literature as being of great importance in the early development of a skill. When the individual perfects a skill pattern through practice, the error response is diminished and feedback becomes less important.

The treatment approaches described below are based on a motor perspective of phonological disorders, and some of the attributes outlined by Ruscello are incorporated in the treatment approaches, sometimes albeit in a rather nonsystematic fashion.

TRADITIONAL APPROACH

The treatment approach that has been in existence the longest, and is best known, is the **traditional approach** to articulation therapy. This approach's foundations were laid during the early decades of the 1900s by the pioneering clinicians of our field. By the late 1930s, Charles Van Riper had assimilated these treatment techniques into a theory of articulation disorders and published them in his text entitled *Speech Correction: Principles and Methods* (originally published in 1939 and modified in subsequent editions). As an outgrowth of his writings, the traditional approach is sometimes referred to as the ''Van Riper method.''

The traditional approach progresses from the identification of error productions to the establishment of correct productions and moves on to transfer and finally to maintenance. Van Riper and Emerick (1984) stated that:

The hallmark of traditional articulation therapy lies in its sequencing of activities for (1) sensory-perceptual training, which concentrates on identifying the standard sound and discriminating it from its error through scanning and comparing; (2) varying and correcting the various productions of the sound until it is produced correctly; (3) strengthening and stabilizing the correct production; and finally (4) transferring the new speech skill to everyday communication situations. This process is usually carried out first for the standard sound in isolation, then in the syllable, then in a word, and finally in sentences (206).

A characteristic of the traditional approach is the emphasis on perceptual training (i.e., speech sound discrimination or ear training). During this part of therapy, the client is not required to produce the sound, but rather, instruction is designed to provide a perceptual standard by which the client can contrast his or her own productions. Thus, perceptual training becomes a precursor to production training. Van Riper and Emerick's (1984) perceptual, or ear, training is outlined as follows.

Perceptual Training/Ear Training. The goal of this phase of instruction is for the client to develop an auditory model that will serve as an internal standard against which comparisons of his or her own productions can be made. Several suggested phases of ear training precede production training. While initially the phases usually proceed in the order listed below, the clinician may wish to reinforce these skills at any point in therapy by going back to earlier ear training activities.

Phases of Ear Training (Perceptual Training)

1. Identification
   a. The clinician demonstrates the sight, sound, and feel of a target sound.
   b. For young children, the sound is often labeled (e.g., /t/ is the ticking sound; /f/ the angry cat sound).
   c. The client recognizes the target sound in isolation from among dissimilar and similar sounds.
2. Isolation
   a. The client is able to indicate when he or she hears (e.g., raise hand, show happy face) or does not hear (e.g., keeps hand down, shows sad face) the target behavior and is able to do so in increasingly complex environments (i.e., words, phrases, sentences).
   b. The client is able to identify the position of a target sound in a word (initial, medial, final).
3. Stimulation
   a. The clinician "bombards" the client with productions of the target sound. This may be accomplished by repetitions of the target sound (e.g., tongue twisters) or variations in the loudness or duration at which target sounds are presented by the clinician.
4. Discrimination
   a. The client makes external discriminations (judgments) of correct and incorrect productions (produced by the clinician) in increasingly complex contexts (i.e., words, phrases, sentences). In this instance the client is comparing someone else's production with his or her own internal image of the correct form of a sound. A clinical narrative that reflects the clinician teaching the client to make an external judgment related to a θ/s substitution is as follows: "Here is a picture of a 'thun.' 'Thun.' Did I say that word right? Did you see my tongue peeking out at the beginning of the word? Can you help me remember to keep my tongue in and say the word right?"

Additional suggestions regarding perceptual training including error detection and error correction have been presented by Winitz (1975). He stated that when the client is unable to imitate the correct form of the target sound or segment, speech sound discrimination is an important prerequisite to motor production. He also speculated that discrimination training can affect changes in production. Winitz (1975) outlined the following principles for discrimination training:

1. The acoustic contrast in discrimination training should at first be large, then the phonemic distance should gradually be narrowed. The target or standard sound and the error sound should be contrasted late in the instructional sequence. It is suggested that the sound error or sound substitution should be contrasted with other sounds before it is contrasted with standard productions of the target sound. It has been demonstrated that training is less efficient when discrimination training is initiated with the target or standard sound contrasted with the sound error (Winitz and Preisler, 1967). Thus, if /θ/ → s/, the /θ/ should be contrasted with other sounds and only later in the instructional sequence should /s/ be contrasted with /θ/. Carefully programmed discrimination training of hierarchically ordered phonemic contrasts is more efficient than contrasting only the error and the target sounds.

2. It could be hypothesized that the most important perceptual contrast the client must learn is the distinction between error and standard productions. If a client is to learn to use a standard production for an error sound, the client must be able to distinguish between the error and the standard production. The client should first learn to discriminate between the clinician's imitation of the client's speech sound error and the standard pronunciation before judging his or her own productions. Obviously, the clinician must be able to produce a good likeness or imitation of the child's error production in order to contrast it with the standard production.

3. Instruction should involve active participation by the client. One way in which the clinician can accomplish this is by contrasting correct and incorrect productions during interaction with the client. For example, when the child misarticulates, wait a few seconds, imitate the child's production, and then respond by repeating the target words correctly several times before handing the object to the child. As training continues, wait for the child to correct him- or herself after you have repeated the child's incorrect production.

4. Once the client can discriminate correct–incorrect productions at the word level, discrimination of sounds in running speech should be trained.

In summary, many of the comments made in this section on traditional perceptual training have emanated from the perspective that speech sound errors are motor based. Later in this chapter we will talk about perceptual training that has stemmed from a cognitive-linguistic orientation. One should keep in mind that at a practical level the clinician may wish to incorporate instructional procedures from both perspectives in clinical instruction that focus on speech sound perception.

Production Training. The second but primary ingredient of traditional instruction is production training. Production training usually includes four sequential instructional phases wherein a target sound is (1) produced in isolation (the target sound is elicited in isolation or, in the case of stops and certain glides, in a CV context such as /pa/); (2) produced in syllables (the sound is produced in CV, VC, and VCV syllables); (3) produced in words (the target sound is produced in a word or lexical context in initial, final, and medial positions); and (4) produced in a meaningful connected speech context. Secord (1989), outlined the following instructional steps for traditional production training:

1. Isolation. An explanation for beginning with production of the target sound in isolation is the assumption that the articulatory gestures of a sound are most easily learned when the sound is highly identifiable and in the least complex context. The goal at this level is to develop a consistently correct response. Specific techniques for teaching sounds are included in the Appendix. It should be pointed out, however, that when a client is able to produce a sound at a more complex level (such as syllables or words), production training should begin at that level.

2. Nonsense syllables. The goal at this step is consistently correct productions in a variety of nonsense syllable contexts. A suggested sequence for syllable practice is CV, VC, VCV, and CVC. It is also suggested that the transition from the consonant to the vowel should be accomplished with sounds that are similar in place of articulation. For example, an alveolar consonant such as /s/ should be facilitated in a high front vowel context, as in [si]. The clinician might also wish to use the target sound in nonsense clusters.

3. Words. Once the client can consistently produce the target sound in nonsense syllables, instruction proceeds to word level productions. Instructions at this level should begin with monosyllabic words with the target consonant (assuming instruction is focusing on consonants as opposed to vowels) in the prevocalic position (CV). Instruction then moves to VC, CVC, CVCV, monosyllabic words with clusters, followed by more complex word-forms. Table 10–1 reflects a hierarchy of phoneme production complexity at the word levels identified by Secord (1989).

Once a core group of words is established in which the client is readily able to produce the target sound, the clinician seeks to expand the small set of core words to a somewhat larger set of training words. Usually target words are selected on the basis of meaningfulness to the client (e.g., family names, places, social expressions, academic curriculum, and so forth), but other factors such as phonetic context and syllable complexity should also be taken into consideration, just as they were for the initial set of core words.

4. Phrases. At this point instruction shifts from single-word productions to practicing a target sound in two- to four-word phrases. This level of production represents a complexity level in-between single words and sentence level productions. This is especially true if carrier phrases are employed. Carrier phrases

TABLE 10–1. **Substages of Word Level Stabilization Training (Secord, 1989).**

SUBSTAGE	SYLLABLES	EXAMPLES FOR /S/
1. Initial prevocalic words	1	*sun, sign, say*
2. Final postvocalic words	1	*glass, miss, pass*
3. Medial intervocalic words	2	*kissing, lassie, racer*
4. Initial blends/clusters	1	*star, spoon, skate*
5. Final blends/clusters	1	*lost, lips, rocks*
6. Medial blends/clusters	2	*whisper, outside, ice-skate*
7. All word-positions	1–2	(any of above)
8. All word-positions	any	*signaling, eraser, therapist*
9. All word-positions; multiple targets	any	*necessary, successful*

involve phrases where only a single word is added with each repetition (e.g., I see the *car*; I see the *cup*; I see the *cane*). Initially in phrase level productions, only the target word should contain the target sound.

5. Sentences. An extension of phrase level productions is sentence level practice. Just as practice at other levels has involved careful sequencing of task complexity, that principle also holds at this level. This includes factors such as phonetic context, syllable structure of words, and number of words in the sentence. Secord (1989) suggested the following sequence of sentence level complexity:

1. Simple short sentence with one instance of the target sound
2. Sentences of various lengths with one instance of the target sound
3. Simple short sentences with two or more instances of the target sound
4. Sentences of various lengths with two or more instances of the target sound

6. Conversation. The final step in production involves using a target sound in everyday speech. At this point the clinician is seeking to facilitate generalization of productions that have already proceeded through more structured production tasks. Initially, generalization situations are structured so that the client produces his or her sound correctly in situations where his speech is monitored. Activities such as role playing, talking about future plans, attempting to get information, interviewing, and oral reading can be used at this level. Structured generalization conversations such as these, then proceed to more free or "off-guard" type conversations. The intent at this point is to provide activities to facilitate transfer that approximate real-life situations. Activities should include speaking situations where the client focuses not on self-monitoring skills but on what he or she says. Telling personal experiences, talking about topics that evoke strong feelings, and taking part in group discussions are appropriate activities. Van Riper (1978) suggested that at this final stage of instruction negative practice helps to stabilize a new response. In negative practice, a client deliberately produces a target sound incorrectly; Van Riper stated that such deliberate error productions increase the rate of learning.

At this point, the clinician also seeks to facilitate the carry-over of conversational usage to situations beyond the therapy environment. It is also suggested that such situational generalization be encouraged once the client can produce a target sound at the word level. By encouraging transfer in earlier stages of instruction, it is assumed that generalization beyond the word level will be significantly enhanced and will perhaps decrease the amount of time needed at the phrase, sentence, and conversational levels.

Van Riper and Emerick (1984) recommended that sensory-perceptual training should be included as production training moves forward from word level productions so that internal perceptions of phonological productions will accompany external perceptions. It is assumed that when the client is able to perceive correct and incorrect productions in another person's speech, such discrimination will facilitate an internal concept of such phonological contrasts. This latter awareness is necessary in order for clients to make judgments about their own error productions.

Facilitating internal or "intra-auditory discrimination" involves helping the client learn how to recall, perceive and predict errors. Detecting one's own phonological errors after they occur, and being able to predict where they may occur are part of what becomes self-monitoring. Unfortunately, techniques for facilitating these skills are not as easy to devise as for external monitoring. Recommended techniques for this type of instruction have been short loop tape recordings, amplification of one's speech, and shadowing of speech by clinician and client.

Summary of the Traditional Approach.

Background Statement. The underlying assumptions of the traditional approach to remediation include the following: (1) Faulty perception of speech sounds is often related to phonological errors, and (2) phonological errors may be viewed as inadequate development of oral motor skills. Thus, the traditional approach relies heavily on motor production combined with activities related to discrimination training (ear training).

Unique Features. The traditional approach to articulation remediation has for many years, constituted the basic framework for articulation instruction and focuses on motor learning of individual speech sounds. The approach provides general instructional guidelines and a sequence for correcting articulatory errors from the establishment phase through the maintenance phase, but it does not provide step-by-step detail. Although some suggested teaching activities are included, no criterion levels are suggested, no reinforcement schedule is recommended, and no data collection system is presented. The approach can be modified to fit the needs of clients of all ages. The perceptual training (ear training) suggested in this approach includes discrimination, identification, auditory stimulation with verbal models, and self-monitoring.

Strengths and Limitations. It may be said that from a historical perspective this is the most widely employed approach to phonological remediation, and one that forms the basis of several treatment approaches. This fact, no doubt, is related to the logical sequence of training tasks, the success that accrues through motor practice, and the adaptability and applicability of the approach. It may not, however, be the most efficacious approach for clients whose phonological problems are not motor based or when client's phonological patterns affect entire sound classes.

Research Support. This approach has stood the test of time because it has "worked" for many clinicians, with many clients. Many investigators have reported phonological change in association with intervention which has been based on this approach; however, comparative studies between the "traditional approach" and others are limited. The emphasis on external discrimination training as part of the treatment process for all children has been questioned because of the lack of data to support its effectiveness.

MULTIPLE PHONEME APPROACH

The **multiple phoneme approach** was designed by McCabe and Bradley (1975) to facilitate instruction on several error sounds during each treatment session and is characterized by a traditional treatment sequence combined with a method for collecting data on articulatory responses. In addition, the approach calls for the application of behavioral principles to treatment and the analysis of sound productions in conversation (Bradley, 1989). The multiple phoneme approach is divided into establishment, transfer, and maintenance phases.

Phase I, called *establishment*, is designed to elicit correct target sound productions in isolation in response to a grapheme (printed letter) or phonetic symbol. Production is initiated first under conditions of auditory-visual-tactile stimulation (the client hears the model, sees the associated grapheme, and receives phonetic placement cues); then follows auditory-visual stimulation (pairing of the grapheme and clinician's model), and finally visual stimulation (the grapheme alone is presented). The goal of establishment is correct production of the target in isolation via visual stimulation on four out of five attempts.

Step 2 of Phase I is called a *holding procedure*, and it is designed as a branching step to maintain correct target productions in isolation. It is to be used if time limitations in a particular training session preclude transfer training on all target segments. For example, consider the client who produces /s, z, ʃ, t, f, v, r, l/ in error in connected speech but has met the criterion for establishment of these sounds in isolation. The clinician may choose for the client to work on transfer /s/, /z/, and /ʃ/ at the word level and /t/, /f/, and /v/ at the syllable level during a particular session. Since time may not allow for transfer training with the /r/ and /l/ in the session, /r/ and /l/ are elicited at least once in isolation. Such elicitations in isolation are reflective of a holding procedure.

Phase II, *transfer*, is designed to facilitate production of sounds along the treatment continuum from isolation to correct production in conversational speech. The transfer phase contains five steps or activities, and clients can be producing different sounds at any of these levels during a single session.

In Step 1 of the transfer phase, an *imitative word probe* is administered to determine whether or not the subject should receive instruction at the syllable or word level. If the client does not produce a target sound in 6 to 10 monosyllabic words, instruction begins at the syllable level. In this step the consonant is produced in combination with all commonly occurring vowels in CV and VC combinations, along with multisyllable sequences in response to presentation of a grapheme and auditory stimuli.

In Step 2 of transfer, target productions are elicited in initial, medial, and final *word-positions* in response to printed words (picture stimuli are used with nonreaders). Care is taken to insure that verbs, adjectives, prepositions, articles, and nouns are utilized as training words, with no more than 25 to 30 total target words. Criterion for moving to the next step is 90 percent accuracy for one session or 80 percent accuracy for two sessions.

Step 3 of transfer involves *phrase and sentence* practice with the goal of having all sounds in words produced correctly. Control of vocabulary and phrase–sentence length is important initially. If a client has established only a limited number of phonemes, the clinician may have to calculate accuracy on the basis of words that actually contain target sounds. At this stage clients are also encouraged to monitor their own productions. Criterion for advancement is the same as that at the word level.

Step 4 of transfer, *reading–storytelling*, has as its goal accurate production of target sounds in connected speech in utterances of four to six word-units. Reading and storytelling are the suggested ways to elicit responses.

Step 5 of transfer, *conversation*, is the final stage of instruction. The criterion level for termination of this stage is 90 percent whole-word accuracy (all sounds articulated correctly within every word) for one entire session or 80 percent for two sessions.

Phase III, called *maintenance*, focuses on whole-word accuracy in various speaking situations. At this stage, accuracy of productions is monitored in various speaking situations by the clinician, the client, and others in the environment.

A primary emphasis in the multiple phoneme approach is placed on counting and charting correct and incorrect responses during a treatment session, with all responses of the client tabulated. Throughout each session the clinician records responses on an Articulation Data Sheet shown in Figure 10–1. The sheet is arranged to record the level and accuracy of production for each sound.

The multiple phoneme approach may be viewed as a structured outline for (1) sequencing training steps and (2) data collection. Specific instructional techniques are left to the judgment and preferences of the clinician.

Summary of the Multiple Phoneme Approach.

Background Statement. This approach was originally developed with clients evidencing severe phonological disorders associated with cleft palate. Reliance on the traditional treatment sequence and the fact that all error sounds are targeted for remediation suggests that with this approach, articulation errors are viewed from a motor perspective.

Unique Features. Unique features of this approach include the following: the structured format for collecting response data; the procedures employed during the establishment phase; the use of graphemes in association with target sounds and words; the use of several parts of speech (e.g., nouns, verbs, adjectives) as training words; and the teaching of several target sounds in each session.

Strengths and Limitations. This approach provides an organized way to teach several sounds simultaneously and to collect data on client performance. Because of the complexity of the data collection system, the approach lends itself to individual rather than group instruction. Preschool children may find simultaneous instruction on all sounds in error to be somewhat confusing and may also find the use of written symbols to be difficult. Even though the approach is designed to focus on the motor production of several error sounds, clinicians can use the data collection system with more linguistically oriented approaches. For example, a clinician may still follow the traditional teaching sequence and utilize this data collection system when teaching exemplars of phonological error patterns.

Research Support. McCabe and Bradley (1975) reported data from 44 clients, ages 5 to 14, who were exposed to the multiple phoneme approach to instruction. They found statistically significant gains on both the Arizona Articulation Proficiency Scale and a specially designed articulation protocol. It should be pointed out, however, that no control group was used in this study. Black (1972) reported an 80 percent dismissal rate of a public school caseload during the first year the multiple phoneme approach was used. Only 20 percent of the caseload had been dismissed the previous year, when a different remediation approach was used. Such data, while supportive, lack scientific rigor due to the lack of control procedures. Van Denmark and Hardin (1986) reported that children receiving multiple

Client _____ Date _____

Clinician _____ Transfer _____

Maintenance _____

Step _____

Date	Session	Activity						Time	Total Response	Total Error	Total Correct	% Correct	Comments
		Isolation	Syllables	Words	Sentences	Reading	Conversation						

FIGURE 10–1. **Articulation Data Sheet.** *Source:* Used with permission of R. McCabe and D. Bradley.

phoneme therapy remained highly motivated to improve speech and maintained treatment gains whereas articulation skills regressed after traditional therapy.

PROGRAMMED CONDITIONING FOR ARTICULATION: MONTEREY ARTICULATION PROGRAM

The **Programmed Conditioning for Articulation** is a behaviorally oriented program authored by Baker and Ryan (1971), based on the traditional approach to articulation remediation. Developed with adherence to the principles of programmed instruction, this program can be adapted to focus on any sound segment the clinician may wish to teach. It consists of an establishment phase, which includes a basic program of 18 steps, 91 branching steps, and several sound evocation programs; a transfer phase of 15 steps; and a maintenance phase of five steps.

Sound evocation programs are intended to teach target productions when such behaviors are not in the client's response repertoire. These programs are available for /s/, /r/, /l/, /θ/, /ʃ/, and /tʃ/. General instructional suggestions and guidelines for teaching other phonemes are presented. Testing is prescribed prior to the initiation of the establishment phase to allow the clinician to select the target sound(s) and determine the appropriate entrance step in the program.

The same basic instructional pattern is followed for all phases of the program: The client responds to a stimulus and is given reinforcement. Verbal modeling, or imitation, is the most frequently used method of stimulus presentation in the program. Pictures, graphemes, and storytelling are also used to elicit responses. The authors recommend that instruction be conducted so that clients produce an average of 300 responses per hour of instruction. Reinforcement for correct responses is presented according to a schedule that begins with continuous reinforcement and shifts to a fixed ratio of 10 to 1 as the student progresses.

The criterion level for advancing from one step to the next in the program is ten correct responses in a row. If errors are consistently produced, then branching activities are initiated. Criteria for shifting to branching is ten consecutive errors or three consecutive sessions with a correct response rate of less than 80 percent.

The establishment phase in this program progresses from sound evocation through production in conversational speech in the instructional setting. Thus, the definition of establishment is broader than the definition used throughout this book. Table 10–2 presents the program outline for the establishment phase. The instructional sequence proceeds from Step A (imitation of the sound in isolation) to Step B (imitation of the sound in syllables) and continues with stimulus and response complexity increasing through the steps. The program delineation includes specific instructions regarding the nature of the stimulus, the expected response, and the schedule of reinforcement.

The transfer phase of the program is designed to facilitate situational transfer. Series A (Table 10–3) of the transfer program is initiated during the establishment phase of the program. When the student reaches certain criterion levels on the establishment program, the instructor gives the client word lists, phrases, and sentences to take home for practice with a parent. The parent is instructed to work with the child during a five-minute period and record his or her responses.

During Series B and subsequent series (see Table 10–3) of the transfer phase, the clinician monitors the client during speaking situations, culminating with the

TABLE 10–2. **Establishment Phase: Programmed Conditioning for Articulation.**

STEP		STIMULUS	RESPONSE	SCHEDULE OF REINFORCEMENT
Series A		Take Criterion Test		
		Placement Start		
	1	Sound in isolation	Sound	
Series B				
	1	Sound in nonsense syllable, random presentation of short vowels (a, e, i, o, u) with X* in initial position (Xa)	Syllable	
	2	Sound in nonsense syllable, random presentation of short vowels (a, e, i, o, u) with X in final position (aX)	Syllable	
	3	Sound in nonsense syllable, random presentation of short vowels (a, e, i, o, u) with X in medial position (aXa)	Syllable	100% (continuous)
Series C				
	1	Word with X in initial position	Word	50%
	2	Word with X in final position	Word	50%
	3	Word with X in medial position	Word	50%
Series D				
	1	Word with X in initial position appearing randomly in 2- or 3-word phrase	Phrase	50%
	2	Word with X in final position appearing randomly in 2- or 3-word phrase	Phrase	50%
	3	Word with X in medial position appearing randomly in 2- or 3-word phrase	Phrase	50%
Series E				
	1	Word with X in initial position appearing randomly in 4- to 6-word sentence	Sentence	50%
	2	Word with X in final position appearing randomly in 4- to 6-word sentence	Sentence	50%
	3	Word with X in medial position appearing randomly in 4- to 6-word sentence	Sentence	50%
Series F				
	1	Contextual reading material (If nonreader, go to series G-2.)	Reads a sentence	100%
Series G				
	1	Story: Instruct to read silently and then tell a story about it.	Reads story silently Tells what he/she reads in phrases and sentences Phrases	100%
	2	Pictures: (Instructor models first picture by telling short story about the picture.)	Tells story about picture in sentences	100%
Series H				
	1	Conversation	Conversation	100%
	2	Conversation	Conversation	10%
		End of Program		
		Stop		
		Take Criterion Test		
		Go to Transfer Program Series B.		
		Begin Program again with New Sound(s).		

* X = target sound
Source: Used with permission of Monterey Learning Systems, 900 Welch Road, Palo Alto, Calif.

TABLE 10–3. **Transfer Phase: Programmed Conditioning for Articulation.**

Series				
A		Child working with parent at home:		
	1	Says word containing X	Repeats word	100%
	2	Says phrase containing word with X	Repeats phrase	100%
	3	Says sentence containing word with X	Repeats sentence	100%
	4	Reading material or pictures	Reads or tells about pictures	100%
	5	Conversation	Conversation	100%
Series				
B		Take Transfer Criterion Test		
		Different physical settings with the clinician:		
	1	Outside clinic (outside the door)	Conversation	100%
	2	Outside clinic (down the hall)	Conversation	100%
	3	Outside clinic (outside the building or in another room)	Conversation	100%
	4	Playground or cafeteria or off school or clinic grounds	Conversation	100%
	5	Outside classroom	Conversation	100%
Series				
C		In the classroom:		
	1	With clinician in classroom	Conversation	100%
	2	With clinician and teacher in classroom	Conversation	100%
	3	Small-group activity	Conversation	100%
	4	Large-group activity	Conversation	100%
	5	"Speech" or "Show and Tell" in front of class	Conversation or monologue	100%
		Take Transfer Criterion Test		
		End of Program		
		Stop		
		Go to Maintenance		

Source: Used with permission of Monterey Learning Systems.

client giving a speech or participating in Show and Tell with his or her peers. During such speaking situations, the clinician must record at least 10 target responses, and the client must produce 90 percent correct responses to proceed to the next step.

The maintenance phase of the program covers a two-month period following completion of the transfer phase. It includes periodic rechecks to help the student maintain the newly acquired sounds. During the first month, the client is seen weekly; during the second month, only once. Criterion for each step in this phase is 10 consecutively produced correct responses. As can be seen in Table 10–4, all steps in the maintenance phase include conversational samples.

SUMMARY OF THE PROGRAMMED CONDITIONING FOR ARTICULATION

Background Statement. This behavioral program views remediation from the perspective that speech sounds are learned motor behaviors. Instruction involves a progression of motor skills and employs behavioral principles that are used in modifying behaviors. In this program, instruction consists of several series of small, sequential steps associated with contingent reinforcement. Thus, it represents a formal programmed approach to instruction that is based on behavioral conditioning.

Unique Features. The detailed step-by-step instructions for correcting misarticulations provide the clinician with what some might call a "recipe" for se-

TABLE 10–4. Maintenance Phase: Programmed Conditioning for Articulation.

STEP	STIMULUS	RESPONSE	SCHEDULE OF REINFORCEMENT
Series			
A			
1	1 weekly meeting	Conversation	100%
2	1 weekly meeting	Conversation	100%
3	1 weekly meeting	Conversation	100%
4	1 weekly meeting	Conversation	100%
5	1 monthly meeting	Conversation	100%
	Dismiss		
	End of Program		
	Stop		

Source: Used with permission of Monterey Learning Systems.

quencing therapy. The scope of the program, which moves from establishment to transfer to maintenance, including a home program, is more comprehensive than most. As with all programmed instruction, the course of treatment is based on data which accrues from tabulation of responses made by the client.

Strengths and Limitations. This program is well suited to those clients for whom a highly structured sequence of motor articulation instruction is desired. Similarly, for clinicians or instructional aides that seek guidance in how to organize therapy, this program provides systematic, step-wise instructional procedures which take a client from establishment to dismissal. The emphasis on numerous responses per session insures much repetition and motor practice. Program methodology relies heavily on imitation, which may become tedious for some clients and clinicians. The inclusion of branching steps allows some individualization of the program, but the basic assumption is that the program is suitable to a wide spectrum of clients.

Research Support. Data to support the program have been reported by Baker and Ryan (1971) and Gray (1974). These investigators reported that significant gains can be achieved by subjects when comparing pretest and post-test scores for all phases of the program. However, experiments that have included control groups or other controls have not been reported.

McDonald's Sensory-Motor Program

The **McDonald Sensory-Motor Program** of articulation remediation was developed by McDonald (1964) and is focused on motor productions in various phonetic contexts. The system assumes that phonetic context can be used to facilitate generalization of target sounds from simple to more complex productions. When first introduced, this system was unique in rejecting notions that (1) perceptual training should precede production training and that (2) the initial step in production training should be production of sounds in isolation. Rather, McDonald pointed out that sounds in conversational speech do not occur in isolation but instead are organized into syllables. Thus, it would follow that if the syllable is assumed to be the basic unit of speech production, instruction should begin at and focus upon production at the syllabic level. He pointed out that traditional discrimination training typically involves external discrimination, a task that differs from the more critical skill of making judgments of one's own speech productions (internal discrimination). The sensory-motor approach uses techniques designed to "heighten auditory, tactile and proprioceptive awareness of the motor patterns" associated with the production of a sound. Thus, management focuses on motor production–oriented tasks.

The initial objective of treatment is to heighten the client's responsiveness to motor productions associated with connected speech. At this point, the client imitates combinations of bisyllables and trisyllables following the presentation of verbal models by the clinician. The stimuli are arranged to follow a hierarchy from simple movements to more complex movements with a variety of stress patterns. The intent of such practice is to enable the client to "listen and then to hear and feel his reproductions of the stimulus."

Practice begins with sounds that the child can produce correctly (non-error sounds) in bisyllable (CVCV) productions. The second CV of the bisyllable is a duplication of the first CV syllable, and each syllable is produced with equal stress. The consonant is then combined with each of the commonly used vowels; as in the example: [titi], [tɪtɪ], [tete], [tætæ], [tʌtʌ], [tutu], [tʊtʊ], [toto], [tata]. Next the client imitates syllables with primary stress on the first syllable followed by practice with primary stress on the second syllable. Following this, the vowels used in each syllable are changed, as in /titɪ/, and then other consonants that the client can produce correctly are substituted in a variety of vowel contexts and stress patterns. Combinations that will produce a variety of movement patterns (i.e., changes in place of consonant-vowel articulation) should be included.

Following practice with bisyllables, imitation of trisyllables, such as [lalala], is initiated. Practice with trisyllables follows the same general pattern presented for bisyllables, including a variety of movement sequences and stress patterns. As a part of bisyllable and trisyllable practice, clients are instructed to describe the placement of the articulators and the direction of the articulatory movements. Some of the error sounds should be included in bisyllabic and trisyllabic contexts, but no effort should be made to remediate these sounds if they are produced incorrectly.

The second treatment objective of this approach is "to reinforce the child's correct articulation of his error sounds." The sensory-motor approach assumes that most error sounds can be produced correctly in at least one phonetic context. If contexts where the target sound is produced correctly cannot be found, McDonald suggested that a deep test for the error sound be administered again after the child has produced a series of bisyllables and trisyllables using non-error sounds.

Instruction for articulatory errors is initiated in a context where the error sound can be produced correctly. McDonald provided an example of a child with a defective /s/ who produced [s] correctly on a deep test in the context of *watchsun*. He suggested the following sequence of instructions after *watchsun* was identified as a context where /s/ was correctly produced: (1) Say *watchsun* with "slow-motion" speed; (2) say *watchsun* with equal stress on both syllables, then with primary stress on the first syllable, and then with primary stress on the second syllable; (3) say *watchs* and prolong [s] until a signal is given to complete the bisyllable with [ʌn]; (4) say short sentences with the same facilitating context such as "Watch, sun will burn you." The sequence is repeated with other sentences and stress patterns. The meaningfulness of the sentence is not important since the primary focus of the activity is the movement sequences.

Remediation Systems and Approaches

The third objective is "to facilitate the correct articulation of the sound in systematically varied phonetic contexts." The client is instructed to alter slightly the movement patterns associated with the correct /s/ by changing the vowel following the segment. For example, when /s/ was correct in *watchsun*, McDonald suggested a sequence such as:

watch–sun	*watch–sat*
watch–sea	*watch–soon*
watch–sit	*watch–sew*
watch–send	*watch–saw*

The next step is to practice words that include a second contextual modification. Using the above example, segments preceding and following /tʃ/ would be altered. Words like *teach, reach, pitch, catch,* and *beach* would be used in combination with one-syllable words beginning with /s/ and followed by a variety of vowels (such as *sand, sun, said,* and *soon*). Practice is then conducted with various combinations of the words that terminate with /tʃ/ in combination with words that begin with /s/ (for example, *teachsun*). Various sound combinations are practiced with different rates and stress patterns and should also be practiced in sentence contexts.

The next phase of instruction is directed toward a phonetic context other than [tʃ] in which the /s/ was correct. A similar series of sequential steps for varying the phonetic context, rate of speech, and syllable stress in alternative contexts would then be practiced. These activities would be designed for correct articulation in sentence contexts. Situational transfer procedures and activities are similar to those used with other treatment systems.

Summary of McDonald's Sensory-Motor Program.

Background Statement. The theoretical concept underlying this approach is that the syllable is the basic unit of speech production and learning to articulate sounds correctly should be based on motor practice of syllabic productions in a variety of different contexts and at several complexity levels. Rather than engaging in perceptual training as a precursor to production training, this approach assumes that with motor practice at the syllable level, one heightens the auditory, tactile, and proprioceptive awareness of the speaker. It is an underlying assumption that speakers will produce correct productions in some contexts, and these are used to initiate syllable practice.

Unique Features. The emphasis on imitated, repetitive syllable productions is a unique aspect of this program. The systematic variation of phonetic contexts and stress patterns in productions of both sounds produced correctly and error sounds targeted for remediation sets this program apart from others. The approach capitalizes on facilitating contexts in a client's repertoire.

Strengths and Limitations. A major strength of this approach is that it builds on behaviors (segmental productions in particular phonetic contexts) that are in a client's repertoire. The concept of syllable practice and systematic variation of phonetic contexts and stress may be useful to any training method that includes syllable productions. Elicitation of a target sound via deep testing may be problematic in some instances, and it has not been shown that bisyllable and trisyllable practice with non-error productions will aid in the elicitation of correct productions for those that are in error. It may be that some clients will need to be taught articulatory productions of certain sounds by other, more direct methods.

Research Support. Although a deep test to facilitate the location of facilitating contexts has been widely used, published clinical investigations which provide support for the efficacy of this intervention approach are lacking.

HOFFMAN-SCHUCKERS-DANILOFF MOTORIC AUTOMATIZATION OF ARTICULATORY PERFORMANCE PROGRAM

Hoffman, Schuckers, and Daniloff (1989) presented a sequenced set of production-based training tasks designed to facilitate the motoric automatization of articulatory performance. The basic assumption behind their suggestions is that "revision of over learned, highly automatic behavior is possible through carefully planned and executed performance rehearsal" (248). They also indicated that once *inappropriate* patterns of a behavior are automatized or habituated the process of revising those behaviors may differ from development of the original behavior. Intervention is seen as involving instruction and extensive practice of motor articulatory adjustments to replace previously learned (incorrect) behavior. The paragraphs that follow present the sequence of tasks and instructional activities these authors suggest.

Stimulability tasks. Prior to working directly on error targets, the clinician elicits, via imitation, sound segments that the client already produces correctly. This provides the client with an opportunity to experience success in a speech task as well as the opportunity to observe and imitate the clinician's demonstrations. It is suggested that the clinician not only model the correct form of sounds in the child's repertoire but also distort such productions through excessive movements (e.g., lip rounding for /m, p, f/) for the purpose of giving the client the opportunity to practice manipulation of the articulators in response to the clinician's model. Such activity will hopefully facilitate the client's skill at identifying, comparing, and discriminating the clinicians and his/her own sound productions.

Rehearsal. Following stimulability tasks, the clinician and client work together to employ the articulatory adjustments necessary for correct target sound production. It is suggested that the clinician be able to repeat sentences using error productions similar to those of the client in order to be aware of the motoric acts involved in the client's misarticulations. Instead of instruction focusing on "correct" or "better" target sound productions, the focus is on doing interesting things with the speech mechanism, with the ultimate goal being the production of a target sound. Activities designed to provide information about the anatomy and physiology of the speech mechanism are suggested at this stage, and children are encouraged to view their productions in the mirror and listen to themselves on audio/video tapes.

Rehearsal involves four levels: nonsymbolic units, words and word pairs, sounds in sentences, and narratives. While initial instruction follows these four complexity levels, once the narrative level is reached, rehearsal can include a mixture of the four levels.

Practice with *nonsymbolic* units (the authors use the term *nonsymbolic* rather than *nonsense syllables*) provides for manipulation of articulatory gestures that were begun during pretraining. Nonsymbolic instruction focuses on target productions in VC, CV, VCV, and VCCV syllables. It is asserted that production of

Remediation Systems and Approaches

TABLE 10–5. **Nonsymbolic Sound Unit Rehearsal Matrices.**

V C	V C V	C V	V C C V
i s	i s i	s i	i t s i
a s	i s a	s a	i t s a
u s	i s u	s u	i t s u
æ s	i s æ	s æ	i t s æ
	a s i		a t s i
	a s a		a t s a
	a s u		a t s u
	a s æ		a t s æ
	u s i		u t s i
	u s a		u t s a
	u s u		u t s u
	u s æ		u t s æ
	æ s i		æ t s i
	æ s a		æ t s a
	æ s u		æ t s u
	æ s a		æ t s a

nonsymbolic units imposes minimal constraints on the speaker by allowing him or her to focus on the speech task rather than also including morphologic, syntactic, and semantic concerns. Table 10–5 reflects nonsymbolic sound unit rehearsal matrices. The authors suggest that motoric success at this rudimentary level facilitates success at more linguistically and socially complex levels.

Word and *word-pair* practice is the next step in the program. Initial targets should reflect a transition from nonsymbolic units to meaningful units that encompass the nonsymbolic syllables already practiced. Target words should reflect the child's age, interests, and social needs. Practice activities at this level may require memory and speed but should be designed to encourage the client to assume responsibility for recognizing and judging the adequacy of personal performance. Table 10–6 reflects a list of words and word-pairs by word-position that might be used at this level.

The next step in the program involves *sound in context rehearsal sentences*. At this stage the client repeats the clinician's model of sentences that includes words practiced at the word level stage. As in target word selection, it is important that sentences selected for imitation are appropriate for the client's age, abilities, and interests.

A second phase of this level consists of presenting a stimulus word containing

TABLE 10–6. **Word and Word-Pair List for [s].**

PREVOCALIC		INTERVOCALIC	POSTVOCALIC	
Initial	Cluster	Medial	Final	Word-Pair
Sam	scat	passing	pass	Jack sat
seed	ski	receive	niece	jeep seat
soup	scooter	loosen	loose	room soon
saw	scar	bossy	toss	cop saw
sit	skit	kissing	miss	lip sip
sign	sky	nicer	mice	right side

the target segment to the client, then requiring the client to repeat the word, and then embed it in a spontaneously generated sentence.

The final step in this program involves using a target sound in *narratives*. In this activity stories that can be illustrated, acted out, or read are employed. Felt boards and figures are particularly recommended. A series of clinician-generated narratives are employed; for example, "This is Poky the turtle. Today is his birthday. He is six years old. He says, 'It's my birthday.' What does he say?" This is followed by the client saying "It's my birthday." Through such narratives, practice of the target sound is embedded in communicative tasks. The clinician may have a client practice individual sentences from these narratives for additional practice at the sentence level.

While this program has been presented as a series of steps or levels, the authors point out that these steps should overlap. Throughout the program the client is the primary judge of productions, describing the movement patterns, articulatory contacts, and adequacy of production of each target sound. For children misarticulating more than a single phoneme, once training on one target has moved from stimulability through rehearsal, a second target can be introduced, while continuing to work on the first.

Summary of Hoffman-Schuckers-Daniloff Motoric Automatization of Articulatory Performance Program.

Background Statement. An underlying assumption behind this program is that the client is sufficiently aware of his or her misarticulations and has sufficient linguistic maturity that he or she can benefit from a motor-oriented direct intervention approach. Treatment is then viewed as the motoric automatization of specific articulatory behaviors.

Unique Features. The emphasis on describing motor movements and articulatory contacts of both "correct" and "incorrect" productions is unique. Encouraging clients to identify and describe physiologic aspects of production (e.g., articulatory contacts, air flow) is an important element of this program.

Strengths and Limitations. Development of motor awareness and self-monitoring skills are strengths of the program. The fact that it follows the traditional therapy sequence adds to its face validity. As the authors acknowledge, the approach is not appropriate for phonological disorders that are linguistically based.

Research Support. The success accorded the traditional approach would support this approach; however, no studies regarding the efficacy of this particular treatment outline have been reported.

PAIRED-STIMULI APPROACH

The **Paired-Stimuli approach** to articulation remediation developed by Weston and Irwin (1971; Irwin and Weston, 1971, 1975) is a technique applicable to the generalization stage of instruction. The basic assumption underlying the approach is that a behavioral reinforcement paradigm will facilitate generalization of the correct production of a target segment from one context to others. More specifically, generalization of a correct sound production can be facilitated from a key word (target sound embedded in a word produced correctly) to other words containing the target sound.

The paired-stimuli technique is used to teach one speech sound at a time

(Irwin and Weston, 1971). After the clinician has selected a target sound for instruction, the clinician must find a key word in which the target sound is produced correctly. The criteria for a key word is 9 out of 10 correct productions on a probe of a given word. For example, if the target sound is /s/ and it is produced correctly in the *cup–sun* context of the *Deep Test of Articulation*, the word *sun* would be tested on the preliminary probe. If the client produced /s/ correctly in *sun* in at least 9 out of 10 attempts, *sun* would meet the criteria as an acceptable key word. In this instance, the target sound is in the initial position of the key word, but it is also acceptable for the target sound to be in the key word's final position.

Once the key word is determined, the clinician selects 10 training words that contain the error sound in the same word-position (initial or final) as the key word. In order to qualify as a training word, the target sound should be misarticulated in two out of three productions. For example, if the client says *thoap, thoap, soap*, the word *soap* would qualify as a training word. If, on the other hand, the client says *sink, sink, shink*, the word *sink* would not qualify as a training word.

If a key word cannot be found in a client's repertoire, then it is suggested that the client be taught to produce the target sound and transfer it to a key word. Since the paired-stimuli procedure uses picture stimuli to elicit responses from the client, both key words and training words must be morphemes able to be illustrated. The authors indicate that the sound-position (initial, final) of the target sound in key and training words need not be the same.

Step 1 of the instructional procedure uses "training strings" and consists of the following procedure: the client is presented a set of pictures with the key word in the center and the 10 training words placed around the key word (see Figure 10–2). The clinician begins by pointing to the picture of the key word and directing the client to "say this." As soon as the client responds, the clinician judges the acceptability of the target phoneme production and, if correct (which in all probability it will be), administers reinforcement. The clinician then points to the first training word and asks the client to name it; appropriate reinforcement follows the response, and then the clinician again elicits the key word. When the key word has been successfully paired with each of the 10 training words, a training string is said to have been completed. Three training strings are included in each training session, and a clinician can usually administer two or three training strings during a half-hour session.

The training sound is not identified for the client, nor is the client provided cues or instruction other than the verbal instruction to name the key and training words. Each training string is preceded by a pre-probe and followed by a post-probe. These probes consist of the production of the key word plus each training word without contingent reinforcement. Such probes serve as a check on whether the client can produce stimulus words without appropriate reinforcement. In Step 2 a question-and-answer technique is used to elicit training words in simple phonetic contexts. In Step 3, spontaneous conversation becomes the context for eliciting the target phoneme (not necessarily in training words).

SUMMARY OF THE PAIRED-STIMULI APPROACH

Background Statement. This approach is based on the psychological principle of stimulus-response generalization as a method to facilitate contextual generalization. It is based on the notion of pairing words, one in which the client produces

Key Word

SUBJECT: *Karen Jones*

PHONEME: /f/   POSITION: Ⓘ F

ORDER: Ⓘ II

FIGURE 10–2. **Paired-stimuli training sheet.** *Source:* Used with permission of National Educator Services, Inc.

a target sound correctly (key word), with several words in which the target sound is produced incorrectly. By reinforcing correct phoneme production in the key word, it is expected that such productions will generalize to the target word. In essence this approach combines learning theory and motor practice.

Unique Features. This technique represents an attempt to employ the principles of paired-stimuli generalization to the process of phonological remediation.

Remediation Systems and Approaches

While key words are sometimes used in other treatment approaches, key words are the focus of this generalization approach. Also included are pictures and recording sheets in "kit" form.

Strengths and Limitations. This approach builds on behaviors already in a client's repertoire and requires minimal time for giving directions and instructions to the client. Thus, clients have opportunity to make numerous responses during a session. If a client does not exhibit a key word, then one must be taught. The approach allows clients to practice sounds in a variety of phonetic contexts, albeit in a seemingly random fashion, since pictures used in the kit are simply a collection of nouns able to be illustrated. Clinicians may, however, choose to use a paired-stimuli procedure with their own training words.

Research Support. Weston and Irwin (1971) reported that this approach was successful in modifying the articulation of three children to the point where generalization of correct production occurred in conversational speech. Irwin and Weston (1975) subsequently reported that mean scores for 338 children on the McDonald Screening Deep Test for a target sound went from 1.76 items correct on the pretest to 6.02 correct on the post-test following paired-stimuli instruction. However, generalization was absent in sounds that had not received paired-stimuli instruction. Such evidence must be considered tentative because control procedures were not utilized in Irwin and Weston's study.

SUMMARY OF MOTOR APPROACHES TO REMEDIATION

The treatment approaches described on the previous pages focus on the development of the motor skills necessary for target sound productions, with the traditional approach to remediation forming the basis of these approaches. An underlying assumption is that motor practice leads to generalization of correct productions to untrained contexts and to automatization of behaviors. Motor approaches to remediation are especially appropriate for phonetically based errors but are also employed by some clinicians with disorders which reflect a cognitive-linguistic basis.

REMEDIATION GUIDELINES FOR MOTOR APPROACHES

1. A motor approach to remediation is recommended as a teaching procedure for clients who evidence motor production problems with individual segments such as lisping for /s/ and /z/. It can also be incorporated into treatment programs for clients reflecting cognitive-linguistic or pattern-based errors, especially if the patterns reflect motor constraints (e.g., prevocalic voicing or certain cluster simplifications). Instruction should be initiated at the linguistic unit level (isolation, syllable, word) at which a client can produce target sounds.

2. Perceptual training is recommended as part of a motor remediation program for those clients who evidence perceptual problems related to their error sounds.

3. A multiple phonemic approach is recommended for clinicians who wish to teach several sounds in the same session or who wish to work simultaneously on several sounds which reflect the same error pattern.

4. For clinicians who wish to follow a detailed treatment protocol, the Programmed Conditioning for Articulation provides such a model.

COGNITIVE-LINGUISTIC APPROACHES TO REMEDIATION

The primary focus of cognitive-linguistic approaches to remediation is the establishment of phonological rules in a client's repertoire. Instruction is oriented toward relationships among sounds (contrasts and other rules), as opposed to the individual sound focus of motor-oriented approaches to remediation.

Treatment programs designed to facilitate acquisition of linguistic rules are not associated with a single unified method; however, two primary characteristics are frequently associated with cognitive-linguistic oriented treatment approaches. The first characteristic relates to the targeting of behaviors for treatment, and the second relates to instructional procedures.

Treatment involves selecting for instruction certain target behaviors (sounds), called exemplars, that are likely to facilitate generalization to an entire class of sounds or sound-positions (e.g., other sounds containing a certain feature; other sounds in the same word-position). By analyzing phonological errors for underlying patterns or rules, exemplars can be selected that are designed to facilitate the acquisition of appropriate sound contrasts and/or sequences.

Most treatment protocols that are based on a cognitive-linguistic model employ minimal contrast word-pairs, which in turn often involve minimal or maximal feature contrasts (Weiner, 1981; Gierut, 1989). For example, minimal pairs such as bus–buck and bus–but represent minimal pairs with greater and lesser contrasts respectively due to the differences in place of articulation between /s/ and /k/ (greater contrast because of the alveolar-velar contrast), and /s/ and /t/ (lesser contrast because both /s/ and /t/ are alveolar consonants).

The remainder of this chapter will focus on treatment approaches that have emanated from a cognitive-linguistic perspective. The primary focus of these approaches has been to (1) establish distinctive feature contrasts and (2) eliminate or reduce phonological processes (simplifications). Cognitive-linguistic approaches have also been concerned with other aspects of the phonological system. Included among these are elimination of homonyms and development of new syllable shapes. In addition, language-based approaches have been recommended for those who have phonological as well as other types of language disorders (i.e., syntax, semantics, pragmatics).

The reader will note that remediation approaches associated with distinctive features and phonological processes stem from a similar theoretical base, and treatment procedures associated with each resemble one another. Since the treatment approaches for distinctive features and phonological processes are similar, a single critique will be presented for these approaches.

Distinctive Feature Therapy

Distinctive features may be considered sub-phonemic elements of phonemes that determine the linguistic contrasts between sounds and sound classes. In other words, unique bundles of distinctive features underlie the distinctions between phonemes in a language. For a review of information concerning distinctive features, refer back to Chapters 1 and 7.

The intent of a remediation program based on distinctive features is to establish feature contrasts that are lacking in a client's repertoire, thus accounting for one or more error patterns. Distinctive feature remediation programs usually focus on the establishment of a feature through teaching a sound containing that feature. It is then assumed that the newly established feature will generalize from the exemplar to other members of the sound class in which the feature may be absent (e.g., + continuant generalizes from target /f/ to /θ/, /s/, and /ʃ/).

Stoel-Gammon and Dunn (1985) identified the following remediation concepts and treatment strategies that evolved from distinctive feature treatment programs:

1. Selection of target phonemes shifted from isolated phonemes to sound classes. The clinician focuses on features which are common to several phonemes, and thus the client learns a feature common to a class of sounds rather than learning unrelated sounds one at a time.
2. The emphasis on facilitation of generalization as a treatment goal requires the clinician to look at the influence treatment may have on a sound class rather than isolated sounds.
3. The emphasis on phonological contrasts as the basis for correcting errors and acquiring the adult sound system.

McReynolds and Bennett (1972) reported data indicating that features established in one sound (the exemplar) will generalize to other sound segments in which the target feature is absent. They inferred from this finding that remediation based on distinctive features should be an efficient treatment approach. Similar to other types of generalization, the nature and extent of feature generalization that takes place is highly variable. Generalization seems to be significantly influenced by the similarity between the segment selected for training and other segments in which the generalization occurs (e.g., segments in the same sound class). In general, the more features two sound segments share, the more potential there is for generalization to occur.

In the paragraphs below, we describe several distinctive feature treatment approaches that have appeared in the literature. The reader will note that distinctive feature approaches to remediation frequently incorporate methodologies that were described above in the motor approaches to therapy. Since the establishment of distinctive feature contrasts often involves production of individual sound segments, remediation frequently follows a similar sequence to that seen in motor approaches.

McReynolds and Colleagues' Approach. McReynolds and Bennett (1972) described instructional procedures used in a distinctive feature training study that investigated the nature of feature generalization. Their approach was designed to teach a feature contrast that was absent in a child's productive repertoire and included two overall teaching phases.

In Phase 1, production focused on nonsense syllables which contained the target feature in the initial position (e.g., *f*a). In Phase 2, the child was taught to produce a sound containing the target feature in the final position of a nonsense syllable. Within each phase there were several steps. In Step 1, the child was instructed to produce a consonant in which this feature was lacking. In Step 2, the child was taught to contrastively produce two consonant sounds in syllables, the segment learned in Step 1, and a second consonant selected to contrast with the first. For example, if [+ continuant] was the feature contained in the first sound taught, [− continuant] was the feature selected for the second or contrast sound ([fi] vs. [pi]). Subsequent steps in Phase 1 consisted of producing the two phonemes, each in the initial position, and in combination with four vowels (e.g., [fi] vs. [pi], [fa] vs. [pa], [fʌ] vs. [pʌ], and [fo] vs. [po]). Phase 2 was identical except for position of the target sound.

In a subsequent monograph, McReynolds and Engmann (1975) recommended that whenever possible, distinctive feature training should be initially restricted to sound units that reflect a single contrast, such as voicing in [p] versus [b]. They also recommend that when sound contrasts involve two or more feature differences, training should focus on segments with the least number of feature differences. For example, if a child uses /g/ for /s/ (e.g., /gʌn/ for /sʌn/), and also uses /g/ for /d/ (/gæd/ for /dæd/), the clinician may wish to focus initially on the /g/–/d/ contrast rather than the /g/–/s/ contrast because of fewer feature differences (i.e., /g/ and /d/ have the same manner and voicing features but differ only in place of articulation, whereas /g/ and /s/ differ in place, manner, and voicing features).

Costello and Onstein (1976) published an extension of the original McReynolds and Bennett (1972) study and developed a distinctive feature remediation approach based on motor and programming principles. The reader will note that while this treatment approach is described as a distinctive feature approach and classified as a cognitive-linguistic approach to remediation, the treatment protocol is motor based. In other words, the target behaviors are selected from a cognitive-linguistic error analysis, while intervention procedures stem from a motor production model.

The program Costello and Onstein outlined was designed specifically to teach young children /t/ versus /θ/ and /t/ versus /s/ contrasts because the [+ continuant] feature was not stabilized and stops were substituted for continuants. Phase 1 was intended to establish production of /t/, /θ/, and /t/ versus /s/ in isolation; Phase 2 involved production of the target sounds in a CV context; and Phase 3 involved production of the target sounds in a VC context. Phases 4 and 5 included imitation of /θ/, /t/, and /s/ in the releasing (initial) position of words, followed by imitation in the arresting (final) position. Phases 6 and 7 included imitation of /t/, /θ/, and /s/ in the releasing and arresting positions in words embedded in phrases and sentences, followed by sentences which were not imitated. Phases 8 and 9 included the production of /t/, /θ/, and /s/ in releasing and arresting positions in stories, conversational speech, and finally in utterances used outside the clinical environment.

Weiner and Bankson's Approach. Weiner and Bankson (1978) published an exploratory program that attempted to teach a feature (i.e., [+ frication]) in specific segments where the feature was not used correctly. Rather than relying on feature generalization from trained sounds to nontrained sounds as did McReynolds and Bennett (1972), they attempted to establish a feature in segments that reflected the feature deletion, without focusing on the correct production of a particular sound segment, but rather on the presence of frication only. Their client was a child who substituted stops (plosives) for fricatives. The first task in the training program consisted of an identification procedure that directed attention to developing awareness of [+ frication] in a number of contexts. The client was then required to contrast production of fricatives and stops. The client imitated fricative sounds and was reinforced for the production of [+ frication] regardless of the correctness of the remaining features in the segments. In other words, the sound imitatively produced might have been in error, but if [+ frication] was present, the response was reinforced. More specifically, [+ frication] was taught in the following instruction sequence:

1. Introduction of the concept of "dripping" sounds (stops) and "flowing" sounds (fricatives)
2. Identification of words that begin with dripping as compared to flowing sounds
3. Imitation of words containing fricatives in the initial position, with such fricatives emphasized through duration of initial sound (e.g., *f-f-f-fish*). Following his or her production, the client was required to judge whether the word began with a dripping or a flowing sound. Feedback was provided for both production and identification.
4. Repetition of Step 3 without exaggeration of the word-initial fricative
5. Presentation of a 20-item picture-naming task in which each item began with a fricative

These investigators reported that as a result of this instructional sequence, their client was able to successfully produce [+ frication] on a 20-item picture-naming task.

Blache's Approach. Blache (1989) published a distinctive feature approach to remediation of phonological delay. The approach is organized into four basic steps:

Step 1. *Discussion of words.* Determine whether or not the child knows the concept of the lexical items to be used in therapy. Once a minimal pair contrast has been selected to teach a distinctive feature, it is important to determine if the child understands both lexical items in the word-pair. For example, if the word-pair selected is the letter *T* and *key*, the child might be asked: "Which one opens the door? Which one is a letter of the alphabet? Which one goes into a lock? Which one do you write?" (See Figure 10–3.)

Step 2. *Discrimination testing and training.* The child is tested to determine if he or she can perceive the feature contrast. The clinician presents one word of a minimal pair, for example, *fan–pan* or *bear–pear*. The child is instructed to point to the picture that the clinician has named. A criterion of seven consecutive correct responses is used to establish perception of the contrasting word-pairs.

Step 3. *Production training.* After the client has demonstrated that he or she perceives the minimal contrast, the next step is to demonstrate the feature in a productive task. In this step, the child is instructed to say the word and the clinician is to point to the picture of the word the client pronounced. The client should always be able to correctly pronounce one word of the pair but may not be able to pronounce the other member of the word-pair; thus, a correct production of an error sound may not be required at this stage.

Step 4. *Carry-over training.* Once the child is able to pronounce the target word, the word is placed in longer and more complex linguistic environments. The word is used with the indefinite article *a* in varied phonetic contexts, two-word expressions, three-word carrier phrases, and the like, until the word is used in meaningful situations, social situations, and in the school and home.

Blache (1989) points out that this distinctive feature approach serves as a program which ". . . provides a context in which learning can occur but does not teach the child how to produce the sounds" (369) since sounds are not taught in isolation but only as contrastive units within words.

The selection of management targets requires the determination of specific sound classes which the child has difficulty producing. Blache divided the sounds

FIGURE 10–3. **Exemplars illustrating six different distinctive feature contrasts (a = front — back lingual; b = labial–lingual; c = voiced–voiceless; d = nasal–nonnasal; e = continued–interrupted; f = strident–mellow.** *Source:* "Minimal Word-Pairs and Distinctive Feature Training" by S.E. Blache, in *Phonological Intervention: Concepts and Procedures* (p. 65), M. Crary (Ed.), 1982, San Diego: College-Hill Press, Inc. Copyright 1982 by College-Hill Press. Little, Brown. (Reprinted by permission.)

of English into six major sound classes that reflect developmental levels: (1) primitive (non-speech sounds), (2) vocalic, (3) stop–nasal, (4) semivowel, (5) continuant, and (6) sibilant. The primitive and vocalic are expected to be acquired by the third year with others following thereafter.

An individual child's level of development is determined by the administration of a 67-item picture articulation test (Quick Test), which includes 25 consonants and semivowels in prevocalic, intervocalic, and postvocalic contexts. The child's performance on individual segments is then compared to sound class norms for children of the same age. Instruction begins with that sound class which is developmentally earliest and includes at least two sounds in error. For example, if a client reflects one sound error in the vocalic class, two in the stop–nasal class,

Remediation Systems and Approaches

TABLE 10–7. Contrast Ordering for Stop–Nasal Sound Class.

NO. PAIR	FEATURE	SAMPLE WORDS
1. [t-k]	front–back lingual	*tea–key, tape–cape, ten–Ken*
2. [n-ŋ]	front–back lingual	*win–wing, fan–fang, ton–tongue*
3. [p-b]	voiced–voiceless	*pea–bee, pig–big, pat–bat*
4. [t-d]	voiced–voiceless	*toe–doe, time–dime, tot–dot*
5. [k-g]	voiced–voiceless	*curl–girl, coat–goat, cap–gap*
6. [b-m]	nasal–nonnasal	*beet–meat, bat–mat, bike–Mike*
7. [d-n]	nasal–nonnasal	*D–knee, deck–neck, dot–knot*
8. [g-ŋ]	nasal–nonnasal	*wig–wing, bag–bang, log–long*
9. [b-d]	labial–lingual	*big–dig, bark–dark, bow–dough*
10. [d-g]	front–back lingual	*deer–gear, date–gate, doe–go*

Source: "A Distinctive Feature Approach" by S.E. Blache, in *Assessment and Remediation of Articulatory and Phonological Disorders* (p. 377). N. Creaghead, P. Newman, and W. Secord, eds., Columbus, Ohio: Charles E. Merrill, 1989.

and four in the semivowel class, the stop–nasal class is targeted for remediation since it develops earliest and reflects two speech sound errors. A therapeutic model has been developed wherein features that comprise the most salient contrasts are focused on first, followed by successive steps to finer distinctions. Blache (1989) identified the following feature comparisons occurring in the stop–nasal sound class, which proceed from larger to finer contrasts and are presented in Table 10–7.

Summary of Distinctive Features Approaches

Background Statement. Distinctive feature approaches to phonological remediation are based on the theory that speech sounds are comprised of individual bundles of features, each phoneme having a unique set of features from the pool of features that characterize segmental productions. Further, if a client has several sounds in error, an efficient strategy in treatment may be to identify or teach an exemplar which contains the absent feature(s), and monitor generalization from that exemplar to other sounds in the same class which are in error.

Unique Features. This approach is designed to capitalize on patterns or commonalities among error productions that the clinician needs to be aware of in planning the most efficacious treatment plan. Although features are taught in segments, feature analysis and remediation represent a more integrated approach than a traditional listing of individual segments in error.

Strengths and Limitations. An attraction of distinctive feature–oriented therapy is that it is designed to assist in the identification of phonological patterns that may underlie individual errors. A major limitation, however, relates to our earlier discussion indicating that distinctive features were not designed to be used for purposes of clinical intervention. Rather, they emanated from a set of features used to classify and identify sound segments among language systems of the world. Features systems have not been developed to classify speech sound errors, and thus not all errors can be described within this framework. In addition, the linguistic feature classification systems which have been applied clinically are easy to use with sound substitutions, but sound omissions and distortions are difficult to describe within such feature systems.

Research Support. Data to support a distinctive feature approach to therapy may be gleaned from studies that reported the treatment approaches described earlier. McReynolds and Bennett (1972) reported that all three of their subjects reflected distinctive feature generalization from the exemplar sounds they were taught to other sounds, although the amount of feature generalization varied across subjects. Similarly, Weiner and Bankson (1978) reported that their subject generalized [+ frication] to non-trained items. Costello and Onstein (1976) also reported that their instructional approach was successful in teaching their subject to generalize the [+ continuant] feature. These data support the finding that feature generalization is seen with distinctive feature approaches to remediation, although the amount of generalization varied considerably across subjects. The number of subjects involved in these studies was small, and additional data regarding the efficiency of this approach are needed.

CONTRAST THERAPY

A remediation approach commonly identified as a cognitive-linguistic approach is known as **minimal pair contrast therapy.** Contrast therapy employs pairs of words that differ only by a single phoneme (e.g., *bat–pat*, *move–mood*, *sun–ton*). The underlying concept of this type of therapy is that by focusing on near identical word-pairs that typically differ by a single phonemic contrast, the client will be taught that different sounds signal different meanings in words. Investigators have reported changes in children's phonological systems (Weiner, 1981; Elbert and Gierut, 1986; Gierut, 1989) following training focused on word-pair contrasts. While contrast therapy usually focuses on reduction in the use of phonological processes, it can also be used for treatment based on distinctive features and/or a traditional approach to substitution errors.

An example of a contrast approach to treatment can be observed through remediation strategies employed with a client who deletes final consonants. In this instance, stops may be produced correctly in word-initial position, but deleted in word-final position (lack of syllable closure). In such a circumstance, the clinician can assume that the final consonant deletions are probably not a production (motor or phonetic) problem. Rather, final consonant deletion in this case likely reflects a process or conceptual problem related to syllable structure (use of the open syllable). Treatment for this problem would focus on getting the client to recognize that the presence of a consonant in word-final position is a necessary contrast to distinguish certain word-pairs in the language (e.g., *two–tooth; bee–beet*). In this instance, the motoric production of a target consonant is already within a child's productive repertoire, and thus motor production of the sound is not the primary focus of instruction. Rather, motor production becomes secondary to the task of developing cognitive awareness of final consonant contrasts/syllable closure.

Contrast treatment may involve word-pairs reflecting minimal or maximal phonemic contrasts. In both instances, word-pairs are employed that differ by a single phonemic contrast. However, they differ in the specific nature of those contrasts. These differences will become clear in the sections that follow.

The most commonly employed type of contrast training typically contrasts a substituted or deleted sound with a target sound. For example, if a client substitutes /t/ for /k/ in word-initial position, contrast training words might include *tea–key* and *top–kop*. Similarly, if a child deletes the final /t/, contrast pairs might

Remediation Systems and Approaches

include *bow–boat* and *see–seat*. Minimal contrast instruction is appropriate when two contrasting sounds in the adult language are collapsed into a single sound unit with the result that no contrast is made (e.g., /t/ replaces /k/), or where segments are deleted, such as in final consonant deletions. Training is designed to establish sound contrasts that mark a difference in meaning. Such contrasts are often selected for remediation because of their relationship to phonological processes or error patterns seen in children's phonology (i.e., they become exemplars to facilitate generalization to other segments).

Minimal contrast instruction may focus on either perception of contrasts or production of contrasts. A training task that focuses on perceptual training utilizing contrast pairs was first proposed by La Riviere, Winitz, Reeds, and Herriman (1974). In the minimal contrast application of this procedure, subjects are taught to identify sound categories where the target sounds and errors are presented in word-pairs. For example, if a child deletes /s/ in /s/ clusters (cluster simplification), the clinician verbally presents minimal pairs like *spool–pool* or *spill–pill* to the client. The client is required to sort each lexical item into one of two categories (/s/ singletons or /s/ clusters).

A production-based task would require the client to verbally produce minimal pairs. For example, a client who deletes final consonants might ask the clinician to give him or her the picture of either a *bee* or a *beet*, then be reinforced by the clinician's response for the appropriate production. In this task, the client must be able to perceive the distinction between *bee* and *beet*, and in addition, be able to produce such a distinction. As stated earlier, the reverse of this procedure (i.e., the clinician asks the client to give him or her certain pictures) can be used to establish perceptual contrasts.

Weiner (1981) reported a study where minimal contrast training was used to reduce the frequency of selected phonological patterns. Weiner used minimal pair words in activities where accurate word productions were required for the child to communicate successfully. For example, Weiner used a game to teach final [t] in a minimal contrast format. He placed into minimal pairs such words as *bow* and *boat*. Sample stimuli consisted of several pictures of *bow* and several pictures of *boat*. The instructions for the game were as follows:

> "We are going to play a game. The object of the game is to get me to pick up all the pictures of the *boat*. Every time you say boat, I will pick one up. When I have all five, you may paste a star on your paper." If the child said *bow*, the clinician picked up the *bow* picture. At times he would provide an instruction, e.g., "You keep saying *bow*. If you want me to pick up the *boat* picture, you must say the [t] sound at the end. Listen, *boat, boat, boat*. You try it. Okay. Let's begin again" (98).

He reported that such training reduced the use of the phonological simplifications (processes) and generalization to nontrained words was observed.

A variety of treatment materials (word lists, pictures) have been published which are oriented toward minimal contrast therapy. An example of such material is *Contrasts: The Use of Minimal Pairs in Articulation Training* (Elbert, Rockman, and Saltzman, 1980), which contains a comprehensive list of minimal pairs designed to facilitate the establishment of phonological contrasts. These minimal pair lists were generated for training production and/or perceptional contrasts between phonemes. In the development of the word stimuli presented in these

TABLE 10–8. Contrasts for /t/–/ʃ/ Initial Position.

A. TRADITIONAL ARTICULATORY CLASSIFICATION
   CATEGORY: MANNER
   CONTRAST: /t/–/ʃ/ INITIAL

/i/	/ɪ/	/e/	/ɛ/	/æ/
T	tip / ship	tape / shape	Ted / shed	tad / shad
tea / she	tin / shin	take / shake	tell / shell	tack / shack
tee	till / shill	tame / shame	tear / share	tax / shacks
teak / sheik	tear / shear sheer	tail / shale		tag / shag
teeth / sheath				tam / sham
teethe / sheathe				tank / shank
tease / she's				
teen / sheen				

/ɑ/	/ʌ/	/u/	/ʊ/	/o/
top / shop	Tut / shut	to /shoe	took / shook	toe / show
tot / shot	tuck / shuck	too / shoe		tone / shone
Tod / shod	ton / shun	two / shoo		toll / shoal
tock / shock		toot / shoot		
tarp / sharp				
tarred / shard				

/ɔ/	/ɝ/	/ɔɪ/	/au/	/aɪ/
tall / shawl	term / Sherm		tout / shout	tie / shy
tore / shore				tine / shine
torn / shorn				
tort / short				

Source: Adapted from M. Elbert, B. Rockman, and D. Saltzman, *Contrasts: The Use of Minimal Pairs in Articulation Training.* Austin, Tex.: Exceptional Resources, Inc. 1980. Used with permission.

materials, all possible combinations of consonants, vowels, and clusters for each English phoneme in meaningful words (initial and final word-positions), together with consonant clusters in the word-initial position, were generated. Lists of minimally paired monosyllabic words are presented for approximately 60 different contrasts. (See Table 10–8 for the /t/–/ʃ/ contrast.) The contrasts are organized according to common classification systems used in assessment and training: (1) traditional articulatory error classification, including place, voice, and manner; (2) distinctive feature classification, including stridency, voicing, and continuancy; and (3) phonological process classification, including final consonant deletion, cluster simplification, fronting, stopping, and gliding. An example of a protocol employing a minimal pair training procedure is as follows:

1. Select a sound contrast to be trained based on the client's phonological errors. For example, if the child substitutes /t/ for /ʃ/ (stopping), one might select *tea–she, toe–show*, and *tape–shape* as target contrast words reflecting the stopping pattern. Select 5 pictures for each of the target words. (In the above example that would include a total of 30 pictures.)

2. Engage the client in minimal contrast training at a *perceptual* level (e.g., ''I want you to pick up the pictures that I name. Pick up _____.'').

3. Pretest the client's motor production of each of the target words containing the error sound, and if necessary instruct him or her in production of the target phoneme.

Remediation Systems and Approaches

4. Have the client imitatively produce each target word.
5. Engage the client in minimal contrast training at a *production* level (e.g., "I want you to tell me which picture to pick up. Every time you say *toe*, I will pick up this picture.").
6. Engage the client in a task designed to incorporate each of the contrast words in a carrier phrase (e.g., "I want you to point to a picture and say 'I found a *tea*'.").
7. Continue the carrier phrase task, only this time incorporate both words into the phrase (e.g., "I found a *tea* and a *she*.").

Clinicians can use their creativity and clinical knowledge to modify a protocol such as that just presented. As stated earlier, there are several descriptions in the literature of minimal pair treatment approaches, in addition to several commercially available sets of materials designed to facilitate this treatment approach.

A variation of contrast therapy is one that employs phonemic contrasts that involve "maximal" as opposed to "minimal" oppositions. In this instance the word-pairs contrast the target sound with a second sound and this second sound contains as many featural differences from the target sound as possible. For example, if a child replaces /ʃ/ with /t/, the target words might be *shoe* and *moo*, rather than *shoe* and *two*. In this case, /s/ and /m/ are more dissimilar than are /s/ and /t/, and thus the phoneme oppositions are greater (maximal opposition) rather than smaller (minimal opposition). A second difference between maximal and minimal oppositions is that in maximal oppositions a target sound is not contrasted with the error sound (an approach characteristic of minimal opposition contrast approaches). An underlying assumption of the maximal contrast approach is that phonological oppositions of greater disparity may be easier to acquire than minimal oppositions and will facilitate the client's acquisition of more feature contrasts. Examples of minimal and maximal oppositions are as follows:

Minimal Oppositions	Feature Differences
*s*un–*t*on	manner of production
*th*umb–*s*um	place of production
*ch*ew–*sh*oe	manner of production

Maximal Oppositions	Feature Differences
*ch*ain–*m*ain	manner of production, nasality, place of production
*c*an–*m*an	manner of production, place of production, nasality
*g*ear–*f*ear	manner of production, voicing, place of production

The usage of maximal oppositions is supported by clinical data from Gierut (1989). Others (Van Riper, 1939; Winitz, 1975), operating from somewhat different clinical frameworks, have also suggested that learning to perceive or discriminate sound contrasts can be facilitated by first focusing on sound contrasts that evidence maximal opposition of features. It appears that linguistic functioning, particularly acquisition of phonemic contrasts at a perceptual or productive level, may be facilitated by first teaching maximal (as opposed to minimal) contrasts.

The treatment methodologies outlined earlier for minimal contrast therapy are applicable to maximal contrast training. The difference between the two types of instruction is the nature of the contrasts in the word-pairs.

Two final notes on contrast therapy: (1) occasionally clinicians employ contrast training at the syllable level (e.g., /sa/–/ʃa/ before moving on to words, in order to reduce interference from meaningful words, and to provide production practice, and (2) for those instances where meaningful minimal pairs cannot be found to reflect a particular contrast, *near* minimal pairs are sometimes used (e.g. [væn-ʃæn].

Suggestions from Ingram. Ingram (1989) offered several suggestions for a cognitive-linguistic approach to phonological delay. He indicated that a major component in the acquisition of phonology is learning to use sounds contrastively (e.g., voicing contrasts, manner contrasts, place contrasts). He recommended that when such contrasts have not been acquired, remediation should focus not only on reduction in the use of phonological processes but also on the establishment of sound contrasts that may be lacking in a client's repertoire. He outlined the following three tasks that may be involved in teaching the phonologically delayed child to utilize additional sound contrasts: (1) elimination of instability in the child's speech (several forms are used for a lexical item); (2) elimination of homonyms (words with different meanings but pronounced the same); and (3) establishment of new contrasts (production of sounds in minimal pairs). Further explanations of what Ingram meant by items (1) and (2) are presented below. Establishment of new contrasts are not discussed here, since Ingram's comments and suggestions for contrast therapy are similar to those in our earlier discussion of this topic.

Elimination of Instability in Children's Speech. Some children with delayed phonological development demonstrate variations in phonetic forms used from one production of a specific word to another. Such inconsistent productions (instability) probably reflect the operation of several different phonological processes that operate simultaneously during a particular stage in a child's phonological productions. Ingram reported on a child who produced 13 different pronunciations of *pencil* (i.e., [bʌbə], [pʌbə], [pítə], [ɛ́tə], [pɛ́ʔtəʔ], [pɛd], [pɛdə], [pɛdza], [pɛtə], [pʰad], [pta], [pɪt], [pʰɛ́ʔtv̆]). The clinician selected one of the 13 pronunciations [pɛtə] as the most similar to the adult form. The stabilization of this form, for the word *pencil*, was an initial target of remediation. Once [pɛtə] was established for *pencil*, the other 12 forms could be contrasted with [pɛtə] and, if appropriate, be assigned to other lexical items. This form, when stabilized as the established form, eliminated the processes of (1) consonant deletion, (2) syllable deletion, (3) vowel variation, and (4) labial assimilation.

Elimination of Homonyms. Homonyms occur when a single phonetic form is used to refer to two or more objects or events. For example, a child may use [wawa] for *water, washcloth,* and *wipe.* The use of homonyms reduces the intelligibility of the child's speech since the same phonetic forms may be used to refer to several different objects or events. There is some evidence that phonologically delayed children may use more homonyms than normal children (Ingram, 1989). The elimination of homonyms is required to establish the standard phonemic contrasts of the language.

In terms of remediation, an alternative word is taught for certain items within a group of homonyms. In the example above, [wawa] might be used only for *water* and then another phonetic form used for *washcloth* and *wipe.* Each new phonetic form the child acquires will refer to one of the words initially labeled with the same phonetic form (homonyms). An example Ingram provided was [dado], which

Remediation Systems and Approaches

was used for *butter, ladder, letter, spider, water,* and *whistle.* By elimination of the process of alveolar assimilation (an alveolar sound is used for the initial segment because of the influence of the /d/ in the second syllable), [bado] was established for *butter, spider, water,* and *whistle,* and [dado] for *ladder* and *letter.* The next step was to reduce the use of "glide stopping" by the establishment of [wado] for *water* and *whistle.*

Summary of Contrast Training.

Background Statement. Contrast training is a cognitive-linguistic approach to phonological remediation and is designed to facilitate acquisition of phonological contrasts. Instruction typically involves perceptual and production tasks related to word-pairs reflecting phonemic contrasts. Contrast training procedures represent techniques to facilitate the reorganization of the phonological system so as to reduce the use of phonological processes, and to establish phonemic contrasts.

Unique Features. A unique contribution of contrast training is that all of the training is communication-oriented. That is, the listener–speaker must perceive–produce a particular phonemic contrast in order to communicate (act or get someone else to act appropriately).

Strengths and Limitations. The approach is designed for those clients who have certain sounds in their repertoire but fail to use them contrastively. This is important for clients with a cognitive-linguistic component to their phonological delay. By focusing on communication-oriented teaching activities, the training steps are generally less tedious than more drill-oriented activities. Clinicians need to be creative when using this approach and must have a plan for how contrast training fits in with other treatment activities.

Research Support. Data to support the efficacy of contrast training, both minimal and maximal are available (Ferrier and Davis, 1973; Weiner, 1981; Elbert and Gierut, 1986; Gierut, 1989). It is anticipated that research in this area will be ongoing and will assist in developing a stronger theoretical base for understanding and treating phonological disorders.

CYCLES APPROACH

The **cycles approach** (Hodson and Paden, 1991) reflects a combination of linguistic and motor-oriented approaches to remediation and was designed for unintelligible children. The cycles approach targets certain phonological patterns for instruction that are lacking in a client's repertoire. The procedures for this treatment method include (1) stimulation (the client is made aware of the auditory, tactual, and visual characteristics of target sounds); and (2) production practice (eliciting sound productions which are incompatible with process occurrence so that the operation of the target processes are reduced in the child's speech).

The remediation plan is organized around *treatment cycles* which can range from 5 or 6 weeks in length to 15 to 16 weeks, depending on the client's number of deficient patterns and the number of stimulable phonemes within each pattern. Hodson's (1989) suggestions for treating behaviors during cycles included the following:

> Each phoneme within a pattern should be targeted for approximately 60 minutes per cycle (i.e., one 60-minute, two 30-minute, or three 20-minute sessions) before progressing to the next phoneme in that pattern and then on to other phonological

patterns. Furthermore, it is desirable to provide stimulation for two or more target *phonemes* (in successive weeks) within a pattern before changing to the next target *pattern* (i.e., each deficient phonological pattern is stimulated for two hours or more within each cycle). Only *one* phonological pattern should be targeted during any one session so that the client has an opportunity to focus, and patterns should not be intermingled (324).

A cycle is complete when all phonological patterns that have been selected for remediation at a given point in time have been treated. Following completion of one cycle, a second cycle begins which will again cover those patterns not yet emerged or targeted or in need of further instruction. Hodson (1989) indicated that 3 to 6 cycles of phonological remediation, involving 30 to 40 hours of instruction (40 to 60 minutes per week) are usually required for a phonologically disordered client to become intelligible. Within each cycle, a pattern is the focus of instruction for 2 to 4 weeks with a different phoneme (selected to reduce the pattern) targeted each week. Processes targeted for remediation should occur in at least 40 percent of the instances in which the opportunity for their occurrence is present, based on a 50-item single-word naming task (Hodson and Paden, 1991).

Phonological patterns are targeted for remediation based on the child's "phonological deficiencies" and those patterns on which he or she is most stimulable. Hodson (1989) identified the following "primary potential target patterns/phonemes": early developing phonological patterns, posterior–anterior contrasts, /s/ clusters, and liquids.

An example follows of how the Hodson-Paden approach works. If fronting of velars occurs at least 40 percent of the time, and if velars are stimulable (can be imitated with auditory and visual cues), fronting would likely be selected as a target pattern for remediation. Following this, a target velar (e.g., /k/) would be selected as an instructional target and the focus of instruction for approximately a week (two to four sessions). Following work on this instructional goal, a second velar (e.g., /g/) would be targeted for the next two to four sessions.

The instructional sequence for each session is as follows:

1. *Review.* At the beginning of each session, the prior week's production practice word cards are reviewed, unless a new pattern is initiated during the session.
2. *Auditory bombardment.* This step requires listening for about 2 minutes while the clinician slowly reads approximately 12 words containing the target sound, including production in sentences. For example: "Shoe. You have brown shoes on today. They look like new shoes." This auditory stimulation typically is done at the beginning and end of each session and frequently includes the use of amplification (auditory trainer). The clinician may also demonstrate the error and contrast it with the target.
3. *Target word cards.* The client draws, colors, or pastes pictures of three to five target words on large index cards. The name of the picture is written on each card.
4. *Production practice.* The client participates in production practice activities through game-based activities. The client is expected to have a very high success rate in terms of correct productions. Shifting experiential-play activities every five to seven minutes helps to maintain a child's interest in repetition of the target words. The client is also given the opportunity to use target words in conversation.

   Production practice includes auditory, tactual, and visual stimulation for correct production at the word level. Usually five words per target sound are used in a single session and the client is instructed to produce the words. A variety of games are used in each session. These activities are the "heart" of an instructional session.

5. *Stimulability probing.* The target phoneme to be focused on in the next session for a given pattern is selected based on stimulability probing (checking to see what words a child can imitate) which occurs at this point in the treatment session.

6. *Auditory bombardment.* Auditory bombardment is repeated using the 12-item word list from the beginning of the session.

7. *Home program.* Parents are instructed to read the 12-item word list used in the auditory bombardment task to the child at least once a day. The 5 cards used during the week for production practice are also sent home for the child to practice daily.

The client is not required to meet a criterion level prior to moving on to treatment of other patterns within a cycle. When patterns persist after a single cycle of training, they may be recycled for treatment at a later time.

Ingram (1986) suggested that a theoretical rationale for this approach may be gleaned from preliminary data from studies in cross-linguistic phonological acquisition. Just as children acquire the sounds that occur most frequently in their language (e.g., French children learn [v] early, American children learn [v] later), so children receiving repeated auditory bombardment may come to acquire speech sounds presented through this approach. In addition, the recurring focus on particular sounds, which occurs with this cyclical approach, may allow for the gradual acquisition of phonological contrasts. He suggested that learning in this treatment approach is not unlike that which occurs in the normal acquisition process wherein children learn the contrasts that they hear most frequently.

Summary of Cycles Approach.

Background Statement. The cycles approach is purported by its authors to be based on the phenomena of gradualness as observed in normal phonological acquisition. The emphasis on acquisition of phonological patterns stems from a cognitive-linguistic perspective of phonological behavior. Production practice of exemplars (target sounds) along with the practice of auditory bombardment are reflective of traditional motor approaches to intervention.

Unique Features. Perhaps the most distinctive contribution of this approach is its focus on cycling of remediation targets. Focusing on pattern (correct rule) *acquisition* rather than on the more usual concept of elimination of developmentally inappropriate patterns is an interesting way to conceptualize intervention. The overall blending of traditional and cognitive-linguistic assessment/treatment methodologies is also unique.

Strengths and Limitations. The attributes identified above as unique features are all strengths of this approach. The approach was designed for unintelligible children, but aspects of the approach can be used with less severely impaired clients.

Research Support. While the authors have a wealth of clinical experience to support this approach to intervention, published data, particularly of a comparative nature, are lacking. This approach, like many others, represents a composite or "package" of various instructional components; however, research support for individual aspects as well as the overall program are lacking.

LANGUAGE-BASED APPROACHES

Children with severe phonological disorders frequently have difficulty with other aspects of language, particularly semantics and syntax (Camarata and Schwartz, 1985; Panagos and Prelock, 1982; Hoffman, Schuckers, and Daniloff, 1989). Severe impairments of phonology that coexist with other language impairments suggest that many children have difficulty with the broader aspects of the language learning process. Although the precise nature of the relationship between phonology and other aspects of language is unknown (Fey, 1986), an idea which is gaining increasing acceptance is that phonological delay, especially when it coincides with other language impairments, is best remediated by employing a language-based intervention approach (Gray and Ryan, 1973; Matheny and Panagos, 1978; Hoffman, Schuckers, Daniloff, 1989). Hoffman, Norris, and Monjure (1990) stated that "descriptive research continues to show the importance of language organization levels that are higher than the word level upon sound production, suggesting that remediation of speech disorders outside of a more generalized context of language development may not be the most efficacious tack" (102). Hoffman, Schuckers, and Daniloff (1989) indicated that "the preschool child who misarticulates many phonemes and deletes consonants is not likely to be a sophisticated enough language user to profit from such [motoric automatization] approaches" (p. 259).

Phonetic Elaboration in Narratives. Hoffman, Schuckers, and Daniloff (1989) have described a language-based approach to phonological intervention based on client generation of narratives. In this approach, preschool children construct verbal stories in response to pictures depicting commonly occurring childhood experiences and share these with a listener(s). The clinician's primary role in this type of treatment is to engage the child in constructing and talking about the pictures. The goal for each child is to produce meaningful linguistic units, syllable shapes, phonemes, and gestures that are shared with a listener. The clinician seeks to expand each child's language-processing ability by asking children to produce utterances that exceed their then current level of functioning.

Norris and Hoffman (1990) also suggested that language-oriented intervention needs to be naturalistic and interactive as the clinician seeks to simultaneously improve semantic, syntactic, and phonological knowledge. Such interactions need to be based on spontaneously occurring events, utterances and communicative situations that arise in the context of daily play routines, and instructional activities. They outline three steps for intervention by the clinician: (1) providing appropriate organization of the environment/stimulus materials for the child to attend to, which enables the clinician to systematically alter language complexity throughout the course of therapy; (2) provide a communicative opportunity including scaffolding strategies that consist of various types of prompts, questions, information, and restatements that provide support to the child as he or she actively engages in the process of communicating a message; and (3) providing consequences or feedback that is directly related to the effectiveness of the child's communication.

Norris and Hoffman (1990) described an "interactive storytelling" technique in which the clinician points to a picture and models language for the client, then gives the child an opportunity to talk about the event. If the child miscommunicates the idea, the adult provides feedback to the child designed to assist the child in reformulating the message. There are three primary responses which the clinician can use with the child:

1. *Clarification.* When the child's explanation is unclear, inaccurate, or poorly stated, the clinician asks for a clarification. The clinician then supplies relevant information to be incorporated in the child's response, restates the event using a variety of language forms, and asks the child to recommunicate the event. Hoffman, Norris, and Monjure (1990) presented the following example of this type of response: If a child described a picture of a man cooking at a grill by saying, "Him eating," the clinician might say:

> No, that's not what I see happening. The man isn't eating yet, he's cooking the food. See his fork, he is using it to turn the food. I see him—he is cooking the food. He will eat when he's done cooking, but right now the food is cooking on the grill. He is cooking the food so that they can eat (105).

Then the clinician provides an opportunity for the child to restate the information (e.g., ". . . so tell that part of the story again"). Thus, feedback is meaning based rather than structure based.

2. *Adding events.* If the child adequately reports an event, the clinician points out another event to incorporate in the story using a variety of language models. The child is then given the opportunity to retell the story. An example of this from Hoffman, Norris, and Monjure (1990) follows. The clinician points to specific features in the picture and says something like:

> That's right, the man is cooking. He is the dad and he is cooking the hamburgers for lunch. Mom is putting plates on the table. Dad will put the hamburgers on the plates. So you explain the story to the puppet (105).

3. *Increase complexity.* If the child adequately describes a series of events, the clinician seeks to increase the complexity of the child's story by pointing out relationships among events such as motives of the characters, cause–effect relationships among the individual events, time and space relationships, and predictions. The child again is given the opportunity to reformulate his or her own version of the story. Another example from these authors is as follows.

If the child said, "The daddy is cooking hamburgers and the mommy is setting the table," the clinician might prompt the child to link these two events in time and space by saying:

> That's right, the mommy and daddy are making lunch for the family. When daddy finishes cooking the hamburgers he will put them on the plates, so tell that part of the story to the puppet (105).

While the concepts expressed by Hoffman, Schuckers, and Daniloff (1989) and Norris and Hoffman (1990) have appeared relatively recently, they are not totally unlike some of the concepts espoused by Backus and Beasley (1951) several decades ago. Backus and Beasley expressed the need to work from whole to part to whole in a social context (i.e., language discourse to specific components of language back to overall communication). More recently, Low, Newman, and Ravsten (1989) have extended the communication focus of Backus and Beasley by developing what they call a communication centered instruction (CCI) approach to articulation remediation. CCI emphasizes the social use of language with the focus on a speech sound in a word that is part of a socially useful communicative utterance. It should be pointed out that CCI is applicable to other disorders besides those of phonology.

Guidelines that Low, Newman, and Ravsten (1989) developed for planning treatment activities based on this approach are as follows:

1. Teaching activities should simulate the client's daily communication experiences.
2. Activities should encourage clients to use correct phonology to clarify communication in preference to teaching them directly (though requiring responses such as imitation may be included in instruction).
3. Positive group interaction is essential to the approach.
4. To facilitate generalization, practice of target behaviors is repeated in several communication-centered activities, all of which are slightly different.
5. Individual therapy should be viewed as a supplement to group therapy that allows for isolating target sounds and engaging in more traditional phoneme-related instruction. Such traditional instruction should be followed by rehearsing the phonemic behaviors in communicative utterances to be used in subsequent group lessons.

Summary of the Language-Based Approaches.

Background Statement. Language-based approaches are generally based on two basic premises: (1) phonology is a part of the overall language system and should be treated in a language context; and (2) improvement in phonological behaviors occurs more rapidly when instruction is focused on the overall use of language as a tool of communication, rather than on specific aspects of language (syntax, semantics, phonology).

Unique Features. Unique features of this approach relate to the heavy emphasis on facilitating overall language improvement as opposed to correction of specific phonemes. The instructional style is different than the traditional practice of working directly on phonology.

Strengths and Limitations. From a theoretical perspective the rationale behind this approach is attractive. It remains to be seen, however, just how and with which clients this approach can be beneficial. The role of traditional phonological intervention in conjunction with this approach has not been adequately explored.

Research Support. Preliminary data from Hoffman, Norris, and Monjure (1990) suggested that a whole language approach was a more efficacious approach to language–phonology intervention than was phonological intervention by itself. In their study, treatment focusing on cluster simplifications was successful in reducing the presence of the process; however, language-based therapy not only improved clusters but also resulted in improvement of other language behaviors.

REMEDIATION GUIDELINES FOR COGNITIVE-LINGUISTIC APPROACHES

1. A cognitive-linguistic approach is recommended when there are multiple sound errors that reflect phonological error patterns.
2. A cognitive-linguistic approach is also recommended when there are few errors but the errors reflect a single phonological rule.
3. Once error patterns have been identified, a review of the child's phonetic inventory will assist in the identification of target sounds (exemplars) and key

Remediation Systems and Approaches

words. This review should include such factors as facilitative contexts, word-position, stimulability, frequency of occurrence, and developmental occurrence.

4. Selection of training words should reflect the syllabic word shapes the child uses. For example, if the child uses only CV and CVCV syllable shapes, multisyllabic target words are inappropriate. Obviously this guideline is not appropriate, however, if the focus of remediation is the unstressed syllable deletion process or other processes focusing on syllable structure simplifications.

5. Treatment efficiency may be increased by selecting target words that facilitate the reduction of two or more processes simultaneously. For example, if a child uses stopping and deletes final fricatives, the selection of a final fricative for training may aid in the simultaneous reduction of the processes of stopping and final consonant deletions.

6. When phonological errors reflect errors in several sound classes (e.g., final consonant deletion may affect stops, fricatives, and nasals), at least one exemplar should be selected for training from each sound class.

7. Instruction related to process reduction should focus on deletion of the process rather than the phonetic accuracy of sounds used in reorganizing the phonological system. For example, if a child deletes final consonants but learns to say [dɔd] for [dɔg], the /d/ for /g/ replacement should be overlooked at the *initial* stage of instruction because the child has begun to change his or her phonological system to incorporate final consonant productions.

8. When using a cognitive-linguistic approach to remediation, the clinician probably will need to devise specific treatment protocols and procedures since few complete remediation programs based on this approach have been published.

9. Minimal contrast therapy, focusing on both perception and production, is recommended as part of a remediation program when phonemic contrasts are collapsed.

10. Treatment focused on other aspects of language frequently results in positive changes in phonology. For example, working on plural and morphological endings may reduce the deletion of final consonants.

11. Teaching behaviors from a cognitive-linguistic perspective may be quite similar to certain methods used in more traditional approaches.

12. Correction of phonological errors based on treatment of overall language behavior is still in an experimental period.

REFERENCES

Backus, O., and J. Beasley, *Speech Therapy with Children.* Boston: Houghton Mifflin, 1951.

Baker, R.D., and B.P. Ryan, *Programmed Conditioning for Articulation.* Monterey, Calif.: Monterey Learning Systems, 1971.

Blache, S., "A distinctive feature approach." In N. Creaghead, P. Newman, and W. Secord (Eds.), *Assessment and Remediation of Articulatory and Phonological Disorders.* Columbus, Ohio: Charles E. Merrill, 1989.

Black, L., "So you want to dismiss 80% of your caseload." Paper presented at the 1972 North Carolina Special Education Conference, Raleigh, N.C., 1972.

Bradley, D., "A systematic multiple-phoneme approach." In N. Creaghead, P. Newman, and W. Secord (Eds.), *Assessment and Remediation of Articulatory and Phonological Disorders.* Columbus, Ohio: Charles E. Merrill, 1989.

Camarata, S., and R. Schwartz, "Production of object words and action words: Evidence for a relationship between phonology and semantics." *Journal of Speech and Hearing Research, 26* (1985): 50–53.

Costello, J., and J. Onstein, "The modification of multiple articulation errors based on distinctive feature theory." *Journal of Speech and Hearing Disorders, 41* (1976): 199–215.

Elbert, M., and J. Gierut, *Handbook of Clinical Phonology Approaches to Assessment and Treatment.* San Diego: College-Hill Press, 1986.

Elbert, M., B. Rockman, and D. Saltzman, *Contrasts: The Use of Minimal Pairs in Articulation Training.* Austin, Tex.: Exceptional Resources, Inc., 1980.

Ferrier, L., and M. Davis, "A lexical approach to the remediation of final sound omission." *Journal of Speech and Hearing Disorders, 38* (1973): 126–130.

Fey, M., *Language Intervention with Young Children.* San Diego: College-Hill Press, 1986.

Gierut, J., "Maximal opposition approach to phonological treatment." *Journal of Speech and Hearing Disorders, 54* (1989): 9–19.

Gray, B., "A field study on programmed articulation therapy." *Language, Speech, and Hearing Services in the Schools, 5* (1974): 119–131.

Gray, B., and B. Ryan, *A Language Program for the Nonlanguage Child.* Champaign, Ill.: Research Press, 1973.

Hodson, B., "Phonological remediation: A cycles approach." In N. Creaghead, P. Newman, and W. Secord (Eds.), *Assessment and Remediation of Articulatory and Phonological Disorders.* Columbus, Ohio: Charles E. Merrill, 1989.

Hodson, B., and E. Paden, *Targeting Intelligible Speech.* Austin, Tex.: PRO-Ed, 1991.

Hoffman, P., J. Norris, and J. Monjure, "Comparison of process targeting and whole language treatments for phonologically delayed preschool children." *Language, Speech, and Hearing Services in Schools, 21* (1990): 102–109.

Hoffman, P., G. Schuckers, and R. Daniloff, *Children's Phonetic Disorders: Theory and Treatment.* Boston: Little, Brown, 1989.

Ingram, D., "Explanation and phonological remediation." *Child Language Teaching and Therapy, 2* (1986): 1–19.

Ingram, D., *Phonological Disability in Children.* London: Cole and Whurr, 1989.

Irwin, J.V., and A.J. Weston, *A Manual for the Clinical Utilization of the Paired-Stimuli Technique.* Memphis, Tenn.: National Education Services, 1971.

Irwin, J.V., and A.J. Weston, "The paired-stimuli monograph." *Acta Symbolica, 6* (1975): 1–76.

La Riviere, C., H. Winitz, J. Reeds, and E. Herriman, "The conceptual reality of selected distinctive features." *Journal of Speech and Hearing Research, 17* (1974): 122–133.

Low, G., P. Newman, and M. Ravsten, "Pragmatic considerations in treatment: Communication centered instruction." In N. Creaghead, P. Newman, and W. Secord (Eds.), *Assessment and Remediation of Articulatory and Phonological Disorders.* Columbus, Ohio: Charles E. Merrill, 1989.

McCabe, R., and D. Bradley, "Systematic multiple phonemic approach to articulation therapy." *Acta Symbolica, 6* (1975): 1–18.

McDonald, E.T., *Articulation Testing and Treatment: A Sensory Motor Approach.* Pittsburgh: Stanwix House, 1964.

McReynolds, L.V., and S. Bennett, "Distinctive feature generalization in articulation training." *Journal of Speech and Hearing Disorders, 37* (1972): 462–470.

McReynolds, L.V., and D. Engmann, *Distinctive Feature Analysis of Misarticulations.* Baltimore: University Park Press, 1975.

Matheny, N., and J. Panagos, "Comparing the effects of articulation and syntax programs on syntax and articulation improvement." *Language, Speech, and Hearing Services in Schools, 9* (1978): 57–61.

Norris, J., and P. Hoffman, "Language intervention within naturalistic environments." *Language, Speech, and Hearing Services in Schools, 2* (1990): 72–84.

Panagos, J., and P. Prelock, "Phonological constraints on the sentence productions of language-disordered children." *Journal of Speech and Hearing Research, 24* (1982): 171–177.

Ruscello, D., "Motor learning as a model for articulation instruction." In J. Costello (Ed.), *Speech Disorders in Children.* San Diego: College-Hill Press, 1984.

Ruscello, D., and R. Shelton, "Planning and self-assessment in articulatory training." *Journal of Speech and Hearing Disorders, 44* (1979): 504–512.

Secord, W., "The traditional approach to treatment." In N. Creaghead, P. Newman, and W. Secord (Eds.), *Assessment and Remediation of Articulatory and Phonological Disorders.* Columbus, Ohio: Charles E. Merrill, 1989.

Stoel-Gammon, C., and C. Dunn, *Normal and Disordered Phonology in Children.* Baltimore: University Park Press, 1985.

Van Denmark, D., and M. Hardin, "Effectiveness of intensive articulation therapy for children with cleft palate." *Cleft Palate Journal, 23* (1986): 215–224.

Van Riper, C., *Speech Correction: Principles and Methods.* Englewood Cliffs, N.J.: Prentice Hall, 1939.

Van Riper, C., *Speech Correction: Principles and Methods,* 6th ed. Englewood Cliffs, N.J.: Prentice Hall, 1978.

Van Riper, C., and L. Emerick, *Speech Correction: An Introduction to Speech Pathology and Audiology.* Englewood Cliffs, N.J.: Prentice Hall, 1984.

Weiner, F., "Treatment of phonological disability using the method of meaningful minimal contrast: Two case studies." *Journal of Speech and Hearing Disorders, 46* (1981): 97–103.

Weiner, F., and N. Bankson, "Teaching features." *Language, Speech, and Hearing Services in Schools, 9* (1978): 29–34.

Weston, A.J., and J.V. Irwin, "Use of paired-stimuli in modification of articulation." *Perceptual and Motor Skills,* *32* (1971): 947–957.

Winitz, H., *From Syllable to Conversation.* Baltimore: University Park Press, 1975.

Winitz, H., and L. Preisler, "Effect of distinctive feature pretraining in phoneme discrimination learning." *Journal of Speech and Hearing Research, 10* (1967): 515–530.

Appendix

Procedures for Teaching Sounds

SPECIFIC INSTRUCTIONAL TECHNIQUES

As a supplement to the establishment procedures presented in Chapter 9, the following methods for teaching sounds are presented. Clinicians must be familiar not only with general approaches to establishment of phonemes but also with specific suggestions for teaching sounds. Sources such as Nemoy and Davis (1954) may be consulted for a more extensive list of ideas regarding phonetic placement and successive approximation approaches to sound teaching; however, the material presented on the following pages represents a potpourri of ideas that may be helpful to those who are beginning to develop a repertoire of techniques for evoking and establishing consonant sounds frequently in error. Clinicians who need word lists or drill material are referred to *Articulation Therapy and Consonant Drill Book* by Goda (1970), *Voice and Articulation Drill Book* by Fairbanks (1960), *Better Speech and Better Reading* by Schoolfield (1951), *Phonetic Context Drillbook* by Griffith and Miner (1979), and *Contrasts: The Use of Minimal Pairs in Articulation Training* by Elbert, Rockman, and Saltzman (1980).

INSTRUCTIONS FOR CORRECTION OF AN INTERDENTAL LISP

It is important to remember that /s/ may be taught by having the client place his or her tongue behind either the upper teeth or the lower teeth (usually preferred).

1. Instruct the client to protrude the tongue between the teeth and produce a /θ/, and then push the tip of his or her tongue inward with a thin instrument, such as a tongue blade. As a variation, instruct the client to slowly and gradually withdraw the tongue while saying /θ/ and, while still attempting to make /θ/, scrape the tongue tip along the back of the front teeth and upward.

2. Instruct the client to produce /t/ in a word like *tea*. Have him or her pronounce it with a strong aspiration after release of the /t/ prior to the vowel. Instruct the client to slowly slide the tip of the tongue backward from the alveolar ridge following a prolonged release. The result should be [ts]. Then prolong the [s] portion of [ts].

3. Instruct the client to say the following word-pairs, pointing out that the tongue is in a similar position for /t/ and /s/.

tea–sea	*teal–seal*	*tell–sell*	*told–sold*	*tame–same*	*tip–sip*
top–sop	*tight–sight*	*too–Sue*	*tub–sub*	*turf–surf*	*till–sill*

4. Instruct the client to open his or her mouth, put the tongue in position for /t/, drop the tip of the tongue slightly, and send the air stream through the passage. The client can sometimes feel the emission of air by placing a finger in front of his or her mouth.

5. Instruct the client to produce /ʃ/ and then retract his or her lips (smile) and push the tongue slightly forward.

6. Instruct the client to say /i/ and blow through the teeth to produce /s/.

7. Insert a straw in the groove of the tongue and have the client blow to produce /s/.

8. If the client can make a correct /z/, take a word such as *zero* and ask him or her to listen carefully and to feel where the tongue is when whispering the word, prolonging the first sound. This sound can then become the client's model.

9. Instruct the client to use the following phonetic placement cues:
   a. Raise the tongue so that the sides are firmly in contact with the inner surface of the upper back teeth.
   b. Groove the tongue slightly along the midline.
   c. Place the tip of the tongue about a quarter of an inch behind the upper teeth.
   d. Bring the teeth together.
   e. Direct the air stream along the groove of the tongue toward the cutting edges of the lower teeth.

INSTRUCTIONS FOR CORRECTION OF A LATERAL LISP

1. Position a straw so that it protrudes from the side of the mouth. When a lateral [s] is made, the straw should resonate on the side of the mouth where the air stream is directed. When the straw is inserted into the front of the mouth and a correct /s/ is made, the straw will resonate in the front of the mouth.

2. Direct attention to a central emission of the air stream by holding a feather, a strip of paper, or a finger in front of the center of the mouth, or have the client tap the incisor gently with his or her forefinger while [s] is being produced. If the sound is being emitted through a central aperture, a break in continuity of the outflow of the breath will be noted. If the sound is being emitted laterally, no break in the continuity of the air stream will be noted. An awareness of central aperture may also be developed by instructing the client to inhale air and directing his or her attention to the cool sensation from the intake of air. Then instruct the client to exhale the air through the same aperture by which air entered upon inhalation.

3. Instruct the client to put a tongue blade down the midline of the tongue in order to establish a groove for the air stream.

4. Instruct the client to retract the lips sharply and push the tongue forward, attempting to say /s/.

5. Instruct the client to make /t/, holding the release position for a relatively long time, then retract the lips and drop the jaw slightly. A [ts] should be heard if

grooving was maintained properly. Then, extend the duration of the [ts], gradually decreasing the release phase of [t] until /s/ is approximated.

INSTRUCTIONS FOR PRODUCTION OF THE /ɝ/

1. Instruct the client to growl like a tiger (grrr), crow like a rooster (r-rr-rr) or sound like a race car (rrrr).
2. Instruct the client to lower the jaw, say /l/ and push the tongue back until [ɝ] is produced. One can also move from [n] to [nɝ] or [d] to [dɝ].
3. Instruct the client to produce /l/. Then, using a tongue blade, gently push the tip of the tongue back until the depressor can be inserted between the tongue tip and teeth ridge so that an /ɝ/ is produced.
4. Instruct the client to imitate a trilled tongue plus /ɝ/ sound with the tongue tip on the alveolar ridge. Stop the trill but continue producing /ɝ/.
5. Instruct the client to produce /a/ as in the word *father*. As he or she produces the [a], instruct him or her to raise the tongue tip and blade, arching the tongue toward the palate but not touching the palate.
6. Instruct the client to produce /i/ and then lift and retract the tongue tip to produce /ɝ/.
7. Instruct the client to place the tongue lightly between the incisors as in /θ/ and then retract the tip quickly into the /ɝ/. Instruct the client to keep the tip of the tongue near the alveolar ridge to avoid the intrusion of a vowel sound.
8. Instruct the client to say /z/ and to continue to do so while dropping the jaw and saying /ɝ/.
9. Instruct the client to position the tongue for /d/ and then retract it slightly, at the same time dropping the tongue tip and saying /ɝ/. Other clusters such as /tr/, /θr/, and /gr/ may also be used.
10. Spread the sides of the child's mouth with his or her finger, then ask him or her to produce a prolonged /n/ and then curl the tongue backward, continuing to make the sound.
11. Contrast pairs of words beginning with /w/ and /r/. This task may make the distinction between these two sounds more obvious for the client who substitutes /w/ for /r/.
    Practice word-pairs might include:

wipe–ripe	*wan–ran*	*woo–rue*	*wing–ring*	*way–ray*	*wake–rake*
wag–rag	*wail–rail*	*woe–roe*	*weep–reap*	*wed–red*	

INSTRUCTIONS FOR PRODUCTION OF /l/

1. Instruct the client to produce /l/ with the mouth open in front of a mirror.
2. Instruct the client to position the tongue for /l/ and then lower it to produce /a/. Alternate these movements. The result should be [la], [la], [la]. This procedure can be varied by using /i/ and /u/ instead of /a/.
3. Instruct the client to imitate the clinician's singing of the nonsense syllables [leɪ], [li], [laɪ].
4. Using a lollipop, peanut butter, or tongue blade, touch the place on the client's alveolar ridge where the tongue tip makes contact to produce a correct /l/. Then tell the client to place the tongue at that point and say /l/.
5. Instruct the client to pretend that the tongue is one part of a bird's beak and the roof of the mouth is the other part of the beak. Tell him or her to put the tongue directly behind the teeth and move it up and down quickly, as a bird's beak might move when it is chirping, and say /a/.

Procedures for Teaching Sounds

Instructions for Production of /f/ and /v/

1. Instruct the client to touch the lower lip with the upper front teeth, and blow. The breath stream may be directed by placing a feather or strip of paper in front of his or her mouth while /f/ or /v/ is being produced.
2. Instruct the client to say [a], place the lower lip under the edge of the upper teeth, and blow the breath stream between the lip and teeth so that frication is audible.

Instructions for Production of /k/ and /g/

1. Press underneath the posterior portion of the child's chin and ask him or her to say [kʌ] in a whisper as the pressure is suddenly released.
2. Hold the tongue tip behind the lower teeth, using a tongue blade if necessary. Instruct the client to hump the back of the tongue and build up oral pressure. The tongue contact should be released quickly, thus releasing the pressure built up behind the constriction.
3. Instruct the client to imitate the clinician as the clinician pretends to shoot a gun, producing a lingua-fricative, as in [ka].
4. Instruct the client to alternate the raising of the back and front of the tongue in a rocking movement from [k] to [t].

Instructions for Production of /t/ and /d/

1. Instruct the client to press the tongue tip firmly against the upper dental ridge in front of a mirror. Then have him or her quickly lower the tongue; air pressure will be released, producing approximations of /t/ or /d/.
2. Instruct the client to make a /p/. Then ask him or her to place the tongue tip between the lips and again to try to say /p/. This gives the tactual sensation of a stop made with the tip of the tongue but is not the correct position for /t/ or /d/. Finally, instruct the client to make a similar sound with the tongue tip in contact with the upper lip only. Repeat with the tongue tip touching the alveolar ridge.

REFERENCES

Elbert, M., B. Rockman, and D. Saltzman, *Contrasts: The Use of Minimal Pairs in Articulation Training*. Austin, Tex.: Exceptional Resources, Inc., 1980.

Fairbanks, G., *Voice and Articulation Drill Book*, New York: Harper & Row, 1960.

Goda, S., *Articulation Therapy and Consonant Drill Book*. New York: Grune and Stratton, 1970.

Griffith, J., and L.E. Miner, *Phonetic Context Drillbook*. Englewood Cliffs, N.J.: Prentice Hall, 1979.

Nemoy, E.M., and S.F. Davis, *The Correction of Defective Consonant Sounds*. Magnolia, Mass.: Expression Company, 1954.

Schoolfield, L.D., *Better Speech and Better Reading*. Magnolia, Mass.: Expression Company, 1951.

Author Index

Edwards, M.L., 67, 96, 122, 241, 242, 244, 274, 275, 331
Eguchi, S., 60
Ehri, L.C., 139, 142
Eilers, R.E., 63, 73, 75, 78, 92, 123, 173
Eimas, P., 71, 170
Ekelman, B., 210
Elbers, L., 79
Elbert, M., 69, 79, 90, 184, 232, 236, 237, 239, 241, 268, 271, 279, 283, 318, 324, 325, 326, 328, 331, 335, 336, 338, 339, 351, 353, 388, 389, 390, 402
Elliott, L.L., 132, 134
Ellis, D., 235
Emerick, L., 232, 316, 319, 326, 361, 362, 365
Engel, D.C., 330
Engmann, D., 270, 384
Erickson, R., 225
Evan, K.E., 132
Everhart, R., 205, 209, 210
Ewanowski, S., 184

F

Fairbanks, G., 177, 179, 345, 402
Faircloth, M., 231
Faircloth, S., 231
Farquhar, M.S., 235, 236
Farwell, C.B., 65, 68, 91, 102, 103
Fee, J., 119
Fenton, A., 205
Ferguson, C.A., 64, 65, 67, 68, 69, 70, 79, 83, 85, 86, 90, 91, 93, 103, 114, 115, 119, 122, 138
Fernald, A., 73
Ferrier, L., 393
Fey, M.E., 123, 204, 290, 351, 396
Fichter, G.R., 205, 331, 353
Fisher, H.B., 230, 240, 268, 269
Fitzsimons, R., 205
Fletcher, S., 179, 188, 190
Fluharty, N., 226
Flynn, P., 206
Folger, M.K., 119, 204, 212, 230
Footo, M.M., 120, 168, 275
Forner, L.L., 59, 60
Foster, D., 270
Fowlow, P.J., 81
Francescato, G., 63
Franklin, M.B., 86
Frauenfelder, U.H., 131
Freebairn-Farr, L., 206
Freilinger, J.J., 115, 208, 263
Frick, J., 174, 316
Fristoe, R., 251
Fry, D.B., 37, 68
Fucci, D., 184
Fudala, J., 260
Fundrella, D., 235, 353
Furbee, C., 205, 210
Furlong, A.K., 331, 353
Furr, M., 163

G

Gaines, F., 179
Gallagher, R., 231
Gammon, S., 185
Gandour, J., 55, 123
Garnica, O.K., 64, 96, 97
Garrett, R., 171
Gavin, W., 73
Geith, A., 171
Gerber, A.J., 235, 327, 345, 353
Gierut, J.A., 232, 279, 282, 283, 284, 328, 331, 351, 382, 388, 391, 393
Gilbert, J.H.V., 84, 123, 129, 136, 137
Giles, S.B., 27
Goda, S., 402
Goldman, R., 171, 251
Goldsmith, J.A., 55
Goldstein, B., 156, 157
Gonzalez, A., 155, 156
Goodban, M.J., 112, 113
Goodsitt, J., 59
Goodstein, L., 214
Gottsleben, R., 199, 200
Graham, L.W., 97
Grahamjones, F., 198
Gray, B., 331, 373, 396
Green, E., 177
Greenlee, M., 94, 117, 118, 120, 121, 122, 125, 127, 128, 129, 133, 317
Griffith, J., 402
Grosjean, F., 131
Gross, G., 202
Groth, L.R., 330
Grunwell, P., 67, 117, 120, 230, 253, 275, 277, 301, 302
Gutierrez-Clellen, V., 155
Guyette, R., 197

H

Hadden, W.B., 196
Haelsig, P.C., 120
Haley, V., 235
Hall, M., 171, 205, 209
Halle, M., 17, 31, 54, 55, 138
Halle, P.A., 69, 89
Halliday, M.A.K., 85, 86
Hammer, M.A., 132
Hand, L., 115, 208, 263
Hansen, B., 171
Hanson, B., 280
Hanson, M.L., 189, 191
Hardcastle, W.J., 49
Hardin, M., 368
Hardy, J.C., 186, 231, 320
Harrington, J., 234
Hatten, J., 232
Hawk, A., 180, 181, 182
Hawkins, S., 137
Hayes, B., 55

Haynes, S., 195, 198
Hedrick, D., 112, 113, 114, 124, 262, 264
Henderson, F.W., 168
Herriman, E., 317, 389
Higgins, R., 234
Hillis, J.A., 184
Hilton, L., 191
Hirsh, I.J., 60
Hixon, T.J., 34, 60
Hoard, J.E., 50, 52, 53
Hockett, C.F., 38
Hodson, B.W., 122, 135, 158, 167, 270, 275, 276, 290, 299, 300, 332, 352, 393, 394
Hoffman, K., 242, 245
Hoffman, P.R., 173, 204, 207, 231, 265, 278, 376, 396, 397, 398
Holland, A., 175, 176
Holloway, M., 201, 204
Hood, L., 129
Horan, E.A., 60
Horii, Y., 186
House, A.S., 97, 184
House, H., 185, 186
Householder, F.W., 72
Howard, B.H., 128
Hull, F., 202, 209
Hulme, C., 136
Humphrey, K., 84
Huntington, D.A., 123, 316
Hustedde, C.G., 59
Hutton, S., 270
Hyman, L.M., 50

I

Iglesias, A., 155
Ingham, J.C., 176, 330
Ingham, R., 197
Ingram, D., 52, 67, 112, 116, 117, 119, 122, 123, 227, 230, 234, 270, 305, 306, 308, 360, 392, 395
Ingram, T., 275
Irwin, J.V., 324, 378, 379, 381
Irwin, R., 174, 236
Itoh, M., 195

J

Jackson, E., 320
Jaeger, J.J., 138, 139
Jaffe, M., 197
Jakimik, J., 132
Jakobson, R., 64, 65, 114
Jann, G., 190
Jann, H., 190
Jenkins, E., 187
Jimenez, B.C., 155
Johns, D., 182, 195, 196
Johnson, A.F., 163, 174, 176, 186, 317, 332
Johnson, C.E., 137
Jones, B., 167
Jong, K.J. de, 37

Jordan, E.P., 231
Jordan, L., 186
Jusczyk, P.W., 59, 71, 74, 75, 170

K

Kamhi, A.G., 128
Kantner, C.E., 27
Karzon, R.B., 73
Keappock, N., 334
Kearns, K.P., 344
Kenney, K., 209
Kent, R.D., 37, 40, 42, 49, 54, 59, 60, 68, 70, 76, 77, 78, 79, 80, 81, 86, 87, 88, 238
Kern, C., 112, 113, 114, 124, 262, 264
Keyser, S.J., 55
Khan, L.M., 262, 266, 270, 276, 277
Kim, C., 185
Kiparsky, P., 65
Kisatsky, T., 235, 236
Klatt, D.H., 58
Kleffner, F., 285
Klein, H., 118, 128, 129
Klich, R., 202, 203
Koch, H., 212
Koch, M.A., 168
Koegel, L.K., 176, 330
Koegel, R.L., 176, 330
Kronvall, E., 171
Kuhl, P.K., 72
Kutz, K., 174
Kwiatkowski, J., 125, 167, 227, 231, 242, 245, 258, 260, 266, 270, 276, 280, 281, 302, 306, 327, 348, 354, 355

L

Ladefoged, P., 23, 29, 33
Landahl, K., 129
Landberg, I., 76, 86
Lapko, L., 174
Lapointe, L., 195
La Riviere, C., 317, 389
La Voie, L., 63
Lawrence, A., 136
Lehiste, I., 38
Leiss, R.II., 235, 353
Leonard, L.B., 84, 91, 119, 204, 212, 230, 336
Leopold, W.F., 68, 117, 121, 204, 212
Lerea, L., 213
Levitt, A.G., 89
Levitt, H., 34, 165
Lewis, B., 206, 210
Lewis, M.M., 83
Lewis, N.P., 262, 270, 276, 277
Li, K., 186
Liberman, I., 206
Liebergott, J., 59
Lieberman, P., 38, 79, 80
Lightbown, P., 129
Lindblom, B.E.F., 35, 36, 58, 69, 70

P

Paden, E.P., 122, 135, 167, 275, 332, 352, 393, 394
Pagan, F., 290
Paletta, R., 181
Palmer, J., 190
Panagos, J., 202, 203, 204, 396
Parker, F., 32, 270
Parlour, S., 210, 214
Parnell, M., 282
Patterson, J., 200
Paul, R., 204
Payne, A.C., 141, 142
Payne, K.T., 157
Paynter, W., 234
Pearson, D., 68
Pegg, J.E., 84
Peizer, D.B., 67, 119
Pendergast, K., 128, 171
Perfetti, C.A., 132, 133, 134, 135
Perkell, J.S., 54
Perkins, W., 209, 212
Peters, A., 129
Picheny, M.A., 35
Picknell, K., 182
Pieczuro, A., 195
Pilberg, M., 174
Poizat, M., 81
Pollack, E., 236, 237
Pollack, K., 240, 311
Pollio, H., 201
Pond, R., 226
Poole, E., 112
Poplack, S., 151, 153
Powell, J., 324, 328
Powell, T.W., 268, 326
Powers, M.J., 212, 316, 353, 354
Prather, E., 112, 113, 114, 124, 209, 262, 263, 264
Preisler, L., 363
Preisser, D.A., 122, 275
Prelock, P., 203, 204, 396
Priestly, T.M.S., 67
Prins, D., 163, 171, 187, 210
Proffit, W.R., 189, 190
Prosek, R., 186
Purves, B.A., 129, 136, 137
Pye, C., 290

Q

Quine, M., 203

R

Rabiner, L., 34
Raeburn, V.P., 60
Ramer, A.L.H., 86, 91
Ramirez-Diaz, M., 157
Rasmus, B., 171
Ratusnik, D., 231
Ravsten, M., 397, 398

Read, C., 37
Reeds, J., 317, 389
Rees, N., 236, 237
Reid, G., 171, 187, 198
Reinhart, R., 199, 200
Revucky, M., 235
Rhodes, F.H., 331, 353
Riley, K., 270
Ringel, R., 184, 185, 186
Robb, M.P., 89
Roberts, J.E., 120, 168, 275
Rockman, B.K., 253, 318, 389, 390, 402
Roe, V., 208, 209, 232
Rose, M., 188
Rosenbek, J., 196
Rosenberg, A., 34
Rosenthal, J., 197
Rosin, M., 200, 201
Roug, L., 76
Roug-Hellichius, L.L., 86
Ruscello, D.M., 186, 202, 325, 361
Ryan, B.P., 370, 373, 396

S

Sagart, L., 63, 69, 81
Sagey, E., 55
Sakuda, M., 46
Saltzman, D., 318, 389, 390, 402
Salyer, K., 182
Sander, E., 113, 124, 262, 263, 264
Sasanuma, S., 195
Saunders, Z.G., 331, 353
Savin, H.B., 317
Sax, M., 112
Saxman, J.H., 89, 202, 241, 331
Sayler, H., 208
Scarborough-Franks, L., 139, 140
Schaeffer, M.H., 353
Schlanger, B., 199, 200
Schmauch, V., 202
Schmitt, J.F., 128
Schmitt, L.S., 128
Schoolfield, L.D., 402
Schreiber, P.A., 37
Schuckers, G.H., 231, 278, 376, 396, 397
Schultz, M., 59
Schutz, R., 175, 331
Schwartz, A., 171
Schwartz, R.G., 55, 84, 91, 119, 204, 212, 230, 396
Scott, C., 184, 185
Scripture, M.K., 320
Secord, W., 239, 364, 365
Selmar, T., 128
Seymour, C.M., 150, 157
Seymour, H.N., 150, 157
Shankweiler, D., 206
Shelton, R.L., 163, 174, 176, 184, 186, 189, 228,
    239, 278, 317, 324, 332, 333, 338, 353, 361
Sherman, D., 171
Shibamoto, J.S., 91

Shore, C., 85
Shoup, J., 280
Shriberg, L.D., 67, 125, 167, 199, 200, 204, 227,
    231, 242, 258, 260, 266, 270, 276, 280, 281, 290,
    302, 306, 310, 321, 327, 348, 354, 355
Shriner, T., 201, 204, 231
Shuy, R.W., 148
Shvachkin, N.K.H., 96, 97
Siegel, R., 234
Silber, R., 68
Silverman, E., 286
Simmons, H., 65
Simon, T., 73
Siqueland, E., 71, 170
Sistrunk, D., 199, 200
Skelly, M., 181
Sloat, C., 50, 52, 53
Slobin, D.I., 103, 140
Smit, A.B., 96, 112, 113, 114, 115, 123, 208, 209,
    210, 240, 263, 265, 331
Smith, A.J., 167
Smith, B.L., 59, 79, 123, 136, 156, 199, 278
Smith, C., 169
Smith, M.W., 234
Smith, N.V., 66, 70, 98
Smith, P., 185
Smith, R., 235
Snow, J., 234, 236
Snow, K., 112, 114, 178
Snyder, L., 129
Soder, A., 128
Solomon, A., 213
Somers, R.K., 199, 200, 205, 235, 236, 335,
    353
Sonderman, J., 175, 176
Spector, D., 181
Spencer, A., 55
Spriestersbach, D., 172, 214
St. Louis, K., 202
Stager, S., 175
Stampe, D., 52, 54, 66, 68, 70, 270
Stark, R.E., 76, 77
Starr, C., 178
Steiner, V., 226
Stelcik, J., 174
Stephens, M.I., 265
Stewart, W.A., 149
Stick, S., 334
Stockman, I., 225
Stoel, C., 63
Stoel-Gammon, C., 64, 78, 79, 88, 91, 123, 125,
    199, 200, 227, 258, 266, 267, 275, 383
Stokes, T.F., 323
Straf, M., 140
Straight, H.S., 101
Strange, W., 99, 173
Streeter, L.A., 74
Streit, H., 209
Stromberg, H., 165
Subtelny, J., 46, 178, 191
Sufit, R.L., 49

Swartzlander, P., 268, 326, 327
Swift, E., 200

T

t'Hart, J., 37
Tabor, T., 180
Taylor, O.L., 157, 159
Taylor, S.H., 50, 52, 53
Tees, R.C., 84
Templeton, S., 139, 140
Templin, M.C., 112, 113, 114, 115, 139, 140, 174,
    209, 211, 225, 232, 243, 240, 262, 263
Terrell, F., 148
Terrell, S.L., 148
Terrell, T.D., 153
Thevenin, D.M., 63
Thompson, A.E., 60
Thompson, E., 59
Thomson, N., 136
Tiffany, W., 188
Tikofsky, R.S., 97
Timmons, R., 209
Tingley, B.M., 60
Tomkins, E.R., 353
Towne, R., 197
Travis, L., 171
Trehub, S.E., 59, 73, 84
Trombetta, M., 236
Turton, L.J., 236, 263, 339
Tyler, A., 202, 204, 241, 331
Tyler, L.K., 131, 133

V

VanDemark, A., 201
Van Denmark, D., 368
Van Hattum, R.J., 352, 353
Van Riper, C., 225, 265, 316, 318, 326, 361, 362,
    365, 391
Van Voy, K., 176, 330
Veach, S., 112, 122
Veatch, J., 171
Velleman, S.L., 173
Ver Hoeve, J., 59
Vetter, D.K., 200
Vignolo, L., 195
Vigorito, J., 71, 170
Vihman, M.M., 63, 65, 68, 69, 79, 81, 84, 85, 86,
    87, 88, 89, 90, 91, 92, 101, 110, 116, 117, 118,
    120, 121, 122, 125, 127, 128, 129, 130, 135, 141
Vincent-Smith, L., 98

W

Wallach, H., 150, 151
Walley, A.C., 134, 135
Walsh, H., 32, 270
Wang, Q., 89
Ward, B., 213
Ward, M., 190

Waterson, J., 67, 68, 70, 102
Watterson, K., 202, 204
Weaver, C., 205, 210
Webster, B., 112, 122
Weeks, T.A., 67, 119
Weinberg, B., 182, 184
Weiner, F.F., 270, 274, 276, 282, 290, 318, 326, 328, 382, 384, 388, 389, 393
Weiner, P., 172
Weismer, G., 241, 331
Wellman, B.L., 112, 113, 124, 212
Wepman, J. 251
Werker, J.F., 84
Wertz, R., 195, 196
West, J., 236
West, R., 27
Weston, A.J., 324, 378, 379, 381
Whalen, D.H., 89
Whitaker, J., 201
Wickwire, N., 180, 247, 248, 250
Widder, C., 199, 200
Wilcox, M.J., 119, 204, 212, 230
Wildgen, P., 200
Wilhelm, C.L., 186
Willeford, J., 209
Williams, A.L., 331
Williams, F., 285
Williams, G., 164, 176, 197, 317
Williams, R., 197

Williams, R.L., 149
Willis, V., 186, 332
Wilson, D., 154
Wilson, F., 199
Wilson, W.R., 74
Winitz, H., 163, 164, 172, 188, 199, 209, 210, 212, 232, 234, 236, 250, 252, 253, 263, 316, 317, 318, 326, 335, 338, 363, 389, 391
Winner, M., 339
Wise, C.M., 27, 159
Wittstruch, M.L., 334
Wolfe, V., 174
Wood, K., 213
Woodcock, R., 251
Woolf, G., 174
Wornall, A., 182
Worth, J., 46
Wright, V., 228
Wynne, M., 311

Y

Yoss, K., 197

Z

Zetterstrom, R., 58
Zimmerman, I., 226
Zlatin, M., 77

Subject Index

A

D

Deaffrication, 273
Deep Test of Articulation, 173–74, 239, 334, 339, 379
Deep testing, 339, 379
Denasalization, 273
Dentition, 170–79, 190, 247–48
Developmental norms, 112–15, 275, 277
Devoicing of final consonants, 30, 123, 272, 275
Diacritics, 242–44
Diadochokinesis, 187–88, 250
Dialectical considerations, 285
Dialects (*see* Nonstandard English dialects; Black English vernacular; Spanish-influenced dialects)
Diphthongs, 16–17, 54
Discrimination (*see* Speech sound discrimination)
Dismissal, 333–37
Distinctive features:
  analysis, 268–70
  classification and description, 17–20, 31–32
  definition, 17
  dismissal, 336
  remediation, 382–88
Distortions, 2, 166, 195, 241
Documentation, 299
Dysarthria, 194
Dyspraxia, 196–98

E

Ear training (*see* Speech sound discrimination)
Elicitation, 289
Epenthesis, 54, 272, 275
Error(s):
  analysis of, 265–68
  categories, 1–2, 166, 241
Establishment phase, 314, 316–23
Etiology (*see* Articulation, related factors)

F

Facilitating contexts, 38–44, 319–20
Feedback, 48–50, 183–87
Final consonant deletion, 117–18, 271, 275
First words, 85
Fisher-Logemann Test of Articulation, 268
Fluharty Speech and Language Screening Test, 226
Frenum, 179, 250
Fricatives, 21–23, 44–48, 371
  acquisition, 114, 122–23, 264
Frontal lisp, 189
Fronting, 116, 121–22, 273, 275, 307
Functional relationship, 341–44
  A-B-A design, 342

G

Generalization, 315, 323–33
  across context generalization, 325–26

across linguistic unit generalization, 326–28
across situations generalization, 329–30
across sound and feature generalization, 328–29
across word position generalization, 324–25
contextual, 325–26
guidelines for, 332–33
linguistic unit, 326–28
parental assistance, with, 331–32
position, 324–25
response generalization, 324
situational, 329–31
sound and feature, 328–29
stimulus generalization, 323
Glides, 21–23, 44–45, 264, 299
Gliding, 121–22, 273, 275
Glottal sounds, 21–22, 30–31, 273
Goldman-Fristoe Test of Articulation, 228
Grandfather passage, 224
Group therapy, 353–54

H

Hard palate, 180, 182, 248
Harmony processes (*see* Assimilation)
Hearing loss, 164–69
  discriminant analysis, 168
  influence on speech, 165–69
  speech intelligibility, 168–69
Hoffman-Schuckers Motoric Automatization, 376–78
Homonomy, 392–93
Horizontal approach, 351
Hypernasality, 182–83

I

Idioms, 102
Idiosyncratic patterns, 63, 85, 102–3
Imitation, 319 (*see also* Stimulability)
Independent analysis, 258
Infant perception, 58–60, 70–75
  categorical, 72–73
  linguistic experience, 74
  methods of study, 71–72
  universals, 73–74
Infant production, 66, 75–82
  consonants, 78–82
  prosodic development, 81–82
  stages of production, 79–80
    canonical babbling, 78
    expansion, 77
    gooing or cooing, 77
    phonation, 77
    variegated babbling, 78–79
  vowels, 79–80
Intelligibility, 259
  assessment of, 227–29
  related to misarticulation, 168–69, 194, 259–61
  interpretation, 259–61
International Phonetic Alphabet, 16, 21, 35, 241–42
Interpretation, 258

Intervention (*see* Therapy)
Intonation, 34

K

Key word, 337–40
Keyboard, 290
Khan-Lewis Phonologic Analysis, 262, 277
Kinesthetic, 48–50, 183–87

L

Language based approaches, 396–98
Lateral, 21–22, 264
Lateral lisp, 285–86, 370–71
Linguistic perception, 93–102
    acquisition, 96–97
    full vs. partial, 97–98
    interaction with production, 98–100
    methods to study, 94–96
Lip(s), 10
    liquids (/r/, /l/), 21–23, 45–46, 264, 370–71
    position for speech sounds, 12–14, 20–25, 42
    structural variations, 177, 181

M

Macroglossia, 179, 249
Maintenance, 313, 333
    guidelines, 337
    retention, 335–36
Management (*see* Remediation systems and
           approaches: Therapy)
Manner of consonant production, 21–23
    affricates, 21–23
    fricatives, 21–23
    glides, 21–23
    lateral, 21–22
    liquids, 21–23
    nasals, 21–22
    stops, 21–22
Markedness, 53
Methathesis, 54
Microglossia, 249, 279
Minimal pairs, 388–93 (*see also* Speech sound
           discrimination)
Morpheme, 6
Motor abilities, 59–60, 187–88
Motor approaches to treatment, 359–81 (*see also*
           Remediation systems and approaches)
Multiple phonemic approach to treatment, 366–70
Multiple rules, 295

N

Nasality, 53, 182–83
Nasals, 21–22, 47–48, 264
Natural phonological processes, 52–54, 66, 265,
    270
Neurological involvement, 193–98
    apraxia, 194–96

developmental apraxia, 196–98
    dysarthria, 194
Nonsense syllables/words, 235, 238, 364
Nonstandard English dialects, 148
    assessment, 157–58
    dialect leveling, 148
    gradient stratification, 150
    intervention, 158–59
    sharp stratification, 150

O

Objectives (*see* Behavioral objectives)
Obstruents, 17–18, 31
Omissions, 1–2, 166, 211
Oral cavity examination, 177–88, 247–50
Oral sensory perception, 183–87
Oral stereognosis, 184
Organic factors, 98–98, 164–83
    neuromotor, 193–98
    sensory, 164–69, 183–87
    structural anomalies, 177–88
Output, 298

P

Paired-stimuli approach to treatment, 278–81
Palatalization, 53
Palate, 180, 182–83, 248–49
Pattern analysis, error, 265–79
    distinctive feature analysis, 268–70
    phonological process analysis, 265, 370–79
    place-manner-voice analysis, 268
Percentage of consonants correct (PCC), 260–61
Perception:
    linguistic (*see* Linguistic perception: Speech
           sound discrimination)
    phonological reorganization, 138–42
        differences in lexical organization, 140–41
        influence of literacy, 138–39
        influence of peer group, 141–42
        influence of spelling, 139–40
    prelinguistic (*see* Infant perception)
    sensory, 183–87
    speech (*see* Speech sound discrimination)
        running speech, 130–31
        word recognition, 132–35
Phoneme, 6
Phonemic errors, 3
Phonetic context:
    assessment, 238–40, 279–80, 282–83
    facilitating correct productions, 38–44, 319–20
    treatment, 373–76
Phonetic placement, 320–22
Phonetic symbols/transcription, 15, 21
Phonological acquisition/development:
    infant perception (*see* Infant perception)
    infant production (*see* Infant production)
    linguistic perception (*see* Linguistic perception)

Remediation systems and approaches, 359–99 (see also Therapy)
  cognitive-linguistic, 259–60, 382–99
    Blache approach, 385–87
    contrast therapy, 388–93
    cycles approach, 393–95
    distinctive features, 382–88
    guidelines, 398–99
    language-based approaches, 396–99
    McReynolds and colleagues approach, 383–84
    phonological processes, 388–93
    Weiner and Bankson approach, 384–85
  motor/perceptual, 360–81
    guidelines, 381
    Hoffman-Schuckers-Daniloff motoric automatization of articulatory performance program, 376–78
    McDonald's sensory-motor program, 373–76
    Monterey articulatory program, 370–73
    motoric automatization, 376–78
    multiple phonemic, 366–70
    paired stimuli, 378–81
    programmed conditioning for articulation, 370–73
Retention, 335–36
Rhotic, 21–23, 240, 264

S

Scheduling of remediation, 180–83, 352–53
Scoring of articulation errors, 1–2, 241–46, 261
  additions, 2, 166
  diacritics, use in, 242–44
  distortions, 2, 166, 241
  International Phonetic Alphabet (IPA), use in, 16, 21, 33, 241
  omissions, 1–2, 166, 241
  substitutions, 2, 98–99, 166, 241
Screening, articulatory/phonological, 223–26
Self-monitoring, 172–75
Semivowels, 21–23
Sensory motor approach to treatment, 373–76
Severity, 260
Shaping, 321–22
Sibilants, 167, 189
Single word productions, 229
Soft palate, 182–83, 248–49
Software, 299 313
Sonorants, 17, 131
Sound inventories (see Articulatory tests)
Sound production task, 338
Spanish-influenced dialects, 151–57
  phonological development, 155–57
  phonology, 152–55
Speech mechanism, 10–12, 76, 177–88, 247–50
  facial patterns, 180
  hard palate, 180, 182, 248
  lips, 10, 170, 181
  nasopharynx, 183
  soft palate, 10, 182–83, 248–49
  teeth, 177

  tongue, 10–11, 149–50, 179–80
  velopharyngeal closure, 10, 44–47, 182–83, 248–49
Speech sound discrimination, 12, 93–102, 169–71
  acquisition (see Linguistic perception: Infant perception)
  discrimination improvement, 175–76
  external vs. internal, 172–75
  relationship between articulation and discrimination, 98–100, 171–72, 175–76
  running speech, 130–35
  testing, 94–96, 251–54
    Locke's speech production perception task, 251–52
    Phonological contrast testing, 253–54
    Winitz's phonological performance test, 252–53
  training, 316–17, 362–63
Spontaneous speech sample, 227–29, 238, 312
Stimulability, 235–38, 280–82
Stopping, 121–22, 273, 275
Stops, 21–22, 44–47, 86–87, 264
Stress, 33–34
  theory of, 37–38
Stridency, 32
Substitutions, 2, 98–99, 166, 241
Successive approximation, 321–22
Suprasegmentals, 33–38, 47–48, 58
  development, 81, 102
  intonation, 34
  juncture, 34–35
  loudness, 34
  pitch level, 34
  rate, 35
  stress, 33–34
  theory of stress, 37–38
  vowel reduction, 35
Syllable:
  development, 58–60, 87
  shape, 20, 125, 203
  structure changes (see Phonological processes)

T

Tabulating responses, 339–40
Tactile feedback, 48–50, 183–87
Templin-Darley Tests of Articulation, 202, 235, 260
Test(s), 232–34, See also Articulatory tests
Therapy/intervention/treatment/remediation, 258–88, 314–55 (see also Remediation systems and approaches)
  administrative considerations, 344
    establishing objectives, 344–46
    individualized education programs, 346–47
    scheduling, 352–53
  baseline measures, 341–44
  cyclical approach, 352
  data tabulation, 339–44
  dialectal considerations, 285
  dismissal criteria, 333–37
  establishment of target behaviors/sounds, 316–23, 396–98

generalization/transfer/carry-over, 315, 323–33
(*see also* Generalization)
group vs. individual, 353–54
guidelines, 286
horizontal approach to treatment, 351
intervention style, 354–55
maintenance, 333–37
measuring changes, 337–44
perception training, 316–18, 362–63
production training, 318–23, 363–81
scheduling, 352–53, 393–95
selection factors for target behavior, 277–82
  age of acquisition, 277
  context, 279–80
  ease of production, 282
  frequency of occurrence, 280–82
  stimulability, 280, 282
social/vocational considerations, 285–86
style, 354–55
treatment models, 342–44
vertically structured program, 351
Tongue, 10–114, 22–29, 76, 179–80, 249–50
frenum, 179, 250
glossectomy, 181
macroglossia, 179, 249
microglossia, 179, 249
position for consonants, 22–29
position for vowels, 12–14
Tongue thrust, 189–93
Traditional approach to treatment, 361–66
Transcription, 16, 21, 241–46
diacritics, 242–44
International Phonetic Alphabet (IPA), 15, 21,
  33–34, 241

phonetic vs. phonemic, 6
reliability, 79, 244–46
Transfer (*see* Generalization)
Treatment approaches, 359–99 (*see also*
  Remediation systems and approaches:
  Therapy)

U

Underlying representation, 278
Unintelligibility, 129, 259–61

V

Velopharyngeal mechanism, 10, 43–45, 76, 182–83,
  218–49
Vertical approach, 351
Vocalizations, infant (*see* Infant production)
Voice onset time (VOT), 72
Voicing, 123
Vowels, 12–20, 47, 53, 76–80, 87, 138–39
acquisition of, 76–80, 87, 113
alternation, 138–39
assessment, 240–41
central, 14–15
diphthongs, 16–17
distinctive features, 17–20
front vs. back, 13–16
high vs. low, 12–15
mid, 15–16
monothongs, 12–16
quadrilateral, 14–17
rounded vs. unrounded, 12–15
tense vs. lax, 16